INNOVATIONS IN CLINICAL PRACTICE: A SOURCE BOOK

Volume 13

Edited by
LEON VANDECREEK
SAMUEL KNAPP
THOMAS L. JACKSON

PROFESSIONAL RESOURCE PRESS
P.O. Box 15560
Sarasota, FL 34277-1560

Published by Professional Resource Press
(An imprint of Professional Resource Exchange, Inc.)
Post Office Box 15560
Sarasota, FL 34277-1560

Copyright © 1994 by Professional Resource Exchange, Inc.

The materials in this volume for which the Professional Resource Exchange holds copyright may be reproduced for use in professional practice and for educational/training purposes. Any reproduction for resale or large scale distribution is strictly prohibited without prior written permission and would be considered unlawful. With the exception of clinical and office forms (not including instruments) which are used with clients, material which is reproduced must contain the following statement:

Reproduced from: *Innovations in Clinical Practice: A Source Book* (Vol. 13) by L. VandeCreek, S. Knapp, and T. L. Jackson (Eds.), Sarasota, FL: Professional Resource Press. Copyright © 1994 by the Professional Resource Exchange, Inc., P.O. Box 15560, Sarasota, FL 34277-1560.

Printed in the United States of America

Looseleaf Edition ISBN: 1-56887-001-9
Hardbound Edition ISBN: 1-56887-002-7
Library of Congress Catalog Card Number: 82-7614
ISSN 0737-125x

The copyeditor for this book was Patricia Hammond, the managing editor was Debbie Fink, and the production coordinator was Laurie Girsch.

PREFACE

This is the thirteenth yearly volume of the *Innovations in Clinical Practice: A Source Book* series. Approximately 550 authors have now contributed to making the *Innovations* series a valued resource for practicing mental health clinicians. All volumes in the series follow the same basic format with five separate sections. No single volume is comprehensive or built around a particular theme. *Innovations* is a wide-ranging clinical resource series that contains topics either selected by the editors, suggested by readers, or, in some cases, based on manuscripts that have been submitted for review. We continue to receive very positive feedback from clinicians who have purchased the volumes, and are pleased that we have apparently played an important role in disseminating information to practicing clinicians.

Peter A. Keller was the senior editor of the series from its inception in 1981 through Volume 10 in 1991. We are all deeply indebted to him for his hard work, outstanding editorial judgment, and insights regarding the types of contributions that mental health practitioners need and want. Lawrence G. Ritt served as co-editor of the first five volumes and continues to consult about the development of subsequent volumes. Steven R. Heyman was co-editor for Volumes 6 through 10.

Beginning with the eleventh volume, Leon VandeCreek assumed the position of senior editor. Samuel Knapp and Thomas L. Jackson have served as assistant editors.

There are two other individuals who have made important contributions to the production of the thirteenth *Innovations* volume. From the onset of this series, Debra Fink has supervised the final production of each volume and insured careful attention to details that others might have missed. Laurie Girsch has ably assisted her since Volume 8. We appreciate their thoroughness and cooperative spirit. Each year they have become more important to the success of the series.

Other contributors to the preparation of this volume include Patricia Hammond and Judy Wariner, who have worked many hours copyediting and proofreading the manuscripts. Without their skilled assistance, this volume would not be a reality. We would also like to thank Mia Coffman, Jean Szegedy, and Dustin Pointer for their help in preparing the volume for distribution.

We believe that the *Innovations in Clinical Practice* series is successful because of its highly applied focus. Our primary audience is mental health practitioners. To insure the continuing value of the series, we need the help of readers, and we invite your ideas and feedback on this volume. We also encourage you to consider the possibility of submitting a contribution.

AN INVITATION TO SUBMIT A CONTRIBUTION

The editors are currently soliciting contributions for future volumes in the *Innovations* series. If you are doing something innovative in your work, please let us hear from you. Contact Dr.

Innovations in Clinical Practice: A Source Book (Vol. 13)

Leon VandeCreek, Senior Editor, School of Professional Psychology, Wright State University, Dayton, OH 45435, if you would like more detailed information on becoming a contributor.

CONTINUING EDUCATION

The Professional Resource Exchange is approved by the American Psychological Association as a continuing education sponsor, and credits may be obtained by readers who are required to participate in CE programs, as well as by those who simply wish to validate their learning. Interested readers are referred to the material at the back of this volume to learn how to obtain home study continuing education credits through the *Innovations in Clinical Practice* series. This service provides an economical means of obtaining continuing education credits while acquiring relevant clinical knowledge. Readers have been consistently positive about the experience of obtaining CE credits through the series.

COPYRIGHT POLICIES

Most of the material in this volume may be duplicated. You may photocopy materials (such as office forms and instruments) or reproduce them for use in your practice or share contributions with your students in the classroom. For materials on which the Professional Resource Exchange holds the copyright, no further permission is required for noncommercial, professional, or educational uses. However, unauthorized duplication or publication for resale or large-scale distribution of any material in this volume is expressly prohibited.

Any material that you duplicate from this volume (with the exceptions mentioned below) must be acknowledged as having been reprinted from this volume and must note that copyright is held by the Professional Resource Exchange, Inc. The format and exact wording required in the acknowledgement are shown on the copyright page of this volume. The only exception to this policy is that clinical and office forms (not instruments) for use with clients in your own office may be reprinted without including the acknowledgement mentioned above.

There are exceptions to our liberal copyright policy. We do not hold copyright on some of the materials included in this volume and, therefore, cannot grant permission to freely duplicate those materials. When copyright is held by another publisher or author, such copyright is noted on the appropriate page of the contribution. Unless otherwise noted in the credit and copyright citation, any reproduction or duplication of these materials is strictly and expressively forbidden without the consent of the copyright holder.

Leon VandeCreek
Wright State University

Samuel Knapp
Pennsylvania Psychological Association

Thomas L. Jackson
University of Arkansas

BIOGRAPHIES

Leon VandeCreek, PhD, Senior Editor, is Dean of the School of Professional Psychology at Wright State University. He was awarded the Diplomate in Clinical Psychology from the American Board of Professional Psychologists in 1989, and he is a Fellow of Divisions 12 (Clinical), 29 (Psychotherapy), and 42 (Independent Practice) of the American Psychological Association. He is the author or coauthor of approximately 50 articles, books, and chapters in psychology. He is a contributing editor for *The Psychotherapy Bulletin* and a member of the editorial board for *Psychotherapy*, both publications of Division 29 of the APA. His interests include professional training, law and psychology, and ethics. Dr. VandeCreek may be contacted at Professional Psychology, Wright State University, Dayton, OH 45435.

Samuel Knapp, EdD, Associate Editor, is the Professional Affairs Officer of the Pennsylvania Psychological Association. He is the author or coauthor of 14 books and numerous articles in psychology. His interests include issues affecting professional psychology, public mental health, and psychopathology. Dr. Knapp can be contacted at 2801 Rumson Drive, Harrisburg, PA 17104.

Thomas L. Jackson, PhD, Associate Editor, is Professor and Director of Clinical Training in the Department of Psychology at the University of Arkansas. He is author or co-author of over 30 articles, chapters, and books, has made over 50 national and international presentations, and serves as a consultant to several national organizations, primarily in the areas of sexual and physical assault. He has directed two American Psychological Association accredited clinical psychology doctoral programs, and has been a member of the Boards of Examiners in Psychology in two different states. Dr. Jackson may be contacted at the Psychology Department, 211B Memorial Hall, University of Arkansas, Fayetteville, AR 72701.

TABLE OF CONTENTS

PREFACE	*iii*
BIOGRAPHIES	*v*
INTRODUCTION TO THE VOLUME	1

SECTION I: CLINICAL ISSUES AND APPLICATIONS

INTRODUCTION TO SECTION 1	3
TREATMENT OF MARITAL VIOLENCE *Amy Holtzworth-Munroe and Gregory L. Stuart*	5
INNOVATIONS IN THE TREATMENT OF MULTIPLE PERSONALITY DISORDER *R. Douglas Smith*	21
TREATMENT OF INCEST AND COMPLEX DISSOCIATIVE TRAUMATIC STRESS REACTIONS *Christine A. Courtois*	37
BEHAVIORAL ASSESSMENT AND TREATMENT OF CHRONIC PAIN IN CHILDREN *Chris A. Coleman, Alice G. Friedman, and Donna Gates*	55
IMAGERY RESCRIPTING: A MULTIFACETED TREATMENT FOR CHILDHOOD SEXUAL ABUSE SURVIVORS *Mervin R. Smucker and Jan L. Niederee*	73
STRATEGIES FOR PARENT TRAINING USING THE ONE-WAY MIRROR *Ron D. Cambias, Jr.*	87
ADOLESCENT SUBSTANCE ABUSE TREATMENT *Eric F. Wagner, Mark G. Myers, and Sandra A. Brown*	97

Innovations in Clinical Practice: A Source Book (Vol. 13)

ASSESSMENT AND TREATMENT OF ATTENTION-DEFICIT/ HYPERACTIVITY DISORDER IN CHILDREN *Gerald McMullen, David T. Painter, and Thomas J. Casey*	123
DEPENDENCY IN PSYCHOTHERAPY: EFFECTIVE THERAPEUTIC WORK WITH DEPENDENT PATIENTS *Robert F. Bornstein*	139
ASSESSMENT AND TREATMENT OF DEPRESSION AND LOSS IN THE ELDERLY *Ruby Takushi Chinen and Linda Berg-Cross*	151
A REVIEW OF SCALES FOR THE BRIEF ASSESSMENT OF ANXIETY *Victoria C. Demos and Maurice F. Prout*	167
CLINICAL GUIDELINES FOR THE TREATMENT OF INSOMNIA *Charles M. Morin and Cheryl A. Colecchi*	179

SECTION II: PRACTICE MANAGEMENT AND PROFESSIONAL DEVELOPMENT

INTRODUCTION TO SECTION II	197
MANAGED CARE: WHAT'S NEXT? *Marc T. Frankel and John M. Feely*	199
DEALING WITH FEES IN PSYCHOTHERAPY *William G. Herron*	223
WORKPLACE HARASSMENT: WHAT MENTAL HEALTH PRACTITIONERS NEED TO KNOW *Lilli Friedland and David Friedland*	237
AN INTERDISCIPLINARY AGREEMENT BETWEEN PSYCHOLOGISTS AND ATTORNEYS: A MODEL FOR PSYCHOLOGY-LAW INTERACTION *William E. Foote*	255

SECTION III: INSTRUMENTS AND OFFICE FORMS

INTRODUCTION TO SECTION III	263
THE DOMESTIC VIOLENCE BLAME SCALE (DVBS) *Patricia Petretic-Jackson, Genell Sandberg, and Thomas L. Jackson*	265
THE VIOLENCE ATTITUDES SCALE (VAS) *Thomas L. Jackson, Richard D. Dienst, Terry L. Efird, Brenda D. Mobley, David A. Schroeder, April D. Hout, Julleah C. Montecillo, and Andrea L. LaBine*	279
A CLIENT SATISFACTION SURVEY *Chris E. Stout*	293

CLINICAL AND ADMINISTRATIVE MANAGEMENT CHECKLIST
John R. Rudisill   299

SECTION IV: COMMUNITY INTERVENTIONS

INTRODUCTION TO SECTION IV   307

A MANUAL FOR TIME-LIMITED GROUP TREATMENT WITH SEPARATED COUPLES
P. Gregg Blanton   309

LITIGATION CONSULTING: PREPARING ATTORNEYS TO CROSS-EXAMINE NEUROPSYCHOLOGISTS
Robert H. Ellis   323

EVALUATION AND TREATMENT OF MOTORISTS CONVICTED OF DRIVING WHILE INTOXICATED
Thomas N. Grant and Mary C. Grant   339

SECTION V: SELECTED TOPICS

INTRODUCTION TO SECTION V   357

A MARITAL THERAPY PROTOCOL
Richard D. Magee   359

CONTEMPORARY ISSUES IN ADOLESCENT GROUP PSYCHOTHERAPY
Beryce W. MacLennan   369

THE CURRENT STATUS OF THE INSANITY DEFENSE
Michael L. Perlin   383

CHINKS IN THE PRISON WALL: APPLYING GRAHAM'S STOCKHOLM SYNDROME THEORY TO THE TREATMENT OF BATTERED WOMEN
Edna I. Rawlings, P. Gail Allen, Dee L. R. Graham, and June Peters   401

DISABLED CLIENTS: WHAT EVERY THERAPIST NEEDS TO KNOW
Sandra K. Brodwin, Leo M. Orange, and Martin G. Brodwin   419

TWELVE MYTHS ABOUT ADOLESCENTS, SEXUALITY, AND AIDS
Samuel Knapp   431

INTRODUCTION TO THE CLIENT HANDOUTS   443

    CONTROLLING ANGER - BEFORE IT CONTROLS YOU
    American Psychological Association   445

    PLAIN TALK ABOUT DEPRESSION
    National Institute of Mental Health   451

SUBJECT INDEX TO VOLUMES 11, 12, AND 13	457
INFORMATION FOR CONTRIBUTORS	467
CONTINUING EDUCATION	469

INTRODUCTION TO THE VOLUME

As in previous volumes, *Innovations in Clinical Practice: A Source Book* (Volume 13) is organized into five sections that reflect the diversity of contributions to the series. This volume includes a subject index for Volumes 11, 12, and 13. Volumes 1 through 5 are indexed in the fifth volume (1986) and Volumes 6 through 10 are indexed in the tenth volume (1991). A cumulative index for all 13 volumes is also available from the publisher.

The first section, CLINICAL ISSUES AND APPLICATIONS, deals primarily with therapeutic concerns. The various contributions, however, go beyond traditional therapeutic issues and also address important questions of assessment, as well as treatment. Issues that relate to a number of different types of clients and situations are covered.

The second section addresses PRACTICE MANAGEMENT AND PROFESSIONAL DEVELOPMENT. This section is included because of the increasing number of clinicians who work independently and require a source of information on practice management and professional development issues. We remain in a period of dramatic changes that affect the nature of our practices. New risks as well as opportunities are constantly emerging in this era of health care reform. In this section, we try to address relevant issues that we believe will be of interest to our readers. Some of our discussions here also should be of interest to students and clinicians who practice in organizations or agencies.

The third section includes assessment INSTRUMENTS AND OFFICE FORMS. The assessment instruments are primarily informal and designed to assist clinicians in collecting information about clients. Our goal is to publish screening instruments and forms that aid in the organization of data, rather than the making of formal inferences. There are some exceptions to this rule; however, we believe all fall within the bounds of accepted professional practice in the format in which they are presented. The materials presented here should be useful to psychologists and other professionals, with minimal potential for misuse. We assume that readers will be thoroughly familiar with any disorders or processes that they attempt to evaluate, and readers are advised to carefully review the introductory materials that accompany contributions to this section.

The fourth section on COMMUNITY INTERVENTIONS reflects our view that mental health practitioners have much to offer in the community beyond traditional clinical services. We trust that the material in this section will be of assistance to those who are interested in mental health consultation, education, prevention, and expanding their services to reach new and broader populations.

The fifth section, SELECTED TOPICS, includes a variety of contributions that do not fit neatly into one of the other sections. We have also included two client handouts in this section dealing with anger control and depression.

ISSUES AND APPLICATIONS

INTRODUCTION TO SECTION I: CLINICAL ISSUES AND APPLICATIONS

The CLINICAL ISSUES AND APPLICATIONS section includes contributions that are primarily related to assessment and treatment. No unifying themes are intended, and the range of topics is quite broad. This section provides a means for practitioners to access current information about new clinical techniques that might be incorporated into their practices, or to learn of new developments in specialized areas.

In the first contribution, Amy Holtzworth-Munroe and Gregory Stuart focus on the topic of marital violence and its treatment. Data suggest that as many as 1.8 million wives are beaten by their spouses, and over 50% of couples seeking marital therapy have experienced spousal violence. But sadly, many clinicians are not alert to the indicators. The authors guide clinicians through the steps of assessment and therapy.

Multiple personality disorder has received increased attention in the literature in the last decade. Traditional approaches to treatment have included several steps including building trust, establishing communication linkages with the alter personalities, and eventually blending the alters toward a single personality. In our second contribution, R. Douglas Smith reviews several of the traditional steps in therapy with these patients and then identifies crucial choice points for therapists where the traditional wisdom may be inadequate or where unique therapeutic strategies will assist clinicians in breaking through treatment barriers.

In recent years, research and clinical observations have suggested that 50% to 70% of adult female psychiatric patients have a history of childhood sexual abuse. In our third contribution, Christine Courtois discusses symptoms and aftereffects of incest in three main diagnostic categories: post-traumatic reactions, dissociative disorders, and characterological disorders. She articulates a treatment model which is directed toward trauma resolution and also addresses issues of personal development, self-management, skill-building, and mastery.

In Volume 12 of the *Innovations* series, Alice Friedman and Cheryl Blau discussed assessment and treatment issues for children with acute pain. In this volume, Alice Friedman has joined with Chris Coleman and Donna Gates to provide similar coverage of chronic pain in children. The authors provide an eclectic perspective on assessment and treatment with a special focus on behavioral strategies.

The fifth contribution, by Mervin Smucker and Jan Niederee, provides a detailed approach to treatment of sexual abuse victims who experience symptoms of Post-Traumatic Stress Disorder (PTSD). The authors suggest that the manner in which abuse memories are encoded is affected by the age of the child when the molestation began. Between the ages of 2 and 7, memories are encoded primarily in the visual system, with verbal representation developing more slowly until adolescence. Therefore, the authors propose that visual imagery techniques are needed to supplement verbal techniques when working with PTSD survivors of sexual abuse.

Ron Cambias provides a guide for parenting skills training through the use of a one-way mirror observation room. Live supervision and intervention from behind the mirror, as with family therapy training, allows for the relatively unobtrusive observation of a family without the therapist's physical presence in the room.

Adolescent substance abuse and its correlates are some of the most prevalent problems facing clinicians involved in the area of adolescent health. Given the risks for later life problems, the early identification and intervention for teen substance abuse is critical. Eric Wagner, Mark Myers, and Sandra Brown provide a theoretical rationale and practical suggestions for assessment and intervention with teens who have alcohol and other drug problems.

Attention-Deficit/Hyperactivity Disorder (ADHD) is one of the most common reasons for referring children to mental health practitioners. Performance problems associated with ADHD manifest themselves in family, school, and other social or work-related situations. Gerald McMullen, David Painter, and Thomas Casey provide an up-to-date overview of ADHD for practitioners.

In the next contribution, Robert Bornstein focuses on the variable of dependency in psychotherapy. The author familiarizes therapists with the clinical features of patients who show exaggerated dependency needs, describes the ways these dependency needs may affect therapeutic process and outcome, and presents strategies for working with dependent patients.

The elderly are the fastest growing segment of the U.S. population. Data suggest, however, that the elderly utilize mental health services proportionately less than other age groups. Ruby Takushi Chinen and Linda Berg-Cross discuss the assessment and diagnosis of depression among the elderly and treatment implications. Their discussion is specifically geared toward the depressed elderly population that lives independently in the community.

Victoria Demos and Maurice Prout examine clinical issues related to the self-report assessment of anxiety in adults and children. They outline the general symptoms of anxiety and then present a survey of the most frequently employed self-report measures to assess the severity of anxiety.

In the last contribution in this section, Charles Morin and Cheryl Colecchi provide guidelines for the assessment and treatment of insomnia. They focus primarily on the nonmedication approaches to treatment.

TREATMENT OF MARITAL VIOLENCE*

Amy Holtzworth-Munroe and Gregory L. Stuart

PREVALENCE AND CONSEQUENCES OF MARITAL VIOLENCE

Marital violence is a serious problem in this country. Data from a recent national survey indicate that each year one out of eight husbands engages in at least one violent act toward his wife and 1.8 million wives are beaten by their spouses (Straus & Gelles, 1990). Examining both husband and wife violence, one out of six American couples experienced violence during the year of the study, leading to estimates that 8.7 million couples experience marital violence each year and 3.4 million couples experience severe violence carrying a high risk of injury (Straus & Gelles, 1990).

Data suggest that such violence may begin early in a relationship and often continues to occur without intervention (e.g., O'Leary et al., 1989). In addition, clinicians working with violent couples believe that violence escalates over time. Although longitudinal data addressing this issue are unavailable, retrospective reports from violent couples (e.g., Walker, 1979) indicate that many couples experience an escalation in the frequency, intensity, and severity of marital violence over time.

The costs of marital violence are staggering in terms of physical injuries, marital dissatisfaction, and psychological problems, including depression, alcohol abuse, and post-traumatic stress disorder (e.g., Hotaling & Sugarman, 1986; Sonkin, Martin, & Walker, 1985). Physical aggression in marriage has also been linked to child abuse and other negative effects on the children of such marriages (e.g., McDonald & Jouriles, 1991).

Although both husbands and wives engage in physical aggression, research has consistently demonstrated that husband-to-wife violence has more negative consequences than wife-to-husband violence. Husband aggression results in more physical injury and more health problems, including stress and depression (Cascardi, Langhinrichsen, & Vivian, 1992; Stets & Straus, 1990). Thus, husband violence is a particularly important problem and is the focus of this contribution.

Given the prevalence of marital violence, the likelihood that it will continue or escalate once begun, and the resulting negative consequences, the problem of marital violence should be of particular interest to marital therapists. Indeed, data indicate that over half of couples seeking marital

---

*Note. Portions of this contribution will appear in "The Assessment and Treatment of Marital Violence: An Introduction for the Marital Therapist" by A. Holtzworth-Munroe, S. B. Beatty, and K. Anglin in *Clinical Handbook of Marital Therapy* (2nd ed.) by N. S. Jacobson and A. S. Gurman (Eds.), in press, New York: Guilford.

therapy have experienced husband violence (e.g., Holtzworth-Munroe et al., 1992). However, couples often do not spontaneously report problems with violence (O'Leary, Vivian, & Malone, 1992). Perhaps as a result, marital therapists often fail to detect the occurrence of marital violence (e.g., Hansen, Harway, & Cervantes, 1991). Thus, *therapists must systematically seek information on violence* through a careful and direct assessment.

ASSESSMENT OF MARITAL VIOLENCE

IS MARITAL VIOLENCE OCCURRING?

Given the prevalence of marital violence among couples seeking therapy, marital therapists must consider the possibility of violence in every case. Because many couples do not spontaneously discuss this problem, therapists must directly assess the occurrence of marital violence. To do so, we recommend that spouses be separated and independently asked about the occurrence of violence, because battered wives may be afraid to speak truthfully in front of their abusers.

The quickest way to screen for the occurrence of marital violence is to administer the Conflict Tactics Scale (CTS; Straus, 1979), the most widely used measure of marital violence. It lists 19 behaviors couples may engage in during conflicts, ranging from nonviolent (e.g., discussed the issue calmly) to violent (e.g., used a knife or gun). Respondents first report whether they or their partner have ever engaged in any of the listed behaviors. If so, they then report how often each behavior has occurred in the past year (i.e., from "never" to "more than 20 times").

Researchers have found low inter-spousal reliability in reports of marital violence on the CTS; partners rarely agree on the occurrence of specific violent behaviors (e.g., Jouriles & O'Leary, 1985), and, relative to wives' reports, husbands tend to underreport their own violence. Thus, therapists should accept either spouse's report of the occurrence of violence and should not ignore wife reports of husband violence even if these are not confirmed by the husband.

ASSESSING THE VIOLENCE IN MORE DETAIL

Although the CTS is a popular measure for identifying violent couples, it suffers from several shortcomings. The number of violent behaviors assessed by the CTS is limited. In addition, the CTS does not assess the context of the violence (i.e., the events leading to the violence, the sequence of events during a violent incident, the intentions behind the violence, or the consequences of the violence); however, such factors are important for understanding the role violence plays in a relationship.

Given these limitations of the CTS, a therapist who detects the occurrence of marital violence will need to conduct clinical interviews to gain additional information about the context, intent, and consequences of the violence. More detailed information should be sought about the severity and frequency of the violence and any resulting injuries (e.g., severity of injuries, what medical attention was sought). In addition, the therapist should assess any involvement of third parties (e.g., police) and the possibility of danger to others (e.g., children).

IS THERE A RISK OF LETHALITY - IS THE WIFE SAFE?

If the therapist establishes that severe or frequent marital violence is occurring, he or she should immediately assess the dangerousness and potential lethality of the situation. Although it is difficult to predict whether, and when, a client will engage in lethal behavior, it is important to be aware that this risk exists among violent couples. Of obvious relevance is information about the severity and consequences of the violence. In addition, the therapist should ask whether guns or other weapons are present in the household; if so, the therapist may require that they be removed from the home (Saunders, 1992). The therapist should investigate whether alcohol or other substance use is associated with the use of violence; such substances may reduce individuals' inhibitions, making lethal behavior more likely.

In many cases, the therapist should also discuss safety planning with the couple, particularly the wife. If the probability of continuing or escalating violence is high, this discussion should take place immediately. The wife should be made aware of local resources (e.g., shelters) and legal options (e.g., restraining orders). The therapist should discuss practical issues such as whether the wife can get herself, and her children, out of the house if she fears for her safety, and where she can go if she decides to leave. She should be helped to develop a plan for such situations (e.g., where the keys and money are in case a quick exit is needed; whether she has access to important documents).

Similarly, the husband should be warned of the dangerous nature of his violence and of the possibility of an escalation in violence. He should be asked to consider methods of stopping himself from using violence (see anger management techniques, below). In some cases, the couple should be asked to temporarily separate to lower the risk of dangerous violence.

ASSESSING OTHER RELEVANT VARIABLES

In addition to a careful assessment of the physical violence, therapists should assess other variables that may be relevant to treatment planning.

Physical violence is often accompanied by *psychological and emotional abuse* of the wife. Such abuse includes actions that denigrate and humiliate the victim (e.g., controlling her behavior, putting her down) as well as threatening behaviors and actions that damage her property (e.g., driving recklessly when she is a passenger in the car; destroying a prized possession). Women often report that these behaviors are equally, or more, harmful psychologically than the physical abuse they suffer. Psychological abuse can be assessed through interviews and/or with several new questionnaire measures (e.g., Psychological Maltreatment of Women Inventory; Tolman, 1989).

Violent husbands describe themselves as experiencing significantly more *anger and hostility* than nonviolent men (e.g., Maiuro et al., 1988). Although anger is not always a precursor for violent behavior, the level of anger experienced by violent husbands is relevant to treatment planning and the assessment of therapy outcome, because many marital violence treatment programs include anger management components. Questionnaire measures of anger and hostility are available (e.g., Novaco's Anger Index, Novaco, 1977; Spielberger's State-Trait Anger Scale, Spielberger, Gorsuch, & Lushene, 1970).

Alcohol is involved in many battering incidents (e.g., Hotaling & Sugarman, 1986; Leonard & Blane, 1992). Thus, practitioners should obtain a detailed history of the couples' *alcohol and drug use* and of the role alcohol and drugs play in the violent episodes. Some violent husbands may require alcohol or substance abuse counseling prior to addressing their problems with marital violence.

Given the psychological consequences of violence, therapists may also wish to assess the presence of other *psychological problems*, including post-traumatic stress disorder among battered wives (Houskamp & Foy, 1991) and depression and risk of suicide among both spouses. Although standard measures of these problems may be employed (e.g., the Beck Depression Inventory; Beck et al., 1961), therapists should keep in mind that these problems may exist solely as a consequence of the marital violence; cessation of the violence may lead to improvements in these problems without the need for further interventions. In addition, a substantial proportion of male batterers have been found to have personality disorders (e.g., Hamberger & Hastings, 1986); obtaining such information may aid treatment planning.

Research has indicated that violent husbands have difficulty with *spouse-specific assertion* (e.g., Rosenbaum & O'Leary, 1981) and lack the skills to generate *competent solutions* in certain types of marital conflicts (e.g., Holtzworth-Munroe & Anglin, 1991). In addition, observational studies have revealed that violent couples have poorer problem-solving skills and more negative *marital interactions* than nonviolent couples (e.g., Margolin, John, & Gleberman, 1988). Thus, therapists may wish to assess the communication and problem-solving skills of violent couples, using either paper-and-pencil measures (e.g., the Spouse-Specific Assertion/Aggression Scale; Rosenbaum & O'Leary, 1981) or direct observation of marital interactions.

Given feminist theories that men may use violence as a means of asserting their domination over women, therapists may choose to assess husbands' and wives' *beliefs about sex roles* and the relationship between men and women, using measures such as the Attitudes Toward Women Scale (Spence & Helmreich, 1972). In addition, practitioners may wish to gather information regarding violent husbands' *beliefs about violence* (e.g., Saunders et al., 1987) to identify batterers who believe that there are situations in which violence is productive and necessary.

Many violent husbands grew up in violent homes, witnessing parental violence and having themselves been the victim of parental aggression (Hotaling & Sugarman, 1986). Both husbands' and wives' past experiences with violence may have influenced their perceptions of their own, current marital violence. Thus, it is often useful to assess each partner's experiences with violence in their family of origin and in past relationships.

TREATMENT OF MARITAL VIOLENCE

TREATMENT GOALS AND FORMAT

Elimination of Violence as the Treatment Goal. Regardless of theoretical orientation or therapeutic modality, the primary goal of therapy when working with violent couples is the elimination of physical aggression. However, this is not always the couple's goal, particularly among couples who have not experienced severe violence. In fact, when marital violence is identified as a problem by the therapist, many couples will disagree, stating their beliefs that the violence is not serious, will not occur again, and so on. Spouses sometimes believe that their use of physical aggression was justified or had positive benefits (e.g., "After I hit her, she finally calmed down, and we were able to have a good discussion") and sometimes deny responsibility for their aggression. Thus, it is the therapist's responsibility to stress the dangerousness of the violence and the importance of targeting violent behavior for therapeutic intervention.

To do so, it is useful to firmly adopt the stance that it is the therapist's expert opinion that the violence is a serious problem, even if the couple does not agree, and that no violent acts are acceptable within the relationship. It should be pointed out that, even if serious consequences have not yet occurred and even if the spouses' intentions do not involve harm, violence always carries the potential for serious injury and destructive outcomes. Examples help to make this point (e.g., a husband pushed his wife, with no intent to hurt her; however, she slipped and hit her head on the kitchen counter, losing consciousness). In addition, it should be pointed out that research and clinical experience suggest that unless it is stopped, marital violence will continue and may even escalate. Finally, the therapist should explain that therapy may actually increase the risk of violence because the couple will be asked to discuss many of their most difficult problems. As a result of these factors, the therapist should explain that he or she has no option but to be concerned about the violence and that therapy must focus on this problem.

It is also necessary to help spouses accept responsibility for their violent actions. The fact that spouses are able to "choose" where, when, and against whom to aggress can be used as proof of their responsibility. For example, many spouses' descriptions of their violence are inconsistent with their claim that they are "out of control" when angry and violent (e.g., a man who beat his wife severely but when asked why he didn't kill her says, "Oh, I couldn't do that," or a man who in a "fit of rage" carefully, and with precise aim, shot every one of his wife's knick-knacks with his gun). In addition, violence can be framed as a learned behavior; this opens the possibility that spouses can learn to choose nonviolent, constructive methods of handling marital conflict.

Conjoint or Individual/Group Treatment. Based upon information gathered during the assessment, the therapist must decide whether to proceed with conjoint marital therapy or refer the individual spouses for relevant marital violence therapy. No firm guidelines have been established for making this decision and no data currently exist regarding the relative efficacy of conjoint versus individual/group therapy for treating marital violence. Thus, at this point in time, common sense and theoretical orientation often dictate the therapist's decision.

Conjoint treatment is generally recommended if the occurrence of past violence is relatively "mild" and infrequent and if the wife is not in immediate or serious danger. In addition, the perpetrator must be willing to acknowledge that the violence has occurred and is problematic and be willing to address this issue in therapy. Thus, conjoint therapy is an option if the violence is not severe, if there is a genuine commitment to avoid physical aggression, and if both partners wish to remain in the relationship.

Others have outlined the potential advantages of conjoint therapy (e.g., Margolin & Burman, 1993). These include giving the therapist a more accurate picture of the violence that is occurring (i.e., husband's and wife's reports often differ significantly) and introducing both spouses to the same information and techniques, thus helping to insure that both understand the therapist's conceptualization of the violence (i.e., the wife is not responsible) and how to implement various procedures. Other advantages include changing interactional patterns that precede the violence, helping the husband to monitor his anger and communicate with his wife, helping the wife to recognize danger cues and take steps to protect herself, and allowing the couple to postpone discussion of emotionally laden issues until therapy sessions.

However, there are potential disadvantages and dangers involved in conjoint treatment (e.g., Margolin & Burman, 1993). These include the fact that the wife's safety may be jeopardized (e.g., if she accurately reports her husband's behavior, he may later retaliate with further aggression). In addition, it may be difficult, with both spouses present, to accurately assess the spouses' desire to continue their marriage. Finally, conjoint interventions and the involvement of the wife in treatment may send the message that the wife is responsible for the violence.

Given these potential disadvantages, conjoint treatment is contraindicated if the wife is in grave danger, if the husband refuses to take steps to reduce the danger (e.g., remove weapons from the house, seek help for alcohol problems), or if the wife is too afraid of the husband to be an equal participant in conjoint treatment. In such cases, the violent husband should be referred to a batterer's treatment program. In these programs, the husband will get extensive interventions targeted specifically at eliminating his violence and abusive behaviors. The wife should be referred to a local battered women's support group, where she will receive access to resources for battered women and support to make her own decisions about the future of her relationship.

After the spouses have sought such help, many marital therapists will treat the couple conjointly, although no data regarding the efficacy of doing so is currently available. To be seen in conjoint therapy, the therapist should require that the husband has completed a batterer's program, accepted responsibility for his violence, and taken steps to reduce it; the therapist should also verify that the wife has made a decision, free of fear, to work on her relationship.

Conjoint Behavioral/Cognitive Therapy With Violent Couples. If the decision is made to offer conjoint marital therapy, the therapist should again note his or her concern about the violence, and the couple should again be cautioned regarding the affective arousal that occurs in marital therapy and the resulting risk of violence. They should be informed that treatment may be terminated if the violence continues and should be asked to make a "no violence" contract with the therapist. Couples experiencing more serious or frequent violence should be told that the violence must be brought under control before work on other issues can begin; therapy should then focus on reducing the violence.

Couples experiencing lower levels of violence can be offered a "two-pronged" therapy approach. These couples are told that, given the potential dangers of the violence, they must learn methods for reducing and managing their destructive conflicts (e.g., time-out; reviewed later). However, focusing only on eliminating negative, aggressive interactions may be frustrating, because it does not provide couples with other, more constructive methods of resolving disputes. To deal with this issue, work on communication and conflict resolution may be done concurrently with the anger management treatment. This dual treatment approach can be explained to the couple by stating that anger control techniques help to prevent the escalation of conflicts, and problem-solving and communication training give the couple skills to use after the time-out to solve problems and to avoid future conflicts.

Given our behavioral/cognitive orientation, we utilize skill-based interventions when teaching couples new ways to handle conflict; these are discussed elsewhere (e.g., Jacobson & Margolin, 1979). Anger and violence management techniques are introduced later in this contribution.

Group Therapy With Violent Husbands. As noted previously, if severe violence is occurring, the husband should be referred to a batterer's treatment group. Although no data on this issue exist, it is widely assumed that group therapy provides the best setting for treating violent men, and most available programs utilize this format. The group provides an opportunity for exchanging social support and reducing the isolation and stigma that violent men might feel. A group is also a vehicle for confrontation, as group members are encouraged to interact with each other in a direct manner, pointing out instances of denial and minimization of violence among others in the group.

The usual format for group therapy involves weekly sessions of approximately 1½ to 2 hours for periods ranging from 8 to 36 weeks. Having a male and a female as cotherapists is generally recommended, because the therapists can model a positive, egalitarian relationship; group members can benefit from the opportunity to relate to an authority figure of each sex who, in turn, treat each other with respect and caring.

Groups for male batterers are usually psychoeducational. They may be run as self-help groups, involving peer counseling, or as therapist-led groups. Although there is much variability across group treatments for male batterers, the primary goal of most available programs is to end the violence. Men are asked to accept responsibility for their abuse and for ending their violence. Many of the programs use behavioral-cognitive interventions for teaching anger management and violence cessation (see below). They also often involve interventions from a feminist perspective, including sex role education, resocialization, and discussions of patriarchal, male power issues. Finally, they often include skills training designed to improve the marital relationship (e.g., assertion training).

Group Therapy With Battered Women. Groups for women who have been victims of marital violence are also available (e.g., Cox & Stoltenberg, 1991), often being offered through battered women's shelters. Such groups typically function as support systems and advocates for women who are working to achieve independence from the men who have battered them. Treatment typically involves the provision of instrumental help, including assistance in dealing with social and legal services (e.g., help obtaining employment and housing, information on legal interventions). In addition, with their nonjudgmental and supportive atmosphere, these groups offer battered women emotional support and the opportunity to build their self-esteem; they are designed to empower women to make their own decisions regarding their relationships.

BEHAVIORAL-COGNITIVE THERAPEUTIC INTERVENTIONS DESIGNED TO ELIMINATE VIOLENCE

Cognitive-behavioral treatments are based upon assumptions that violent husbands have difficulty controlling their anger, combined with deficits in relationship and communication skills. It is assumed that as an unskilled husband encounters marital conflicts and is unable to effectively handle the conflict and his anger, he is at increased risk to engage in violence. His use of violence may be inadvertently reinforced (e.g., it ends the conflict and decreases his anger), increasing the probability that he will choose violence again in future marital situations and decreasing the probability that he will learn more constructive methods for handling anger and conflict.

Available data support many of these theoretical assumptions (see Holtzworth-Munroe, 1992, review). For example, research indicates that violent husbands experience more anger than other men (e.g., Maiuro et al., 1988), especially in marital situations (e.g., Margolin et al., 1988). In observations of marital interactions, violent couples have been found to lack communication skills and to engage in more negative behaviors than other couples (e.g., Margolin et al., 1988); violent husbands have also been found to provide less competent responses in problematic marital situations than nonviolent men (Holtzworth-Munroe & Anglin, 1991).

Given these data, therapists trained in the behavioral-cognitive orientation teach violent husbands anger managements skills. They also teach violent men and couples other communication and conflict resolution skills (e.g., listening, expressing feelings, problem-solving).

Anger Control Strategies. A variety of behavioral-cognitive interventions are available to help violent spouses recognize and reduce their anger and choose nonviolent actions even when angry (e.g., Novaco, 1975; Sonkin & Durphy, 1989). These interventions often teach clients to recognize the cues that they are experiencing anger and then to implement responses incompatible with violence when angry.

Anger Recognition. Anger recognition strategies allow the client to identify the physiological, behavioral, and cognitive cues of anger that precede acts of violence. Examples of physiological cues are a racing heart, feeling flushed or tense, and clenched jaw or fists. Behavioral cues may involve such activities as standing up, pacing, and exaggerated gestures. Cognitive cues include thoughts or statements to oneself that result in increasing anger levels (e.g., ruminating about how one was wronged).

Cue recognition can be facilitated by having clients self-monitor their feelings, thoughts, and behaviors during experiences in which they felt angry. This is often done with anger logs on which clients record a description of incidents in which they felt angry, including the time, place, people involved, and their thoughts, behaviors, emotions, and physical reactions in these situations. Situational analyses of clients' anger experiences are then reviewed with the therapist; common elements are identified as specific anger cues (e.g., for one client, a flushed face was a consistent sign that he was close to using violence) and high-risk situations are identified (e.g., one couple realized that their most destructive arguments occurred during exam week at school).

Once high-risk situations are identified, the clients and therapist can plan ways to avoid or prevent high-risk situations from occurring. In addition, once anger cues are identified, clients can be taught to implement responses that are incompatible with violence when anger cues occur. These responses may be behavioral, such as taking a time-out or using relaxation techniques, and/or cognitive, such as changing one's self-talk.

Time-Out Procedures. Time-out procedures are almost universally used in marital violence programs. These procedures are designed to help a violent spouse leave an escalating argument before violence occurs; they involve recognizing and acknowledging one's anger, removing oneself from the situation before violence occurs, and returning after one is calmed down.

Many couples initially object to the use of time-outs. These procedures may, at first, seem undesirable to couples, given our culture's emphasis on the cathartic benefits of "getting it all out" and never leaving issues unresolved. Thus, the therapist must remind the couple that, given their past use of violence, such immediate emotional expression is ill-advised and that it is better to temporarily leave issues unresolved than to engage in further physical violence. Time-out can be framed for the clients as a way to stop themselves from engaging in destructive behavior that they will later regret.

The basic time-out procedure is as follows: When clients first recognize that they are angry, they make a statement such as, "I feel angry and am going to take a time-out." They then state a specific and reasonable amount of time for the time-out and say that they will be back after that time period; this can range from 15 minutes to 2 hours, depending on the individual, the level of anger experienced, and the danger of violence. The person who called the time-out then leaves the interaction and, preferably, the setting (e.g., house, apartment) altogether. During the time-out, the individual should engage in techniques designed to decrease his or her anger. These may include nonaggressive physical exercise (e.g., running) and other calming techniques such as deep breathing, positive self-talk, and relaxation. Activities that may escalate one's anger or endanger the person, such as alcohol or drug use, aggressive exercise, ruminating about the anger-provoking interaction, or driving, should be avoided. At the conclusion of the time-out period, the individual should return to the partner. If the couple can *calmly* resume their discussion, they may do so; if not, such a discussion should be postponed until it can be conducted safely, perhaps in the presence of the therapist. If anger levels are still high, another time-out should be implemented.

Each step in the time-out must be reviewed carefully with the couple. First, stating that one is angry and needs a time-out necessitates taking responsibility for one's feelings (i.e., as opposed to "you make me angry") and for one's behaviors when angry. It should be emphasized that each individual is responsible for his or her own time-outs. Telling the other person to take a time-out is *not* allowed. Similarly, each partner must respect the other's right to take a time-out; we have encountered problems as one partner tries to stop the other from leaving. To avoid this, the couple must be prompted to remember the function and importance of the time-out - to stop destructive arguments.

Second, setting a limited length of time for the time-out is important, as is the couple's agreement to resume communication after the time-out. The qualitative difference between this and the "unilateral cessation of an argument" (Margolin, 1979, p. 17) should be stressed. Without attention to this issue, many husbands will simply use time-out as one more abusive technique (e.g., one man said he needed a time-out and then left home for 3 days). Similarly, the couple must be reassured that therapy will teach them the skills necessary to constructively resolve their unfinished discussions.

Finally, one's actions during the time-out must be directed at reducing, rather than escalating, the anger. The first impulse of many men is to jump in the car, go get a drink, or punch a punching bag. The potential dangerousness of these actions should be discussed (e.g., Is it safe to drive when so angry? Can one calm down when punching a bag and envisioning revenge?).

Time-out procedures are often initially difficult for couples to incorporate into their interactions; with practice, couples become increasingly proficient. After practicing the procedures during a therapy session, couples should be asked to take several practice time-outs per week, even if they do not really need one or feel only mildly irritated. Practicing these skills greatly increases the likelihood that the couple will have learned the time-out procedures and use them when they are truly needed. It also allows the therapist to troubleshoot problems the couple encounters when using the procedure. If a couple has had difficulty using time-outs, we ask them to enact a time-out in the therapy session. This provides an opportunity to examine what is interfering with the couple's execution of this procedure (e.g., one spouse is telling the other to leave; one spouse is concerned that the issue will never be resolved).

Self-Talk. Self-talk strategies are grounded in the belief that self-statements and thoughts play a critical role in the initiation and intensification of anger. Several writers have discussed cognitions that are related to anger (e.g., Ellis, 1977; Novaco, 1975). For example, Deffenbacher (1988) suggests that different types of thoughts lead to an increase in anger. These include catastrophizing thoughts, demanding/coercing thoughts (i.e., those that change desires into necessities), and the tendency to consistently personalize the reasons for a particular situation occurring. Following identification of the types of thoughts clients have, they can be trained to engage in more productive thoughts that, in turn, enable them to deal more appropriately with frustrating situations.

Relaxation Training. Relaxation training can also be implemented to help violent spouses calm down during an angry incident or during a time-out. Detailed descriptions of relaxation procedures can be found elsewhere (e.g., Sonkin & Durphy, 1989).

OTHER TREATMENT/THEORETICAL APPROACHES DESIGNED TO ELIMINATE MARITAL VIOLENCE

Cognitive-behavioral treatments for marital violence, such as those introduced previously, are widely used. However, other approaches exist as well.

Another major approach includes programs based upon *feminist theories* of marital violence. For example, Pence (1989) has developed treatment programs for violent men derived from feminist theories. These programs view marital violence as a sociopolitical issue; they assume that male violence toward women is based in, and supported by, our patriarchal society, which allows men to dominate women through a variety of economic and institutional mechanisms. Men are assumed to be more powerful than women, physically, politically, and economically. Thus, the husband's use of physical violence is simply one of the many methods he uses to control his wife's actions; others include psychological abuse, control of economic resources, and sexual abuse. Such tactics are supported by society, both directly (e.g., peer support of violence; the stated doctrine of some religious groups) and indirectly (e.g., lack of police response to domestic violence calls; lack of training of physicians to recognize the needs of battered women).

Feminist intervention programs target men's views of women and their belief that they should be able to control their wives. Therapy focuses on helping men to examine their sexist assumptions and their beliefs about relationships between men and women. Men are asked to examine the various methods they use to control their wives and how society sanctions those actions. The critical dimensions in feminist treatment are power and control; a didactic approach is often used to help violent men explore the sociopolitical meaning of abuse.

In addition, feminist programs emphasize the need for community support of marital violence intervention programs. These programs are ideally only one part of active, coordinated efforts by all relevant community agencies (e.g., police, prosecutors, probation, judges, battered women's advocates); such coordination is designed to provide a consistent message that abuse will not be tolerated and that the violent husband is responsible for his actions. Through such efforts, it is hoped that changes can be made in societal norms and attitudes toward male domination and marital violence.

Treatment programs derived from *family systems* theories of marital violence also exist (e.g., Lane & Russell, 1989; Madanes, 1990). According to systems theory, relationship violence is seen "as a symptom of dysfunctional interactions in a couple's relationship. Violent episodes are seen as part of an interactional sequence in which both batterer and victim contribute to an escalation of tension that ends in a violent outburst" (Harris et al., 1988, p. 148). This approach views marital violence as a relationship issue, as the function of the couple's interactional patterns; the causation of violence is believed to be circular, not linear, with both partners contributing to the escalation of conflicts.

This treatment approach usually includes the wife in therapy. It is designed to help each spouse identify his or her role in relationship processes and to break the couple's rigid patterns of interaction, allowing constructive change to take place. Specific therapy techniques that are systemic in nature include behavioral prescriptions, paradoxical interventions, use of a treatment team, and triangulation interpretations; these may be helpful in countering the resistance and avoidance of violent men (Madanes, 1990).

Systems therapy has been extensively criticized (e.g., Bograd, 1984; Margolin & Burman, 1993). Critics charge that this approach implies that the abused wife is, in some way, responsible for the solution to the problem and, perhaps, for the violence itself (i.e., blaming the victim). There is also concern that the wife's safety may be jeopardized by requiring her to actively participate in therapy (e.g., the husband may retaliate, with violence, if the wife discusses issues that he believes should not have been discussed with the therapist). In general, systems theory is criticized for ignoring gender issues and the inherent power of the men in our society, thus confusing the issue of who is responsible for male violence.

CLINICAL ISSUES FOR MARITAL VIOLENCE THERAPISTS

THERAPIST'S EMOTIONAL REACTIONS TO MARITAL VIOLENCE

Marital violence is a complex, emotionally charged, and potentially dangerous problem. The intensity of spouses' emotions during violent conflicts and the despicable nature of some batterers' behaviors may elicit intense emotional responses in therapists. In addition, given the prevalence of marital violence in our society, many therapists will have experienced physical aggression themselves, either in their own adult relationships or in their family of origin. Such experiences may color and shape a therapist's reactions to reports of violence among his or her clients. Sometimes therapists become particularly concerned about their own safety when working with violent couples or batterers.

Therapists beginning work in this area should be aware of the potential for a variety of strong reactions to couples' reports of marital violence and should seek consultation and supervision as needed. Therapists' fears regarding their own safety should be dealt with by receiving training in the treatment of marital violence; such training should help the therapist to conduct better assessments of the level of danger in each case and to develop contingency safety plans for the protection of all involved parties.

THERAPIST'S BELIEFS ABOUT MARITAL VIOLENCE AND RELATED ISSUES

Therapists who work with violent clients often need to examine their personal beliefs about family violence. It is impossible to offer "value free" therapy for marital violence (Margolin & Burman, 1993); every choice made by the therapist will reflect and convey his or her own beliefs about domestic violence.

It is essential that therapists are clear, in their own minds, as to which behaviors are violent and which are not (e.g., Is an occasional push or shove "violence"? When, if ever, should conjoint treatment be terminated because the violence has become too severe?). In addition, marital therapists need to consider whether they believe that violence is simply an extreme version of marital conflict in general, or whether violence qualitatively differs from other marital conflict (e.g., by involving possible injury, by altering the power structure of the relationship). Confusion on such matters will lead to an inconsistent therapy approach with violent cases.

Similarly, personal beliefs regarding male power and control should be confronted. Does the therapist view violence in the context of our patriarchal society and our culture's assumptions of male domination? Is the therapist sensitive to the terror felt by the female victim of violence? Is he or she aware of gender differences in our culture and how these are translated into various power structures within marital relationships?

Finally, it is important that therapists carefully consider their goals when working with violent couples. Is the primary goal to end the violence, as we have suggested? If so, marital therapists used to working with nonviolent couples may find it difficult to shift, and maintain, their attention on the violence; they may find themselves ignoring the violence, believing that relationship improvement is the major treatment goal. Again, seeking additional training in the treatment of marital violence should help the clinician to consider such issues.

THERAPEUTIC ALLIANCES

Therapeutic alliances are always an issue when conducting conjoint therapy, but are perhaps a more prominent issue when working with violent couples. The therapist must insure the safety of the wife. However, it is also critical that therapists working with violent men be able to accept them as human beings deserving of respect. Batterers may enter therapy anticipating rejection or punishment from therapists and thus adopt a resistant posture. Therapists can circumvent this dynamic by emphasizing their acceptance of the batterer *and* their concurrent rejection of his violent behavior. This nonjudgmental status regarding the batterer's worth as a person must be balanced against a condemnation of his violence. We have encountered therapists who simply state that they cannot work with violent men, given their anger at such men's behavior; such personal awareness is necessary.

In addition, marital therapists often serve as an advocate for the marital relationship, rather than for either spouse. In fact, marital therapy, by definition, is designed to preserve and improve the marriage. However, in the case of violent couples, a marital therapist must reconsider this assumption. For example, at what point is it better for a violent relationship to be dissolved? Can one be an advocate for the relationship, for the wife, and for the husband?

LEGAL ISSUES

Therapists must bear in mind the legal, ethical, and moral responsibilities involved in working with violent couples. Mandatory reporting laws for child abuse exist in all states; any knowledge or reasonable suspicion of child abuse must be reported to a child protective agency. Although there are no such regulations concerning wife abuse, legal rulings regarding the duty to warn and protect potential victims are relevant (e.g., *Tarasoff v. Regents of University of California,* 1976), as reviewed elsewhere (Hart, 1988; Sonkin, 1986; Sonkin & Ellison, 1986).

RESEARCH ON INTERVENTIONS FOR MARITAL VIOLENCE

METHODOLOGICAL PROBLEMS

Assuming that a violent husband seeks treatment, one must examine whether the available treatments serve as effective means of eliminating marital violence. Unfortunately, at this time, few methodologically sound studies have been conducted to examine the efficacy of treatment for marital violence. The majority of studies conducted to date examined group treatment for male batterers, although a few researchers have studied conjoint treatment. However, interpretation of the results of these studies is difficult, because a variety of methodological problems plague the marital violence treatment outcome literature. These problems have been discussed in detail elsewhere (Hamberger & Hastings, 1993; Rosenbaum, 1988; Rosenfeld, 1992).

TREATMENT OUTCOME FINDINGS

Despite these methodological limitations, two recent reviews of the currently available data regarding treatment outcome have been conducted. Hamberger and Hastings (1993) reviewed 28 outcome studies, while Rosenfeld (1992) reviewed 25 studies of treatment programs for marital violence.

Hamberger and Hastings (1993) concluded, "After reviewing much of the research literature, what do we 'know' about the short- and long-term effects of treatment on spouse abuse? The answer, unfortunately, is 'not much' . . . We cannot confidently say whether 'treatment works' . . . While there are some moderately good studies, many have one or more significant methodological or conceptual flaws which render them unhelpful at best, and at worst, misleading. Taken together, these studies are so varied in their make-up, process, and reporting as to make cross-study generalization impossible" (p. 220).

Rosenfeld (1992) acknowledges the same limitations in the currently available data; however, he chooses to make conclusions based upon these data. Across the studies, Rosenfeld found an average recidivism rate, weighted by study sample size, of 27%; in other words, by the time of the follow-up assessment in each study, 27% of the men had been violent, at least once, since treatment. Based on this figure, Rosenfeld (1992) concludes that men who complete treatment have only slightly, and often nonsignificantly, lower recidivism rates than men who refuse treatment, drop out of treatment, or remain untreated. He also notes that studies examining the efficacy of treatment in reducing psychological abuse have demonstrated "only modest gains."

Focusing on the efficacy of court-ordered treatment for marital violence, he concludes, "Although men and couples completing a treatment program (whether court-ordered or voluntary) report renewed violence at rates lower than those found when no form of intervention has occurred, men arrested but not referred to treatment appear to resume their violent behavior no more frequently than men arrested *and* treated. In addition, court-ordered men withdraw from treatment as often as do voluntary subjects, indicating that legal-system involvement may not be sufficient to motivate men who would otherwise be unmotivated to change their behavior" (Rosenfeld, 1992, p. 221).

Others have suggested that some treatment programs for violent husbands may not only be ineffectual but actually may be detrimental (e.g., programs that focus exclusively on anger control rather than recognizing that violence is used to control women; Gondolf & Russell, 1986). In addition, Gondolf (1988) has demonstrated that whether a batterer has sought counseling is the most influential predictor of whether his wife will return to him after leaving a shelter. Given the current lack of evidence demonstrating the efficacy of marital violence treatment programs, these data suggest that the very existence of such programs may actually increase the wife's risk, by leading to a false sense of security among battered women whose husbands have sought treatment.

Questions have also been raised regarding whether it is reasonable to assume that the currently available short-term interventions for marital violence can effectively treat what is often a chronic and severe problem; suggestions for incorporating relapse prevention interventions into treatment programs have been made (Jennings, 1990). In addition, at the present time, virtually no information is available regarding which batterers or violent couples are most likely to benefit from treatment or how to match clients to the appropriate treatment approaches.

In summary, the efficacy of treatment programs for marital violence has not been well researched, since past studies have been plagued by methodological problems. Thus, it is difficult to interpret the currently available data; however, these data do not indicate great success of available programs in reducing either physical or psychological abuse. In addition, questions regarding the possible detrimental effects of marital violence treatment programs have recently been raised. Thus, we concur with Hamberger and Hastings' (1993) and Rosenfeld's (1992) conclusion that questions regarding the efficacy of these programs remain unanswered until more, and better, research is conducted to clarify these issues.

Amy Holtzworth-Munroe, PhD, is an Assistant Professor in the Psychology Department at Indiana University. She has extensive experience in marital therapy and the treatment of marital violence and has published chapters and led workshops on these topics. Her research compares the skills of violent and nonviolent husbands, using a social information processing model; she has published numerous research articles on the topic of marital violence. Dr. Holtzworth-Munroe may be contacted at the Department of Psychology, Indiana University, Bloomington, IN 47405.

Gregory L. Stuart, BA, is an advanced doctoral student in clinical psychology at Indiana University. He has been studying marital violence since 1991. He is particularly interested in the treatment of marital violence and marital distress. Mr. Stuart can be contacted at Indiana University, Department of Psychology, Bloomington, IN 47405.

RESOURCES

Beck, A. T., Ward, C. H., Mendelson, M., Mock, J., & Erbaugh, J. (1961). An inventory for measuring depression. *Archives of General Psychiatry, 4*, 53-63.

Bograd, M. (1984). Family systems approaches to wife battering: A feminist critique. *American Journal of Orthopsychiatry, 54*, 558-568.

Cascardi, M., Langhinrichsen, J., & Vivian, D. (1992). Marital aggression: Impact, injury, and health correlates of husbands and wives. *Archives of Internal Medicine, 152*, 1178-1184.

Cox, J. W., & Stoltenberg, C. D. (1991). Evaluation of a treatment program for battered wives. *Journal of Family Violence, 6*, 395-414.

Deffenbacher, J. L. (1988). *A Cognitive-Relaxation Approach to Anger Reduction: A Treatment Manual*. Fort Collins, CO: Colorado State University.

Ellis, A. (1977). *How to Live With- and Without-Anger*. New York: Reader's Digest Press.

Gondolf, E. W. (1988). Who are those guys? Toward a behavioral typology of batterers. *Violence and Victims, 3*, 187-203.

Gondolf, E. W., & Russell, D. (1986). The case against anger control treatment programs for batterers. *Response to the Victimization of Women and Children, 9*, 2-5.

Hamberger, L. K., & Hastings, J. E. (1986). Personality characteristics of men who abuse their partners: A cross-validation study. *Journal of Family Violence, 1*, 323-341.

Hamberger, L. K., & Hastings, J. E. (1993). Court-mandated treatment of men who batter their partners: Issues, controversies, and outcomes. In Z. Hilton (Ed.), *Legal Responses to Wife Assault* (pp. 188-229). Newbury Park, CA: Sage.

Hansen, M., Harway, M., & Cervantes, N. (1991). Therapists' perceptions of severity in cases of family violence. *Violence and Victims, 6*, 225-234.

Harris, R., Savage, S., Jones, T., & Brooke, W. (1988). A comparison of treatments for abusive men and their partners within a family-service agency. *Canadian Journal of Community Mental Health, 7*, 147-155.

Hart, B. (1988). Beyond the "duty to warn": A therapist's "duty to protect" battered women and children. In M. Bograd & K. Yllo (Eds.), *Feminist Perspectives on Wife Abuse* (pp. 234-248). Newbury Park, CA: Sage.

Holtzworth-Munroe, A. (1992). Social skill deficits in maritally violent men: Interpreting the data using a social information processing model. *Clinical Psychology Review, 12*, 605-617.

Holtzworth-Munroe, A., & Anglin, K. (1991). The competency of responses given by maritally violent versus nonviolent men to problematic marital situations. *Violence and Victims, 6*, 257-269.

Holtzworth-Munroe, A., Waltz, J., Jacobson, N. S., Monaco, V., Fehrenbach, P. A., & Gottman, J. M. (1992). Recruiting nonviolent men as control subjects for research on marital violence: How easily can it be done? *Violence and Victims, 7*, 79-88.

Hotaling, G. T., & Sugarman, D. B. (1986). An analysis of risk markers in husband to wife violence: The current state of knowledge. *Violence and Victims, 1*, 101-124.

Houskamp, B. M., & Foy, D. W. (1991). The assessment of posttraumatic stress disorder in battered women. *Journal of Interpersonal Violence, 6*, 367-375.

Jacobson, N. S., & Margolin, G. (1979). *Marital Therapy: Strategies Based on Social Learning & Behavior Exchange Principles*. New York: Brunner/Mazel.

Jennings, J. L. (1990). Preventing relapse versus "stopping" domestic violence: Do we expect too much too soon from battering men? *Journal of Family Violence, 5*, 43-60.

Jouriles, E. N., & O'Leary, K. D. (1985). Interspousal reliability of reports of marital violence. *Journal of Consulting and Clinical Psychology, 53*, 419-421.

Lane, G., & Russell, T. (1989). Second-order systemic work with violent couples. In P. L. Caesar & L. K. Hamberger (Eds.), *Treating Men Who Batter: Theory, Practice, and Programs* (pp. 134-162). New York: Springer.

Leonard, K. E., & Blane, H. T. (1992). Alcohol and marital aggression in a national sample of young men. *Journal of Interpersonal Violence, 7*, 19-30.

Madanes, C. (1990). *Sex, Love, and Violence: Strategies for Transformation.* New York: W. W. Norton.

Maiuro, R. D., Cahn, T. S., Vitaliano, P. P., Wagner, B. C., & Zegree, J. B. (1988). Anger, hostility, and depression in domestically violent versus generally assaultive men and nonviolent control subjects. *Journal of Consulting and Clinical Psychology, 56*, 17-23.

Margolin, G. (1979). Conjoint marital therapy to enhance anger management and reduce spouse abuse. *American Journal of Family Therapy, 7*, 13-23.

Margolin, G., & Burman, B. (1993). Wife abuse versus marital violence: Different terminologies, explanations, and solutions. *The Clinical Psychologist, 13*, 59-73.

Margolin, G., John, R. S., & Gleberman, L. (1988). Affective responses to conflictual discussions in violent and nonviolent couples. *Journal of Consulting and Clinical Psychology, 56*, 24-33.

McDonald, R., & Jouriles, E. N. (1991). Marital aggression and child behavior problems: Research findings, mechanisms, and intervention strategies. *The Behavior Therapist, September*, 189-192.

Novaco, R. W. (1975). *Anger Control: The Development and Evaluation of an Experimental Treatment.* Lexington, MA: Lexington Books.

Novaco, R. W. (1977). Stress inoculation: A cognitive therapy for anger and its application to a case of depression. *Journal of Consulting and Clinical Psychology, 41*, 600-608.

O'Leary, K. D., Barling, J., Arias, I., Rosenbaum, A., Malone, J., & Tyree, A. (1989). Prevalence and stability of physical aggression between spouses: A longitudinal analysis. *Journal of Consulting and Clinical Psychology, 57*, 263-268.

O'Leary, K. D., Vivian, D., & Malone, J. (1992). Assessment of physical aggression against women in marriage: The need for multimodal assessment. *Behavioral Assessment, 14*, 5-14.

Pence, E. (1989). Batterer programs: Shifting from community collusion to community confrontation. In P. L. Caesar & L. K. Hamberger (Eds.), *Treating Men Who Batter: Theory, Practice, and Programs* (pp. 24-50). New York: Springer.

Rosenbaum, A. (1988). Methodological issues in marital violence research. *Journal of Family Violence, 3*, 91-104.

Rosenbaum, A., & O'Leary, K. D. (1981). Marital violence: Characteristics of abusive couples. *Journal of Consulting and Clinical Psychology, 49*, 63-71.

Rosenfeld, B. D. (1992). Court-ordered treatment of spouse abuse. *Clinical Psychology Review, 12*, 205-226.

Saunders, D. G. (1992). Woman battering. In R. T. Ammerman & M. Hersen (Eds.), *Assessment of Family Violence: A Clinical and Legal Sourcebook* (pp. 208-235). New York: John Wiley and Sons.

Saunders, D. G., Lynch, A. B., Grayson, M., & Linz, D. (1987). The inventory of beliefs about wife beating: The construction and initial validation of a measure of beliefs and attitudes. *Violence and Victims, 2*, 39-57.

Sonkin, D. J. (1986). Clairvoyance vs. common sense: Therapist's duty to warn and protect. *Violence and Victims, 1*, 7-22.

Sonkin, D. J., & Durphy, M. (1989). *Learning to Live Without Violence: A Book for Men.* Volcano, CA: Volcano Press.

Sonkin, D. J., & Ellison, J. E. (1986). The therapist's duty to protect victims of domestic violence: Where we have been and where we are going. *Violence and Victims, 1*, 205-214.

Sonkin, D. J., Martin, D., & Walker, L. E. A. (1985). *The Male Batterer: A Treatment Approach.* New York: Springer.

Spence, J. T., & Helmreich, R. L. (1972). The attitudes toward women scale: An objective instrument to measure attitudes toward the rights and roles of women in contemporary society. *JSAS Catalogue of Selected Documents in Psychology, 2*, 66.

Spielberger, C. D., Gorsuch, R. L., & Lushene, R. E. (1970). *Manual for the State-Trait Anxiety Inventory.* Palo Alto, CA: Consulting Psychologist Press.

Stets, J. E., & Straus, M. A. (1990). Gender differences in reporting marital violence and its medical and psychological consequences. In M. A. Straus & R. J. Gelles (Eds.), *Physical Violence in American Families: Risk Factors and Adaptations to Violence in 8,145 Families* (pp. 151-165). New Brunswick, NJ: Transaction Publishers.

Straus, M. A. (1979). Measuring intrafamily conflict and violence: The conflict tactics (CT) scales. *Journal of Marriage and the Family, 41,* 75-88.

Straus, M. A., & Gelles, R. J. (1990). How violent are American families? Estimates from the national family violence resurvey and other studies. In M. A. Straus & R. J. Gelles (Eds.), *Physical Violence in American Families: Risk Factors and Adaptations to Violence in 8,145 Families* (pp. 95-112). New Brunswick, NJ: Transaction Publishers.

Tarasoff v. the Regents of the University of California, 17 Cal.3d. 425, 551 P.2d 334 (1976).

Tolman, R. M. (1989). The development of a measure of psychological maltreatment of women by their male partners. *Violence and Victims, 4,* 159-177.

Walker, L. E. A. (1979). *The Battered Woman.* New York: Harper & Row.

INNOVATIONS IN THE TREATMENT OF MULTIPLE PERSONALITY DISORDER

R. Douglas Smith

Multiple Personality Disorder (MPD) is a dissociative disorder characterized by the presence of two or more alternate ego states, identities, or "alters" within the same person. At any given time, one or more of these alters may emerge to assume executive control of consciousness, behavior, and identity. The primary or host personality is often amnestic for the emergence and actions of these alters, who have their own separate motivations and goals. Amnesia, memory deficits, auditory hallucinations, depression, and a multitude of psychopathological symptoms may be concurrently present, often confusing attempts at accurate diagnosis (Coons, 1980; Kluft, 1985; Putnam, 1989). Several diagnostic assessment instruments assist in the recognition of MPD and other dissociative disorders (Bernstein & Putnam, 1986; Chu, 1991; Frischholz et al., 1991). The etiology of MPD is usually found in a background history of physical, emotional, or sexual abuse (Putnam, 1989).

The principles and goals of treatment with this population involve the following important issues: (a) the establishment of trust in the therapeutic relationship; (b) the identification of the various alters and their repressed abusive memories; (c) the appropriate use of specific therapeutic techniques and strategies; (d) the gradual weakening of amnestic barriers between the alters, enhancing communication and movement toward system-wide cooperation; (e) the gradual blending and possible integration of all alters into one identity; and (f) appropriate follow-up to assist the patient in dealing with normal adjustment issues as a single personality. In general, the goal is the integration, restructuring, or reorganization of the patient's sense of unity by recovering and working through abusive memories such that the patient assimilates and "owns" them in a psychological sense.

Traditional treatment approaches have been described by Braun (1986) and Kluft (1980) and generally consist of the following steps: (a) the development of trust via a strong therapeutic alliance, both global and with each individual alter; (b) sharing the MPD diagnosis with all the personalities; (c) establishing communication linkages with the alters; (d) contracting with the alters to attend the therapy sessions and avoid self-harm to the body they share; (e) gathering a historical overview of each alter to determine its origins, functions, and relationships with the others; (f) solving the various alters' specific problems; (g) understanding the structure of the personality system; (h) encouraging and facilitating interpersonality communications between the alters; (i) blending the alters toward a unity; (j) helping the patient (once integration begins) develop new and more realistic defenses and coping mechanisms to deal with stress; (k) solidification of the gains by continual working through and support; and (l) follow-up to insure that the therapeutic gains are maintained.

Complications arise in following these steps for a variety of reasons. The different alter personalities may not be aware of each other. Varying degrees of awareness are not uncommon: some personalities are aware of and supportive of others, some are in direct and often hostile conflict, and some may exist in isolation with no awareness of the others. Typically only one personality interacts with the external environment at any given time, although others inside may try to passively influence the dominant alter personality. During certain periods, the other personalities may "listen in" on what is happening, or there may be a total amnestic barrier. The personalities typically express awareness of the amnestic barrier as lost periods or distortions in their experience of time. Several studies (Braun, 1983; Putnam, 1989; Smith, Titus, & Carr, 1989) have demonstrated that alter personalities may have quite different physiological and psychological characteristics, such as different eyeglass prescriptions, strikingly different responses to the same medication, and different IQ levels. Most of the personalities can be identified by specific names. They may describe themselves as being of a different age or sex than the patient and will exhibit behavioral characteristics appropriate to that age and sex.

Differentiating multiple personality from other associated disorders such as schizophrenia, psychogenic amnesia, fugue states, and borderline personality disorder may be difficult. The comprehensive analysis described by Kluft (1980) in diagnosing MPD is helpful in this regard. As a general guideline, the existence of multiple amnestic episodes together with the presence of alternating separate and distinct identities will often distinguish it from other psychiatric syndromes.

One of the primary purposes of therapy is to assist the patient to face and work through some significant and disruptive trauma of the past. In the typical treatment process, a mutually agreed-upon traumatic memory is selected by the patient and therapist, generally followed by emotional abreaction of the traumatic memory via imagination and subsequent working-through procedures. This is generally considered to be a generic and traditional approach. However, the alters typically strongly resist the disclosure of those abusive experiences because they fear the pain or cannot distinguish between the memory and the original trauma. Sometimes the perpetrators of the abuse have threatened the alters with death or revenge if they disclose the abuse. Unfortunately, conventional treatment for MPD and the dissociative disorders is often long and arduous. There are numerous crises, resistances, spontaneous regressions, and self-abusive and self-destructive behaviors. Trust that varies among the alters and denial contribute to this most difficult and complex disorder. Typical treatment duration for MPD may average 3 to 5 years (Kluft, 1980), although treatment may well extend beyond that for cult survivors or for other idiosyncratic reasons. In addition, the literature provides little guidance to the therapist as to which memory to process; several sessions may be necessary to process a single traumatic memory (Putnam, 1989). It is difficult to judge progress - or lack of it - under such conditions. Therapists bound to a single orientation or rigid in their approach may lack practical tools for dealing with the massive dissociation and resistances encountered.

The time now appears appropriate for exploring the skillful blending of both traditional and nontraditional treatment approaches in an attempt to describe more systematic approaches to this disorder. A description of practical therapeutic techniques and the timing of their use, embedded in a more systematic conceptual framework, appears necessary if we are to approach a more efficient resolution of MPD. This contribution will address a variety of therapeutic strategies arbitrarily divided into beginning, middle, and end phases. Each phase includes specific tasks for the therapist and suggested procedural techniques. However, as in any therapeutic endeavor, certain alters may require beginning-phase approaches while others are functioning at a middle or ending phase. In this pragmatic conceptual system, the beginning phase consists primarily of diagnosis and treatment planning. The middle phase involves the actual work of the therapist, and the end phase prepares the patient for unity and follow-up support.

THE BEGINNING PHASE: DIAGNOSIS AND TREATMENT PLANNING

The beginning phase of treatment involves the accurate diagnosis of the patient. It is obvious that the concerned clinician must be familiar with the criteria listed in *DSM-IV*, as well as diagnostic criteria problems described by a variety of researchers (Bloch, 1988; Putnam et al., 1986; Young, 1988).

Diagnostic problems arise because, almost invariably, the clinical manifestations are embedded within a polysymptomatic presentation suggestive of one or more commonplace conditions such as depressive, phobic, borderline, or somatoform disorders. Depressive symptoms are nearly universal, as are hallucinations, which may be misdiagnosed as schizophrenia. In addition, such patients often withhold or are amnestic for crucial information needed for a correct diagnosis. A number of dissociative disorder and MPD scales have been developed to assist the clinician in diagnostic assessment (Bernstein & Putnam, 1986; Chu, 1991; Frischholz et al., 1991).

Once the diagnosis has been established, it is then necessary to share the diagnosis, implications, and treatment procedures with the patient. Some patients are relieved to understand their amnestic periods, unusual behaviors, and other dissociative experiences. Others may be frightened and refuse to acknowledge the presence of a condition that permits several personalities in one shared body. It is important to be supportive and empathic with this latter patient, pointing out a positive outlook for the future with adequate treatment. Sharing written literature, booklets, or other material in which other MPD patients describe their awareness and treatment is often helpful. If the patient has sufficient ego-strength and curiosity, a videotape of one or more alters emerging may be a useful teaching tool. Nonabusive relationships, such as with a spouse or friend, can provide a very useful adjunctive support. With the patient's permission, the "significant other" may be educated as to the nature of MPD, can be instructed as to methods of support and in-home crisis management, and can report on the patient's progress or problem areas between sessions. Often partners of MPD patients become skillful in the management of spontaneous flashbacks and crisis situations.

INNOVATIVE METHODS OF DATA GATHERING

As much data as possible must be gathered prior to beginning treatment. This is especially difficult with MPD patients who have periods of amnesia, memory lapses, denial, and resistance to revealing past abuse. Many such patients have been threatened with harm if they reveal their "secrets." Therefore, a therapist should use a simple and nonthreatening approach that respects the defenses of the patient whenever possible. An initial approach is to have the host personality simply draw or write about a family tree, listing the names and relationships of all family members, relatives, and even outside individuals as they exist. It is preferable to present this information in a genogram in which all relationships are graphically drawn on a blackboard or poster board. The second step is to have the patient go to the board and indicate, perhaps by marking with a colored marker, all individuals for whom he or she has a "bad or negative feeling" but *without* revealing the source or cause of that feeling. The patient may identify several or only a few who fall into that classification. Nevertheless, this information provides the baseline of conscious awareness of possible past abuse and defines where the patient's limits of awareness begin and end. The task of simply identifying those individuals with whom the patient has a "bad feeling" without discussing the cause or nature of that feeling is less threatening, does not reveal any protected "secrets," and minimizes defenses of denial and repression. It is a subtle but effective approach to gaining essential data.

The next step is to attempt to identify and call out the patient's Inner Self Helper (ISH) alter. The ISH is typically an alter who functions as an objective observer of all that occurs with the patient and the various other alters involved. The ISH usually possesses judgment, objectivity, and insight and can be asked to serve as a consultant to the therapist. Putnam (1989) suggests that the helpful ISH can provide guidance and direction in therapy and warn of danger or impending crisis situations. Comstock (1985) offers a number of therapeutic suggestions in working with the ISH in therapy. The therapist can request assistance in resolving problems and can even ask the ISH to write comments on the effectiveness of therapy between sessions.

Once the ISH has been identified, it is necessary to have it go to the board or genogram and specifically identify all those with whom "bad memories" are associated. This may yield a similar but often quite different list of individuals, because the ISH may have memories of experiences unknown to the host personality. Other cooperative alters are individually called forth and asked to complete the same task. Each alter should be given a different-colored marker to indicate persons on the board. Once all the alters willing to participate in this task have finished, the therapist has what has been called an "alter genogram." This noninvasive approach has a number of significant advantages: (a) At a glance it identifies all the potentially abusive individuals associated with the patient recalled by the host personality at a conscious level; (b) it further identifies other individuals associated with abuse toward specific alters; (c) because each alter used a specific color to identify an abuser, those alters who share memories of a common abuser can be readily identified by the number of colors on that abuser's name on the genogram; and (d) with this approach a very rich amount of valuable data can be gathered in a relatively short period of time without having discussed a single traumatic memory. This systematic alter genogram has been developed by Titus (Smith et al., 1989).

A subsequent approach, based upon the preceding, is to establish a "trauma hierarchy" in which each alter cooperates by listing all those individuals associated with an abusive memory, from "most abusive" to "least abusive." The name of the most abusive individual goes at the top of the list and the least abusive at the bottom. The therapist assists the alter by a "paired comparison" of each name with every other name to come up with a systematically ranked trauma hierarchy. Each alter is asked to complete this task. All of this data is collected without the patient describing any abuse or any memories associated with these individuals. This is less threatening to the alters and less likely to mobilize resistances. At the end of this procedure, the therapist now possesses a systematically arranged series of individuals associated with traumas; the therapist may begin processing lesser traumas and gradually work up to the more emotionally threatening traumas. This procedure allows the therapist to have a series of "benchmarks" with which to gauge progress while allowing the patient to gain a sense of self-control by working with more manageable traumas first and more disruptive ones later. Although this does not prevent spontaneous abreactions, flashbacks, or sudden emergence of abusive memories, it nevertheless provides a more systematic approach than simply trying to deal with a multitude of memories, or the "memory of the moment" in any given session. As therapy progresses, other information will spontaneously emerge and will be added to this data bank.

More traditional methods of gathering information involve having the host personality and all the alters communicate by writing in a journal, sending letters to the therapist, drawing pictures of past abusive memories or recurrent flashbacks, or working with a sand tray. These techniques are especially valuable for patients unable to verbally communicate. Although Kaliff (1980) is generally credited with introducing the sand play technique, different therapeutic uses of sand play have been discussed by Bradway (1979) and Sachs and Sweig (1993). A number of human figures, houses, cars, and furniture are constructed by the patient in a small sandbox. The patient then describes the sand play creation and the feelings it elicits. The sand tray technique appears to function like an implicit, rather than explicit, memory test (Sachs & Sweig, 1993). Hypnosis and guided imagery are also frequently used in the elicitation of alters as well as in the processing of abusive memories; it is assumed the therapist will be skilled in these areas prior to treatment. Hypnotic suggestions and metaphors have been comprehensively discussed by Hammond (1990).

The final step in the beginning phase, following adequate data gathering, is to share the treatment plan with the patient and elicit as much cooperation through interactions with as many alters as possible. Those alters who are identified as helpful as well as those who are potentially abusive to self or others should be identified as early as possible. Therapists who need to remember a large number of alters may establish a card file, a diagram that connects all the alters, or another type of quick-reference index of names and personality characteristics. Large numbers of the inner population may be handled by asking the group to nominate one specific alter to speak for the rest or by simply assigning the task to a designated alter after some negotiation by the therapist.

At this point in the beginning phase of treatment the therapist should have made the appropriate diagnosis, shared that information with the patient and others with permission, identified the significant abusive individuals in each of the initial alter's past, established a beginning trauma hierarchy as a baseline, and informed the patient of the necessity of recovering and reintegrating past abusive experiences as part of the therapeutic process. It is further assumed that the issue of trust will continue to be an important factor that will emerge time and again, to varying degrees with each alter. However, although trust is necessary, it is not sufficient for successful treatment. Effective therapeutic techniques and strategies that help patients resolve their abusive disorder are equally important. A sense of safety and protection is the third leg of successful treatment. All three will continue to require attention throughout the middle phase of treatment.

MIDDLE PHASE: TREATMENT APPROACHES

PRINCIPLES OF TREATMENT

This phase begins the most difficult and time-consuming part of therapy with the MPD patient. During this phase the therapist may be faced with a widely disparate group of alters, ranging from children to adults. The most flexible and creative talents of the therapist will be needed to constantly shift focus, deal with different levels of maturity and self-control between alters, negotiate the demands of each for expression, conduct effective abreactions, and control self-abusive or suicidal alters. Because of past traumatic histories, the patient may attempt to manipulate, seduce, or betray the therapist by attempting to encourage countertransference feelings.

In addition, the important work of abreaction is further complicated by the tendency of the patient to confuse the past traumatic memory as if it were happening again, with the therapist being perceived as perpetrator (Comstock & Vickery, 1992). Pacing of the therapy is also important in order to avoid overwhelming and retraumatizing the patient. In general, the therapist must pace memory work to the patient's ego-strength and available internal resources. Uncovering traumatic content too early or without regard to these factors may overwhelm the patient or threaten the therapeutic alliance (Calof, 1991).

Maintaining personal and professional boundaries is also important, but this always remains a matter of personal judgment. Although many therapists agree with the conventional belief that boundaries should be kept rigid and firm, it would seem more appropriate that boundaries must remain firm but flexible. It is often necessary to modify boundaries to meet the needs of the patient while keeping in mind the dynamic and transference/countertransference implications. Putnam (1989), for example, described the unusual method of treating a client at a zoo in order to elicit certain alters.

Therapists bound to a single orientation or rigid in their approach may lack practical tools for dealing with the massive dissociation and denial of traumatic memory in multiple and dissociative disorder clients. Without a variety of alternative strategies and techniques for confronting patient memories and repression, therapy may drag on indefinitely and therapists may succumb to a countertransferential resentment toward clients.

In the early stages of therapy, it is important to gain some degree of cooperation by establishing an atmosphere of trust, safety, and competence. Identifying an Inner Self Helper (ISH) as well as one or more alters to begin the process is a necessary first step. Referring to the alter genogram, the previous history given, the journals, or other information will identify the alter to be considered, while the trauma hierarchy will establish a memory more easily accessible to work. In general, the successful resolution of less traumatic abusive memories gives the patient a sense of accomplishment while demonstrating the effectiveness of the therapeutic approach. This may provide the patient with a groundwork of courage to face even more abusive memories in the future. To the extent that the therapist and client can progress up a trauma hierarchy, there will be benchmarks for progress regardless of often-necessary diversions to deal with crisis situations from time to time.

Once an alter and an abusive memory associated with some past individual has been chosen, the therapist should consult the ISH regarding which alter should directly participate in the memory retrieval, who might profit more by just listening or observing, and who should be nowhere in the vicinity at the time - or asleep. Frequently, several alters share specific involvements in the past event. Special needs of each alter must be anticipated in advance of the process. At a minimum, the therapist must convey the reasons for the proposed experience, the proposed safeguards, and the expected outcome. The patient must come to the process with some hope and trust of its efficacy and thus some emotional investment.

It must be kept in mind that the normal existential assumptions we all take for granted have been shattered or distorted for MPD patients, who no longer believe in invulnerability or that the world makes logical sense. They often verbalize, "If God loved me, then he would protect me. Therefore I must be bad," and responsibility is transferred incorrectly by the abuser through statements such as, "It is your fault this is happening to you." Guilt, fear, and shame are often the result of such abusive assumptions. These false underlying assumptions will emerge in one form or another with every alter who is confronted, and the therapist must work to assist the client in regaining normal, healthy assumptions instead.

METHODS AND STRATEGIES

Abreactive work is often the most effective method of regaining and effectively processing the abusive memory until resolution is accomplished (Van Der Hart & Brown, 1992). Abreaction is the process of vividly reliving and reexperiencing an intensely emotional experience of traumatic abuse which had previously been repressed and dissociated. In spontaneous abreactions, the patient relives a past traumatic experience several times with no effective resolution, as in "flashbacks." In typical therapy for the MPD patient, a mutually agreed-upon traumatic memory is selected by the patient and therapist, safety procedures are discussed, and this is generally followed by emotional abreaction of the traumatic memory via imagination and subsequent working-through procedures. This is considered to be a generic and traditional approach in dealing with most MPD patients. Each alter typically has one or more traumatic memories to be processed in this manner. Prior to the establishment of the alter genogram and trauma hierarchy, the literature gave little guidance to the therapist as to which memory to process.

The therapeutic value of abreaction lies in the careful presentation of the trauma in a manner the patient can handle without being overwhelmed or left with retraumatization. The postabreaction cognitive work reframes and reinterprets the traumatic event in order to leave the patient not with just a sense of victimization but also with a sense of empowerment. The therapist must provide constant emotional support during the abreaction, modulating the amount of emotional discharge, providing an anchor to the present by reminding the patient of the current reality and the fact that it is a memory being recalled, and deciding when to terminate the memory recall. Hypnosis and guided imagery are often the treatments of choice in the elicitation and management of traumatic memories in abreactive work. When used by a therapist trained and experienced in clinical hypnosis, it is a valuable therapeutic tool with this population and can be used in a number of ways as described by Kluft (1982), Watkins (1980), and Braun (1984). Typical abreactive work is to be found in Comstock (1986), Putnam (1989), and Watkins (1980).

Following are several approaches therapists can use to elicit and manage abreactions.

Fragmentation. In fragmentation the therapist asks the patient to recall only parts of the abusive memory, such as the first third, second third, or last third, while simultaneously hypnotically blocking other portions of the memory until a given individual portion is discussed and assimilated. This allows the patient to discuss events leading up to the abuse, the act of the abuse, and the subsequent events in a manageable manner. With minor or secondary abusive memories, this is often effective. However, with more intensely emotional memories, patients have great difficulty partializing it out and the abreaction tends to run its full course.

Time-Limited. Time-limited techniques involve hypnotically conditioning patients to accept that they will reexperience the trauma while the therapist is counting to 10, or some other arbitrary number, at which time the emotional abreaction reaches its peak expression, followed by counting backwards from 10 to 1, at the end of which suggestions that the memory is fading away, becoming "weaker," or leaving entirely are given to the patient. The abusive memory is thus contained within a specified time period and can be repeated as often as necessary.

Journaling, Drawing, and Working With Clay. These techniques are other effective methods for working through abusive memories. Journal entries kept by specific alters can be read aloud during the abreaction to increase the vividness of recall of the abusive memory, drawings of the event can be used as specific "visual triggers" to elicit the event, and clay can be modeled to represent individuals associated with the memory. It is often helpful to have the patient redraw an abusive memory, following an abreaction, placing the abuser in the role of victim; this allows a healthy expression of anger on the part of the patient reframing the event.

Age Progression. Age progression is often used with child alters or adolescent alters fixated upon some specific abusive period in their life and unable to progress further. Some alters are too young to verbally express the trauma and the trauma is "frozen" in some body memory. It is appropriate to seek the approval of the alter involved to rapidly age the alter over a specified period of time. The process of hypnotically aging a young alter has two major advantages: It subjectively places more emotional distance between the patient and the abusive memory as the age progresses, and it allows more accurate, objective verbalizations from an "older" alter once the process is completed. Typically, hypnotic suggestions are given to grow to a specified age by a mutually agreed-upon date. At that time both the alter and the abusive memory may be more easily accessed.

Transposition of Abilities. This is a process in which one or more alters can be called upon to assist an alter undergoing an abreaction or being worked with in therapeutic recall. For example, with vocally impaired alters who were possibly "gagged" or smothered during a traumatic event, the therapist may ask a second alter to "lend" its voice to the alter who cannot speak so that communication can be restored. If there is too much body pain associated with a past abusive memory, such that abreactive work is blocked, the therapist may ask one or more other alters to temporarily divide up and "hold" the pain taken from the blocked alter until the abusive episode has been faced and described by the original alter.

Transposition of affect is also quite helpful in dealing with an alter who is normally passive, feels helpless, and is lacking in normal assertiveness. At such times, the therapist can make prior arrangements with another alter in the system who carries a good deal of anger and aggressiveness to assist in the abreactive work with the passive alter. At the appropriate time during the abreactive work, usually toward the end of the process, the therapist may ask for the passive alter to be filled with anger, resentment, and assertive feelings "borrowed" from another alter and directed toward the perpetrator of the abuse. This serves to model a more healthy response to the abuse, allows the alter to externalize self-directed anger, and facilitates closer cooperation between alters.

Cognitive information may be shared in a similar manner. Skill in carrying out a job or technical task can often be accomplished by assisting the ISH in transferring knowledge from one alter, who may be unable to function for a number of reasons, to another alter to carry on the job function. It is assumed, of course, that the alter system has reached a point of reasonable trust and cooperation with the therapist and the goals of therapy.

Slow-Leak Approach. This approach involves the suggestion that certain abusive memories will not be recalled all at once but that the memory will slowly come into conscious awareness a bit at a time, consistent with how much the patient is able to tolerate over an extended period of time. This prevents the patient from feeling overwhelmed and allows greater management of unpleasant affect. The suggestion is usually given to the alter under hypnosis and the memory may be leaked slowly from another alter who has that memory or from the individual alter's own memory banks. This approach is often helpful when two alters share opposite and seemingly incompatible behavior patterns due to unique abusive histories. One alter may be promiscuous and have a strong but indiscriminate sex drive, while a second alter may be phobic for any type of physical contact and frightened of sexual feelings. Within appropriate guidelines, the first alter may agree to allow a gradual, slow leak of those feelings in a nonthreatening manner. Although this does not resolve the problems of the promiscuous alter, it does selectively share appropriate feelings and assists in resolving the problems of one alter.

Time Distortion. Time distortion is a technique in which the amount of time a patient subjectively experiences recalling an abusive memory or part of that memory is made shorter by hypnotic suggestion. This means that an abusive memory reexperience that lasted objectively for an hour could be experienced in 10 minutes subjectively by the patient. In a similar manner, a brief period of time set aside for rest or processing the abusive memory could be made to seem much longer.

Memory Combinations. This method involves the therapist combining all memories with a similar theme, for example, cutting or burning episodes, such that one overall memory issue is abreacted and processed with all involved alters participating. Whenever possible, the therapist should try to categorize by issues, themes, age, sex, or other relevant dimensions to expedite the process. It is often not necessary to address every abusive memory of each alter. Furthermore, alters not involved in the abusive memory, or who may be vulnerable, should be asked to go to "sleep" or to a safe place until the abreaction is completed. The ISH is quite helpful in bringing this about.

Hypnotic Dream Suggestions. Hypnotic dream suggestions is a procedure in which the patient is hypnotically induced to have a dream that may involve one or more alters, the abusive perpetrator, the setting for the abuse, and even a metaphorical story that describes the events. The patient is also given the suggestion to discuss this dream with the therapist. The various techniques utilized in this dream-work approach have been carefully evaluated by Paley (1992).

Time-Limited Blending. In time-limited blending, two alters are temporarily blended together into one alter to carry out some mutually agreed-upon, time-limited task that no single alter could complete. For example, an assertive alter may agree to be temporarily blended with a passive, inhibited alter who is knowledgeable in order to deliver an important required speech. Mutual agreement, preparation, and prior rehearsal of the blending is necessary, and the alters may be separated following the event.

Memory Repression Technique. This technique is sometimes used when the patient is anticipating a stressful crisis situation that could not ordinarily be managed due to the spontaneous emergence of flashbacks or abreactions. During such times, the patient and therapist may agree to temporary total repression of all abusive memories until the crisis has passed. This can only be used when the alters have developed enough trust in each other to cooperate fully. For example, a patient about to undergo traumatic surgery, in which cooperation is essential, may agree to be placed in a deep hypnotic state and have all the abusive memories sealed away in a secure place or symbolically buried deep in the ground with all the alters "throwing in" their memories. Alternatively, all alters who may potentially abreact or become disruptive during the operation could be placed in a deep sleep or become dormant with their cooperation. This is obviously only a temporary measure designed for only a brief period of time. The buried issues will need to be continuously addressed by the therapist at a later date.

Negative Addictive Feedback. Negative addictive feedback is a procedure of cooperation between two alters, one of whom has an addictive disorder such as drugs or other compulsive habits. With prior agreement, a second, healthier alter may agree to "feed" negative, unpleasant physical sensations to the addicted alter after the ingestion of the substance. Although this technique does not address the underlying dynamics of the addiction, it does provide a useful behavioral control over the frequency and amount of the substance abuse until it is more fully resolved.

Eye Movement Desensitization Response (EMD). Another specialized technique for dealing with post-traumatic events is gaining increased recognition. Eye movement desensitization response is a procedure developed by Shapiro (1989) designed to eliminate the conditioned emotional responses to traumatic memories. The procedure requires that the patient create a visual image of the disturbing event and rate the subjective level of disturbance. This is often termed a "SUD" level with the patient reporting a number representing the "Subjective Unit of Disturbance" ranging from low to high on an arbitrary scale of 1 to 10. The patient is then required to hold that image while the therapist generates sets of 25 to 30 eye movements by having the patient track the therapist's finger as it moves back and forth laterally across the patient's field of vision approximately 18 inches in front of the patient's face. After each set of eye movements the patient is asked to rate again the SUD level of the disturbing image. Although only a limited number of studies have been published thus far (Marquis, 1991; Puk, 1991; Wolpe & Abrams, 1991), the resolution of trauma is usually quite rapid, often requiring few sessions. The underlying rationale and factors that both explain and account for this effect remain unclear. Marquis (1991), in a study of 78 cases, has addressed some of these technical questions but feels that "the adoption of this important technique has priority over its explanation" (p. 192). Further study of this procedure and the underlying explanatory mechanisms will be needed to more fully assess its importance and its lasting value to MPD patients.

DEALING WITH RESISTANCES

Chu (1988) has carefully identified four basic areas of resistance in the treatment of MPD patients: (a) resistance to uncovering repressed trauma, (b) resistance to trust in the therapist and to the treatment itself, (c) resistance to giving up the defense of dissociation and repression, and (d) resistance to integration. Resistance is an expression of the client's fear, and considerable work must be accomplished by the therapist in the areas of trust and safety with the patient. The wise therapist must strike a balance between respecting that resistance and knowing when it is time to confront it more directly if therapy is to progress and be effective. It is also important to remember that successfully dealing with resistances with one alter has ramifications for other alters, because the therapist is essentially dealing with a dynamic system that is interrelated. Resolving one alter's problems and then having that alter communicate those events and feelings to other alters inside accelerates the degree of overall cooperation and trust. An effective therapist will move between strong empathic sensitivity to the needs of the patient and professional judgment as to moving the patient past resistance by various confrontational approaches.

Because dissociation is a psychological process that defends and protects the patient from disruptive and, at times, destructive abusive memories, it is natural for a great deal of resistance to surface. The amount of resistance will vary with the specific nature of the relationship with the therapist, the severity of the past abuse, and the willingness of the patient to reexperience the past traumatic memory. As Bloch (1988) has stated, "disclosure and uncovering of those experiences can be resisted strongly by protective alters who cannot distinguish between the memory and the original trauma, and who were threatened by the abuser with death or severe retribution if the abuse were ever disclosed" (p. 58). It is equally obvious that patience, empathic support, encouragement, and technical success is necessary over a period of considerable time before some alters are willing to relinquish their resistance to change. Good clinical judgment is needed to determine when to confront the resistance and when to postpone further progress toward integration.

Establishing sound safety procedures for the patient often serves to both reassure and reduce the degree of resistance. Contracting for the safety of the body with abusive alters, encouraging other alters to report potentially dangerous or threatening situations, starting and stopping sessions on time, insuring that a "safe" or protective alter is out before the patient leaves the office, sealing unfinished memories away in a box or container between sessions, allowing a frightened alter to go to sleep between sessions, and being available for reasonable telephone consultation are all designed to encourage cooperation. In general, successful early abreactions with less traumatic material improve the chance for success with more difficult and complex abusive memories. Consistent use of both verbal and physical hypnotic signals to terminate an abreaction and bring the patient back to the present, as well as permissible holding the hands of the patient to anchor in the here-and-now, establishes a sense of security. A very vulnerable child alter who is subject to unhealthy influences or suggestions for self-harm by another abusive alter may be temporarily protected by the therapist offering to symbolically "adopt" the child with the understanding that the child alter will obey only the requests of the "good parent" and ignore any previous loyalty to a threatening alter.

Other methods of effectively dealing with resistances involve obtaining the "resistive secret" that one alter is fearful of discussing from a second, more cooperative alter who is aware of that specific traumatic memory. The therapist can even request that the resistive alter first disclose the traumatic memory to another trusted alter inside and then have the trusted alter write about the experience in a journal which is then shared among all concerned.

Temporary removal or blocking of the somatic aspect of body pain may allow a method of effectively sidestepping the resistance and discovering the structure of the trauma. For example, if severe nausea and the probability of throwing up prevents an alter from talking about a past traumatic memory, the therapist has the option of hypnotically attempting to block the symptoms of nausea by constructing an "affect wall" in which none of the nausea and fear can penetrate to stop the discussion, or, if sufficient cooperation has been established with one or more alters, hypnotic imagery can be used to sweep the feelings of nausea and fear into a distant, interior corner of the self for a specified period of time until the primary alter can discuss the situation. At other times, the pain or discomfort may be shared among several alters, each assuming a small portion of the pain until the primary alter can discuss it. This is, of course, a temporary measure allowing the therapist to have the behavior and knowledge of what transpired. At some point it is necessary to have the primary alter acknowledge and experience the emotions as he or she relives the traumatic memory, so that affect, behavior, and knowledge can be experienced and worked through completely. All of these methods assume that therapy has progressed to the point where the therapist has the cooperation of at least several alters in the system.

A more direct method of dealing with the extremely resistive patient when other methods have not been successful is hypnotic personalization/confrontation (HP/C; Smith & Titus, 1993). The HP/C approach emerged out of a need to face patient issues in a more immediate, convincing, and effective manner. Within certain limits and guidelines, trauma seems best handled when the original event can be made as realistic as possible. There is certainly historic precedent for this approach. Janet, as reported by Ellenberger (1970), provided external cues or would play roles to facilitate induction of abreaction in his patients. Maoz and Pincus (1979) reported on the use of sound effects and on therapist participation in the drama of the patient's battle by playing the role of comrade or officer. Putnam (1989) points out that the most useful external cues for the induction of abreaction are situation-specific, relatively commonly experienced, or associated with traumatic events. Putnam goes on to add, "in MPD patients, the effort of an external cue is frequently to trigger the emergence of a specific alter personality who embodies the traumatic material. This alter will usually vividly recall the traumatic experience" (p. 238).

In the HP/C approach, the patient is hypnotically assisted to reenact a past traumatic relationship or event with a co-therapist who role plays (by prior arrangements) the patient's perpetrator. Patients play themselves during the abreaction. The primary therapist functions as patient advocate, facilitator, and process observer to insure objectivity and provide support for the patient in the process. HP/C is proposed as an effective, direct, and often briefer means of working through traumatic material than traditional imaginary recall or uncontrolled abreaction. It is one method of staging a symbolic confrontation between perpetrator and patient in a manner that not only provides abreaction but also a more successful resolution. It enables therapists to work directly and more immediately in the client's internalizations and projections of his or her historical relationships. This approach has also been described as "hypnotic psychodrama" in its concept. This new approach is consistent with the conclusions of Dietz and Button (1991) who state, "symbolic confrontations with perpetrators and others can often effectively accomplish the necessary discharge of pent-up emotions. Many survivors have accrued the benefits of a confrontation without actually involving the other party" (p. 28).

Because the therapists will be assuming the perpetrator's posture, verbalizations, and stance, they need to gather knowledge about the perpetrator and, to the extent possible, the details and nature of the abusive event such as triggers, perpetrator's key words and sentences, tone of voice, sounds, and so on. Consultation with the ISH, the patient's journals, the drawings, and other material usually provide clues in this regard. During typical HP/C abreactions, adequate safeguards are hypnotically imposed for the safety of both the patient and therapist. For example, the patient is clearly informed that the perpetrator will not be allowed to harm him or her, that the office is a safe place with a "safe chair" that the patient cannot leave, and that the therapist will protect the patient. The patient is then hypnotized and the alter to be worked with is informed that the perpetrator will be present and that the patient needs to confront the perpetrator in a safe and protected setting. The alter is then awakened to face the symbolic perpetrator, who begins slowly but gently to remind the alter of the abusive acts between them. As needed, the perpetrator then gradually escalates the description of the abuse, using specific triggering words or phrases. During this time the co-therapist reflects and reframes the situation, suggesting appropriate ways to respond to the perpetrator and supportively prodding the patient into the necessary abreaction.

In treating self-mutilating or self-destructive alters, the HP/C strategy externalizes and redirects the patient's self-anger and recriminations toward the symbolic perpetrator within adequate safeguards that have been described elsewhere (Smith & Titus, 1993). The direct discharge of emotion toward the symbolic perpetrator appears to result in more rapid and effective resolution of traumatic events. This is usually the first time an alter has had the opportunity and courage to safely confront an abuser. The patient, at the end of this confrontation, is also encouraged to symbolically banish the perpetrator from the room and from his or her life - at which time the second therapist may physically leave the situation. This effective procedure assists the patient in moving from a "helpless victim" stance to one of appropriate assertiveness and empowerment.

A similar nonhypnotic approach with MPD patients in a group psychodrama session has been described by Altman (1992). In an illustrative case example of confrontation in a group psychodramatic session, "Sandy's angry alter directly confronted her mother, strongly expressing long withheld angry feelings about physical abuse, abuse of her younger sister and forced sex with her mother's male friends" (p. 107).

A related approach is now being used by therapists using hypnosis as the framework for reenacting effective abreactive traumas symbolically. A hypnotic psychodrama approach appears to offer three distinct advantages over conventional abreaction techniques:

1. When necessary, strong resistances to recovery of traumatic memory can be successfully negotiated and rather quickly resolved using this approach. It is considerably more difficult for the patient to resist uncovering memories when confronted with the sounds, verbalizations, and emotions in role-playing scenarios.
2. The patient, often for the first time, is able to be empowered to confront the "perpetrator" of the abuse, externalize and express appropriate rage and anger, and not be punished. This is extremely liberating for the patient in terms of discovering his or her own inner strength.
3. The patient, through the action phase of the process, is able to move out of identification with the role of "helpless victim" and into a proactive role of appropriate assertiveness.

Continued research is needed to carefully evaluate the effectiveness of this approach in comparison with other techniques.

SPECIAL PROBLEM AREAS

Of special concern are those clients who present with such complex and difficult problems that immediate and consistent attention must be paid to their control and resolution. A representative listing would include clients with one or more alters who are self-abusive, suicidal, or a threat to others; alters who have a serious eating disorder or addiction to substances such as alcohol or drugs; alters who engage in sexually promiscuous behavior or place the body in dangerous situations and then retreat to allow other alters to face the consequences; and alters sworn to secrecy upon threat of death. Patients who have reportedly been victims of satanic or ritualistic abuse require special procedures beyond the scope of this discussion.

It is a relatively common experience to have one or more alters express self-abusive and self-destructive behaviors. The dynamics of that situation typically vary between patients but may involve introjection of guilt and shame with a need to be punished, identification with a sadistic perpetrator, displacement of anger, belief that the body cannot be harmed, a need to relieve a build-up of internal pressure, a sense of "psychic numbness" that can only be relieved by cutting or hurting oneself, alters who wish to punish one another, or any combination of these factors.

An obvious first step is to attempt to contract with the self-destructive alter(s) to agree not to harm the body accidentally or on purpose. Difficulties arise, however, when the alter is unwilling or unable to contract or when the alter agrees to contract but is often overwhelmed with being flooded with a past traumatic memory and cannot control the resulting self-destructive impulses. Whenever possible, the therapist should attempt to establish a therapeutic bonding or empathic relationship with the abusive alter with a goal toward redirecting the anger toward the original perpetrator. As described previously, the HP/C approach is quite useful in this regard. Over a period of time the self-abusive acts are curtailed and the alter often comes to redefine its function as helpful rather than abusive.

If contracting is not possible for any number of reasons, and the other alters are sufficiently helpful, it may be necessary to hypnotically put the self-destructive alter to sleep, awakening it only to work on specific problems. The ISH can also be trained and empowered to hypnotically place any destructive alter into a dormant state when it is dangerous to the system of alters. Working through self-destructive traumatic memories may take several sessions, and the alter in question is often awakened and put back to sleep several times after a session. Due to the high level of suggestibility present in this disorder, it is possible to feed the positive emotional experiences and feelings of a more healthy alter into a dormant alter without awakening it. In a similar manner, hypnosis can be used to induce a "therapeutic dream" in which the problem alter can be placed in a dream state that involves solving a metaphorical problem similar to the actual traumatic memory but sufficiently different so as to prevent triggering an abreaction.

Another strategy is to plant the hypnotic suggestion that any attempt to, for example, cut oneself will be satisfied by using a red marker on the wrist rather than a cutting instrument, or having the destructive alter lose control of arms or legs so that no such intended act can be completed. These, of course, are temporary strategies designed to prevent immediate danger to the body and, as such, must take precedence over normal work with other alters.

With addictive alters it is often useful to attempt to trace the symptom back to its origin, discover the basic premise or dynamic, and then reverse or reframe the response for the alter. For example, an alter who is anorexic and determined to lose weight down to life-threatening levels may be found to have a strong motivation to become so thin as to be no longer sexually desirable to an abusive father. If the therapist, through role-playing or other cognitive-behavioral means, can convince the alter that the abusive father is actually more attracted to thin, underweight females and that safety and control requires maintaining a certain positive weight level, it may be possible to bring about a shift in the alter's paradigm of thinking. Therapists have often been able to reduce this self-destructive behavior pattern in a relatively short period of time (Smith & Titus, 1993).

Contracting with helpful alters to monitor the behavior of alters who engage in dangerous sexually promiscuous behavior is often possible, asking the ISH or others to assume executive control when such behaviors begin to emerge. The alter system can often be sensitized by imaginary "red flags" or an "alarm system" when a self-defeating alter emerges to carry out some act.

Some alters have such violent abreactive symptoms when trying to discuss some abusive memory that progress is often impossible. Alters who, in discussing some past abuse, trigger vomiting or such severe pain that they cannot talk, require specialized approaches. One approach involves guided imagery in which the alter is to stand outside a door with a window that looks into a darkened room. Beside the door is a red button that starts and stops a movie projector in the room that describes the abuse. The alter is told that the solid door is an emotional barrier that prevents any feelings, emotional or physical, from being experienced while the door is closed. At the same time the red button allows the movie to start or stop at the sole control of the alter. The alter is thereby given several methods of "emotional distancing" such that the abusive memory can be described with that scene and the door can be made to open to varying degrees allowing a more controlled outpouring of emotion. Previously described techniques of fragmentation or time-limited abreactions are useful in modulating the affect as well as sealing away the memory between sessions so as to minimize the possibility of spontaneous flashbacks between sessions.

Through guided imagery or hypnosis, it is often possible to seal up traumatic memories in a safe place constructed by the ISH and other cooperative alters. This may take the form of suggestions that the memory be placed in a strong box, in a bank vault, inside a cavern, or even in a concrete reinforced soundproof room to which only the therapist or ISH has the key. These are temporary control measures to provide a sense of safety and control until the memories can be more fully processed.

The opposing problem sometimes occurs with alters who are so completely repressed and blocked that they refuse to confront the abusive memory regardless of the empathy and support of the therapist. This is essentially a very frightened and traumatized alter who is figuratively "frozen in time" and who cannot begin to reexperience or describe any past abuse. Resolving this particular resistance can often be accomplished by consulting with other alters who have pieces of that memory or the ISH who can supply the therapist with certain "trigger words" or key phrases that were used by the perpetrator in the actual abuse. The therapist can then guide the alter into a relaxed, hypnotic state and can begin to read a description of the abuse aloud, using the appropriate trigger words and key phrases. This is usually sufficient to engage a full abreactive episode, because it is difficult for the alter to avoid such direct stimulation.

An often disturbing event occurs when, toward the end of a successful period of therapy, a previously unknown alter emerges, as if one had simply exposed another layer or system of one or more alters. This can be discouraging to the therapist as well as frightening to those alters who felt the alter system was fully mapped and understood. Although the same strategies are applied as before, it is necessary to reassure the patient that with time this system will also be processed and integrated with the existing system. Encouraging communication between the two systems, and discussing the functions and perceptions of other alters, is often the initial step in ultimate resolution. If the newly discovered alter is malevolent and bent on self-destruction due to commands given by a past abusive perpetrator, the creative and effective therapist can sometimes symbolically assume the role of that perpetrator or another controlling figure and impose new nonabusive commands upon the alter.

THE END PHASE: PREPARATION FOR UNITY

As the successful patient continues to discover, face, and work through all of the significant past abusive experiences, there will be a movement toward unity or integration. Along that pathway, various alters may decide to blend with others as they finish their therapeutic work. The usual criteria for integration involves the alter(s) having completed enough of the abusive memory work to feel relatively free from the symptoms of the abuse, an expressed desire or curiosity about joining with another alter who is compatible, and a thorough discussion by all concerned as to the expectations of that joining. Some alters, even though their work is completed, may resist integration for fear of losing their separate sense of self or identity - of being "swallowed up" into a larger entity with a sense of personal anxiety. This is, of course, an interesting ethical and philosophical situation the literature has not adequately addressed. In such instances, it is often helpful to propose a "temporary blending" of the alters involved that is time limited, for example, 1 day, 1 week, and so on, to help the alters decide whether the integration is appropriate and a satisfactory arrangement for both. If it is, the blending or integration may remain. If it is not, the alters may separate to do more work prior to a final joining.

Ritual and ceremony appear to be very important to patients going through an integration. Although some alters, along the way, may blend or integrate with others without the assistance of the therapist, many alters insist on a more formal ceremony. Ritual and ceremony have always been cornerstones that identify and proclaim significant events in our lives, and it is not surprising that patients require a symbolic event. The first step, after determining that integration is desired and appropriate, is to assist the involved alters in choosing the form of the ceremony if they have not already done so. Common rituals or ceremonies may involve the two alters symbolically using guided imagery or hypnosis to imagine walking into a beautiful meadow together, facing each other, and stepping forward to embrace and blend together, or perhaps a golden light coming down to blend and integrate both of them. Other alters may request a more religious ceremony such as imagining being in a church or being supported by a priest or wise man. The nature of the ritual is limited only by the creativity of the therapist and patient. Kluft (1982) and Putnam (1989) have discussed such rituals. Greaves (1989) has also discussed the prelude to integration with indicators of treatment success or failure.

Little has been written concerning the criteria for a successful ritual leading to a complete integration of two or more alters. In general, therapists have reported that the "new" integrated alter reports a more vivid and intense experience of sensory awareness (e.g., lights seem brighter, colors more saturated, sounds more distinct and less muffled). There may be some slight unsteadiness in movement or balance that is similar to becoming more comfortable with the new body sensations. The voice tone and inflection may seem to be more of a blend of the original two voices than either one predominating. If the two alters have different handedness, the resulting integrated alter may be ambidextrous or have difficulty deciding whether to write with the left or right hand. Continuous monitoring and follow-up by checking for any further splitting or difficulties by the therapist should yield no evidence of the two separate alters if successful. Alters who integrate, only to split apart soon afterwards, suggest unresolved traumatic issues not fully resolved by either alter, or possibly some unexpected trauma or stress the alter was not prepared to face. Behavioral criteria for success varies in the literature but typically involves a specified period of post-therapy evaluation without subsequent symptoms of splitting or MPD and no eliciting of new alters via hypnotic inquiry.

The integrated patient may still be sensitive and vulnerable to certain times of the year that mark events or anniversaries that once held traumatic significance, such as birthdays, holidays such as Halloween, the full moon, or even telephone calls or correspondence from past abusers. The therapist must be aware of and sensitive to such occasions or "triggers" and provide the necessary additional support.

The importance of post-therapy follow-up cannot be underestimated. Following complete integration or resolution of the major difficulties of the patient, the therapist is faced with a "single personality disorder" rather than a multiple personality. The single personality must now be assisted in learning new coping skills instead of dissociation and splitting. The unity of the personality structure needs to be reinforced and the teaching of skills such as stress management, assertiveness training, relaxation with continuous modeling, and education is paramount.

R. Douglas Smith, PhD, is currently Deputy Director of the Central Georgia Mental Health Center in Macon, Georgia. His training is in Clinical Psychology with special interests in hypnosis, the innovative treatment of trauma, and other altered states of awareness. He is the author of three books, has published several articles related to treatment of Dissociative Disorders, and has presented workshops on both a national and international level. Dr. Smith may be contacted at 1910 Forsyth Street, Suite 102, Macon, GA 31201.

RESOURCES

Altman, P. A. (1992). Psychodramatic treatment of multiple personality disorder and dissociative disorders. *Dissociation, 5,* 104-108.

Bernstein, E. M., & Putnam, F. W. (1986). Development, reliability, and validity of a dissociation scale. *Journal of Nervous and Mental Disease, 174,* 727-735.

Bloch, J. P. (1988). *Assessment and Treatment of Multiple Personality and Dissociative Disorders.* Sarasota, FL: Professional Resource Press.

Bradway, K. (1979). Sandplay in psychotherapy. *Journal of Psychotherapy, 6,* 85-93.

Braun, B. G. (1983). Psychophysiological phenomena in multiple personality and hypnosis. *American Journal of Clinical Hypnosis, 26,* 124-137.

Braun, B. G. (1984). Uses of hypnosis with multiple personality. *Psychiatric Annals, 14,* 34-40.

Braun, B. G. (1986). Issues in the psychotherapy of multiple personality disorder. In B. G. Braun (Ed.), *Treatment of Multiple Personality Disorder* (pp. 1-28). Washington, DC: American Psychiatric Press.

Calof, D. L. (1991). Protecting the therapeutic framework. *Treating Abuse Today, 1,* 10-12.

Chu, J. A. (1988). Some aspect of resistance in the treatment of multiple personality disorder. *Dissociation, 1,* 34-38.

Chu, J. A. (1991). On the misdiagnosis of multiple personality disorder. *Dissociation, 4,* 200-204.

Comstock, C. M. (1985, October). *Internal Self Helpers or Centers.* Paper presented at Second International Conference on Multiple Personality and Dissociative States, Chicago, IL.

Comstock, C. M. (1986, September). *The Therapeutic Utilization of Abreactive Experiences in the Treatment of Multiple Personality Disorder.* Paper presented at the Third International Conference on Multiple Personality and Dissociative States, Chicago, IL.

Comstock, C. M., & Vickery, D. (1992). The therapist as victim: A preliminary discussion. *Dissociation, 5,* 155-158.

Coons, P. M. (1980). Multiple personality: Diagnostic considerations. *Journal of Clinical Psychiatry, 41,* 330-336.

Dietz, A., & Button, B. (1991). The challenges of survivors of childhood sexual abuse in adult relationships. *Treating Abuse Today, 1,* 26-40.

Ellenberger, H. F. (1970). *The Discovery of the Unconscious: The History of Evolution of Dynamic Psychiatry.* New York: Basic Books.

EMDR Network, Inc., P.O. Box 51010, Pacific Grove, CA 93950-6010.

Frischholz, E. J., Braun, B. G., Sachs, R. G., Hopkins, L., Shaeffer, D. M., Lewis, J., Leavitt, F., Pasquotto, J. N., & Schwartz, D. R. (1991). The dissociative experiences scale: Further replication and validation. *Dissociation, 3,* 151-153.

Greaves, G. B. (1989). Precursors of integration in multiple personality disorder. *Dissociation, 2,* 224-230.

Hammond, C. (1990). *Handbook of Hypnotic Suggestions and Metaphors.* New York: W. W. Norton.

Kaliff, D. (1980). *Sandplay: A Psychotherapeutic Approach to the Psyche.* Santa Monica, CA: Sigo Press.

Kluft, R. P. (1980). The treatment of multiple personality disorder. *Directions in Psychiatry, 5,* Lesson 24, pp. 1-10. Washington, DC: American Psychiatric Press.

Kluft, R. P. (1982). Varieties of hypnotic interventions in the treatment of multiple personality. *American Journal of Clinical Hypnosis, 24,* 230-240.

Kluft, R. P. (1985). The natural history of multiple personality disorder. In R. P. Kluft (Ed.), *Childhood Antecedents of Multiple Personality* (pp. 197-238). Washington, DC: American Psychiatric Press.

Maoz, B., & Pincus, C. (1979). The therapeutic dialogue in narco-analytic treatments. *Psychotherapy: Theory, Research and Practice, 16,* 91-97.

Marquis, J. (1991). A report on seventy-eight cases treated by eye movement desensitization. *Journal of Behavior Therapy and Experimental Psychiatry, 22,* 187-192.

Paley, S. (1992). Dream wars: A case study of a woman with multiple personality disorder. *Dissociation, 5,* 111-116.

Puk, G. (1991). Treating traumatic memories: A case report on the eye movement desensitization procedure. *Journal of Behavior Therapy and Experimental Psychiatry, 22,* 149-151.

Putnam, F. W. (1989). *Diagnosis and Treatment of Multiple Personality Disorder.* New York: Guilford.

Putnam, F. W., Guroff, J. J., Silberman, E. K., Barban, L., & Post, R. M. (1986). The clinical phenomenology of multiple personality disorder: Review of 100 recent cases. *Journal of Clinical Psychiatry, 47,* 285-293.

Sachs, R. G., & Sweig, T. L. (1993). Applications of sandtray in the treatment of multiple personality disorders. In R. P. Kluft (Ed.), *Expressive and Functional Therapies in the Treatment of Multiple Personality Disorder* (pp. 189-199). Springfield, IL: Charles C. Thomas

Shapiro, F. (1989). Eye movement desensitization method: A new treatment for post traumatic stress disorder. *Journal of Behavior Therapy and Experimental Psychiatry, 20,* 211-217.

Smith, R. D., & Titus, E. (1993). Hypnotic personalization/confrontation: A controlled abreaction technique for multiple personality disorder. *Treating Abuse Today, 2,* 6-10.

Smith, R. D., Titus, E., & Carr, M. (1989). An integrative treatment technique in multiple personality disorder. *Journal of Medical Psychotherapy, 2,* 1-10.

Van Der Hart, O., & Brown, P. (1992). Abreaction re-evaluated. *Dissociation, 5,* 127-140.

Watkins, H. H. (1980). The silent abreaction. *International Journal of Clinical and Experimental Hypnosis, 2,* 101-113.

Wolpe, J., & Abrams, J. (1991). Post-traumatic stress disorder overcome by eye movement desensitization: A case report. *Journal of Behavior Therapy and Experimental Psychiatry, 22,* 39-43.

Young, W. C. (1988). Psychodynamics and dissociation: All that switches is not split. *Dissociation, 1,* 33-38.

TREATMENT OF INCEST AND COMPLEX DISSOCIATIVE TRAUMATIC STRESS REACTIONS

Christine A. Courtois

This contribution discusses symptoms and aftereffects of incest in three main diagnostic categories: post-traumatic reactions and disorders, dissociative disorders, and characterological disorders. These diagnoses are presented as logical consequences of incestuous abuse. Many adult survivors are polysymptomatic and thus may pose a formidable treatment challenge to the clinician. This contribution offers a treatment model which consists of three stages and includes strategies and techniques for effective management and therapeutic gain. Transference and countertransference issues particular to a dissociative, post-traumatic relational field are also discussed.

INCEST AND ITS POTENTIAL FOR DAMAGE

Incest is, on average, a particularly virulent and severe form of child sexual abuse with high potential for serious psychological sequelae, both in childhood and adulthood (Chu & Dill, 1990; Courtois, 1988). Defined as sexual contact or behavior occurring between relatives and quasi-relatives, incest is considered a form of child abuse when the perpetrator is older or holds a position of power or authority over the victim. This power differential as well as the victim's age and level of maturity also make informed consent impossible. Unfortunately, incest is not a rare occurrence as was believed as recently as the 1950s (Weinberg, 1955) and 1960s. The prevalence studies of the 1970s and 1980s (Finkelhor, 1984; Russell, 1986; Wyatt, 1985) suggest that it may affect as many as one in three girls and one in seven boys in the United States. According to Butler (1978), incest is "relentlessly democratic" in that it occurs at all socioeconomic levels, in different ethnic and cultural groups, and in urban, suburban, and rural locales.

Incest is a stressor with many traumatizing characteristics which put the victim at risk for serious initial and long-term aftereffects. These include its occurrence within the family perpetrated by a relative, a quasi-relative, or someone in close proximity or relationship on whom the child depends. Most often, its occurrence is aided and abetted by particular family dynamics, many of which are dysfunctional. These include other forms of family violence, chemical dependence and codependence (often across generations), and ensuing patterns of denial, secrecy, and shame (Fossum & Mason, 1986). Parental discord and immaturity are common. Children often become the caretakers of their parents and essentially raise themselves in the absence of functional parenting. Neglect and abandonment as well as betrayal are implicated in the occurrence of incest. These aspects, above and beyond the sexual transgression, also damage the victim. In some cases they may actually be more damaging (Alexander, 1992).

Variables in how the incest occurs, that is, the age of the child at onset and termination, the duration of the abuse, and any escalation in severity, are related to its likely impact. The average duration of incest is 4 years; however, it can range from a one-time occurrence to multiple episodes spanning decades. In recent years, evidence has accumulated that in some cases the abuse has never stopped and continues into adulthood.

Incest usually begins with a mild form of sexual behavior or contact. In the most common scenario, the child is gradually enticed and "groomed" into sexual activity which is misrepresented. Outright coercion and violence are not the norm, yet are not uncommon. However the abuse takes place, the child is blackmailed into shame and secrecy. Without disclosure and especially without intervention, incest flourishes and, over time, may escalate to more severe forms of sexual behavior ultimately involving physical penetration.

The child caught in such a situation is virtually powerless to stop it without outside help. He or she is trapped and dependent (especially when the incest is within the nuclear family, that is, with parents, parent substitutes, or siblings) and must cope however possible. Most, if not all, victims come to believe *they* are the cause of the abuse, a belief which paradoxically allows them to maintain an image of having good parents. Denial and disavowal on the part of other family members and the lack of assistance even when the incest is observed or disclosed, consolidates the child's self-blame and sense of badness. Additionally, child victims often cope by emotionally distancing themselves from the abuse as it occurs. They step outside of themselves in whatever way possible and otherwise distort reality and self-perceptions to accommodate ongoing incest (Courtois, 1988; Summit, 1983).

Victims suffer other dissociative and acute post-traumatic reactions such as depression, anxiety, guilt, self-blame, shame, and rage (Cole & Putnam, 1992; Courtois, 1988; Herman, 1981) which interact with their psychosexual development and personality formation. Hence, the seeds are sown for a variety of maturational and traumatic difficulties across the life span. Although research has shown great variability in aftereffects and damage attributable to incest (Courtois, 1988; Herman, 1981; Kendall-Tackett, Williams, & Finkelhor 1993; Russell, 1986) and that a child's genetic makeup and personality resilience can insulate effects (Sanford, 1989) as can other moderating variables (Wyatt & Newcomb, 1990), incest holds great potential for severe episodic and/or lasting effects.

In recent years, research studies and clinical observation have yielded data documenting a history of childhood sexual abuse in 50% to 75% of adult female psychiatric patients in both inpatient and outpatient settings (Bryer et al., 1987; Chu & Dill, 1990). Research on the aftereffects of child sexual abuse has documented a host of nonspecific effects such as depression, anxiety, low self-worth, and relationship problems. A more specific pattern has emerged when samples of abused versus nonabused individuals are compared. Abused subjects report more depression and sleep disturbance, irrational guilt, anxiety reactions, dissociation, somatization, suicidality and other forms of self-harm, revictimization and other relational disturbances, substance abuse and other addictive-compulsive patterns and behaviors, and polarities of behavior (Kendall-Tackett et al., 1993; National Institute of Mental Health [NIMH], 1990). It should be noted that several confounding methodological issues impact these findings: (a) These studies rely on retrospective self-reports of abuse, most without corroboration; (b) nonabused samples contain an unknown percentage of individuals who in reality have been abused, but who do not disclose or know of (i.e., are amnestic for) its occurrence; and (c) research studies have not, until recently, routinely utilized true experimental designs or comparison samples (Briere, 1992; Kendall-Tackett et al., 1993; NIMH, 1990).

Severe childhood trauma is increasingly recognized as correlated with three (and possibly more) main areas of psychological distress, the first two on Axis I and the third on Axis II of the *DSM-III-R* (American Psychiatric Association, 1987): post-traumatic stress symptoms (acute, chronic, and delayed); dissociative symptoms (with multiple personality disorder as the most severe and extreme manifestation); and characterological difficulties due to maturational disruption (as most commonly identified by the diagnosis borderline personality disorder) (Briere, 1989; Chu, 1992; Courtois, 1988; Herman, 1992b). (Also see *DSM-IV*; American Psychiatric Association [APA], 1994.) As discussed previously, great variability in response is possible; however, it is of note that incestuous abuse correlates with the most severe effects including the triad mentioned before (Cole & Putnam, 1992; Courtois, 1988; Strick & Wilcoxon, 1991). Also noteworthy is the fact that many of the symptoms, whether fitting Axis I or Axis II diagnoses, pertain to an alteration of the individual's sense of self including an absence of self-reference, an inability to modulate affect, and an alteration in the ability to relate effectively and intimately with others.

Survivors of severe child sexual abuse, with their wide variety of symptoms and diagnoses as well as their relational difficulties, present many treatment challenges. This contribution now expands the discussion of complex dissociative traumatic stress reactions including characterological manifestations to set the stage for outlining a sequenced plan of treatment with suggestions for therapeutic strategies and management.

COMPLEX DISSOCIATIVE POST-TRAUMATIC STRESS REACTIONS

Clinicians and researchers have come to understand that the post-traumatic stress reactions common to chronic abuse and other forms of repeated, prolonged trauma (i.e., hostage situations, concentration camps, political torture) differ from those of more circumscribed and time-limited traumatic events such as rape, accidents, and natural disasters (Herman, 1992a, 1992b). A condition of captivity including ongoing contact with and subordination to the captor/perpetrator often characterizes the former. Paradoxically, the captor/perpetrator is the source of both safety and danger to the victim who is thus dependent upon the very person who does harm. This situation creates what Spiegel (1986) described as a "macabre double-bind" of love-hate and dependence-terror between victim and perpetrator.

Victims of chronic trauma have a wide array of initial and long-term psychological symptoms which Herman (1992a, 1992b) and other clinician-researchers have organized into a diagnosis of "Complex Post-Traumatic Stress Disorder" or alternately "Disorders of Extreme Stress, Not Otherwise Specified" (DESNOS), to differentiate them from generic post-traumatic stress disorder (PTSD) as currently defined in *DSM-III-R* and *DSM-IV* (American Psychiatric Association, 1987, 1994). Although this diagnostic formulation has not been included in *DSM-IV* (APA, 1994), it provides a very useful conceptual model for understanding and planning the treatment of the complex symptom picture presented by incest survivors and other victims of prolonged trauma.

According to Herman (1992a), three broad areas of psychological disturbance have been identified in this formulation which transcend the symptoms of simple PTSD. The first has to do directly with the various symptoms and their complexity, diffuseness, and tenacity. The second is characterological. Survivors of prolonged abuse develop changes in their personalities including disturbances in their identity, their emotional functioning, and their ability to relate to others. Third, survivors are vulnerable to repeated harm or revictimization, either self-inflicted or caused by others. Chu (1992) puts additional emphasis on dissociation as a common coping mechanism of child victims of chronic trauma. The three main areas of distress - complex post-traumatic stress disorder (including the increased risk for revictimization), dissociative disorders, and characterological disturbances - are described in more detail below.

POST-TRAUMATIC STRESS DISORDER

Post-traumatic stress disorder, whether acute, chronic, or delayed, encompasses a wide array of symptoms alternating between those that cause a recollection or reexperiencing of the trauma and those that give respite by blunting or numbing it. Studies have documented that post-traumatic symptomatology is often characteristic of adult survivors of incest (Donaldson & Gardner, 1985; Lindberg & Distad, 1985), but clinicians and researchers such as Armsworth and Holaday (1993), Finkelhor and Browne (1985), and Gelinas (1983) have noted that the fit between symptoms of child-onset PTSD (due to abuse) and those of adult-onset PTSD is less than perfect.

According to Herman (1992a), it appears that chronic childhood trauma involving captivity creates a unique form of PTSD with intensified symptoms especially affecting personality development. Because the trauma occurs over the course of the child's physical and psychological maturation, both are impacted. Researchers are now identifying neurological and other biological consequences of traumatic stress which form a physical substrate to the individual's psychological development (van der Kolk, 1987).

A chronic, characterological depression with complications and atypical impulsive and dissociative features is very common in incest survivors (Gelinas, 1983) as in other chronically traumatized populations (Herman, 1992b). They also further experience other intense affects such as shame, excessive responsibility and guilt, self-blame, and rage which underscore and become entangled with the depression. They are further prone to a host of anxiety disorders including panic, agoraphobia, and the range of simple phobias (often directly or symbolically related to the original trauma). Self-destructiveness in the form of suicidality, self-mutilation, and revictimization due to repetition compulsions, reenactments, naïveté, personal disregard, and risk taking is very evident in this population. Chemical dependence and many forms of compulsive behaviors aimed at alleviating distress are common. Further, the trauma causes existential crises for survivors who often suffer profound damage to their self-esteem; a loss of faith, personal meaning, and safety in the world; and a mistrust in the beneficence of other human beings and in a just and loving God (Russell, 1986).

Physical aftereffects and symptoms are also characteristic of PTSD. The victim may have been physically injured or may have psychosomatic manifestations of the trauma. Among incest survivors, an abbreviated list of some of the most common physical symptoms include gastrointestinal and genitourinary disorders, headaches and other neurological problems, muscular and skeletal pain, nausea and gag responses, eating disturbances, sexual dysfunction and reproductive distress, and dissociation of various physical sensations (Courtois, 1988).

DISSOCIATIVE DISORDERS

At present, PTSD is categorized within *DSM-III-R* (APA, 1987) and *DSM-IV* (APA, 1994) as an anxiety disorder; however, many clinicians and researchers now conceptualize post-traumatic reactions as inherently dissociative as well. Research is supporting the hypothesis that dissociative phenomena are utilized as defenses both during and after traumatic experiences (Putnam, 1985; Spiegel, Hunt, & Dondershine, 1988), are common in response to childhood physical and sexual abuse (Chu & Dill, 1990), and are perhaps most likely to develop from severe abuse (Putnam et al., 1986; Ross, Norton, & Wozney, 1989) and particularly from early incestuous abuse (Pribor & Dinwiddie, 1992; Strick & Wilcoxon, 1991). Spiegel and Cardena (1991), in their review article on the dissociative disorders, caution that although a relation between trauma and dissociation is strongly suggested by the clinical literature, it is not clear whether trauma is a necessary and sufficient condition or an incidental correlate of dissociative disorders. Nevertheless, it is reasonable to conclude that individuals with dissociative disorders frequently have histories of prior abuse and traumata.

Dissociation is generally defined as involving a separation of mental processes which are normally integrated (such as thoughts, emotions, identity, and memory). A number of clinical researchers have placed dissociation on a continuum ranging from normal reactions to everyday events (e.g., daydreaming, "highway hypnosis") at one pole to extremely abnormal reactions (e.g., amnesia, lack of or changing personal identity) found in the most compartmentalized forms of multiple personality disorder at the other. Post-traumatic stress disorder is approximately at the midpoint of this continuum of dissociation.

CHARACTEROLOGICAL DISTURBANCES

According to Herman (1992a), "Survivors of childhood abuse develop . . . complex deformations of identity. A malignant sense of the self as contaminated, guilty and evil is widely observed. Fragmentation in the sense of self is also common, reaching its most dramatic extreme in multiple personality disorder" (p. 386). A number of researchers have posited and are now documenting the damaging characterological consequences of incest as those which impact the development of a sense of self, the regulation of affect and of self-integrity, and the ability to trust others and to develop intimacy in relationships (Briere, 1989; Cole & Putnam, 1992).

Many of these issues are characteristic of the diagnosis of borderline personality disorder, and a number of clinicians have speculated about (Briere, 1989; Courtois, 1988) and documented (Herman & van der Kolk, 1987) an impressive overlap between a history of abuse and symptoms of borderline personality. Additionally, an overlap between borderline personality and post-traumatic stress disorder is increasingly acknowledged (Kroll, 1993; Waites, 1993) as is a relation to multiple personality disorder (Horevitz & Braun, 1984; Ross, 1989). Severe abuse often precludes the development of a cohesive sense of self, engenders the use of the most primitive ego defenses, and interferes with the development of normal interactions with others and of effective coping strategies.

It should be noted that not all adults with a history of significant childhood abuse and trauma develop such personality, dissociative, and post-traumatic disorders; however, many of these reactions are not evident either to clinicians or to survivors, having long been hidden or dissociated in the interest of survival or not recognized or diagnosed because they appeared in disguised fashion. The clinician should not anticipate that every client with a history of abuse automatically has this symptom triad, yet it is very often evident in the most chronic and disabled populations with serious and complicated symptomatology and should therefore be given consideration (Chu, 1992).

The remainder of this contribution articulates a treatment model for clients for whom this triad is in evidence. The model is directed toward a sequenced, titrated treatment for trauma resolution which also addresses issues of personal development, self-management, skill-building, and mastery on the part of the survivor/client. Because abuse occurs in an interpersonal context, the personal and interpersonal "lessons of abuse" are projected onto the therapeutic relationship. Their skillful interpretation and management holds the potential for growth and healing. The treatment model presented next incorporates a strong emphasis on the relational dimensions of both the abuse and the resolution of its effects in the therapy. This model is generic. It provides sequenced treatment applicable to the aftereffects experienced by the majority of adult survivors. Although it addresses dissociative behaviors and issues, it is not specialized enough for the multiple personality client. Therapists treating multiple personality can use this model as the foundation for their treatment but, of necessity, need additional information and training. They are referred to texts by Putnam (1989) and Ross (1989) for such information.

A TREATMENT MODEL FOR COMPLEX DISSOCIATIVE PTSD

The issue of therapist training to work with traumatized individuals is a very salient one. Because the study of trauma, its consequences, and treatment is rarely covered in the training of most mental health professionals, therapists need to avail themselves of additional training, consultation, and supervision to effectively organize their work with this treatment population. Therapists are hard-pressed to *not have* abuse survivors in their caseloads because of the high percentage of abuse histories in both outpatient and inpatient populations. Despite this fact, not all therapists should treat abuse survivors (i.e., some are not suited by temperament or choice, others by their own personal history of abuse which is not worked through or by other life stresses which make it hard for them to have the emotional resources necessary for the demands of the work). It is now well recognized that work with trauma, especially of a human-induced, premeditated, repetitive sort, is vicariously traumatizing to the helper, causing personal changes in perceptions of self and others and in life assumptions similar to those experienced directly by the victim/client (McCann

& Pearlman, 1990). Therapists doing trauma work benefit by instituting strategies for self-care including personal and professional support and opportunities for ventilation or discharge of affect.

Certain perspectives on the part of the therapist have been found helpful to the successful treatment of adult survivors with complex symptoms. Once an abuse history is suspected through the client's symptom picture and behavioral style or is disclosed, the trauma must be seen as a core issue and a focus in treatment, although not the only one. Because of the wide-ranging impact of sex abuse trauma, treatment incorporates characterological, developmental, life-skill, and relational work as discussed below.

The therapist treating this population must be capable of recognizing the reality of abuse as well as its high potential for damage and distress. Because an abuse of power and a loss of control are central to victimization, a therapeutic goal is to empower the client. The therapist assumes strength and resilience on the part of the client and starts from the position that the client, not the therapist, is responsible for the healing process. A major treatment trap with this population is for the therapist to assume an overly fragile and helpless client - an understandable reaction given what many of these clients have experienced and how they present for treatment. However, such an assumption can set the therapist up as a rescuer or compensator for the losses of the past rather than as a helper who assists in the hard work of identifying and grieving the losses.

In order to progress, this treatment relies upon the development of safety and security in both the therapeutic relationship and, more globally, in the survivor's life. The clinician must strive to create a safe therapeutic environment by being personally reliable and consistent in order to counter the interpersonal inconsistencies characteristic of abusive and dysfunctional families. The therapist is responsible for the establishment, communication, and maintenance of clear limits and boundaries and, as just noted, should avoid creating a rescue norm. Therapists doing trauma work must be personally responsive to the client rather than abstinent in style and must be patient, because the work often progresses slowly. Therapists are further required to model relational honesty and respect to counter the disrespect and disregard of abuse and, at times, to admit mistakes and to show themselves as human beings capable of error. Such a stance challenges the client's expectation that the therapist as an authority figure is perfect and above reproach, a perspective often taught by abusers and other family members. Many survivors, used to being scapegoated in their families, expect the same of their relationship with the therapist. They might present as totally compliant and acquiescent and have minimal expectations of a relationship that is mutual and respectful of their needs.

The therapist must regard the client's defenses as having been important to psychological survival and therefore not to be dismantled wholesale without regard to client readiness or the development of alternative methods of coping and self-soothing. The therapist is ethically and professionally bound not to exploit the client for his or her own gratification and should be especially vigilant to sexual interactions with this population. Sexual abuse often conditions its victims to anticipate or precipitate a sexual interaction. This may occur in the context of the therapeutic relationship and is critical to be discussed but not acted upon. To sexually transgress with a client with such a history compounds the original injury and is nothing short of professional incest.

Finally, the therapist must also maintain respect and boundaries in working with the traumatic content *per se*. When the client is directly recounting the trauma, the therapist must strive to elicit details of the abuse and its attendant emotions, carefully, with attention to the client's shame, and using methods that minimize retraumatization. The therapist must be willing to hear the story but must not be voyeuristic nor express overly strong reactions which might be further shaming or overwhelming. At times, however, the therapist will need to function as an alter ego and react and label feeling states when the client is unable to do so. The therapist must also be prepared to accept all feelings about abuse experience, not only those that are negative. Sexual abuse can cause a wide variety of ambivalent responses and attachments on the part of the victim with which the clinician should be familiar. These include but are not limited to such issues as attachment to and love for the abuser, rage toward the nonabusing or nonprotective parent (usually the mother), sexual arousal and orgasm during the abuse or desire for the sexual contact, perpetration against others, and patterns of sexual arousal linked to sadism and deviancy. Many survivors are guilty, ashamed, and disgusted with themselves for these responses and express their emotions through acts of self-directed aggression.

A CONCEPTUALIZATION OF THE THERAPY PROCESS

Although the therapy process should be tailored to the needs and goals of each client, a number of conceptualizations of the goals, phases, and tasks of the therapy process have been suggested, with a fair degree of consistency between them (Braun, 1986; Briere, 1989; Chu, 1992; Courtois, 1988, 1991; Gil, 1988; Herman, 1992b; Jehu, 1988; S. Kirschner, D. A. Kirschner, & Rappaport, 1993; Meiselman, 1990; Sgroi, 1989). Little outcome data is as yet available on the efficacy of these treatment models; thus, these recommendations are made largely on clinical reports and findings (NIMH, 1990).

In general, the therapy process for the resolution of complex dissociative post-traumatic reactions associated with child sexual abuse is long-term rather than short-term, although some short-term treatments and interventions have been described, as have episodic, sequenced treatment packages (Courtois, 1993; Gil, 1988; Herman & Schatzow, 1987; Jehu, 1988; Johnson, 1989; Sgroi, 1989). Therapists must be aware of the client's motivational and financial resources and plan therapy accordingly (Chu, 1988; Turkus, 1991). A treatment dilemma of major proportions is being created by managed care limitations, because adult survivors often need longer and more intensive treatment than is allowed by many plans. Both therapist and client must monitor resources throughout the process. It goes without saying that the client is not assisted if treatment is predicated upon resources which are no longer available and the client is unable to afford to continue. This is especially problematic if the client is in the trauma-resolution phase of treatment when the need for consistency and availability is the greatest.

Long-term treatment is generally acknowledged as necessary due to the pervasive effects of abuse, the compounding of effects over time (due to the absence or limited effectiveness of previous treatment), and the complexities and tenacity of the symptoms. Uncovering of the intense affect associated with long-term trauma response must proceed at a pace that is tolerable to the client and that does not precipitate decompensation. Optimally, uncovering follows a period of time devoted to the stabilization of the client's life and defenses and to the development of a reasonably strong therapeutic alliance. Once the trauma is approached, however, it is likely that both therapist and client will experience one or more phases of "things getting worse before they get better" (Briere, 1989; Chu, 1992; Courtois, 1988; Gil, 1988; Herman, 1992b; Jehu, 1988; Meiselman, 1990).

Before undertaking treatment, the therapist should provide the client with information about both post-traumatic reactions and the treatment process. Information-giving and psychoeducation are beneficial throughout the treatment as they function to provide the client with a general map of the process, and, with informed consent, a degree of control. Such a strategy is recommended for traumatized clients to counter their lack of control during the victimization and to somewhat lessen their anxiety about the treatment.

The therapy process encompasses the following goals, phases, and issues:

1. *The Decision to Heal and Make a Commitment to Treatment.* The client must be motivated to seek treatment for his or her life difficulties, be willing to do the work necessary to identify antecedent conditions (including but not limited to the abuse), experience painful affect, and make concrete changes. A corollary commitment involves developing a therapeutic alliance in which to do the work.
2. *Life Stabilization.* Many clients enter treatment in considerable life chaos and/or are having intense post-traumatic reactions (either intrusive or numbing) which they subjectively experience as "going crazy." Of necessity, these issues must be addressed and managed before proceeding. Special supports and strategies are put in place in this stage to restabilize the client.

3. *Disclosure and Remembering.* In this stage, the abuse is discussed in whatever detail available. Secrecy surrounds sexual abuse, allowing for its recurrence and engendering shame. Breaking the silence may be quite difficult (especially if the child was threatened for talking) but is essential to "break the spell" and to contradict feelings of stigma and isolation.

   Some survivors retain clear memories of their abuse which they may or may not have previously disclosed. The client is encouraged to disclose to whatever degree possible and to experience the associated affect. Similarly, for those clients with little or no direct recall, available clues in the affective, behavioral, perceptual, and somatic domains and the identification of triggers are assessed as to their possible meaning. It is very important that therapists not determine the client's experience, make the assumption that the client's symptoms could only be caused by sexual abuse, or be overzealous in uncovering such a history by excessive, intrusive, or suggestive questioning. Hypnosis should be used only by therapists well-trained and experienced in its use and only with the client's consent and understanding that hypnotically refreshed memory may be inadmissible in court proceedings (Scheflin & Shapiro, 1989) and that memories "retrieved" under hypnosis may be no more or less accurate than memories recalled without it.

4. *Determining What Is Real.* It is the client's sole responsibility to determine the meaning of these various clues and reactions to his or her autobiographical history. The client in this stage must struggle with denial and dissociation to arrive at acceptance of a personal abuse reality. In the case of abuse, this involves recognition and acceptance of betrayal on the part of significant others and thus is very painful and involves grieving. A quote from Chu (1992) is very pertinent here:

   > Patients have sometimes asked therapists to validate or deny the reality of their past abuse when patients themselves have inadequate information to make such a determination. Although it seems quite appropriate for a therapist to acknowledge or even raise the issues of abuse when the history seems relatively clear, it is difficult to respond to all inquiries of "Do you believe me?" In situations where patients are uncertain about the reality of past events, therapists should respond to these inquiries by acknowledging only the patient's uncertainty and the painfulness of not knowing. Patients and therapists should assume the responsibility of sifting through known facts, likely conclusions, fantasy, and conjecture until such time as patients themselves can be reasonably clear about their personal realities. (p. 365)

5. *Resolving Issues of Responsibility, Self-Blame, and Complicity.* Sexual abuse by its very nature and dynamics causes reactions of guilt, shame, and self-blame. The client must resolve these issues and must understand reactions in the context of helplessness, power differentials, and the conditioning inherent in chronic abuse to arrive at self-forgiveness and to place the major responsibility on those who perpetrated or did not protect. This part of the process also involves the pain and disillusionment of facing the betrayal and selfishness of significant others.

6. *The Recognition, Labeling, and Expression of Feelings.* Clients must learn about the emotions that were suppressed or dissociated at the time of the abuse and later. Many strong feelings must emerge and be accepted and catharted including grief, anger and rage, and pain.

7. *Cognitive Restructuring of Distorted Beliefs and Behavior Change.* Distorted and negative beliefs resulting from the abuse and its effects must be restructured based on new information derived from the resolution of issues mentioned previously and the experience of the therapeutic relationship. These in turn allow for behavioral and relational changes. The client learns to connect the abuse and its aftermath to current behaviors and relationships and lessen the use of maladaptive defenses and survivor skills. The abuse is not forgotten, but its effects no longer play havoc with the survivor's life and he or she no longer feels

"crazy," out of control, or at the whim of spontaneous traumatic reactions and reenactments.

The therapist basically assists this process by being empathically attuned to the client but also by the strategic use of empathic confrontation (Chu, 1992) or what the present author has labeled as "nudge" therapy. The client must be nudged, enjoined, supported, and otherwise encouraged to risk changing long-ingrained beliefs, learned behaviors, assumptions, and so on. Titration of the therapeutic tasks and change process is described in more detail below.

8. *Disclosure, Confrontation, and Other Issues Involving the Perpetrator and Others.* The survivor must decide about disclosing abuse to others, about confronting the perpetrator and others, about maintaining contact with family members or other individuals involved in the abuse, about reporting ongoing abuse, and about forgiveness of any of the involved parties. It is usually best for these decisions to be made toward the end of treatment and with adequate discussion and preparation after the survivor has assessed the abuse and its impact and has tested whether safe, healthier relationships are possible with family members and significant others.

THE SEQUENCING OF THERAPY AND THE CHOICE OF STRATEGY

These goals and issues suggest a general chronology of interventions; yet, additional attention to sequencing is necessary. In particular, a treatment progression must be established and the therapist must guard against "jumping into" the trauma work prematurely, without adequate assessment, preparation, and stabilization. Some issues precede the work on others and, in the typical case, issues may become evident only after other work has been accomplished (Jehu, 1988). For example, the building of a modicum of trust in the therapist and the development of a working alliance often precede disclosure of shame-based issues (e.g., the abuse itself, secondary secrets associated with the abuse, eating disorders, self-mutilation or other dangerous behaviors, etc.).

The treatment of adult survivors is generally considered to encompass three phases which should be considered dynamic and fluid rather than static, each with a variety of therapeutic tasks and strategies. Treatment is planned according to the needs and available emotional and financial resources of the individual client (Chu, 1992; Courtois, 1991; Gil, 1988; Herman, 1992b; S. Kirschner et al., 1993; Meiselman, 1990).

The Preliminary Phase. Of foremost importance at this stage is the development of a working alliance involving a consistent, reliable, and stable therapeutic relationship. Survivors often are mistrustful of others, authority figures in particular; therapists are no exception and can expect to be tested throughout the treatment. Therapists best handle this reaction by expecting it, not taking it personally, and providing the conditions for the development of an honest, trustworthy relationship. They must also take care not to distance from the client during times of transference crises, during the discharge of intense affect, or during traumatic recall, as such a response will disrupt any alliance that has been developed (Chu, 1988).

Other preliminaries include intake, assessment, and diagnosis; treatment planning based on diagnosis; treatment negotiation and contracting; and informed consent. As noted earlier, the client may present for treatment with a disclosure of a sexual abuse history (a much more common event in the last decade with widespread acknowledgement of the reality and prevalence of child abuse and incest) or may make a "disguised presentation" (Gelinas, 1983) of symptoms with little or no memory that abuse occurred or that it has any relevance to the presenting symptoms. It is recommended that therapists ask clients about any sexual contact or trauma in childhood and about family functioning as part of their routine psychosocial screening at the initiation of treatment. Such inquiries, whether verbal or written, signal the client that these issues are pertinent and that the therapist is open to hearing about them. If, however, the client does not identify such a history but the symptom picture corresponds to the description presented earlier in this contribution, or if the therapist observes certain behavioral and response patterns associated with trauma (such as dissociation or microamnesias in the session or intersession amnesia), then the therapist can inquire about possible abuse and trauma. Even in the face of a client's denial or lack of knowledge, the therapist must ethically continue to explore the possibility and to provide treatment that allows for it. As mentioned previously, however, the therapist must avoid being overzealous in trying to identify an abuse history or in assuming that sexual abuse is the only possible causative explanation of symptoms.

A number of questionnaires and screening instruments specific to trauma symptoms and dissociation are now available to supplement more standard psychological assessment tools and batteries (Bernstein & Putnam, 1986; Briere, 1989; Courtois, 1988; Jehu, 1988; Loewenstein, 1991; Ross, 1989; Steinberg, Rounsaville, & Cicchetti, 1990).

The therapist should expect that the client's history might unfold throughout the course of treatment according to the client's readiness and should therefore not push disclosure prematurely or without regard for the client's defensive structure and ego capacities. This is in keeping with standard therapeutic practice but especially with guidelines for the treatment of trauma. According to McCann and Pearlman (1990), "self-work precedes memory or trauma work" and early-phase work should include the assessment of the client's schemata about self and others, defenses and ego resources, and life management and stability. Gil (1988) and Horowitz (1986) further recommend assessing the client's personality style and defensive pattern, adjusting the pace of exploration to the individual's style and readiness with a recognition that some clients are able to move more quickly than others.

In this subphase, it is useful to assess the client's self-care and quality of life and to institute stress-management, self-nurturing, and self-regulating strategies as needed. For example, it is well recognized that traumatized individuals are frequently depressed and deficient in the basics of self-care. They may eat and sleep poorly, overwork and function either excessively well or poorly, and neglect their medical health and physical care. These deficiencies may provide a preliminary focus of therapeutic intervention and provide issues that allow for therapeutic interaction and testing. A stress management contract involving adequate nutrition, exercise, rest and sleep, recreation, and dental and medical care can be established. Relaxation through deep breathing, guided imagery, auto-hypnosis, or exercise can counteract chronic body tension and armoring.

The highly dissociative client or the client who spontaneously reexperiences the trauma through flashbacks or other reenactments can be taught to recognize episodes of "spacing out." This response is frequently unconscious and goes unrecognized without specific inquiry and attention. Clients can be taught substitute strategies for coping with triggers to dissociative or reexperiencing responses as well as techniques for emotional containment, grounding, and personal safety. The reader is referred to Dolan (1991) for a variety of creative techniques useful in refocusing a client caught in dissociative or reexperienced trauma responses.

Any current life crises should, of necessity, receive treatment attention at this time. They can, however, be expected to occur concurrently throughout the treatment process since crises tend to wax and wane over time in this population. Likewise, anything life-threatening - including addictions and compulsions, eating disorders, self-mutilation, or revictimization (such as being battered or sexually assaulted in a relationship) - and debilitating degrees of dissociation and reenactment/reexperiencing must be addressed early, if not treated first. Lethality and severe addictive patterns must be assessed and controlled so that therapy can proceed. Difficulty with sequencing arises because these very symptoms may well have developed to cope with the trauma and its painful aftermath; dismantling or otherwise lessening them usually means that the client feels what had been avoided. In many cases, this has resulted in relapse to the same or new means to cope or escape. Survivors of child abuse have been found to have a high rate of relapse for all types of addictions and compulsions and are hypothesized to have become addicted to their own endogenous opioids, released in response to increased arousal (Carnes, 1991; van der Kolk, 1988). Sobriety often has the effect of calling up suppressed memory and avoided affect. Thus, relapse prevention must take the return of post-traumatic reactions into consideration to offset jeopardizing sobriety (Carnes, 1991).

The best strategy in working with these issues is to treat anything life-threatening first and then allow enough time for the client to stabilize without self-destructive coping strategies before proceeding with trauma work. The therapist should anticipate and prepare the client for relapse to some of the old coping methods when the trauma is addressed directly. Such a relapse does not mean failure; rather, the client is returning to the "tried and true" coping methods of old. Throughout this phase, clients learn to substitute the new ways of coping and self-regulating they have been taught.

Also in this phase, the client must be encouraged and assisted in the development of a support system besides the therapist. This is another "chicken and egg" treatment dilemma with this population: how to get interpersonally traumatized and generally mistrustful survivors to find and develop a support system of trustworthy others. Some clients come with rather intact social networks and supportive spouses, partners, families, and friends. These are to be capitalized on and can be brought into treatment early (of course with the client's permission and if such a strategy suits the therapeutic orientation of the therapist) to educate them about post-traumatic conditions, the likely course of therapy, and their roles and responsibilities with regard to the survivor. They can be encouraged to read books such as *Allies in Healing* by Laura Davis (1992), written especially for supportive others, for supplementary information. Clinicians experienced in working with this population have come to recognize the wisdom in incorporating the survivor's support system early in the treatment. For a detailed discussion of this rationale as well as a comprehensive treatment strategy, the reader is referred to S. Kirschner et al. (1993).

A totally different problem arises with those clients for whom relationships are chronically absent, stormy, short-lived, abusive, or otherwise problematic. Much therapeutic time must be spent in working on the skills and attitudes necessary to develop healthy, interdependent relationships. In all likelihood, these were not taught or learned in the abusive family. The relational rules that were taught need to be unlearned and replaced with others more conducive to trust and mutuality. The therapeutic relationship hopefully models a healthy relationship from which the client can learn and apply skills. In any event, relational work is likely to proceed slowly with many false starts and stops. It is important for the therapist to teach the utility of relationships with supportive others and further to insist that the survivor develop supports other than the therapist. Group therapy may be especially useful to address these issues; yet, here again, the client may not be able to productively engage in a group until some preliminary relational work has been accomplished. If a group is used at this juncture, it is best that it be a highly structured, theme, or issue-focused psychoeducational support group as opposed to an open-ended therapy group (Courtois, 1988). See Courtois (1993) for a model of such a group.

Many other practicalities are addressed in this treatment phase including the client's level of functioning and employment and financial stability and resources. Many adaptive patterns might be identified in assessing how the client functions and manages financially. In some cases, such as the chronically financially chaotic client, wholesale intervention is needed, while in others, clients have self-management under good control.

This phase is also the time to assess the client's mood including depressive and anxiety symptoms and any degree of impairment. Jehu (1988) recommends specific cognitive-behavioral interventions with this population as a preliminary strategy in treating mood disturbances. Should such techniques prove inadequate, the client can be evaluated for medication. Specific antidepressants and anxiolytics have been found effective with this population (Schwartz, 1990); however, the clinician must prepare the client adequately for their use and must simultaneously guard against overmedication of the client, a not uncommon occurrence because of the complexity and intensity of many of these clients' symptoms.

Obviously, the depth and duration of this phase varies considerably. Some clients move through it rapidly while others literally require years of stabilization and alliance-building before trauma resolution work is undertaken. For others, the work is done episodically, with time-outs to build personal resources for the work, to deal with other life issues and life stresses, during times of symptomatic stabilization, or until symptoms recur. For still others, this phase satisfies their needs, energy level, and motivation for treatment and they go no further. Although the therapist, of necessity, must assess and interpret resistances, it is the survivor's choice whether to continue or discontinue treatment. Chu (1988) cautions about the type of treatment trap in which the therapist is overinvested in the client's remaining in treatment and takes on too much responsibility, does too much of the work, and becomes increasingly resentful as a result.

The Incest/Trauma Resolution Phase. This phase is also shaped according the needs and defenses of the individual client. As a general rule, uncovering and working with traumatic material proceeds slowly and carefully, with continuous attention to the client's capacities and defenses. An approach-avoid paradigm has been suggested by Horowitz (1986) to parallel the phasic alterations of the trauma response with the deliberate intent of increasing the client's ability to approach and tolerate the traumatic material while simultaneously lessening avoidance and numbing.

In this phase, the client is encouraged to remember and talk about the specifics of the trauma and to reconnect whatever has been previously dissociated. Many traumatized individuals "know more than they know they know" (Herman & Schatzow, 1987) and with specific inquiry and encouragement their story emerges. The titration provided by the approach-avoid paradigm paces recollection at tolerable levels so that the client is neither emotionally overwhelmed nor inadvertently retraumatized. According to Horowitz, the therapist titrates by deliberately employing triggers when the client is in the denial/numbing phase of the trauma response. These might include such strategies as verbally describing or journaling what is known about the abuse, creating artwork to express the story and associated feelings, examining memorabilia such as photographs and medical and school records from childhood, talking to relatives or neighbors about family characteristics or abuse-related issues, and involvement in a trauma-related support or therapy group. If, in response to these triggers and the resultant material, the client signifies an inability to tolerate the material through an increase in dissociative/denial/numbing or reexperiencing, the therapist titrates the treatment by diluting or removing the trigger and by encouraging the client to approach the material more slowly while applying specific coping strategies that had previously been taught in Phase 1.

An alternative strategy is used when the client is in the intrusive/reexperiencing phase of the trauma response. Then, the therapist encourages the deliberate removal of whatever trigger is generating the overwhelming response (e.g., resulting nightmares, flashbacks, startle responses, sleep disturbance, urges to self-harm, etc.). Instead, strong external support and deliberate dosing and containment strategies are utilized until the client restabilizes. In this stage, the therapist might encourage the client to get away from the traumatic content or might encourage staying with it but utilizing previously learned coping, self-soothing, or cognitive techniques.

It is this back-and-forth strategy that produces gradual reconstruction of the story along with its associated affect. A therapeutic challenge is to find methods to successfully control the pace of recall and the intensity of affect. Very strong emotions emerge as the trauma along with its betrayals and losses is faced. Numerous therapeutic strategies are utilized during this phase according to the needs and capabilities of each client and in a cooperative effort between therapist and client. Nonverbal strategies hold a special place in the resolution of trauma. They provide the means to symbolize and communicate what the survivor may not be able to verbalize. Common reasons for the inability to verbalize child abuse trauma include that it occurred when the child was preverbal, or that the child was threatened with dire consequences for ever disclosing, or simply that the client has no words with which to verbalize his or her story.

Emotional ventilation gives way to assimilation and new meaning later in this phase. Once the survivor has faced the abuse directly and experienced associated emotions, assimilation occurs as he or she expands personal understanding for what happened in childhood and why, and attaches new meaning to the experience and its personal implications. At its most basic, the client resolves issues of self-blame in response to a deeper understanding of the abuse scenario including the abuser's motivations and contributory family dynamics and characteristics. Resolution is furthered by addressing any related issues and by determining future courses of action. At this time, some survivors choose to disclose their abuse to or to confront the perpetrator or others. Some choose to try to work out a new relationship with the family while others choose separation. Forgiveness is considered by some, spirituality issues addressed, and sometimes public disclosure and education is undertaken. All of these issues are best resolved as part of the therapy - but after the most arduous of the trauma work is completed. An exception to this is provided by the S. Kirschner et al. (1993) treatment model which incorporates relational work with significant others and with family members (as available and according to dictates of safety) during this phase.

Group therapy specific to sexual abuse trauma is especially useful in this phase of treatment (Herman & Schatzow, 1987) because it relieves isolation and hence stigmatization; encourages disclosure and the recognition of commonalities among members; serves as a catalyst for the exploration of memories, beliefs, cognitions, and emotions; and offers a unique forum for grieving and a safe context for exploring and changing abuse-related interpersonal dynamics. Group members assist and support others and, in turn, are supported and helped (Courtois, 1988).

The Postresolution or Reconnection Phase. The third phase builds on the work of the first and second. Treatment of problems that first require significant resolution of the trauma occurs in this phase. Most of these problems have been attended to previously; their resolution is now more possible with the amelioration of the traumatic content and effects. They include relational difficulties and imbalances (including intimate relationships, parenting, other family relationships, friendships, and social and work relationships); sexual difficulties and dysfunctions; mood disturbances; substance abuse and eating disorders; obsessive-compulsive difficulties; and personality disorders and disturbances. Any other problems or psychological symptoms receive attention at this time. This phase, in contrast to the previous two, is easier and provides more satisfaction to both therapist and client. The hard work of the therapy becomes abundantly obvious as the progress is observable and felt.

As in the previous phase, many standard therapeutic strategies and techniques are available to treat these symptoms and problems, but they too might need some modification as they are applied to the aftermath of traumatic circumstances. For example, sex therapy for the sexually traumatized client requires specific modification concerning issues of control and pacing (Maltz, 1991; Westerlund, 1992).

The final task of this phase is to prepare the client for the termination of treatment. Sufficient time should be allotted to review the course and progress of the therapy, to grieve its end, and more specifically, to grieve the loss of the ongoing relationship with the therapist. As mentioned earlier, the relationship between therapist and survivor is the foundation of the work and may have been the first truly beneficial and trustworthy relationship experienced by the survivor. Its loss therefore must be addressed and reactions ventilated. Although the therapist aims for a clearly demarcated termination of this phase of the treatment, return in the future should not be precluded with this population unless warranted for a specific reason. The client might need to return for an occasional "tune-up" or "check-in" due to a resurgence of symptoms, because of a relapse due to a developmental stage or issue, or due to an unanticipated trigger or crisis. Of necessity, the therapist must scrupulously guard against the development of dual relationships and blurred boundaries after formal treatment has ended. Survivors more than any other therapeutic population must be assured that the therapeutic relationship is "clean," that is, unencumbered by conflicted roles, so that a return to the "safe place" is assured if needed (Herman, 1992b).

TRANSFERENCE AND COUNTERTRANSFERENCE ISSUES

The treatment of clients with complex dissociative post-traumatic reactions poses a number of challenges for the clinician, some of which play out in the therapeutic process and relationship through the transference and countertransference. Rather than dismiss these reactions as bothersome or insignificant, the therapist must assess them for their thematic content and for how the trauma might be reenacted in either a coded or direct relational form (Courtois, 1988). The client is not only likely to reenact issues in the transference but to experience them and to cause the therapist to experience them in a process colored by dissociative and post-traumatic reactions and distortions. For example, the therapist is likely to be transferentially mistrusted as an authority figure (a post-traumatic response to which the client reenacts scenarios from the abuse). This reaction is compounded by a dissociative response in which the client misperceives the therapist as the actual abuser.

A detailed discussion of these issues is beyond the scope of this contribution, but the therapist is well advised to anticipate the most common transference and countertransference issues and to become familiar with strategies for their therapeutic management. (Several of these have been given as examples throughout this contribution, e.g., client mistrust or compliance, therapist lack of boundaries, overcompensation, rescue, resentment, and sexualization.) Failure to attend to these issues has resulted in many therapeutic blunders, misalliances, and misadventures. Although many of these, if caught early and managed therapeutically, do not do substantial harm and sometimes actually enhance the process and the relationship due to the way that they are resolved, others recapitulate elements of the abuse and its aftermath and further damage the client. The therapist must remain vigilant to the treatment traps and dilemmas with this population and the potential for both very positive and very negative outcomes depending upon their management (Chu, 1988, 1992).

In general, the client can be expected to project upon and reenact with the therapist salient issues from past relationships, including the relational messages of the abuse and the family environment. Many of these are similar to those identified with such personality disturbances as borderline personality disorder (Herman, 1992b). Thus, the client might be superficially compliant and nonassertive, mistrustful, disillusioned, overdependent and overidealizing, sexualized, rageful, aggressive, demanding and entitled, shamed, highly defended, fearful, and anxious in all combinations and permutations. Some clients are somewhat modulated while others swing widely between extreme relational patterns, as is often found in borderline personality.

A transference reaction quite particular to this population was labeled "traumatic transference" (Spiegel, 1986) and refers to the client's projection that the therapist is just like the abuser and, at some point sooner or later, will be gratified by using and abusing the client in some way. Traumatic transference can be very upsetting for the therapist who has worked mightily to provide a healthy and healing relationship for the client and who then feels both attacked and incompetent. As noted earlier, the therapist must have enough observing ego and ego strength to depersonalize these responses and must interpret them with the client in order to correct and defuse them. In general, the therapist must refuse the role of victimizer or rescuer while refusing to be victimized by the survivor. Traumatized clients play out the "victimization triangle" of victim-victimizer-rescuer roles which are often projected against and played out with the therapist. Major therapeutic gains are made when the client is able to function outside of these three roles and hence has many more degrees of freedom in interpersonal relationships. Repeated interpretation and analysis along with the challenging of cognitive distortions and the teaching and modeling of new relational skills contribute to these gains.

Common countertransference issues can be organized under the three categories of avoidance, attraction, and attack (Renshaw, 1982) which the therapist engages in due to the client's issues (objective countertransference) or due to his or her own issues (subjective countertransference). In terms of avoidance, therapists might disbelieve, deny, dismiss, or discourage disclosure of any material that appears to be abuse related. This position is rather codified in some theoretical orientations which hold that such events constitute fantasy formation on the child's part. The therapist working with this population must modify this theoretical orientation lest it interfere with the ability to encourage disclosure and exploration.

Avoidance is also implicated when the therapist dreads hearing about the client's experience due to personal horror or the inability to tolerate the material. Such a stance often leads to defensive maneuvering on the part of the therapist who may minimize its importance, change the subject, urge the client to "put it behind him or her," transfer the client to another therapist, and so forth. Some therapists also minimize by using imprecise language (e.g., "when your father did those things to you" versus "when your father forced you to have oral sex or sodomized you"). Finally, some therapists are so personally overwhelmed by the material, by burnout or by the demands of an overly large or demanding caseload or other personal and professional stresses, that they numb out or use post-traumatic numbing strategies similar to those used by the victim (e.g., denial, dissociation, intellectualization, minimization, detachment, etc.) or they maintain an overly rigid professional stance and are largely unavailable and unempathetic.

Some therapists have just the opposite reaction, of being attracted by the client's plight and by the abuse. Countertransference errors of overidentification and overprotection often result when the therapist tries to "make up for the abuse" and attempts to reparent the client. The loss of limits and gross boundary violations often ensue. This rescuing response usually results in the therapist giving or doing far too much and encouraging a position of entitlement or overdependence and helplessness on the part of the client. Sooner or later, the therapist resents the demands and becomes angry and withholding. In this scenario, the therapist goes from rescuer to victim to victimizer offsetting each complementary role in the client.

In some cases, the therapist is attracted and even aroused by the abuse. Incest has historically been taboo. The transgression of such a taboo and the very sexual nature of the abuse may cause the therapist to become fascinated with the sexual dimensions of the client to the exclusion of others and to have a position of privileged voyeurism. Obviously, obsessive sexual interest repeats the sexual objectification of the client and is therefore retraumatizing rather than healing. The most blatant and damaging countertransference response in this category occurs when the therapist becomes sexually involved with the client to provide a "corrective emotional experience" or due to the therapist's own pathology or sadism. As noted previously, such a response constitutes professional incest, a direct reenactment of the earlier betrayal by someone who is in a position of providing assistance and protection, and is thus retraumatizing.

Sexual involvement is but one way that the therapist might attack or victimize the client. Therapists might be pulled into reenactments of the abuse scenario by clients who are in perpetual victim/masochistic roles. The projections directed toward the therapist might invite him or her to play out complementary roles. The therapist must guard against revictimizing the client but must also be free to recognize when his or her anger is being piqued, not an uncommon occurrence. Work with abuse survivors is arduous with many difficult stories, interactions, and emotional storms and with numerous crises involving such demanding issues as self-harm, revictimization, regressions, and so on. Additionally, therapists find themselves enraged at the abuser, the family, coworkers who do not understand or offer assistance, the agency, the system, and so forth. Therapists who are able to acknowledge their anger and work it through, whether directly with the client or more commonly in supervision or consultation, are less likely to act it out. Their relationship therefore stays on a more honest footing with the client and they are less prone to directly express or defend against their hostility.

SUMMARY

To summarize, many treatment traps, and many transference, countertransference, and vicarious traumatization issues affect the clinician working with the population of adult survivors of severe childhood abuse. The work is very rigorous and requires patience and perseverance on the part of both therapist and client. The vagaries and complicated issues of this work make it both compelling and challenging. This therapy has the potential for major therapeutic gains for these clients who have the opportunity to move beyond their dissociative post-traumatic symptoms and lifestyle to one which is substantially better. Much remains to be learned about this population, the triadic symptom aftermath, and treatment methodologies. Nevertheless, a preliminary model is offered here to assist the clinician working with adult survivors. The model suggests therapist perspectives found useful in conducting this treatment along with goals and sequencing/strategic guidelines. Finally, the relational demands of this work are great. Therapists must constantly assess the relational field with its transference and countertransference challenges as "grist for the mill" wherein much of the therapeutic work will be conducted.

Christine A. Courtois, PhD, is a psychologist in private practice in Washington, DC, and Clinical Director of the Center for Abuse Recovery & Empowerment, The Psychiatric Institute of Washington, Washington, DC. She conducts workshops nationwide on the treatment of incest and other forms of sexual assault. She has authored two books, with a third in process, and has coedited the 1988 issue of *The Counseling Psychologist* on the topic of victimization and its aftermath. Dr. Courtois received her doctorate from the University of Maryland, College Park, in 1979. She is a member of the Program Committee, Eastern Regional Conference on Abuse and Multiple Personality Disorder, and was appointed to the American Psychological Association Working Group on the Investigation of Childhood Memories and the President's Task Force on Family Violence. She is a Fellow of APA Divisions 17 and 29. Dr. Courtois may be contacted at Three Washington Circle, Suite 206, Washington, DC 20037.

RESOURCES

Alexander, P. C. (1992). Application of attachment theory to the study of sexual abuse. *Journal of Consulting and Clinical Psychology, 60,* 185-195.

American Psychiatric Association. (1987). *Diagnostic and Statistical Manual of Mental Disorders* (3rd ed. rev.). Washington, DC: Author.

American Psychiatric Association. (1994). *Diagnostic and Statistical Manual of Mental Disorders* (4th ed.). Washington, DC: Author.

Armsworth, M., & Holaday, M. (1993). The effects of psychological trauma on children and adolescents. *Journal of Counseling and Development, 72,* 49-72.

Bernstein, E. M., & Putnam, F. W. (1986). Development, reliability, and validity of a dissociation scale. *Journal of Nervous Mental Disorders, 174,* 727-735.

Braun, B. G. (1986). *Treatment of Multiple Personality Disorder.* Washington, DC: American Psychiatric Press.

Briere, J. (1989). *Therapy for Adults Molested as Children: Beyond Survival.* New York: Springer.

Briere, J. (Ed.). (1991). *Treating Victims of Child Sexual Abuse.* San Francisco: Jossey-Bass.

Briere, J. (1992). Methodological issues in the study of sexual abuse side effects. *Journal of Consulting and Clinical Psychology, 60,* 196-203.

Bryer, J. B., Nelson, B. A., Miller, J. B., & Krol, P. A. (1987). Childhood sexual and physical abuse as factors in adult psychiatric illness. *American Journal of Psychiatry, 144,* 1426-1430.

Butler, S. (1978). *Conspiracy of Silence: The Trauma of Incest.* New York: Bantam Books.

Carlson, E. B., Putnam, F. W., Ross, C. A., Torem, M., Coons, P., Dill, D. L., Loewenstein, R. J., & Braun, B. G. (1993). Validity of the dissociative experiences scale in screening for multiple personality disorder: A multicenter study. *American Journal of Psychiatry, 150,* 1030-1036.

Carnes, P. (1991). *Don't Call It Love: Recovery from Sexual Addiction.* New York: Bantam Books.

Chu, J. A. (1988). Ten traps for therapists in the treatment of trauma survivors. *Dissociation, 1,* 24-32.

Chu, J. A. (1992). The therapeutic roller coaster: Dilemmas in the treatment of childhood abuse survivors. *Journal of Psychotherapy Practice and Research, 4,* 351-370.

Chu, J. A., & Dill, D. L. (1990). Dissociative symptoms in relation to childhood physical and sexual abuse. *American Journal of Psychiatry, 147,* 887-892.

Cole, P. M., & Putnam, F. W. (1992). Effect of incest on self and social functioning: A developmental psychopathology perspective. *Journal of Consulting and Clinical Psychology, 60,* 174-184.

Courtois, C. A. (1988). *Healing the Incest Wound: Adult Survivors in Therapy.* New York: W. W. Norton.

Courtois, C. A. (1991). Theory, sequencing, and strategy in treating adult survivors. In J. Briere (Ed.), *Treating Victims of Child Sexual Abuse* (pp. 47-60). San Francisco: Jossey-Bass.

Courtois, C. A. (1993). *Adult Survivors of Child Sexual Abuse*. Milwaukee: Families International.

Davis, L. (1992). *Allies in Healing: When the Person You Love Was Sexually Abused as a Child*. New York: Harper Perennial.

Dolan, Y. M. (1991). *Resolving Sexual Abuse: Solution-Focused Therapy and Ericksonian Hypnosis for Adult Survivors*. New York: W. W. Norton.

Donaldson, M. A., & Gardner, R. (1985). Diagnosis and treatment of traumatic stress among women after childhood incest. In C. R. Figley (Ed.), *Trauma and Its Wake: The Study and Treatment of Post-Traumatic Stress Disorder*. New York: Brunner/Mazel.

Finkelhor, D. (1984). *Child Sexual Abuse: New Theory and Research*. New York: The Free Press.

Finkelhor, D., & Browne, A. (1985). The traumatic impact of child sexual abuse: A conceptualization. *American Journal of Orthopsychiatry, 55,* 530-541.

Fossum, M. A., & Mason, M. J. (1986). *Facing Shame*. New York: W. W. Norton.

Gelinas, D. (1983). The persisting negative effects of incest. *American Journal of Psychiatry, 46,* 313-332.

Gil, E. (1988). *Treatment of Adult Survivors of Childhood Abuse*. Walnut Creek, CA: Launch Press.

Herman, J. L. (1981). Father-daughter incest. *Signs: Journal of Women in Culture and Society, 2,* 735-756.

Herman, J. L. (1992a). Complex PTSD: A syndrome in survivors of prolonged and repeated trauma. *Journal of Traumatic Stress, 3,* 377-391.

Herman, J. L. (1992b). *Trauma and Recovery: The Aftermath of Violence - From Domestic to Political Terror*. New York: Basic Books.

Herman, J. L., & Schatzow, E. (1987). Recovery and verification of memories of childhood sexual trauma. *Psychoanalytic Psychology, 4*(1), 1-14.

Herman, J. L., & van der Kolk, B. (1987). Traumatic antecedents of borderline personality disorder. In B. van der Kolk (Ed.), *Psychological Trauma* (pp. 111-126). Washington, DC: American Psychiatric Press.

Horevitz, P. P., & Braun, B. G. (1984). Are multiple personalities borderline? In B. G. Braun (Ed.), *Psychiatric Clinics of North America, 7,* 69-87.

Horowitz, M. J. (1986). *Stress Response Syndromes* (2nd ed.). Northvale, NJ: Jason Aronson.

Jehu, D. (1988). *Beyond Sexual Abuse: Therapy With Women Who Were Childhood Victims*. New York: John Wiley.

Johnson, S. (1989). Integrating marital and individual therapy for incest survivors: A case study. *Psychotherapy, 26,* 96-103.

Kendall-Tackett, K. A., Williams, L. M., & Finkelhor, D. (1993). Impact of sexual abuse on children: A review and synthesis of recent empirical studies. *Psychological Bulletin, 113,* 164-180.

Kirby, J. S., Chu, J. A., & Dill, D. L. (1993). Correlates of dissociative symptomatology in patients with physical and sexual abuse histories. *Comprehensive Psychiatry, 34,* 258-263.

Kirschner, S., Kirschner, D. A., & Rappaport, R. L. (1993). *Working With Adult Incest Survivors: The Healing Journey*. New York: Brunner/Mazel.

Kroll, J. (1993). *PTSD/Borderlines in Therapy: Finding the Balance*. New York: W. W. Norton.

Lindberg, F. H., & Distad, L. J. (1985). Post-traumatic stress disorders in women who experienced childhood incest. *Child Abuse and Neglect, 9,* 329-324.

Loewenstein, R. J. (Ed.). (1991). *Psychiatric Clinics of North America* [Special issue on Multiple Personality Disorder], *14*.

Maltz, W. (1991). *The Sexual Healing Journey*. New York: HarperCollins.

McCann, I. L., & Pearlman, L. A. (1990). *Psychological Trauma and the Adult Survivor: Theory, Therapy, and Transformation*. New York: Brunner/Mazel.

Meiselman, K. C. (1990). *Resolving the Trauma of Incest: Reintegration Therapy With Survivors.* San Francisco: Jossey-Bass.

National Institute of Mental Health, Division of Biometry and Applied Sciences, Antisocial and Violent Behavior Branch. (1990, April). *Research Workshop on Treatment of Adult Victims of Childhood Sexual Abuse,* Washington, DC.

Pribor, E. F., & Dinwiddie, S. H. (1992). Psychiatric correlates of incest in childhood. *American Journal of Psychiatry, 149,* 52-56.

Putnam, F. W. (1985). Dissociation as a response to extreme trauma. In R. Kluft (Ed.), *Childhood Antecedents of Multiple Personality* (pp. 65-98). Washington, DC: American Psychiatric Press.

Putnam, F. W. (1989). *Diagnosis and Treatment of Multiple Personality Disorder.* New York: Guilford.

Putman, F. W., Guroff, J. J., Silberman, E. K., Barban, L., & Post, R. M. (1986). The clinical phenomenology of multiple personality disorder: Review of 100 recent cases. *Journal of Clinical Psychiatry, 47,* 285-293.

Renshaw, D. (1982). *Incest: Understanding and Treatment.* Boston: Little, Brown.

Ross, C. A. (1989). *Multiple Personality Disorder: Diagnosis, Clinical Features, and Treatment.* New York: John Wiley & Sons.

Ross, C. A., Norton, G. R., & Wozney, K. (1989). Multiple personality disorder: An analysis of 236 cases. *Canadian Journal of Psychiatry, 34,* 413-418.

Russell, D. E. H. (1986). *The Secret Trauma: Incest in the Lives of Girls and Women.* New York: Basic Books.

Sanford, L. (1989). *Strong at the Broken Places.* New York: Random House.

Scheflin, A. W., & Shapiro, J. L. (1989). *Trance on Trial.* New York: Guilford.

Schwartz, L. S. (1990). A biopsychosocial treatment approach to post-traumatic stress disorder. *Journal of Traumatic Stress, 3,* 221-238.

Sgroi, S. M. (1989). *Vulnerable Populations.* Lexington, MA: Lexington Books.

Spiegel, D. (1986). Dissociation, double binds, and post traumatic stress in multiple personality disorder. In B. G. Braun (Ed.), *Treatment of Multiple Personality Disorder.* Washington, DC: American Psychiatric Press.

Spiegel, D., & Cardena, E. (1991). Disintegrated experience: The dissociative disorders revisited. *Journal of Abnormal Psychology, 100,* 366-378.

Spiegel, D., Hunt, T., & Dondershine, H. E. (1988). Dissociation and hypnotizability in post-traumatic stress disorder. *American Journal of Psychiatry, 145,* 301-305.

Steinberg, M., Rounsaville B., & Cicchetti, D. (1990). The structured clinical interview for DSM-III-R dissociative disorders. *American Journal of Psychiatry, 147,* 76-82.

Strick, F. L., & Wilcoxon, A. (1991). A comparison of dissociative experiences in adult female outpatients with and without histories of early incestuous abuse. *Dissociation, IV,* 193-199.

Summit, R. (1983). The child sexual abuse accommodation syndrome. *Child Abuse and Neglect, 7,* 177-193.

Turkus, J. A. (1991). Psychotherapy and case management for multiple personality disorder. In R. J. Loewenstein (Ed.), *Psychiatric Clinics of North America* [Special issue on Multiple Personality Disorder], *14,* 649-660.

van der Kolk, B. (1987). *Psychological Trauma.* Washington, DC: American Psychiatric Press.

van der Kolk, B. (1988). The trauma spectrum: The interaction of biological and social events in the genesis of the trauma response. *Journal of Traumatic Stress, 1,* 273-290.

Waites, E. A. (1993). *Trauma and Survival: Post-Traumatic and Dissociative Disorders in Women.* New York: W. W. Norton.

Weinberg, K. (1955). *Incest Behavior.* New York: Citadel Press.

Westerlund, E. (1992). *Women's Sexuality After Childhood Incest.* New York: W. W. Norton.

Wyatt G. E. (1985). The sexual abuse of Afro-American and white women in childhood. *Child Abuse and Neglect, 9,* 507-519.

Wyatt, G. E., & Newcomb, M. (1990). Internal and external mediators of women's sexual abuse in childhood. *Journal of Consulting and Clinical Psychology, 58,* 758-767.

BEHAVIORAL ASSESSMENT AND TREATMENT OF CHRONIC PAIN IN CHILDREN*

Chris A. Coleman, Alice G. Friedman, and Donna Gates

INTRODUCTION

Although exact epidemiological evidence is lacking, it is estimated that up to 10% of school-aged children experience chronic pain at some point (P. J. McGrath, Unruh, & Branson, 1990). For many of these children, the etiology is easy to determine, such as in the case of sickle cell anemia, hemophilia, and arthritis. For others, the organic basis of the pain is less clear, as in the case of recurrent abdominal pain (RAP), chronic headaches, and bone pain ("growing pain"). Psychological interventions have shown utility for decreasing distress associated with both types of chronic childhood pain. It is therefore increasingly likely that mental health service providers in traditional mental health settings will be called upon to provide services to children who experience chronic pain. This contribution is designed to acquaint the practitioner in nonprimary-healthcare settings with basic information about assessment and treatment of children with chronic pain. In the first section we discuss definitions, common sources of pediatric pain, and general issues associated with the management of pediatric pain. We review these issues because they underlie the rationale for approaching assessment and treatment in the manner outlined in the following two sections. In the second section we discuss assessment strategies that pertain directly to pain-related behaviors. In the third section we discuss intervention strategies.

CHILDREN WITH CHRONIC PAIN

Children who are referred to a psychologist to learn pain management strategies typically have pain that is resistant to medical treatments, deemed as disproportionate to the organic cause, or is interfering with the child's age-appropriate activities and the family's functioning. Common medical complaints are headaches and recurrent abdominal pain, although we have recently been seeing an increasing number of children with chronic fatigue syndrome. Parents are often alarmed by the referral because they infer that the pediatrician either does not fully understand the severity of the pain or has decided that the child has a "psychological" rather than a "physical" problem. It is not surprising, therefore, that one of the most common initial questions among parents of children with chronic pain is, "Is the pain real or is it psychological?"

The very nature of pain makes this question difficult if not impossible to answer. The task of the psychologist is to help the family better understand the factors exacerbating the pain and to

---

*Preparation of this manuscript was supported by a grant from the Prospect Group awarded to the second author, and the Graduate Research Initiative, a SUNY grant designed to promote treatment outcome research. We gratefully acknowledge their support.

lessen the negative impact of the pain. Children with chronic pain are rarely "faking it," and this point should be discussed with the family. On the other hand, even in cases of obvious organic etiology, psychological factors may play a significant role in the lives of children with chronic pain.

DEFINITION OF CHRONIC PAIN

Pain is a subjective experience which is determined by the complex interaction of neurochemical, sensory, cognitive, affective, motivational, behavioral, and historical factors (Katz, Varni, & Jay, 1984). The amount of distress a child expresses is influenced by the specific conditions surrounding the pain incident interacting with a complex array of factors, including (a) the child's previous experience with pain; (b) the presence and type of illness associated with the pain; (c) the response of others to the child's distress during the present incident as well as the past; (d) the anticipated duration of pain; (e) the child's general level of anxiety, and anxiety regarding the pain; and (f) the child's understanding of the cause of the pain and his or her general cognitive and maturational level.

The interaction of these complex factors contribute not only to the amount and degree of distress a child experiences but also the manner in which he or she expresses that distress. As a result, there is no clear relationship between the extent of measurable tissue damage and expression of pain. Seemingly identical injuries can produce pain that differs markedly, both qualitatively and quantitatively. This further complicates matters as the child's pain responses are affected by the behavior of those around him or her, sometimes leading adults to speculate that the pain is not really as severe as the child is reporting.

SOURCES OF CHILDHOOD PAIN

Pain may be classified as either acute or chronic. Acute pain is characterized by rapid onset, often results from a known trauma or insult, and generally runs a predictable course. Chronic pain is persistent but follows a less predictable course than acute pain. The pain may be either recurrent or continuous. It may undermine the individual's health, diminish energy, and interfere with quality of life. According to Varni, Walco, and Wilcox (1990), children with chronic pain typically do not exhibit high levels of anxiety, as they do with acute pain. Instead they may appear depressed, avoid age-appropriate activities, fall behind peers developmentally, and spend much of their time inactive. These behaviors may persist after medical evidence of the disorder appears to have subsided.

There are some medical conditions, such as sickle cell anemia, that almost inevitably are associated with chronic pain. How children cope with pain varies considerably. Some children are able to minimize its negative impact by continuing to engage in age-appropriate activities, attending school when able, and participating in social and recreational activities. However, children referred for psychological services are apt to be those for whom the pain has negative impact on many aspects of life. In many cases, the pain becomes a "distinct clinical entity" rather than a secondary symptom of an underlying disease or injury (D. M. Ross & S. M. Ross, 1988). In these children, the pain is maintained by factors other than the actual disease. These factors may include psychological or emotional difficulties as well as reinforcement of pain behavior by family members and friends. Other aspects of the syndrome include preoccupation with the pain, failure to engage in age-appropriate activities, social isolation, narrowing range of interests, and depression. Some researchers have speculated that certain pain difficulties in childhood may predispose an individual for chronic pain syndrome in adulthood (D. M. Ross & S. M. Ross, 1988; Routh, Ernst, & Harper, 1988). Therefore, a child who has chronic pain that is interfering with age-appropriate activities in a manner that is disproportionate to the injury or disease may be at risk for continued pain-related difficulties.

COMMON TYPES OF REFERRALS

The most common types of pain that are not associated with a specific disease are headaches, recurrent abdominal pain (RAP), and limb (growing) pain. Although each of these complaints can be a symptom of an underlying serious illness, that is rarely the case. An identifiable organic etiology is found in only 5% to 7% of these cases (Schecter, 1984). It is possible that subtle physiological changes or impairments may play a part in development of most instances of chronic pain (Elliot & Jay, 1987), while psychological factors contribute to their development and maintenance. For example, children with recurrent abdominal pain exhibit more problems of emotional adjustment than do well children (Walker, & Greene, 1989).

It is important to note that nearly 20% of children with RAP undergo surgical or medical treatments that may be unnecessary (Dolgin & Jay, 1989). Furthermore, these children show an increase of gastrointestinal ailments and pain into adulthood compared to children without the condition (Christensen & Mortensen, 1975). Although research shows clear differences between RAP and well children (Walker, Garber, & Greene, 1993), these groups tend to score similarly on measures of emotional adjustment. Therefore, attempts to classify the abdominal pain as either organic or psychological are not clinically useful and thus should be avoided (Walker, Greene, et al., 1993). Several factors have been linked to the development of RAP. Stress, parental pressures for academic and athletic achievement, avoidance of demanding tasks, and modeling parental pain behaviors have all been implicated (Adler, Katz, & Bongar, 1982; Berger, Honig, & Liebman, 1977; Robinson, Alverez, & Dodge, 1990).

Children experiencing chronic headaches are also common referrals. Childhood headaches have been divided into two categories: migraine and tension-type headaches. Classic migraines are recurrent headaches that may be preceded by sensory, motor, and mood disturbances (called prodromal symptoms) and are often accompanied by nausea or vomiting (Williamson, Baker, & Cubic, 1993). Common migraines, on the other hand, are not preceded by prodromal symptoms but tend to last longer than the classic type. Approximately half of children with migraines will continue to experience headaches as adults (Billie, 1981). Many children who experience migraines show a positive family history of headaches, usually in parents or first-degree relatives. Similar to children with RAP, children with chronic headaches have scored higher on psychological measures of anxiety, depression, and somatic complaints than do well children (Andrasik et al., 1988). However, the authors note that because this data is correlational, it is impossible to say whether these problems were a cause or a result of their headaches.

Tension headaches (also known as muscle contraction, psychogenic, or nervous headaches), are the second type of common referrals and result from sustained levels of tension in the skeletal muscles. These headaches are most frequently associated with stress and are described as a tightness in the forehead, neck, or head (Williamson et al., 1993).

Compared to the other two complaints, relatively little has been written about back, limb, and chest pain in children. These conditions appear to emerge in early to middle adolescence and are rather transient in nature (Barr, 1989). Nevertheless, it is important that children with these complaints receive a proper medical evaluation in order to rule out any serious conditions.

ASSESSMENT OF CHRONIC PAIN IN CHILDREN

Assessing a child with a chronic pain condition is similar to assessing a child with a chronic behavioral problem. In the case of childhood pain, assessment has several goals:

1. Provide an index of the child's pain to serve as a baseline from which to gauge improvement during and following treatment.

2. Identify factors that are contributing to pain-related behaviors, and clarify the function that the pain may be serving.
3. Determine how the pain is interfering with the child's age-appropriate activities and the family's functioning.
4. Identify deficits in the child's behavioral repertoire that may be interfering with the child's ability to exhibit more appropriate behaviors.

Because of the nature of pain, it is critical that the psychologist remain in close contact with the physician. Communication should be maintained throughout the treatment so the clinician is aware of changes in the child's medical status and treatment regime. Likewise, it is important that the pediatrician be aware of the goals of the psychological intervention so that all involved professionals are consistent in the message they convey to the child and family. It is also desirable to do a thorough and global assessment of the child rather than focusing narrowly on the pain behavior. The assessment of pain should be accomplished in the context of an assessment of the child across the domains of behavior one would assess if the presenting complaint were of a more traditional behavioral nature.

The nature of the child's pain and the resulting impact on school, family, and social functioning will undoubtedly influence the type and amount of information collected. As most psychologists are familiar with the major tools for measuring childhood depression, anxiety, and other areas of assessment, general issues of childhood assessment will not be reviewed here. Instead the focus will be on pain assessment.

The most common method for obtaining information about the child's pain is through reports from the child and parents. Information from the child can be derived from interviews or questionnaires, depending upon the age of the child. Obviously, the specific manner in which information is collected will depend upon how the psychologist generally conducts evaluations. However, certain information should be obtained during the initial sessions. The major goals for the first interview, adapted from Karoly's (1985) delineation of the clinical objectives in the nonmedical assessment of chronic pain, are as follows:

1. *Medical History.* Obtain a thorough medical history and gather information about the impact of the history on the child's current functioning. Making sure that you have received and reviewed all medical records prior to the initial meeting with the family will expedite things considerably. It will be helpful to get the parent's and child's perspective about the effectiveness of medical interventions as well as their understanding of and fears about the medical condition. Review their perceptions of the effectiveness of previous medical interventions. Discuss their plans for future medical interventions or consultations with other health professionals. Pay attention to the family's attitude toward health professionals. Extreme distrust of or overdependence upon the health professional will influence the family's motivation to cooperate with psychological interventions.
2. *Onset of the Pain Condition.* Obtaining information pertaining to the onset of the pain condition may be useful. Also note any recent changes in the family situation or changes that may have occurred in conjunction with the first pain episode.
3. *Advantages and Disadvantages of the Pain.* Compare the disruption versus the benefits of the pain for the child and family. Determine in what ways the family views the pain as having been helpful (e.g., bringing the family closer together, enabling the child to help with baby-sitting during the day) and harmful (e.g., falling behind in schoolwork, missing after-school activities). Avoid implications that the pain is motivated by the "benefits."
4. *Changes in Family Dynamics.* Review changes in the child and family that have accompanied the pain. How were the child and family different prior to the beginning of the child's pain? This may also be covered by asking how things would be different if the child did not have pain. What would be different for the parents/child/sibling? What would be better/worse? Also note if there have been any changes in the family routines to accommodate the child's pain condition.

tiveness of any proposed treatments. This is usually accomplished through daily monitoring of all painful episodes and recording them on a "pain diary" (see p. 69). This may represent the most important aspect in the assessment of pediatric pain and should be conducted through the entire course of treatment.

DAILY MONITORING AND THE PAIN DIARY

Retrospective reports of behavior are not usually as accurate as information observed and recorded at the time of the event. Home monitoring by the parents and child can be helpful for determining usual antecedents and consequences of recurrent pain. This is a particularly useful method for learning more about the frequency, duration, and intensity of the pain; factors associated with pain onset; and usual outcome of the pain episodes. In short, the psychologist can learn more about the possible functions the pain serves for the child and family. It is typically informative to have parents and the child record this information separately and independently. School-aged children can record information in a "diary" consisting of preprinted sheets. A sample of a pain diary sheet adapted from Masek, Russo, and Varni (1984) and designed for school-aged children 9 years and older is presented on page 69.

Parent monitoring forms can include similar items. Parents may record their perceptions of the child's pain prior to school, in the early evening, and at night. In addition, parents may record more detailed information about the mood of the child, response of others, and level of interference with other activities. Disagreement between parents and the child may reflect pain episodes that the parents were unaware of or differences in the perceptions of parents and child. It is important that the monitoring include other outcome measures than simply pain level, because improvement may be noted in other areas while pain persists at pretreatment levels. Parents should record school attendance (full day, partial day specifying when the child left, and absent), amount of time spent in the nurse's office, medication usage, and, if applicable, bedtime behaviors (when in bed, whether slept through the night, etc.). If the pain occurs most often when the child is in school, it is usually worthwhile to have teachers record incidents of pain, activities occurring in the classroom when the pain began, response of others to the pain, and whether the child continued the activity, went to the nurse, or went home.

One aspect of daily monitoring to keep in mind is that it generally causes changes in the behaviors being observed (Barlow, Hayes, & Nelson, 1984). The data collected for the first couple of weeks will usually underestimate the problem. Unfortunately, reactivity to monitoring generally does not persist for more than a couple of weeks without further intervention (Kazdin, 1989). The result is that early improvement may not be detectable, because reactivity usually results in baselines that document fewer pain incidents than usual for the child.

TREATMENT OF CHRONIC PAIN IN CHILDREN

In contrast to treatment for adults, clinical intervention for the management of chronic pain in children is a recent endeavor. As a result, many of the treatments now available for children are downward extensions of those that have been successfully used in adults. Because pain perception is associated with various physical, familial, emotional, situational, and behavioral factors, the goal of intervention is altering children's pain by targeting and modifying these factors (P. A. McGrath, 1991). The types of interventions that have shown the most promise are those that have used multidimensional cognitive-behavioral approaches (Varni, 1990).

There are two primary approaches used in the management of chronic pain in children. The first has two components: teaching the child various self-regulatory skills aimed at influencing the child's perception of pain, and teaching self-initiated coping strategies such as distraction, imagery, thought stopping, hypnosis, and psychotherapy to help with painful episodes. The second approach is aimed at modifying the contingencies operating within the child's environment that may be maintaining the expression of pain behavior.

PAIN PERCEPTION MANAGEMENT

Self-Regulation Techniques. Perhaps the most widely used technique in the management of pediatric pain involves teaching children self-regulatory strategies. Because chronic pain often causes muscle tension, irritability, and arousal, the aim of these strategies is to reduce the negative impact of these physiological changes. The goal is to have children monitor their physiological state and to produce a relaxation response that is incompatible with arousal. Progressive muscle relaxation training, biofeedback, and meditative breathing are the most widely used self-regulatory strategies.

Progressive Muscle Relaxation Training. Progressive muscle relaxation is a specific training procedure in which children are taught to tighten and relax muscle groups. Although the exact mechanisms by which the relaxation response reduces pain are unknown, it is believed that physiological changes produced by relaxation can effectively decrease sympathetic nervous system activity (Benson, Pomeranz, & Kutz, 1984). Many of these relaxation procedures are revisions of Jacobson's (1938) original technique which was designed to help adults recognize and control even the slightest of muscle contractions. In an earlier volume of this series, Culbertson (1990) described a set of relaxation procedures designed specifically for the school-aged child which are appropriate for chronic pain management.

Before beginning, it is important that the physical environment be conducive to relaxation, such as a quiet, softly lit room which minimizes outside noises. The child should be quiet and comfortably seated in a reclining chair or couch. An age-appropriate explanation about relaxation is presented to the child, emphasizing that people learn to be tense and they can also learn to relax. As with any new skill, the child is told that it will be necessary to practice relaxation. A simple rationale for its use might include its helpfulness in reducing tension and anxiety and a discussion about the situations when these feelings arise. The specific suggestions used to teach children about the pain-reducing effects of relaxation depend on the child's age, cognitive level, and pain source. P. A. McGrath (1991) suggests that children younger than age 7 receive concrete examples and coaching assistance when they use relaxation to reduce pain. She suggests that children may benefit from listening to music or interesting stories, or having them imagine they are a favorite character with special powers.

A progressive muscle relaxation program as described by Culbertson (1990) involves 11 tension-releasing actions. The sequence for each muscle group includes (a) tensing the muscles, (b) scanning the muscles and noticing how they feel, (c) relaxing the muscles, and (d) enjoying the pleasant relaxed feeling. The script for this program is reproduced in Culbertson (1990).

Biofeedback. Biofeedback is a technique by which physiological activity of the body is electronically detected, amplified, and translated into salient auditory or visual signals (Jessup, 1984; P. A. McGrath, 1991). The idea is that children can be trained to voluntarily modify the internal processes believed to be associated with the pain condition. Visually stimulating graphics can now be added to the biofeedback procedure through computer hookups which can be an added attraction for children. Although biofeedback has been used to treat many pain conditions in adults, it has also been used to treat headaches in children. Andrasik et al. (1982) reported the results of a case study of an 11-year-old girl who received 12 sessions of biofeedback over a 9-week period. The results showed a 66% reduction in the frequency of headache at the end of treatment as well as at the 17-week follow-up.

The biofeedback session involves the placement of electrodes on the surface of the skin to record a targeted physiological response. In introducing the technique to children, the following explanation can be given:

> How would you like to play a game? The object is for you to change the speed of these blinking lights on the screen. When the lights are blinking really fast, it means that your body is tense and uncomfortable. When the lights are blinking slow, it means that your body is more relaxed. Your job is to let your body become as relaxed as possible and slow down the blinking lights.

The clinician may need to spend considerable time explaining the rationale and simplifying the procedures so that adequate comprehension is achieved (Gagnon, Hudnall, & Andrasik, 1992). Also, it may be useful to have a parent participate during initial sessions to help reduce any anxiety the child may have concerning the procedure. The therapist can assist the child by providing feedback and encouragement and setting realistic expectations. Typically, practice sessions are assigned with the idea of weaning the child from dependency on the biofeedback machine and exploring additional methods (i.e., progressive muscle relaxation) of maintaining control over physiological functions in natural settings. Although biofeedback is a widely accepted treatment, research has shown little relationship between the control of physiological functions and reductions in pain intensity (Flor & Turk, 1989). Therefore, it is possible that the effectiveness of biofeedback may be related to factors not directly associated with the procedure.

Meditative Breathing. Meditative breathing is often incorporated into the relaxation approaches described previously. Frequently, breathing exercises begin the progressive muscle relaxation training. For example a child may be asked to take a deep breath and hold it for to up to 10 seconds. Omizo, Lofferedo, and Hammett (1982) offer an example of meditative deep breathing:

1) Relax muscles in the diaphragm (demonstrate) and the stomach area. Draw air in through the nose, allowing the stomach area to balloon out and fill completely. [Exhale.]
2) As you inhale again, direct your attention to the rib cage. Let your ribs expand sideways. Close your eyes and imagine an accordion expanding. Begin with your lower ribs, but keep the chest and shoulders motionless. Exhale, relax the rib cage and let the air flow out. Repeat two or three times.
3) Now inhale as you would with a normal breath. The air now fills only the upper chest area. Exhale. (p. 603)

Developmental Considerations. As previously noted, many of the techniques used in the management of chronic pediatric pain are those strategies that have been successfully employed in adults. However, one must be cautioned not to apply such techniques directly to children without regard to developmental considerations. Compared with adults, studies on the treatment of childhood pain are still limited. Therefore, a child's perception of pain may be very different from that of adults. In addition, children's conceptualization of pain may differ according to their stage of cognitive development, and this will influence the approach to treatment (Thompson & Varni, 1986). For example, the self-regulatory techniques may be most effective for children over the age of 7. According to Piaget's theory of intellectual development, this age represents the period during which children begin to develop concrete thinking (Piaget, 1930). Studies employing this theoretical approach appear to support this age distinction (Gaffney & Dunn, 1986, 1987). A study investigating coping strategies for pain among hospitalized children found that children between the ages of 7 and 13 were better able to describe cognitive coping strategies than children aged 4 to 7 (Reissland, 1983). The younger children tended to rely more heavily on their parents to help them cope with their pain. This suggests that for younger children in particular, parents play an important role in the treatment process.

Self-Initiated Coping Strategies. The second approach involves teaching self-initiated coping strategies such as distraction, guided imagery, and thought stopping to help children actively cope with their pain. The aim of these approaches is to assist children in becoming selectively focused on novel stimuli in order to alter and modify their perception of pain. Again, due to individual and developmental differences, the particular technique employed should be appropriate to the maturity level of the child.

Distraction. Parents and health professionals readily employ distraction techniques to help children cope with pain and distress. The goal is to distract children's attention from their pain and divert it to a task or an event not associated with the pain. Distraction techniques may include listening to music, recalling stories, counting ceiling tiles, repeating phrases, or interacting with others (P. A. McGrath, 1991). For younger children, parents can play an important role in helping children with this technique. One study used a distraction procedure for children receiving routine injections. The group of children distracted by their mothers during the injections showed less overall distress than children whose mothers gave them simple reassurance (Armstrong, Routh, & Gonzalez, 1993). Although generally effective, distraction techniques can be quite exhausting and are best suited for intermittent or short-lived painful episodes. Therefore, distraction should be used in conjunction with other strategies when treating chronic pain.

Guided Imagery. Although imagery is a popular tool used in pediatric populations, the term has been used to define a variety of techniques. For example, hypnosis, distraction, and emotive imagery have all been considered forms of the technique. Guided imagery, in the traditional sense, refers to a procedure in which an individual concentrates on an image of an experience or situation not associated with pain. Successful programs using imagery techniques have been developed for use in children undergoing acute medical procedures for such conditions as cancer and sickle cell anemia (Kellerman et al., 1983; Zeltzer, Dash, & Holland, 1979; Zeltzer & LeBaron, 1982).

Using another form of imagery, children can be taught to identify and manipulate a painful episode (Krueger, 1987). Here children are asked to describe specific details of a previous pain episode and apply visual and sensory attributes to the experience such as the colors, size, and feel of the experience. Next, they are encouraged to alter these attributes (i.e., decrease the vividness of the image) and told that this decrease represents a decrease in their pain. The following is a imagery procedure developed by Korn and Johnson (1983) that can be adapted for use in children with chronic pain. Please note that the language may need to be adjusted according to the child's age.

1. *Validate Child's Pain.* Explain that sometimes people have sensations that are unpleasant such as pain, discomfort, and tension.
2. *Acknowledge Possible Concerns.* Express the difficulties people have in identifying and describing their pain.
3. *Encourage a Collaborative Relationship.* Explain that together you will try to identify and label their pain to make it easier to make it go away.
4. *Explain Rationale.* Explain that you will teach them a special (magic) skill designed to substitute unpleasant sensations with pleasant ones.
5. *Imagery Formulation.* Ask the child to give his or her pain a shape (e.g., a round ball), a color (e.g., red), and a size (e.g., large). Explain that this new shape is now a symbol of his or her pain.
6. *Imagery Associations.* Explain that the larger and more vividly colored the object, the more pain and discomfort it represents. For example you might explain that when your ball is big, and bright red, it means that you are in pain, and when your ball is really small and a dim red it means that there is no pain.
7. *Practice and Help Guide Imagery Associations.* Help guide the child in changing the various characteristics of his or her object and associate these changes with the corresponding changes in pain perception.
8. *Probe.* Offer suggestions if it becomes apparent that the child is having difficulties in forming the imagery/pain associations. For example, encourage the child to make the object smaller and kick it away or make it bigger like an airplane and let it fly away.

9. *Practice.* Explain that this is a special skill that requires practice. The more they practice the more powerful their skill becomes.

The effectiveness of the technique depends on the child's ability to concentrate fully on the generated image. Because children typically have creative imaginations, a variety of imagery scenes can be generated (P. A. McGrath, 1991). Although not much research has been focused on the use of imagery as a coping technique, the available studies suggest that it may be an effective clinical strategy for reducing childhood pain (Krueger, 1987).

Thought Stopping. According to Wisocki (1992), "thought stopping is a self-control procedure developed for the elimination of perseverative thought patterns which are unrealistic, unproductive, and/or anxiety arousing and either inhibit the performance of a desired behavior or serve to initiate a sequence of undesirable behaviors" (p. 219). Persistent thoughts and feelings regarding the child's condition may influence the child's perception and experience of pain. For example, in a study with adult headache sufferers, Demjen and Bakal (1986) found that thoughts and feelings prior to and during a headache episode were significantly correlated with headache severity. Therefore, the primary goal behind thought stopping is to interrupt the pervasive nature of these thoughts by verbally stating "stop" as soon as they begin to think about their pain. D. M. Ross (1984) successfully utilized a form of this technique to reduce anticipatory anxiety in children undergoing painful medical procedures. The children memorized a list of positive self-statements and were instructed to recite them as soon as they began to think of the upcoming procedure. Similar to the distraction technique, thought stopping may be more effective with acute conditions. Its effectiveness with chronic pediatric pain has yet to be determined.

PAIN BEHAVIOR MANAGEMENT

Altering Environmental Contingencies. The notion that pain expression is a learned behavior is based on operant and classical conditioning models of learning (Fowler, Fordyce, & Berni, 1969). Operant approaches to pain management tend to stress the importance of environmental consequences or contingencies that either promote, maintain, or increase pain behavior. Pain behavior includes grimacing, moaning, complaining, or lying down. Classical conditioning models of pain emphasize antecedents or stimuli that precede pain behavior. Through classical conditioning, specific stimuli (i.e., the sight of a needle, school, etc.) acquire the ability to elicit the pain behavior (Gentry & Bernal, 1977). As such, interventions aimed at altering the environmental conditions associated with the expression of pain behavior are paramount in designing treatment programs for children.

As previously stated, a child's behavior in response to pain is inevitably shaped by the reactions of significant others such as parents, siblings, and teachers. Pain behaviors may be inadvertently reinforced via increased attention, empathy, comfort, or reductions in expectations (P. A. McGrath, 1991). As a result, the child becomes dependent on external methods of pain reductions (i.e., parents or medications) instead of on more self-reliant and independent methods of coping. Thus it is clear that people in the child's immediate environment play a key role in the management of pain behaviors.

Masek et al. (1984) reviewed the essential principles of operant conditioning techniques used in the management of chronic pediatric pain. They stress the importance of identifying all pain behaviors (verbal and nonverbal) and evaluating the responses of significant others (i.e., parents, medical staff, siblings, school personnel, etc.) to the child's pain. Secondly, a plan is designed to modify the responses of these significant persons to minimize maladaptive pain behaviors and maximize adaptive behaviors that reduce pain.

P. A. McGrath (1987) designed a comprehensive operant-conditioning treatment program to monitor and modify both parent's and children's pain behaviors:

1. Thoroughly assess not only the child's pain and pain behaviors but assess the relevant emotional, situational, and familial factors associated with these behaviors.

2. Identify the most disruptive or pain-increasing behavior(s) for modification.
3. Select appropriate positive coping behaviors according to the child's age, sex, and pain problem.
4. Design a reward system that will effectively motivate the child such as stickers, points toward a treat, special time with parents, or increased social activities with peers.

P. A. McGrath (1987) also emphasized the following as critical to the success of the program: the need for all involved in treatment (i.e., significant others) to respond in a consistent manner; that the rewards be contingent on the child fulfilling well-defined behavioral criteria; the child's ability to achieve the behavioral criteria; and that only one maladaptive behavior at a time be targeted.

Summary of Treatments. This is offered solely as a general outline, as specific goals of individualized treatment programs will differ. Clinicians will develop their own techniques which may require adjustments depending on the child and family functioning as well as the nature and location of the child's pain. The interventions reviewed here should be viewed as tools to enhance the practitioner's therapeutic effectiveness in treating children with chronic problems. Given proper assessment, training, and cooperation with family members, these techniques can be valuable in helping to alleviate the discomfort and distress of children and families experiencing chronic pain.

CASE ILLUSTRATION*

The following is an illustrative account of a child experiencing chronic abdominal pain. It is a composite of several children we have assessed and treated clinically.

PRESENTING COMPLAINT

Steven is a 9-year-old boy who was referred by his physician for an evaluation regarding recurrent abdominal pain. After a thorough evaluation, his physician could find no organic explanation for Steven's condition. During the initial meeting, both Steven and his parents were interviewed to discuss the circumstances surrounding Steven's condition. Steven described his stomachaches as a bloated, queasy sensation that sometimes made him vomit. Steven's family had tried a number of methods of pain alleviation including taking medications and letting him lie down when he wasn't feeling well. Recently, the frequency of Steven's stomachaches has caused him to leave school early and to miss several days of school. While at home, Steven watches television or plays video games until he feels better. Assessment of Steven's social life shows that despite his absenteeism he still receives high marks from most of his teachers. Steven is also very active; he reports having many friends, and he is a member of a community baseball and soccer team. Steven's medical history revealed that 1 year previously he had had a severe case of chicken pox that caused him to miss several weeks of school. However, Steven's pediatrician explained that the complications surrounding his chicken pox were unrelated to his current condition. Steven's mother reports no significant behavioral problems at school or at home. Steven has one older sister, age 14, and his parents report a happy family life. His mother is an accountant and his father is a lawyer, and both expressed concern about their son's condition.

ASSESSMENT

Steven and his mother were asked to keep separate pain diary self-monitoring forms for a 2-week period. His mother was the chosen parent, because she spent more time with Steven than his

---

*Identifying characteristics have been changed to protect the confidentiality of the individuals cited in the case illustration.

father. He and his mother were instructed to complete the information on the diary form each time Steven experienced stomach pains. It was explained to the family that once we could identify situations associated with pain, we could develop strategies aimed at avoiding or reducing the pain. The school was contacted, and his teachers were asked to monitor Steven's attendance. His teachers indicated that Steven was rather shy and participated in few activities. After reviewing Steven's forms, it was found that he was experiencing pain most frequently at school and late in the evening. Steven reported an average of seven stomachaches per week. He was leaving school early an average of three times per week and was experiencing on average four nightly stomachaches. He indicated that taking medication and lying down was helpful in alleviating his pain. His mother's forms revealed that when Steven experienced pain, his parents would remove him from school and at night allow him to stay up past his bedtime and watch television.

TREATMENT

The goals of treatment (which were discussed and agreed upon by the family) were to decrease the frequency and intensity of Steven's stomach pain, return him to regular school attendance, and increase his activities with peers. The family was reminded of the importance of monitoring and instructed to continue completing the pain diary throughout treatment. Progressive relaxation was introduced to help reduce the intensity of Steven's stomach pain. Steven received a total of 10 relaxation sessions over a 5-week period. He was instructed to use relaxation at the first sign of any stomach discomfort. In addition to these sessions, he was instructed to practice the technique once a day at home for 15 minutes.

Role plays were also implemented in sessions in an attempt to increase Steven's conversational skills with peers. The focus of treatment was on initiating and maintaining appropriate conversations. In addition, Steven was taught how to identify potential friends whose interests were similar to his. Some of the skills practiced included introducing himself to others, giving compliments, discussing mutual interests, initiating activities, and keeping regular contact.

An operant behavioral approach was used to reduce the frequency of Steven's pain and to reinforce regular school attendance. His parents were educated on how their responses to Steven's pain, although normal, may actually have been reinforcing the expression of his condition. Environmental contingencies identified for change included getting rides to come home early from school and staying up late and watching television. As an alternative to coming home from school, arrangements were made for him to go to the nurse's office to lie down and return to class after feeling better. If too ill to remain in school, he was to call a parent to pick him up from school. While at home, Steven was to rest in his room and was allowed only to do homework. He was not allowed to watch television or play video games during this period. Also, when Steven experienced his stomach pain at night, he was to remain in his room without the television. Furthermore, his parents were instructed to minimize their attention to Steven when he expressed pain-related behaviors (such as moaning) and were provided with guidelines on how to reinforce more appropriate behaviors. For example, they were instructed to verbally praise Steven for regular school attendance, for going to bed on time, and for practicing and using his relaxation strategies. Also, if Steven remained in school for the entire week, he was rewarded by being able to rent a "Nintendo" game from the local video store.

At the end of the 5-week treatment period, the frequency of Steven's stomach complaints decreased from an average of seven per week to only an occasional ache. He was also attending and remaining in school and reported using the relaxation techniques when he didn't feel well. His teachers reported he was participating more in activities and that he had made new friends. A 4-week follow-up revealed that Steven's stomachaches had all but been eliminated and that he was functioning well.

CONCLUSION

Chronic pain generally presents a diagnostic and therapeutic dilemma for all involved. Parents are often unsure about when to stop seeking further diagnostic tests. The child's pain is usually obvious and rarely as clearly related to stress and environmental contingencies as the literature would suggest. We have treated children with RAP who have shown little improvement despite consistent efforts on the part of the parents and therapist. We have watched children make substantial progress only to see the family resort to further intrusive diagnostic tests. On the other hand, many children do improve with behavioral strategies. When the family is satisfied that the medical options have been exhausted and the parents are willing to make changes, improvements are usually noted in the child's quality of life.

PAIN DIARY

Check the day of the week:

☐ Sunday ☐ Monday ☐ Tuesday ☐ Wednesday ☐ Thursday ☐ Friday ☐ Saturday

Time:_____

Check intensity:

☐ Very Severe (You can't do anything)
☐ Severe (It bothers you a lot)
☐ Moderate (It bothers you some)
☐ Mild (You can feel it but it's not too bothersome)

Who was with you when the pain started? _____

Where were you when the pain started? _____

What were you doing when the pain started? _____

What medicine did you take for the pain? _____

What other symptoms did you have? _____

Check the statements that apply:

☐ I could not go to school.
☐ I stayed in the classroom.
☐ I had to leave school.
☐ I went to the nurse's office.
☐ I spent time in bed.
☐ I missed activities (list them):_____

What did you do to stop the pain? _____

Was it helpful (check)?   ☐ Not At All   ☐ A Little   ☐ Some   ☐ A Lot

What did you do after the pain began? _____

When did the pain stop? _____

What did you do after the pain stopped? _____

Chris A. Coleman is currently a senior graduate student in the clinical psychology doctoral program at the State University of New York at Binghamton. His research and clinical interests are in pediatric psychology and health promotion in children. Mr. Coleman may be contacted c/o Department of Psychology, SUNY at Binghamton, Binghamton, NY 13902.

Alice G. Friedman, PhD, is currently an Assistant Professor of Psychology at the State University of New York at Binghamton. She completed her graduate training in clinical psychology at Virginia Polytechnic Institute and State University, an internship in behavioral medicine at West Virginia University Medical Center, and a National Institute of Mental Health fellowship in pediatric psychology at University of Oklahoma Health Science Center. She was on the faculty at St. Jude Children's Research Hospital prior to her current position. She has published papers and chapters in the area of childhood fear and anxiety, and psychological factors associated with childhood illness. Dr. Friedman can be contacted at the Department of Psychology, SUNY at Binghamton, Binghamton, NY 13902.

Donna Gates, MA, is currently a senior graduate student in the clinical psychology doctoral program at the State University of New York at Binghamton. Her research and clinical interests are in pediatric headaches and the integration of psychology in primary health care settings. Ms. Gates may be contacted c/o Department of Psychology, SUNY at Binghamton, Binghamton, NY 13902.

RESOURCES

Adler, R., Katz, E. R., & Bongar, B. (1982). Psychogenic abdominal pain related to excessive parental pressure in childhood athletics. *Psychosomatics, 23,* 1021-1023.

Andrasik, F., Blanchard, E. B., Edlund, S. R., & Rosenblum, E. L. (1982). Autogenic feedback in the treatment of two children with migraine headache. *Child and Family Behavior Therapy, 4,* 13-23.

Andrasik, F., Kabela, E., Quinn, S., Attanasio, V., Blanchard, E. B., & Rosenblum, E. L. (1988). Psychological functioning of children who have recurrent migraine. *Pain, 34,* 43-52.

Armstrong, D. F., Routh, D. K., & Gonzalez, J. C. (1993). Effects of maternal distraction versus reassurance on children's reaction to injections. Special section: Family issues. *Journal of Pediatric Psychology, 18,* 593-604.

Barlow, D. H., Hayes, S. C., & Nelson, R. O. (1984). *The Scientist Practitioner.* New York: Pergamon.

Barr, R. G. (1989). Pain in children. In P. D. Wall & R. Mezlack (Eds.), *Textbook of Pain* (pp. 568-588). New York: Livingstone.

Benson, H., Pomeranz, B., & Kutz, I. (1984). The relaxation response and pain. In P. D. Wall & R. Mezlack (Eds.), *Textbook of Pain* (pp. 817-822). Edinburgh: Churchill-Livingstone.

Berger, H. G., Honig, P. J., & Liebman, R. (1977). Recurrent abdominal pain: Gaining control of the symptom. *American Journal of Diseases in Children, 131,* 1340-1344.

Bibace, R., & Walsh, M. E. (1980). Development of children's concept of illness. *Pediatrics, 66,* 912-917.

Billie, B. (1981). Migraine in childhood and its prognosis. *Cephalagia, 1,* 71-75.

Christensen, M. F., & Mortensen, O. (1975). Long-term prognosis in children with recurrent abdominal pain. *Archives of Disease of Childhood, 50,* 110-114.

Culbertson, F. M. (1990). Relaxation strategies for the school-aged child: Theory, research, and practice. In P. A. Keller & S. R. Heyman (Eds.), *Innovations in Clinical Practice: A Source Book* (Vol. 9, pp. 183-191). Sarasota, FL: Professional Resource Exchange.

Demjen, S., & Bakal, D. A. (1986). Subjective distress accompanying headache attacks: Evidence for a cognitive shift. *Pain, 25,* 187-194.

Dolgin, M. J., & Jay, S. M. (1989). Pain management in children. In E. J. Mash & R. A. Barkley (Eds.), *Treatment of Childhood Disorders* (pp. 383-404). New York: Guilford.

Eland, J. M. (1981). Minimizing pain associated with prekindergarten muscular injections. *Issues in Comprehensive Pediatric Nursing, 5,* 327-335.

Elliot, C. H., & Jay, S. M. (1987). Chronic pain in children. *Behavior Research and Therapy, 25,* 263-271.

Flor, H., & Turk, D. C. (1989). The psychophysiology of chronic pain: Do chronic pain patients exhibit symptom-specific psychophysiological responses? *Psychological Bulletin, 105,* 215-259.

Fowler, R. S., Fordyce, W. E., & Berni, R. (1969). Operant conditioning in chronic illness. *American Journal of Nursing, 69,* 1226-1228.

Gaffney, A., & Dunn E. A. (1986). Developmental aspects of children's definitions of pain. *Pain, 26,* 105-117.

Gaffney, A., & Dunn E. A. (1987). Children's understanding of the causality of pain. *Pain, 29,* 91-104.

Gagnon, D. J., Hudnall, L., & Andrasik, F. (1992). Biofeedback and related procedures in coping with stress. In A. M. La Greca, L. J. Siegel, J. L. Wallander, & C. E. Walker (Eds.), *Stress and Coping in Child Health* (pp. 303-319). New York: Guilford.

Gentry, W. D., & Bernal, G. (1977). Chronic pain. In R. Williams & W. D. Gentry (Eds.), *Behavioral Approaches to Medical Treatment* (pp. 173-182). Cambridge, MA: Ballinger.

Holroyd, K. A., Penzien, D. B., Hursey, K. G., Tobin, D. L., Rogers, L., Holm, J. E., Marcille, P. J., Hall, J. R., & Chila, A. G. (1984). Change mechanisms in EMG biofeedback training. Cognitive changes underlying improvements in tension headaches. *Journal of Consulting and Clinical Psychology, 52,* 1039-1053.

Hughes, M. C., & Zimin, R. (1978). Children with psychogenic abdominal pain and their families: Management during hospitalization. *Clinical Pediatrics, 17,* 569-573.

Jacobson, E. (1938). *Progressive Relaxation.* Chicago: University of Chicago Press.

Jessup, B. A. (1984). Biofeedback. In P. D. Wall & R. Mezlack (Eds.), *Textbook of Pain* (pp. 776-786). Edinburgh: Churchill-Livingstone.

Karoly, P. (1985). The assessment of pain: Concepts and issues. In P. Karoly (Ed.), *Measurement Strategies in Health Psychology* (pp. 461-515). New York: Wiley.

Karoly, P. (1991). Assessment of pediatric pain. In J. P. Bush & S. W. Harkins (Eds), *Children in Pain* (pp. 59-82). New York: Springer-Verlag.

Katz, E. R., Varni, J. W., & Jay, S. M. (1984). Behavioral assessment and management of pediatric pain. *Progress in Behavior Modification, 18,* 163-193.

Kazdin, A. E. (1989). *Behavior Modification in Applied Settings.* Pacific Grove, CA: Brooks Cole.

Kellerman, J., Zeltzer, L., Ellenberg, L., & Dash, J. (1983). Adolescents with cancer: Hypnosis for the reduction of acute pain and anxiety associated with medical procedures. *Journal of Adolescent Health Care, 4,* 85-90.

Korn, E. R., & Johnson, K. C. (1983). *Visualization: The Uses of Imagery in the Health Profession.* Homewood, IL: Dow Jones-Irwin.

Krueger, L. C. (1987). Pediatric pain and imagery. *Journal of Child and Adolescent Psychotherapy, 4,* 32-41.

Masek, B. J., Russo, D. C., & Varni, J. W. (1984). Behavioral approaches to the management of chronic pain in children. *Pediatric Clinics of North America, 31,* 1113-1131.

McGrath, P. A. (1987). The multidimensional assessment and management of recurrent pain syndromes in children. *Behaviour Research and Therapy, 25,* 251-262.

McGrath, P. A. (1991). Intervention and management. In J. P. Bush & S. W. Harkins (Eds.), *Children in Pain* (pp. 83-115). New York: Springer-Verlag.

McGrath, P. J., Unruh, A. M., & Branson, S. M. (1990). Chronic nonmalignant pain with disability. In D. C. Tyler & E. J. Crane (Eds.), *Advances in Pain Research and Therapy* (pp. 255-271). New York: Raven.

Omizo, M. M., Lofferedo, D. A., & Hammett, V. L. (1982). Relaxation exercises for the LD and family. *Academic Therapy, 17,* 603-608.

Perrin, E., & Gerrity, P. S. (1981). There's a demon in your belly: Children's understanding of illness. *Pediatrics, 67,* 841-849.

Piaget, J. (1930). *The Child's Conception of Physical Causality.* London: Routledge and Kegan Paul.

Reissland, N. (1983). Cognitive maturity and the experience of fear and pain in hospital. *Social Science and Medicine, 17,* 1389-1395.

Robinson, J. D., Alverez, J. H., & Dodge, J. A. (1990). Life events and family history in children with recurrent abdominal pain. *Journal of Psychosomatic Research, 34,* 171-181.

Ross, D. M. (1984). Thought-stopping: A coping strategy for impending feared events. *Issues in Comprehensive Pediatric Nursing, 7,* 83-89.

Ross, D. M., & Ross S. M. (1988). *Childhood Pain: Current Issues, Research, and Management.* Baltimore: Urban & Schwarzenberg.

Routh, D. K., Ernst, A. R., & Harper, D. C. (1988). Recurrent abdominal pain in children and somatization disorder. In D. K. Routh (Ed.), *Handbook of Pediatric Psychology* (pp. 492-504). New York: Guilford.

Savedra, M., Gibbons, P., Tesler, M., Ward, J., & Wegner, C. (1982). How do children describe pain? A tentative assessment. *Pain, 14,* 95-104.

Schecter, N. L. (1984). Recurrent pains in children: An overview and an approach. *Pediatric Clinics of North America, 31,* 949-991.

Thompson, K. L., & Varni, J. W. (1986). A developmental cognitive-biobehavioral approach to pediatric pain assessment. *Pain, 25,* 283-296.

Varni, J. W. (1990). Behavioral management of chronic pain in children. In D. C. Tyler & E. J. Krane (Eds.), *Advances in Pain Research Therapy* (Vol. 15, pp. 215-224). New York: Raven.

Varni, J. W., Thompson, K. L., & Hanson, V. (1987). The Varni-Thompson Pediatric Pain Questionnaire: I. Chronic musculoskeletal pain in juvenile rheumatoid arthritis. *Pain, 28,* 27-38.

Varni, J. W., Walco, G. A., & Wilcox, K. T. (1990). Cognitive-biobehavioral assessment and treatment of pediatric pain. In A. M. Gross & R. S. Drabman (Eds.), *Handbook of Clinical Behavioral Pediatrics* (pp. 83-97). New York: Plenum.

Walker, L. S., Garber, J., & Greene, J. W. (1993). Psychosocial correlates of recurrent childhood pain: A comparison of pediatric patients with recurrent abdominal pain, organic illness, and psychiatric disorders. *Journal of Abnormal Psychology, 102,* 248-258.

Walker, L. S., & Greene, J. W. (1989). Children with recurrent abdominal pain and their parents: More somatic complaints, anxiety, and depression than other families? *Journal of Pediatric Psychology, 14,* 231-243.

Walker, L. S., Greene, J. W., Garber, J., Horndasch, R. L., Barnard, J., & Ghishan, F. (1993). Psychosocial factors in pediatric abdominal pain: Implications for assessment and treatment. *The Clinical Psychologist, 46,* 206-213.

Williamson, D. A., Baker, J. D., & Cubic, B. A. (1993). Advances in pediatric headache research. In T. H. Ollendick & R.J. Prinz (Eds.), *Advances in Clinical Child Psychology* (pp. 275-304). New York: Plenum.

Wisocki, P. (1992). Thought stopping. In A. S. Bellack & M. Hersen (Eds.), *Dictionary of Behavior Therapy Techniques* (pp. 219-222). New York: Pergamon.

Zeltzer, L., Dash, J., & Holland, J. P. (1979). Hypnotically induced pain control in sickle cell anemia. *Pediatrics, 64,* 533-536.

Zeltzer, L., & LeBaron, S. (1982). Hypnosis and nonhypnotic techniques for reduction of pain and anxiety during painful procedures in children and adolescents with cancer. *Journal of Pediatrics, 101,* 1032-1035.

IMAGERY RESCRIPTING: A MULTIFACETED TREATMENT FOR CHILDHOOD SEXUAL ABUSE SURVIVORS

Mervin R. Smucker and Jan L. Niederee

The alarming prevalence of childhood sexual abuse and its long-term deleterious effects on adult survivors has been well documented in the literature in recent years. Clinical symptoms frequently cited include chronic depression and anxiety, suicidality, self-destructive behaviors, relationship disturbances, sexual difficulties, and post-traumatic stress disorder (Briere, 1989, 1992; Finkelhor et al., 1989; Russell, 1986). In addition, survivors often experience chronic guilt, self-blame, self-disgust, self-hatred, low self-esteem, inferiority and powerlessness, mistrust of others, and fear of intimacy (Briere, 1989; Browne & Finkelhor, 1986; Herman, 1981, 1992; Jehu, Gazan, & Klassen, 1984-1985; Jehu, Klassen, & Gazan, 1985-1986; McCann, Sackheim, & Abrahamson, 1988).

A number of writers have attributed these effects, in part, to maladaptive beliefs about the self and the interpersonal world that became part of the child's cognitive schemata when the trauma occurred (Briere, 1989, 1992; McCann & Pearlman, 1990). The pathogenic effects of abuse-related beliefs have also been proposed as a significant component of post-trauma reactions (Jehu et al., 1985-1986).

As the effects of abuse-related cognitions receive increasing attention in the literature, clinical interventions designed to address this aspect of post-abuse pathology are becoming more prevalent as well (Fallon & Coffman, 1991; Jehu, Gazan, & Klassen, 1988; Resick & Schnicke, 1992; Staton, 1990). This cognitive focus is reflected in Fallon and Coffman's contention that treatment of abuse survivors must address the cognitions affected by the abuse experience.

Although the restructuring of abuse-related beliefs thus appears to be a necessary component of therapy with this population, recent studies also indicate that the majority of abuse survivors in clinical samples meet diagnostic criteria for post-traumatic stress disorder (PTSD) and would benefit from treatment of post-traumatic symptomatology (Donaldson & Gardner, 1985; Lindberg & Distad, 1985). As defined by the Fourth Edition of the *Diagnostic and Statistical Manual of Mental Disorders* (American Psychiatric Association, 1994), a combination of features from four core criteria comprise the PTSD syndrome: (a) The person has been exposed to a traumatic event, (b) the traumatic event is persistently reexperienced in the form of recurrent and intrusive recollections, dreams, flashbacks, or physiological reactivity, (c) the patient persistently avoids stimuli associated with the trauma and experiences emotional numbing, and (d) the patient experiences symptoms of increased arousal such as difficulty falling or staying asleep, hypervigilance, irritability, and exaggerated startle response.

The concurrent presence of PTSD symptomatology and maladaptive schemas in this population suggests the need for a multifaceted treatment approach which simultaneously addresses PTSD symptoms and abuse-related beliefs. The value of one such approach has recently been noted by Foa et al. (1991), who advocate a combination of prolonged exposure and stress inoculation training in treatment of rape victims. Similarly, in their critique of PTSD interventions, Resick and Schnicke (1990) conclude:

> It may be most advantageous to implement a therapy that will activate memories of the event and also provide corrective information for faulty attributions or expectations that interfere with complete processing of the event or cause other symptoms (depression, low self-esteem, fear). A combination of exposure and cognitive techniques might prove to be a more effective approach than either type of therapy alone. (p. 500)

With a combined treatment approach, the goal of therapy would be to (a) decrease physiological arousal, (b) decrease intrusive PTSD symptoms such as recurring flashbacks or nightmares, and (c) facilitate cognitive change in the meaning of the event and the beliefs about self and relationships.

Consistent with theories of emotional processing (Foa & Kozak, 1986; Lang, 1979) and state-dependent recall (Bower, 1981), abuse-related beliefs/schemas could most readily be accessed and modified when the client is in an emotional state similar to that which occurred during the abuse experience. Thus, it would seem therapeutically useful to evoke the abuse images and responses experienced by the victim and develop alternative imagery and interpretations when the abuse memory is accessed.

THE NATURE OF TRAUMATIC MEMORY AND IMPLICATIONS FOR THERAPY

A number of writers (Briere, 1989, 1992; Herman, 1992; van der Kolk & van der Hart, 1991) have argued that understanding the nature of traumatic memories (e.g., how they are encoded and accessed, how they differ from nontraumatic memories) would enable the clinician to more effectively treat this population. In research with traumatized children and adults, van der Kolk and van der Hart (1989, 1991) suggest that, in contrast to narrative memory, traumatic memories (a) lack verbal narrative and context, (b) are state dependent, (c) are encoded in the form of vivid sensations and images that cannot be accessed by linguistic means alone, (d) are difficult to assimilate and integrate, in that they are stored differently and are often dissociated from conscious awareness and voluntary control, and (e) often remain "fixed" in their original form and unaltered by the passage of time. (Thus, flashbacks or nightmares may be reexperienced over and over without modification or resolution.)

In addition to the characteristics noted previously, the manner in which abuse memories are encoded is affected by the age of the child when the molestation began (Staton, 1990). According to Bruner (1973), a child's earliest memories are encoded in the sensorimotor system, with visual representation becoming dominant between the ages of 2 and 7. Linguistic representation, by contrast, develops more slowly and may not be fully integrated with the kinesthetic and visual modes of representation until adolescence (Bruner, 1973).

Factors specific to sexual abuse further constrain the child's ability to linguistically process the trauma. Because the abuse itself is primarily physical, it is most likely to be encoded in memory through visual or sensorimotor modalities. Moreover, the language spoken during the incident(s) is often minimal, which would lessen the probability of verbal encoding and recall (Staton, 1990).

These characteristics of trauma have profound implications for treatment of survivors. If early abuse memories are encoded primarily in images, it would seem advantageous to utilize imagery in transforming their meanings. Lacking corrective imagery, abusive images may be retained no matter how much "talk" occurs (Staton, 1990). As noted by Beck and Freeman (1990):

Simply talking about a traumatic event may give intellectual insight about why the patient has a negative self-image, for instance, but it does not actually change the image. In order to modify the image, it is necessary to go back in time, as it were, and recreate the situation. When the interactions are brought to life, the misconstruction is activated--along with the affect--and cognitive restructuring can occur. (p. 92)

Likewise, Edwards (1989, 1990) argues for the clinical use of imagery to identify and restructure cognitions, including those resulting from childhood sexual abuse.

It thus appears from the current literature that therapeutic effectiveness with this population is enhanced when (a) both imagery and verbal modalities are employed in recall, desensitization, and cognitive restructuring; and (b) the affect and level of arousal during initial exposure are similar to that which occurred at the time of trauma. Imagery Rescripting was developed to integrate these visual, verbal, and affective components.

IMAGERY RESCRIPTING

Imagery Rescripting is a multifaceted, imagery-focused treatment designed to alleviate PTSD symptomatology and alter abuse-related beliefs and schemas (e.g., powerlessness, unlovability, inherent badness) of childhood sexual abuse survivors. The therapy combines *imaginal exposure* (visually recalling and reexperiencing the images/thoughts and associated affect of the traumatic event) with *imaginal rescripting* (changing the abuse imagery to produce a more favorable outcome). The aim of rescripting is to replace victimization imagery with mastery imagery, thereby enabling the survivor to experience herself* responding to the abuse scene as an empowered individual no longer "frozen" in a powerless state of victimization. Through the rescripting process, the abuse images are modified and the maladaptive beliefs are identified and challenged. The use of imagery allows these abuse-related schemas to be addressed directly through the eyes of the traumatized child and then reprocessed through the eyes of the empowered adult.

Imagery Rescripting was initially developed by Mervin R. Smucker in 1990 and is described in detail by Smucker, Dancu, and Foa (1991). Numerous case examples as well as outcome data from a pilot study (Dancu, Foa, & Smucker, 1993) offer preliminary empirical support for the efficacy of the procedure in reducing PTSD symptoms, eliminating recurring flashbacks and repetitive nightmares, and modifying traumagenic schemas. The treatment program consists of eight sessions ranging in length from 90 minutes to 2 hours each, and is described in the following section. (See Table 1, p. 76.)

IMAGERY RESCRIPTING: EIGHT-SESSION TREATMENT FORMAT

PRETREATMENT EVALUATION: INFORMATION GATHERING

A clinical interview is conducted that includes demographic information, current life situation, family history, history of traumatic experiences, current psychological adjustment, health status, alcohol and drug use, and severity of post-traumatic symptoms. In probing these areas, it is crucial that the therapist show sensitivity to the emotional state of the patient as well as to potential areas of vulnerability and issues of privacy. Patients who meet diagnostic criteria for PTSD and who are experiencing recurring abuse-related flashbacks or nightmares are selected for Imagery

---

*Although Imagery Rescripting has been used successfully in treating both men and women, we have used the female pronoun in this contribution, as the majority of patients seeking treatment to deal with the aftereffects of childhood sexual abuse are women.

TABLE 1: IMAGERY RESCRIPTING: BASIC TREATMENT OUTLINE*

Pretreatment Evaluation (2.0 hours):	Information gathering Clinical interview Administration of assessment battery Must meet diagnostic criteria for PTSD
Session 1 (2.0 hours):	Explain treatment rationale Reexperience in imagery the sexual abuse scene (reexperience in the present the entire abuse memory) Develop mastery imagery: Rescript abuse scene to include coping strategies in which the patient visualizes her ADULT self today rescuing the CHILD and driving out the perpetrator After completion of mastery imagery, facilitate "adult-nurturing-child" imagery Assign homework
Session 2 (1.5 hours):	Review homework Reexperience abuse imagery Develop mastery imagery Develop "adult-nurturing-child" imagery Explain letter rationale Assign homework
Session 3 (2.0 hours):	Review homework and discuss letter Reexperience abuse imagery Develop mastery imagery (include any new information from the letter if appropriate) Develop "adult-nurturing-child" imagery Assign homework
Session 4 (1.5 hours):	Review homework Reexperience abuse imagery Develop mastery imagery Develop "adult-nurturing-child" imagery Assign homework
Session 5 (1.5 hours):	Review homework ADULT "check in" with CHILD Develop "adult-nurturing-child" imagery Assign homework
Session 6 (1.5 hours):	Review homework ADULT "check in" with CHILD Develop "adult-nurturing-child" imagery Assign homework
Session 7 (1.5 hours):	Review homework ADULT "check in" with CHILD Develop "adult-nurturing-child" imagery Discuss termination issues Assign homework
Session 8 (1.5 hours):	Review homework ADULT "check in" with CHILD Develop "adult-nurturing-child" imagery Review termination issues

*Note: Revised from Smucker, Dancu, and Foa (1991).

Rescripting. Prior to beginning rescripting, patients are fully informed about the procedure and the potential for short-term affective distress when traumatic images are evoked.

SESSION 1

Education and Presentation of Treatment Rationale. During the first 20 minutes of this session, the therapist describes the treatment program and educates the patient about the symptoms she is experiencing. The therapist presents the rationale for treatment to the patient in the following manner (revised from Smucker et al., 1991):

> When we undergo a trauma, we experience a sense of extreme danger, whether physical, emotional, or both. The natural response to such an event is intense fear, which involves urges to fight, flee, or freeze. These responses are normal, automatic reactions to danger. They can affect our *physical bodies* (e.g., such as heart pounding, sweating), our *thoughts* (e.g., thinking we are in danger), and our *actions* (e.g., trying to escape from or fight off an attacker). These intense responses can recur years after the trauma if something in our lives triggers memories of the event.
>
> Childhood sexual abuse is a major trauma that can be extremely painful and terrifying. All the circumstances surrounding childhood sexual abuse - including your thoughts and feelings about the abuse - exist in a network of memories. Body sensations, odors, time of day or night, or location of the abuse may all become part of this memory. It is like a "fear network" in your mind. If you think about the abuse or see something that reminds you of it, you may experience intense feelings of fear, disgust, guilt, shame, rage, or sorrow - much like what you felt at the time of the abuse. Reexperiencing these feelings causes great distress, which is why most people try to push away these painful memories or ignore them. You may tell yourself things like, "I should just forget about the whole thing and not let it bother me anymore"; "If I don't think about it, it will eventually go away." Some people may try to convince you that using such avoidance techniques is the best way to cope with trauma. Friends, relatives, or even partners may feel uncomfortable hearing about your experience and discourage you from talking about it. Unfortunately, ignoring your feelings and fears *does not* make them go away. Often the abuse comes back to haunt you through flashbacks, nightmares, or painful recurring memories because it is "unfinished business."
>
> As you know from your own experience, it is not easy to recover from the trauma of child abuse. Your views of the world in general, especially of men and sex, have been dramatically affected by your trauma. You may find it difficult even today to trust anyone. We are here to help you with this.
>
> The purpose of our work together here is to help you work through, and move beyond, your abuse memories. We have found that this treatment not only helps individuals overcome abuse-related memories, it also helps them develop a healthier self-image and move forward with their lives.
>
> Much of the work we will be doing here involves the use of imagery. Initially, I will ask you to visualize the abuse experience in your imagination. Then we will go back over the abuse scene and change the imagery to create a better outcome for you, one which leaves you feeling more empowered and in control.

Following presentation of the treatment rationale, the therapist teaches the patient how to use a SUDS rating (subjective units of discomfort) to describe the degree of discomfort she is experiencing. The therapist may explain this as follows:

This treatment involves asking you to confront memories and scenes which will generate some anxiety and discomfort. We will ask you to monitor and rate the degree of discomfort you experience on a scale from "0" to "100." A rating of "100" would indicate that you are extremely upset, the most distressed you've ever felt. A rating of "0" would indicate that you are experiencing no discomfort or distress at all. How much discomfort might you be feeling at this moment, using this scale?

Imaginal Exposure: Reexperiencing the Abuse Scene. Initially, the patient is asked to visualize and describe the abuse scene in the present tense. (If the patient is experiencing more than one recurring abuse flashback or nightmare, generally the most distressing one is chosen.) The following instructions are given to the patient:

> I'm going to ask you to recall the memories of the abuse. It is best if you close your eyes so you won't be distracted. I will ask you to recall these painful memories as vividly as possible. It is important that you describe the abuse in the present tense, as if it were happening now, right here. We will work together on this. If you start to feel too uncomfortable and want to leave the image, I will help you to stay with it and regain a sense of safety. Every 10 minutes or so I'll ask you to rate your discomfort level on a scale from "0" to "100." Please answer quickly and do not leave the image. Do you have any questions before we start?
>
> I'd like you now to close your eyes and visualize the beginning of the abuse scene, and describe in detail what you experience, including thoughts and feelings you have about what is happening.

During exposure, the therapist's role is facilitative rather than directive. The therapist does not intervene other than to ask the patient for more details of the abuse scene or to elaborate on her thoughts and feelings.

Rescripting the Abuse Scene: Developing Mastery Imagery. Immediately after the patient has reexperienced the abuse scene, the rescripting phase begins. During rescripting, the patient again visualizes the beginning of the abuse memory and describes her experience in the present tense. This time, however, as the molestation begins, the patient is asked to visualize her ADULT self today entering the abuse scene. The therapist may facilitate this through such questions as:

- "Can you now visualize your ADULT self today entering the scene?"
- "Does he (the perpetrator) see you?"
- "How does he respond to your presence in the room?"
- "What would you, the ADULT, like to do at this point? . . . Can you see yourself doing that?"
- "And how does he (the perpetrator) respond?"
- "And what's happening now?"

Essentially, the role of the ADULT during rescripting is to (a) "rescue" the CHILD and protect her from any further abuse, (b) "drive out" the perpetrator (or take the CHILD away to a safe place) so the CHILD is no longer in the presence of the perpetrator, and (c) "nurture" the CHILD. During the initial phase of rescripting, the ADULT uses whatever means necessary to rescue the CHILD from the abuser and provide protection for her. If the ADULT is unable to visualize herself "driving out" the perpetrator, she may bring additional support people (e.g., a spouse, therapist, police officer) into the abuse scene to help her accomplish this task. During the rescripting phase, the therapist continues to record the patient's SUDS level approximately every 10 minutes.

Throughout the rescripting phase, the therapist remains largely nondirective and is careful *not* to tell the patient what to do, or suggest what should be happening, or push her beyond that which she is willing or able to do. The therapist's role is thus primarily facilitative, as the patient is encouraged to decide for herself what coping strategies to use in the mastery imagery.

Following completion of the mastery imagery, the therapist fosters "adult-nurturing-child" imagery, in which the ADULT is encouraged to interact directly with the traumatized CHILD. The therapist facilitates this by asking the ADULT such questions as:

- "What would you, the ADULT, like to say to the CHILD? . . . Can you see yourself saying that to the CHILD?"
- "How does the CHILD respond?"
- "What does the CHILD need at this point?"

In many instances the ADULT will begin to hold or hug the CHILD, reassure the CHILD that the abuse will not happen again, promise not to abandon the CHILD, and so on. If, however, the ADULT has difficulty nurturing the CHILD, or blames the CHILD for the abuse and wants to abandon or hurt the CHILD, it is often helpful to ask the patient:

- "How far away are you, the ADULT, from the CHILD?"
- "When you look directly into the CHILD'S eyes from up close, what do you see?"
- "Might you be able to go up close to the CHILD and tell her why you feel she is to blame for the abuse?"
- "And how does the CHILD respond?"

Generally, as the ADULT moves closer to the CHILD, she becomes more affected by the CHILD'S pain and finds it more difficult to continue blaming, hurting, or abandoning the CHILD. Such intense interactions with the CHILD tend to heighten the patient's level of affect and evoke strong feelings toward the CHILD that are often empathic, apologetic, or conciliatory in nature.

Once it appears that the ADULT has offered sufficient nurturance to the CHILD and the patient may be ready to bring the "adult-nurturing-child" imagery to a close, the therapist asks: "Is there anything more you, the ADULT, would like to do or say to the CHILD before coming out of the imagery?" When the patient has indicated her readiness to terminate the imagery session, the therapist concludes with, "When you are ready, you may let the imagery fade away and open your eyes." (Up to 90 minutes should be allowed for the exposure and rescripting segments described previously.)

As soon as the imagery has ended, the therapist asks the patient to rate on a 0 to 100 scale (a) how difficult it was to drive away the perpetrator, (b) how difficult it was for the ADULT to nurture the CHILD, (c) how angry the ADULT felt toward the CHILD, (d) how angry the ADULT felt toward the perpetrator, and (e) how vivid the imagery was for the patient. The remainder of the session (the last 15 minutes or so) is spent processing the patient's reactions to the imagery session and discussing homework.

It is important to allow sufficient time for the patient to gain control over her emotions prior to leaving the session. The patient is encouraged to call the therapist between sessions if difficulties arise.

Homework. An audiotape of the entire imagery session (the exposure as well as the rescripting) is given to the patient for review twice daily as a homework assignment. The patient is asked to record on a standardized homework sheet her subjective units of discomfort (SUDS) each day (see sample homework sheet on page 83), prior to and after listening to the imagery tape. The patient also records in a journal her reactions to the tape as well as any PTSD symptoms (e.g., nightmares, flashbacks) she may experience between sessions. The patient is encouraged to bring her journal for review at the beginning of each subsequent session.

SESSION 2

The first 15 minutes of this session are spent reviewing the patient's general mood, shifts in mood since last session, and homework assignment (including journal entries). The next 60 minutes or so involves exposure to the abuse imagery and development of mastery imagery and "adult-nurturing-child" imagery. In the remaining 15 minutes, the therapist and patient discuss the patient's reactions to the session and the homework assignment.

As part of her homework assignment, the patient is asked to write a letter to the perpetrator (which she does *not* mail) in which she expresses her thoughts and feelings about the abuse. The rationale behind writing such a letter is explained to the patient in the following manner:

> Many abuse survivors find it useful to express their thoughts and feelings by writing a letter to the perpetrator. Doing this often helps them to work through their painful memories and emotions, and put the past in a healthier perspective. How would you feel about writing such a letter to [the perpetrator] this week as a homework assignment? (Allow sufficient time to discuss reactions to the assignment, and make sure the patient understands that the letter is not to be sent.) In our next session, you will have the opportunity to read your letter and discuss your thoughts and feelings, if you wish to do so.

Even if the patient has written such a letter to the perpetrator in the past, it can be beneficial for her to write another letter in conjunction with Imagery Rescripting.

Homework. Listen to the audiotape of the entire imagery session twice daily and record SUDS on standardized homework sheet. Continue to record in the journal reactions to the audiotape as well as any PTSD symptoms experienced between sessions. Write a letter to the perpetrator (letter *not* to be mailed).

SESSION 3

During the first 45 minutes of this 2-hour session, the patient is encouraged to read her letter aloud and discuss her reactions. In the next 60 minutes, the patient again experiences the abuse imagery, and develops mastery imagery and "adult-nurturing-child" imagery. (During her imagery work, the patient may wish to incorporate information from the letter.) In the remaining 15 minutes, the reactions of the patient to the session are discussed and homework is assigned.

Homework. Listen to the audiotape of the imagery session twice daily and record SUDS on standardized homework sheet. Continue to record in the journal reactions to the audiotape as well as any PTSD symptoms experienced between sessions.

SESSION 4

The first 15 minutes of this session are spent reviewing the patient's general mood, shifts in mood since last session, and homework assignment (including sharing from her journal). During the next 60 minutes, the patient again experiences the abuse imagery, and develops mastery imagery and "adult-nurturing-child" imagery. In the remaining 15 minutes, the reactions of the patient to the session are discussed and homework is assigned.

Homework. Listen to the audiotape of the imagery session twice daily and record SUDS on a standardized homework sheet. Continue to record in the journal reactions to the audiotape as well as any PTSD symptoms experienced between sessions.

SESSIONS 5 THROUGH 8

During the last four sessions, the entire focus of the imagery work is on "adult-nurturing-child" imagery. The patient no longer repeats or rescripts the abuse imagery.

The first 15 to 20 minutes of each session are devoted to reviewing the patient's general mood, shifts in mood since last session, and homework assignment (including sharing from her journal). Next, the therapist asks the patient to close her eyes and visually "check in" with the CHILD. During the next hour or so, the therapist facilitates the "adult-nurturing-child" imagery by asking such questions as:

- "Where is the CHILD now?"
- "What is she doing?"
- "How is she feeling?"
- "What are her needs?"
- "Where are you, the ADULT? . . . How far are you, the ADULT, from the CHILD?"
- "How does the CHILD respond to your presence?"
- "When you look directly into the CHILD'S eyes, what do you see?"
- "What would you like to say to the CHILD? . . . Can you say that to her directly?"
- "And how does the CHILD respond?

In the remaining 10 to 15 minutes, the reactions of the patient to the session are discussed and homework is assigned.

Homework. Listen to audiotape of the "adult-nurturing-child" imagery twice daily and record SUDS on standardized homework sheet. Continue to record in the journal reactions to the audiotape as well as any PTSD symptoms experienced between sessions. In addition, "check in" daily with the CHILD and engage in self-initiated "adult-nurturing-child" imagery. Record reactions to this self-nurturing imagery in the journal as well.

In the last 20 minutes of *sessions 7 and 8 only,* the therapist and patient review the progress made during treatment and prepare for termination. This includes identifying and discussing stressors in the patient's life, and rehearsing coping strategies.

Although the eight-session format is standard, it is open to adjustment according to patient need. In the event that after eight rescripting sessions, the patient reports experiencing other recurring abuse flashbacks or nightmares, the therapist is advised to use the format described in Table 2 (p. 82) for each additional abuse memory.

If the patient continues to be suicidal after the eight sessions, additional "adult-nurturing-child" imagery sessions may be indicated until the patient's ability to self-nurture is enhanced and suicidality is significantly diminished.

Throughout the rescripting sessions, interactions between the ADULT and CHILD provide an opportunity to identify, confront, and modify abuse-related cognitions and underlying schemata (e.g., powerlessness, mistrust, inherent badness, unlovability) at a child's level of representation and understanding. The early origins of the traumagenic beliefs are clarified and, through interactions between the ADULT and CHILD, the patient is encouraged to develop healthier, more adaptive schemas.

SUMMARY

Imagery Rescripting is proposed as an efficacious treatment for alleviating post-traumatic stress symptoms and altering abuse-related beliefs and schemas of adult survivors of childhood sexual abuse. The rationale for the use of Imagery Rescripting is presented in a brief literature review. It is noted that traumatic memories are often encoded in images rather than words, and therefore can be better accessed and modified through the use of imagery as a primary mode of in-

TABLE 2: IMAGERY RESCRIPTING FORMAT FOR ADDITIONAL ABUSE FLASHBACKS OR NIGHTMARES

Sessions 1-2:	Reexperience the abuse scene (imaginal exposure) Develop mastery imagery Develop "adult-nurturing-child" imagery Assign homework (same homework assignment as in Session 1 of standard protocol)
Session 3	ADULT "check in" with CHILD Develop "adult-nurturing-child" imagery Assign homework (same homework assignment as in Session 6 of standard protocol) Discuss termination issues (if applicable)
Session 4	ADULT "check in" with CHILD Develop "adult-nurturing-child" imagery Discuss termination issues (if applicable)

tervention. The application of Imagery Rescripting is described in a session-by-session format with specific instructions for facilitating exposure, rescripting abuse memories, and fostering adult-child interactions.

Additional information on the use of Imagery Rescripting, including training programs and recent outcome data, may be obtained from Mervin R. Smucker. Correspondence should be directed to him at the address on page 84.

HOMEWORK RECORD

NAME OF THERAPIST:_____ DATE:_____

NAME OF CLIENT/PATIENT:_____ SESSION NUMBER:_____

Homework Assignment: Listen daily to audiotape of entire imagery session (exposure and rescripting).

Record Subjective Units of Distress (SUD: 0-100) at the beginning and end of listening to the tape.

DAY	1	2	3	4	5	6	7
Date and Time							
SUDS Beginning							
SUDS Ending							

DAY	8	9	10	11	12	13	14
Date and Time							
SUDS Beginning							
SUDS Ending							

Mervin R. Smucker, PhD, is Associate Clinical Professor in the Department of Psychiatry at the Medical College of Wisconsin, Director of the Cognitive Therapy Institute of Milwaukee, and Clinical Research Director of an inpatient trauma unit at Milwaukee Psychiatric Hospital. From 1983 to 1985, Dr. Smucker was a post-doctoral fellow at the University of Pennsylvania Medical School, where he also served as Director of Education and Clinical Training at the Center for Cognitive Therapy. Dr. Smucker has lectured widely in the United States and abroad on the treatment of borderline personality disorders and dissociative disorders, and the use of Imagery Rescripting with post-traumatic stress disorder. He is senior author of a recently developed manual for the treatment of adult survivors of childhood sexual abuse suffering from PTSD, and has authored numerous publications on this topic. Dr. Smucker may be contacted at Cognitive Therapy Institute of Milwaukee, 1220 Dewey Avenue, Wauwatosa, WI 53213.

Jan L. Niederee, PsyD, is a doctoral student in clinical psychology at the Illinois School of Professional Psychology. She completed her internship at the North Chicago Veterans Administration Medical Center, specializing in the treatment of post-traumatic stress disorder in combat veterans. She is currently a post-doctoral fellow at the Center for Cognitive Therapy, University of Pennsylvania. Together with Dr. Smucker, Dr. Niederee has authored several articles and presented workshops on the use of Imagery Rescripting with abuse survivors, and is involved in ongoing research on this topic at the Cognitive Therapy Institute of Milwaukee. Dr. Niederee can be contacted through the first author.

RESOURCES

American Psychiatric Association. (1994). *Diagnostic and Statistical Manual of Mental Disorders* (4th ed.). Washington, DC: Author.

Beck, A. T., & Freeman, A. (1990). *Cognitive Therapy of Personality Disorders.* New York: Guilford.

Bower, G. H. (1981). Mood and memory. *American Psychologist, 36,* 129-148.

Briere, J. N. (1989). *Therapy for Adults Molested As Children: Beyond Survival.* New York: Springer.

Briere, J. N. (1992). *Child Abuse Trauma: Theory and Treatment of the Lasting Effects.* Newbury Park, CA: Sage.

Browne, A., & Finkelhor, D. (1986). Impact of child sexual abuse: A review of the research. *Psychological Bulletin, 99,* 66-77.

Bruner, J. (1973). *Beyond the Information Given.* New York: Norton.

Dancu, C. V., Foa, E. B., & Smucker, M. R. (1993, November). *Treatment of Chronic Post-traumatic Stress Disorder in Adult Survivors of Incest: Cognitive-Behavioral Interventions.* Paper presented at the annual meeting of the Association for the Advancement of Behavior Therapy, Atlanta, GA.

Donaldson, M. A., & Gardner, R. (1985). Diagnosis and treatment of traumatic stress among women after childhood incest. In C. R. Figley (Ed.), *Trauma and Its Wake* (Vol. 1, pp. 356-377). New York: Brunner/Mazel.

Edwards, D. J. A. (1989). Cognitive restructuring through guided imagery: Lessons from Gestalt therapy. In A. Freeman, K. M. Simon, L. E. Beutler, & H. Arnkowitz (Eds.), *Comprehensive Handbook of Cognitive Therapy* (pp. 283-297). New York: Plenum.

Edwards, D. J. A. (1990). Cognitive therapy and the restructuring of early memories through guided imagery. *Journal of Cognitive Psychotherapy: An International Quarterly, 4,* 33-51.

Fallon, P., & Coffman, S. (1991). Cognitive behavioral treatment of survivors of victimization. *Psychotherapy in Private Practice, 9,* 53-64.

Finkelhor, D., Hotaling, G., Lewis, I. A., & Smith, C. (1989). Sexual abuse and its relationship to later sexual satisfaction, marital status, religion, and attitudes. *Journal of Interpersonal Violence, 4,* 279-299.

Foa, E. B., & Kozak, M. J. (1986). Emotional processing of fear: Exposure to corrective information. *Psychological Bulletin, 99,* 20-35.

Foa, E. B., Olasov-Rothbaum, B., Riggs, D. S., & Murdock, T. B. (1991). Treatment of posttraumatic stress disorder in rape victims: A comparison between cognitive-behavioral procedures and counseling. *Journal of Consulting and Clinical Psychology, 59,* 715-723.

Herman, J. L. (1981). *Father-Daughter Incest.* Cambridge: Harvard University.

Herman, J. L. (1992). *Trauma and Recovery.* New York: Basic Books.

Jehu, D., Gazan, M., & Klassen, M. (1984-1985). Common therapeutic targets among women who were sexually abused. *Journal of Social Work and Human Sexuality, 3,* 25-45.

Jehu, D., Gazan, M., & Klassen, C. (1988). *Beyond Sexual Abuse: Therapy With Women Who Were Childhood Victims.* New York: John Wiley & Sons.

Jehu, D., Klassen, C., & Gazan, M. (1985-1986). Cognitive restructuring of distorted beliefs associated with childhood sexual abuse. *Journal of Social Work and Human Sexuality, 4,* 49-69.

Lang, P. J. (1979). A bio-informational theory of emotional imagery. *Psychophysiology, 16,* 495-512.

Lindberg, F. H., & Distad, M. A. (1985). Post-traumatic stress disorder in women who experienced childhood incest. *Child Abuse and Neglect, 9,* 329-334.

McCann, I. L., & Pearlman, L. A. (1990). Constructivist self-development theory as a framework for assessing and treating victims of family violence. In S. M. Stith, M. B. Williams, & K. Rosen (Eds.), *Violence Hits Home: Comprehensive Treatment Approaches to Domestic Violence* (pp. 305-329). New York: Springer.

McCann, I. L., Sakheim, D. K., & Abrahamson, D. J. (1988). Trauma and victimization: A model of psychological adaptation. *The Counseling Psychologist, 16,* 531-594.

Resick, P., & Schnicke, M. K. (1990). Treating symptoms in adult victims of sexual assault. *Journal of Interpersonal Violence, 5,* 488-506.

Resick, P., & Schnicke, M. K. (1992). Cognitive processing therapy for sexual assault victims. *Journal of Consulting and Clinical Psychology, 60,* 748-756.

Russell, D. E. H. (1986). *The Secret Trauma: Incest in the Lives of Girls and Women.* New York: Basic Books.

Smucker, M. R., Dancu, C. V., & Foa, E. B. (1991). *A Manual for the Treatment of Adult Survivors of Childhood Sexual Abuse Suffering from Posttraumatic Stress.* Unpublished manuscript.

Staton, J. (1990). Using nonverbal methods in the treatment of sexual abuse. In S. M. Stith, M. B. Williams, & K. Rosen (Eds.), *Violence Hits Home: Comprehensive Treatment Approaches to Domestic Violence.* New York: Springer.

van der Kolk, B. A., & van der Hart, O. (1989). Pierre Janet and the breakdown of adaptation in psychological trauma. *American Journal of Psychiatry, 146,* 1530-1540.

van der Kolk, B. A., & van der Hart, O. (1991). The intrusive past: The flexibility of memory and the engraving of trauma. *American Imago, 48,* 425-454.

STRATEGIES FOR PARENT TRAINING USING THE ONE-WAY MIRROR

Ron D. Cambias, Jr.

This contribution is meant to serve as a guide for clinicians in the training of parenting skills through the use of a one-way mirror observation room. Live supervision from behind the one-way mirror, as with family therapy training, allows for the relatively unobtrusive observation of and intervention with a family in a more naturalistic setting (i.e., without the therapist's/observer's physical presence). Use of an overhead speaker, telephone, or bug-in-the-ear device allows the therapist in the observation room to communicate directly with the family in the therapy room. Such an approach more closely creates the impression for the children that any comments or commands directed to the parents by the therapist are coming from their parents. In essence, an illusion is created in which commands and feedback are physically seen as coming from the parents and not from the mouth of the therapist.

There are a number of structured parent training programs available today. Two of the best known programs are Parent Effectiveness Training (PET; Gordon, 1975, 1976) and Systematic Training for Effective Parenting (STEP; Dinkmeyer & McKay, 1989). These two programs utilize approaches common to many parent training programs. However, these programs are specifically geared toward the parent, not the clinician working directly with the parents and child in the office, although they obviously can be adapted by the clinician for use in the office.

Guidelines for use of the one-way mirror in teaching parenting skills are almost nonexistent in the literature. Gross, Shuman, and Magid (1978) describe an approach to teaching foster parents about child development through use of a one-way mirror. However, there is no teaching in vivo of parenting skills reported with this approach. Another approach in which the one-way mirror is used is the Filial Therapy approach (Guerney, 1976) and its derivatives (e.g., Child Parent Relationship Training; Landreth, 1991). Perhaps the best example to date of a systematic approach to parent training which incorporates the one-way mirror is the training program developed by Rex Forehand and his colleagues at the University of Georgia. Forehand and McMahon (1981) describe a program which incorporates practice sessions with parents using a bug-in-the-ear device. Parents enter the playroom, and the therapist behind the mirror "talks them through" the various parenting techniques which are used in the approach. Although this approach appears closest to the one discussed in this contribution, the biggest difference lies in the degree to which the one-way mirror is used. Forehand's approach uses the one-way mirror as one facet of training parents to more skillfully employ behavioral techniques, while the approach offered here employs the one-way mirror as a more extensive component of an approach to working with noncompliant children.

The length of time needed for this type of approach depends upon several variables: the severity of the behavioral problem, the ability of the parents to integrate the techniques, the consistency of the parents in implementing the techniques both within the session and at home, and the degree of marital unity (which will impact on the parents' ability to work as a "team"). Some parents will be able to demonstrate proficiency in utilizing the parenting skills and a consequent lessening of behavioral problems with their children within a relatively short period of time (e.g., a few sessions). Other parents will require a much longer period of time and may require adjunctive family and/or marital therapy in order for gains to be made. It is my belief that this approach may be used by itself, with at least some minimum contact at the beginning or end of the session to "touch base" and problem-solve, or can be used as an adjunct to some other treatment modality (e.g., individual therapy with the child, family therapy, marital therapy, etc.). In whatever way this type of parent training is used, I believe it represents a relatively efficient form of training in that it is both educational and experiential in its approach. After all, there is no better way to learn than by doing.

SETUP

Since the 1950s, family therapists, followed by other types of therapists, have used live supervision incorporating the use of one-way mirrors as an integral part in the training of novice therapists (I. Goldenberg & H. Goldenberg, 1985; Haley, 1976). The approach toward parent training endorsed in this contribution proposes that such skills can be taught to parents in the same live supervision format in which other therapists have been trained through the use of a one-way mirror observation room. In essence, the parents become the trainees, and the therapist becomes the supervisor.

Obviously, this approach is used in facilities where one-way mirror observation rooms exist. Such facilities include hospitals, community mental health centers, family therapy institutes, and university-based therapy training centers. One might argue that parent training need not take place in such a formal manner. Indeed, I agree. Those clinicians in settings lacking such facilities, especially those clinicians in private practice where one-way mirror observation rooms are the exception rather than the rule, need not go to the expense of building an adjoining observation room replete with mirror and state-of-the-art communication system. However, this contribution points out ways in which the advantages of such facilities can be maximized. With simple modifications, these advantages might also be adopted in regular parent-training sessions. For instance, clinicians who do parent training, but have no one-way mirror available, could create an "artificial boundary" in their sessions by sitting in the corner of the room and directing their comments directly to the parents while the child is also present. However, such modifications, while approximating the situation created by use of a one-way mirror, can never take full advantage of the approach.

I believe that this approach is best suited for parent training involving children ranging in age from toddlers to young adolescents (roughly, ages 2 to 13 years). The rationale for this recommended age range is twofold. First, children under the age of 2 years do not have the rudimentary language and cognitive skills necessary to respond to the comments and commands inherent in this particular approach. Second, children older than age 13 are inevitably involved in the complex trials and tribulations of adolescence, especially issues regarding separation and autonomy and the subsequent tug-of-war battles between parent and child. Such issues, if severe enough, are best addressed in the context of family and/or individual therapy where the "tangles" can be combed out by the therapist and family members. However, some basic techniques, such as limit setting and positive and negative consequences, are germane to both age groups as well.

Indications for this approach are the same as for any parent-training program. These include the typical behavioral problems of childhood, such as temper tantrums, defiance, fighting, and noncompliance. Contraindications include behavior reflective of more severe psychopathology, such as fire setting, conduct disorder, and psychosis.

Who should be involved in the parent-training sessions? In an intact nuclear family, both parents should ideally be included in the training. In single-parent families, the single parent and any other significant caretaker (e.g., grandmother or grandfather, aunt or uncle, etc.) should be included. In essence, any person who has significant contact with the child in a caretaker or parenting capacity should be included. The absence of one or more significant caretakers from the training sessions increases the possibility, or in some cases the probability, that parenting techniques will not be implemented in a consistent fashion. Having all significant caretakers present decreases that possibility.

As for the child or children, the identified patient (i.e., noncompliant child) should be included as part of the sessions. Whether other children in the family are included should be based upon the severity of the presenting problems (less severe problems may allow for a greater number of siblings to attend), the need to assess the greater family dynamics in the case, and whether other children are also exhibiting behavioral problems to some degree. It should be remembered, however, that the fewer people in the room, the more likely the training program will be focused rather than diffused through interruptions and the need to address multiple issues within the session.

Most sessions will last for the standard 50 to 60 minutes. However, 90 minutes is not an unreasonable amount of time. The usual frequency of sessions will be weekly. Length and frequency of sessions will more likely be a function of a number of different variables, such as therapist's schedule, severity of presenting problem, and both therapist's and parents' preferences.

THE FIRST SESSION

Prior to initiation of parent training using the one-way mirror, the parents and child should be told about the special procedure in which they will take part. They should be notified of the one-way mirror, the observation room, any other observers who may be watching, and details of the parent training procedures. Any questions or reservations should be addressed ahead of time. If the child or parents appear anxious, you might ask them if they wish to view the observation room to see where you will be for part of the time. Anxieties about being viewed from behind a mirror are normal and should be addressed as such. After beginning the session, most families adjust quickly to the presence of the mirror. However, a family's ultimate refusal to take part should be respected.

The therapist and observer (if present) should enter the waiting room and greet the family members. If any of the family members expresses interest or reservations about the "mysterious" observation room, feel free to show them the room and how it is set up. Answer any questions concerning what you are doing freely and straightforwardly. The greatest anxiety the family is likely to face is at the beginning of the training sessions just prior to walking into the room. Once in the therapy room, explain issues regarding the confidentiality of the sessions and the purpose of having to observe through a one-way mirror. For example, you might say something like, "The reason I will be observing from behind the one-way mirror is to try to recreate as natural a family environment as possible. I may call in from time to time and may even stop and enter the room to speak to you. If you have any questions, please let me know." The therapist then proceeds to answer any questions the family may have.

Although this approach assumes that a thorough intake evaluation has already been conducted to gather details about parenting techniques and styles, the therapist should explore in further detail with the parents early in the first session how the parents handle the tasks of discipline and specific techniques which have proven helpful or unhelpful.

GUIDELINES FOR INTERVENTIONS

Usually during the first session and portions of sessions thereafter, the parents and child are asked by the therapist to engage in a period of free play. Free play means allowing the child to decide what and how to play. The parents are asked to step back and pretend they are radio announcers and simply narrate the actions of their child. They are not to command the child (unless instructed to do so), nor are they to make interpretations or judgments of the child's play behavior.

This type of approach is very similar to the child-centered or Axlinian approach in play therapy (Axline, 1947) and to the "attends" component of Forehand's parent training model (Forehand & McMahon, 1981). This part of the parent training is therapeutic in itself by offering a time in which the family meets in a fun activity and in which no judgments by parents are made of the child. The child feels valued for the attention received and feels more able to express himself or herself freely.

From time to time, parents may need to be reminded by the therapist in the observation room that they are simply to reflect back what their child is doing or feeling. It is easy for parents to fall back into a teaching or directive mode. This is especially true with parents who tend to be overprotective or controlling. Comments such as, "Just sit back and let Billy take the lead and narrate for him what he is doing," may be sufficient to get a parent back on track. For example, the parent might follow Billy's lead in play and narrate in the following manner: "Now, I see you are putting this block on top of this block and then you're getting the policeman and making him jump off the top block." The parent's narration should continue in this same nondirective style.

The question may arise, What does a parent do if the child requests that one or more of the parents participate in the play or assist in the child's activity? In this case, the parent should be instructed to join in but follow the child's lead. The parent should continue narrating the child's play and only participate when and in the manner the child wishes the parent to play, essentially allowing the child to "run the show."

By allowing the child to "run the show" in the beginning of the session, the child begins to feel valued by his or her parents. A certain degree of autonomy and self-confidence is engendered by taking this approach. Later on, the parents will take back control of the session when they command the child to clean up or perform some other task for the sake of "precipitating a crisis." The precipitation of a crisis allows the team of parents and therapist to work, in vivo, on problem behaviors which are similar, if not identical, to those seen in the home.

Periodic positive feedback to the child over the speaker or telephone for compliant behavior and cooperative play is essential for reinforcing "good" behavior and providing proper modeling to parents. The parents should be directed to praise their child if they do not spontaneously do so. Likewise, positive feedback to the parents for good reflection of their child's play activity is also essential for building the parents' confidence in their ability to interact in a therapeutic manner with their child.

Some children, depending on the severity of their behavioral problems and pervasiveness of situations in which their misbehavior is exhibited, will act up during the session without prompting from parents or therapist. However, some children will behave well as if proving wrong their parents' claims of misbehavior. In this case, it may become necessary to give directives to the parents which serve to induce misbehavior or "precipitate a crisis." The purpose of precipitating misbehavior is to provide an opportunity to demonstrate parenting techniques in vivo with the parent and child. Actually, this creates a "win-win" situation in terms of therapy goals: If the child complies with the parent's commands then the parents are getting what they want; if the child does not comply, the opportunity arises to coach the parents through various parenting techniques.

If the child remains compliant for the majority of the session, the therapist in the observation room may ask the parents to command the child to perform certain tasks, especially those tasks similar to ones which the parents might have the child perform at home. For example, the parents might ask the child to pick up a magazine from the other side of the room or pick up some of the toys from the floor. Clean-up time at the end of the session is a frequent time that misbehavior will take place, since the child, for most of the session, has taken part in an enjoyable activity (playing) with his or her parents' undivided attention. In essence, misbehavior is usually precipitated at the point in which the control is shifted from the child back to the parents.

Inevitably, the child will misbehave, and it is at this point that the major therapeutic task takes place. The therapist now has the opportunity to see how the parent actually handles the child's misbehavior and can coach the parents on specific parenting techniques, such as time-out procedures, ignoring of behavior, praise and positive reinforcement, and immediate and long-term consequences.

For example, after directing the parents to tell their young boy to clean up, the therapist may observe that the child has decided to throw a temper tantrum. The parents may be directed to ignore the behavior and have a conversation between themselves which is unrelated to the situation at hand. Perhaps the child becomes combative, attempting to hit one or both of the parents. The therapist in the observation room may direct the parents to explain to the boy that hitting is not allowed and that should he try to hit them again he will be placed in time out. The child responds by hitting one of the parents. The therapist immediately coaches the parents through the time-out procedure, in the process giving both positive and negative feedback to the parents. The parents may correctly explain to the child why they are placing him in time out but then continue giving attention to the child's demands to get out of time out. The therapist would remind the parents not to give attention to the child during the time that he is in the time-out chair. After doing this correctly for the allotted amount of time, the parents may be given praise by the therapist from refraining from talking to their child and reminded that the time is up. The child would then be let out of time out, with the parents reminding the child why they disciplined him. The live supervision format allows for immediate corrective feedback, compared to anecdotal and sometimes distorted parental reports in traditional parent-training sessions.

During time-out procedures, the child may refuse to stay in the time-out chair. (This scenario is not uncommon.) In this case, the parents should be directed to gently hold the child in the chair and look away so as not to appear to be paying attention to the child. If it is too awkward to stand by the chair and prevent the child from getting off the chair, then one of the parents might be encouraged to sit in the chair and hold the child on his or her lap. When working with more than one parent, it is important to have both the parents exchange roles of playing "the bad guy" (i.e., the one holding the child on his or her lap), in order to avoid "vilifying" one parent over the other.

The preceding scenario clearly exemplifies the use of time out (for combative behavior), ignoring behavior (for throwing a temper tantrum), and immediate consequences (time out occurred as an immediate consequence of hitting). However, what would be examples of praise, positive reinforcement, and long-term consequences? Using the same scenario, the therapist might instruct the parents to praise their child for heeding the warning not to hit or for adherence to the time-out procedure (if the boy actually complied with either). Praise is a form of positive reinforcement. Other examples of positive reinforcement might be to give the boy some small reward, like an inexpensive toy or a small amount of money, for each day he is compliant (i.e., for each day the parents do not have to use time out). This particular example also demonstrates use of a long-term consequence in that the reward is given at the end of the day rather than immediately consequent to discrete acts of compliant behavior.

Parents should be encouraged to practice at home what they learn during the training sessions. Consistency should be emphasized as one of the keys to successful parenting. The beginning or end of the session can be reserved for finding out how things have gone at home and any difficulties encountered in handling the child's behavior. If difficulties were encountered, the therapist has the opportunity to explore with the parents what went wrong and ways in which the situation can be handled in the future. Plans for follow-up or referral can be made for more serious concerns which might arise, such as marital problems or family crises.

Approximately 10 to 15 minutes at the end of the session should be reserved to "debrief" the parents. The parents should be given both positive and constructive feedback about their performance during the session. Parents should be encouraged to give their child positive and constructive feedback as well.

There is a tremendous need for flexibility in this (as well as any) therapeutic approach. For example, a trainee and I were working with a 5-year-old boy and his parents. The boy, who had been cooperative for most of the session, became oppositional when we directed the parents to ask the boy to write his numbers. A crisis was precipitated when the boy became upset and refused to write any further. Rather than directing the parents to address his opposition by putting him in time out, we decided to stop the session and asked the boy to wait outside the therapy room. When it was determined by speaking with the parents that the boy's opposition was more out of frustration over remembering his numbers and not oppositional behavior, we decided to forego discipline and had the parents tell the boy that it was all right not to know his numbers and that he need not continue if he wished. Had we continued to treat this incident as a behavioral problem, we might have adversely affected the boy's academic self-esteem, turning number-writing into a punishing task rather than recognizing his struggles with his fledgling number-writing skills.

TERMINATION

Termination involves the same considerations as with any other therapeutic modality. The therapist should ask himself or herself, "Have the parents learned the parenting techniques? Have they demonstrated sufficient skill using the techniques during the training sessions? Has the child responded in session and at home to the parents' discipline?" If the answer to these questions is in the affirmative, then the therapist and parents should discuss the topic of terminating therapy. Termination is an ongoing process, beginning with the first session. From the first session onward, termination is the obvious goal. The therapist wants the parents to function autonomously, using the techniques and skills that have been taught during the course of the parent-training sessions.

The last session offers the opportunity to discuss the gains which have been made over the course of therapy. Credit and praise should be given the parents for the new parenting skills they have learned and the consequent decrease in their child's behavioral problems. Responsibility for change should be placed with the family, not with the therapist. The parents should be encouraged to remain as consistent as possible in implementing the parenting techniques.

Those areas which might not have progressed as much as hoped should also be addressed. For example, a specific technique, such as ignoring certain behaviors, may not have been learned to satisfaction. The therapist might wish to suggest future "booster" sessions to smooth out rough edges. Further sessions might also be indicated if the child's behavior escalates for some reason.

CASE EXAMPLE*

This case example involves a 5-1/2-year-old boy (who will be called "Scott") who was referred for temper tantrums, difficulty getting along with family members, and trouble expressing anger. Scott was quite shy with the therapist and demonstrated difficulty separating from his parents and adjusting to changes in his environment in general. He was angry with his parents, who were undergoing marital difficulties of a longstanding nature and which had not yet been adequately addressed by the couple. In addition to Scott, the family included an 8-year-old sister and 2-year-old brother.

Scott's behavioral problems developed when he was about 2 years old and generally coincided with the time that his parents first separated. When Scott was 3 years old, he and his parents briefly saw a psychologist for help for the behavioral problems and found that Scott's symptoms subsided but that his behavior got worse after they stopped therapy. History appeared to be repeating itself in that, at this latest time help was sought for Scott, his parents had recently separated for a second time.

An intake evaluation was conducted by me with the assistance of a psychology trainee (a predoctoral intern). The parents reported having attempted to use ignoring, time out, reasoning, and what they referred to as "special time" (presumably, special time alone with one or both parents for good behavior). At the end of the initial session, the trainee and I recommended marital therapy, parent training, and play therapy. However, the initial sessions would consist of parent-training sessions in which the one-way mirror observation room would be incorporated.

The beginning of the sessions, and sometimes entire sessions, usually involved conversations concerning how Scott behaved the previous week, how the other children were behaving, and how

---

*Names and other identifying characteristics have been altered to protect the confidentiality of the individuals.

the parents were managing their own relationship in terms of working on marital issues and taking turns watching the children since the father had moved out of the house.

Other parts of sessions entailed observation of family play, which usually included Scott, his mother, and his father. However, during one early session, all three of the children were present. Although the family interacted well together, the youngest boy (age 2) had difficulty complying with the command to clean up. The parents were instructed to put him in time out and performed this task fairly well except for the fact that they spoke to him and, thus, did not refrain from giving their son attention while he was in time out. Toward the end of the session during "debriefing," the parents were reminded not to give attention to their child while the child was in time out. Even though time out was initially performed with Scott's sibling, the parents' modeling the time-out procedure for noncompliant behavior in front of Scott served the purpose of demonstrating to Scott that noncompliance would not be tolerated and that any family member could be disciplined, not just him.

Free play during sessions generally went fairly well. Initially, the mother needed some reminders about reflecting back Scott's actions rather than commenting on or directing such actions. The father seemed to have a good sense of how to do "free play" and demonstrated a close relationship with Scott. This close relationship was likely what Scott angrily missed in his life, because his father was no longer living in the same house. Scott seemed to genuinely enjoy the times of free play alone with both of his parents.

Scott's compliance within the sessions was generally good. Most of the time, he complied well with commands from his parents to clean up or perform some other task. However, one incident in which he did not comply required intervention by the parents with the therapist's and trainee's help. Toward the end of one session, Scott responded to one of his mother's comments by putting his hands over his ears. He would not obey simple verbal requests to take his hands off his ears. Compliance was achieved only after two time-out procedures were performed and Scott's Nintendo was taken away for a specified period of time (this approach demonstrated the use of both immediate and long-term consequences). Both parents were praised for how well they performed these parenting techniques.

Throughout the sessions, one point which was repeatedly underscored to Scott's parents was the importance of seeking marital therapy. It was clear to the trainee and me that the parents' inability to "act as a team" and resolve their marital differences would continue to encourage Scott's oppositional behavior and the anger Scott had towards his parents for not providing a secure enough home environment in which parents could be trusted to stay home to love and protect him. Scott's anger, as well as his anxiety over what would happen to his parents, would not resolve until his parents explored their commitment to each other and came to some sound resolution regarding their relationship.

At the time of the writing of this contribution, therapy had progressed to individual play therapy sessions with Scott in order to allow him an opportunity to express his anger and anxiety in a safe, accepting environment. His parents, who had demonstrated they were quite competent in the use of parenting techniques, had finally decided to seek marital therapy. Although Scott's behavior and ability to manage his anger had only tentatively improved, the stage appeared set for greater therapeutic strides to be made. Therapy for this family, as with most patients and families, was an ongoing process requiring flexibility and a number of different approaches in order to best serve the needs of the entire family.

This case is a good example of how parent training using the one-way mirror can be taught as an adjunct to other types of therapy, in this case marital therapy and individual play therapy.

TRAINING ISSUES

Parent training using the one-way mirror is an ideal format for training mental health trainees. The trainee is able to work directly with the supervisor in the observation room and, at times, in the therapy room itself. The supervisor can direct the student, when ready, to give commands or make comments to the family in the other room. Once the trainee has developed enough competence and confidence, this type of approach allows for immediate and ongoing feedback to the student who has taken charge of the sessions.

Consideration needs to be given to the student's skill level and confidence level in determining how much autonomy should be given to the student during the sessions. This process parallels that of the therapist and parents in the adjoining room. Just as the therapist learns when to step in and assist the parents, the therapist learns when to step in and assist the trainee. Again, flexibility is the key.

CONCLUSION

Parent training using the one-way mirror is one approach to the broad area of teaching parenting skills. Although it shares many basic components with most parent training programs, the usefulness of this approach lies in benefits derived from the presence of a one-way mirror observation room. These benefits include an experiential, "hands-on" component, less distortion through direct observation of parent-child interactions rather than on reliance of parental reports of what takes place at home, and allowance for immediate corrective feedback and reinforcement. Although the techniques of parent training remain the same, I believe the effectiveness of these techniques is enhanced through their in vivo use and the feedback given by an observing therapist. The therapist's general presence in the observation room, not the therapy room, provides some degree of normalcy which is not provided by the therapist's continual presence in the room. In the language of research, reactivity of subjects is kept to a minimum. When necessary, the therapist can enter the therapy room and address the family face to face. The advantages of both relatively unobtrusive observation and face-to-face contact can be exploited. This cannot be done in traditional parent-training sessions which are usually conducted in the therapist's office.

Unfortunately, there is currently no research available on the effectiveness of this technique. Research is needed to assess the effectiveness of this form of parent training as compared to more traditional methods.

Ron D. Cambias, Jr., PsyD, is currently a Staff Psychologist at Children's Hospital in New Orleans, Louisiana, where he is also Co-Director of Clinical Training and Director of the Family Therapy Clinic. Dr. Cambias received his doctorate in clinical psychology from Nova University and completed his predoctoral internship at the Children's Psychiatric Center in Miami. He has special interests in the areas of apperception testing, pediatric hematology-oncology, and family therapy. Dr. Cambias may be contacted at Children's Hospital, Department of Psychology, 200 Henry Clay Avenue, New Orleans, LA 70118.

RESOURCES

Axline, V. (1947). *Play Therapy*. Boston: Houghton.

Crary, E. (1979). *Without Spanking or Spoiling: A Practical Approach to Toddler and Preschool Guidance*. Seattle, WA: Parenting Press.

Dinkmeyer, D., & McKay, G. D. (1989). *The Parent's Handbook: Systematic Training for Effective Parenting* (2nd ed.). Circle Pines, MN: American Guidance Service.

Forehand, R. L., & McMahon, R. J. (1981). *Helping the Noncompliant Child: A Clinician's Guide to Parent Training*. New York: Guilford.

Forehand, R. L., Sturgis, E. T., McMahon, R. J., Aguar, D., Green, K., Wells, K. C., & Breiner, J. (1979). Parent behavioral training to modify child noncompliance: Treatment generalization across time and from home to school. *Behavior Modification, 3,* 3-25.

Gartner, R. B., Bass, A., & Wolbert, S. (1979). The use of the one-way mirror in restructuring family boundaries. *Family Therapy, 6,* 27-37.

Goldenberg, I., & Goldenberg, H. (1985). *Family Therapy: An Overview* (2nd ed.). Monterey, CA: Brooks/Cole.

Gordon, T. (1975). *P.E.T., Parent Effectiveness Training: The Tested Way to Raise Responsible Children.* New York: New American Library.

Gordon, T. (1976). *P.E.T. In Action.* New York: Putnam's Sons.

Gross, B. D., Shuman, B. J., & Magid, D. T. (1978). Using the one-way mirror to train foster parents in child development. *Child Welfare, 57,* 685-688.

Guerney, L. F. (1976). Filial therapy program. In H. L. Benson (Ed.), *Treating Relationships* (pp. 67-91). Lake Mills, IA: Graphic Publishing.

Haley, J. (1976). *Problem Solving Therapy.* San Francisco: Jossey-Bass.

Landreth, G. L. (1991). *Play Therapy: The Art of the Relationship.* Muncie, IN: Accelerated Development.

Minuchin, S. (1974). *Families and Family Therapy.* Cambridge, MA: Harvard University Press.

ADOLESCENT SUBSTANCE ABUSE TREATMENT

Eric F. Wagner, Mark G. Myers, and Sandra A. Brown

INTRODUCTION

Adolescent substance abuse and its correlates are some of the most prevalent problems facing clinicians involved in the area of adolescent health. By some estimates, between one-quarter and one-third of adolescents will have experienced alcohol- or drug-related problems by age 18 (Johnston, O'Malley, & Bachman, 1991; National Institute of Drug Abuse [NIDA], 1990). Given the high levels of experimentation and risks for later life problems (Newcomb & Bentler, 1988), early identification and intervention for teen substance abuse is critical in arresting a negative trajectory that includes unstable academic and work patterns, greater health service utilization and poorer outcomes, and poorer family functioning.

This contribution is designed to provide a theoretical rationale and practical suggestions for assessment and intervention with teens who have alcohol and other drug problems. The first section focuses on the approach and process of substance abuse assessment with teens. We highlight many of the unique features of teen assessment from both developmental and biobehavioral perspectives. The second section provides an approach to designing and implementing personalized cognitive-behavioral interventions with teens. The client-matched skills-building approach may be used in the context of individual or group interventions (e.g., 12-step approaches) or operate autonomously, depending on the needs of the adolescent client.

ASSESSMENT OF ADOLESCENT SUBSTANCE ABUSE

OVERVIEW

A good assessment of any adolescent problem is grounded in sound theory with an appreciation for developmental factors. We believe that adolescent substance abuse problems are best conceptualized as resulting from interactions among biological, psychological, and social factors (see Donovan & Marlatt, 1988). Oftentimes, failure to consider the role of one of these dimensions in the development and perpetuation of substance abuse may result in a worse clinical course (Brown, 1993). Thus, ideally, teen substance abuse assessment should include evaluation of (a) the substance use behavior itself, (b) the type and severity of psychiatric morbidity that may be present and whether it preceded or followed the substance use disorder, (c) cognition, with specific attention to neuropsychological functioning, (d) family organization and interactional patterns, (e) social skills, (f) vocational adjustment, (g) recreation and leisure activities, (h) personality, (i) school adjustment, (j) peer affiliation, (k) legal status, and (l) physical health (Tarter, Ott, & Mezzich, 1991).

The biobehavioral conceptualization of adolescent substance abuse also suggests the need for a broad-spectrum assessment process (Donovan, 1988). Whenever possible, information should include teens' self-reports (gained through self-monitoring, clinical interview, and/or structured reporting forms), significant others' reports (e.g., parents, teachers), psychometric testing, direct observation of adolescents' behavior, and biological measures. In actual clinical practice, however, the reports of the adolescents and their parents are often the only data available to the clinician.

It is also important to consider how results from an adolescent substance abuse assessment may be used. Most commonly, substance abuse assessment is needed to screen for problems, establish a diagnosis, establish eligibility and appropriateness for treatment, understand the individual more comprehensively, and determine which form of treatment, if any, is most appropriate. Miller and Rollnick (1991) offer two additional purposes for assessment which we believe deserve special note: to provide baseline (pretreatment) information for subsequent comparison with status on these same dimensions after treatment in order to assess and document improvement, and to build motivation (i.e., increase the probability that a person will enter into, continue, and adhere to a specific change strategy) and strengthen commitment for change.

DIFFICULTIES IN ASSESSMENT

The assessment of adolescent alcohol and drug abuse is not a simple task. A number of factors strain attempts to accurately and comprehensively assess adolescent substance abuse, among them: (a) significant gaps in scientific knowledge concerning substance abuse among adolescents, (b) more adolescents in need of treatment than there are treatment slots available, (c) inappropriate labeling of certain individuals as "chemically dependent" because parents and/or treatment facilities view such a diagnosis as less stigmatizing and pejorative than "mentally ill" or "delinquent," (d) watchdog groups raising questions about the ethics of adolescent treatment providers and the cost of treatment, and (e) inherent difficulties in assessment of adolescents due to rapid developmental changes (Brown, Mott, & M. A. Stewart, 1992; Winters, 1990).

A more general factor that complicates the assessment of teen substance abuse is the varied nature of substance abuse among adolescents (Farrell & Strang, 1991). Teens who abuse substances differ from one another in the type and frequency of substances used, the actual and anticipated effects and consequences resulting from that use, the contexts and motivations in which use occurs, and the factors that have contributed to or accompany their involvement with substances (Henly & Winters, 1989). Moreover, it is important for substance abuse professionals to realize that, just as there may be a variety of paths into alcohol and drug abuse among adolescents, there are different paths leading away from substance involvement (Brown, 1993).

DIAGNOSTIC ISSUES

Criteria for the diagnosis of substance use problems among adults are fairly well developed. In contrast, procedures and criteria for diagnosing substance abuse or dependence among adolescents are not as well standardized (Harrell & Wirtz, 1989; Winters, 1990). Although criteria from the *Diagnostic and Statistical Manual of Mental Disorders* (*DSM-III-R, DSM-IV*; American Psychiatric Association, 1987, 1994) are often used with adolescents, a number of the diagnostic criteria are inappropriate or inaccurate for teens (D. G. Stewart & Brown, 1993). For example, the progressive nature of the disorder, medical complications, and other consequences of protracted use are less common among adolescent substance abusers than among adult substance abusers (Blum, 1987; Brown et al., 1992; Kaminer, 1991). Furthermore, teens sent for treatment may use a greater number of different types of substances than adults, resulting in more complicated withdrawal and dependency patterns than suggested by the *DSM-III-R* (D. G. Stewart & Brown, 1993). An additional difference between adult and adolescent substance abusers is that adolescent substance use occurs in the context of rapid developmental changes which may mimic or exacerbate drug effects (Brown et al., 1992). It should be noted that substantial proportions of teens who abuse substances mature out of their problem-use patterns by early adulthood without formal intervention or treatment (Blum, 1987; Winters & Henly, 1989). Thus, pronounced developmentally related behavioral changes in conjunction with normal experimentation add to the complexity of diagnosing substance use problems among adolescents (Blum 1987; Brown, 1993).

When this contribution was written, *DSM-IV* criteria for the diagnosis of Substance-Related Disorders were available (American Psychiatric Association, 1994). Because the proposed *DSM-IV* diagnosis of Psychoactive Substance Dependence is based primarily on clinical manifestations of tolerance and withdrawal, the progressive nature of the disorder, medical complications, and symptoms of chronic use, teens are less likely to meet criteria for this diagnosis. However, adolescents with substance use problems may more often meet the proposed Psychoactive Substance Abuse diagnostic criteria, which involve "a maladaptive pattern of substance use manifested by recurrent and significant adverse consequences related to the repeated use of substances" (p. 182). "A maladaptive pattern of substance use" is defined by at least one of the following occurring at any time during the same 12-month period: (a) recurrent substance use resulting in a failure to meet major role obligations, (b) recurrent substance use in situations in which it is physically hazardous, (c) recurrent substance-related legal problems, or (d) continued substance use despite persistent or recurrent social or interpersonal problems caused or exacerbated by the effects of the substance. Adolescents are also likely to meet the proposed diagnostic criteria for Substance Intoxication, which involves clinically significant yet reversible behavioral or psychological changes due to the recent ingestion of a substance.

When making a diagnosis of substance abuse within the adolescent population, timing and developmental context considerations are critical. The diagnostic criteria should be considered in light of major developmentally specific roles (e.g., student) and within a supportive context. Recent evidence suggests that teens may experience more withdrawal and dependency symptoms than previously appreciated (D. G. Stewart & Brown, 1993) if queried later rather than earlier in the assessment process.

PERFORMING THE ASSESSMENT

Setting the Stage. A substance abuse assessment begins with the preparation of adolescents and their parents for the evaluation. The purpose of evaluation should be explained in a clear, forthright manner. The referring clinician should clarify his or her ongoing relationship with the adolescents and their family, and facilitate contact with the clinician who will actually perform the assessment. It is often preferable to meet first with the parents, and then have the parents share the preparatory information with the adolescents. The assessing clinician should be prepared to help the parents with this task and should make sure the purpose of evaluation is clear to the adolescents before evaluation begins. Important points to emphasize are that the evaluation is being done in an effort to provide relevant interpersonal or educational help, and that the assessing clinician is a "talking doctor" who will not perform any physically invasive procedures.

Approaches to Assessment. Donovan (1988) notes that a clinician is likely to take one of two approaches to evaluating substance abuse. One approach, termed *clinical hypothesis testing*, begins with the clinician generating a number of hypotheses about the identified problem. Consistent with a biobehavioral conceptualization of adolescent substance abuse, these hypotheses should cut across biological, psychological, and social domains. Once such hypotheses have been established, the clinician examines each in turn. The clinical hypothesis-testing approach is appropriate when it is relatively certain prior to the assessment that the adolescent is experiencing substance use-related difficulties. A second approach, called sequential evaluation, begins with the administration of a substance abuse screen, is followed by a more comprehensive substance use assessment if the screen is positive, and may be extended into a specialized assessment (e.g., neuropsychological evaluation) if indicated. The sequential evaluation approach is best when little, prior to the assessment, is known about whether the adolescent has been involved with substances.

Collecting Data. In regard to actual evaluation, clinicians have tended to rely upon clinical judgment or locally developed procedures to diagnose substance use problems among teens (Owen & Nyberg, 1983). This is beginning to change, however, as standardized and clinically valid instruments are introduced into the literature. Standardized assessment offers several advantages over more traditional approaches: It provides a benchmark against which clinical decisions can be compared and validated, it is much less vulnerable to rater bias and inconsistencies, it provides a common language for treatment professionals, and it permits the pooling of data from descriptive and evaluation studies (Henly & Winters, 1989).

Table 1 (pp. 102-103) lists and describes a number of different standardized self-report instruments for assessing adolescent substance abuse. The six screening measures are best utilized in a sequential evaluation approach to the assessment of teen substance abuse. Among the screening measures, the Personal Experience Screening Questionnaire (Winters, 1991) is notable for its biobehavioral theoretical grounding and psychometric strengths. Multidimensional measures are best utilized in a clinical hypothesis testing approach. Both of the multidimensional measures included in Table 1 originate from a biobehavioral conceptualization of teen substance abuse and each possesses good psychometric characteristics.

Several additional self-report measures of adolescent substance use have been developed primarily for research purposes (e.g., the Youth Experience Questionnaire [Dunnette et al., 1980]; the Institute of Social Research's Annual High School Senior Survey Questionnaire [Johnston et al., 1991]; the National Household Survey [NIDA, 1990]; American Drug and Alcohol Survey [Oetting & Beauvais, 1986]; and The Customary Drinking and Drug Use Record [CDDR; Brown, Vik, & Creamer, 1989]). These measures tend to be quite lengthy and have limited utility from a clinical perspective. However, there are several briefer research-oriented measures that may have more applicability in clinical settings. These instruments include a measure developed by M. Cohen, Karras, and Hughes (1977), which evaluates drug use severity and includes the assessment of the history, effects, usage pattern, utility, and social basis for substance consumption; a 6-item questionnaire developed by Smart and Jones (1970), which measures the frequency of drug use, availability, source, and history of professional contacts for drug use problems; and the Client Substance Abuse Index (Moore, 1980), which focuses on drug use severity within the *DSM-III* diagnostic scheme.

Table 2 (p. 103) lists and describes five different standardized interview-based measures of adolescent substance abuse, each of which examines several domains of functioning related to substance abuse. With the exception of Home, Education, Activities, Drug use and abuse, Sexual behavior, and Suicidality and depression (HEADSS; E. Cohen, MacKenzie, & Yates, 1991), which is intended to be used as a primary care screening interview, these interview measures are designed to be used when it is relatively certain that teens are experiencing problems resulting from their use of substances (i.e., the clinical hypothesis testing approach). Of the interviews listed here, the Teen Addiction Severity Index (T-ASI; Kaminer, Bukstein, & Tarter, 1991; Kaminer et al., 1993) and the CDDR are the only interviews for which psychometric data are available. Furthermore, the T-ASI has the advantage of being conceptually and procedurally linked to the Addition Severity Index (McLellan et al., 1980), a widely used substance abuse interview for adults.

Many standardized semistructured psychiatric diagnostic interviews are currently available which can aid in the assessment of adolescent substance abuse. Several of these interviews have sections devoted to the diagnosis of Psychoactive Substance Use Disorder, and several have complementary versions that can be administered to parents or other collaterals. However, it should be noted that these interviews require specialized training and monitoring for appropriate administration and are very time-consuming to administer, score, and interpret. As a result, such interviews are often impractical for use in clinical settings and should be used only when diagnostic precision is more important than diagnostic efficiency (e.g., research projects). The most prominent of these instruments include the Diagnostic Interview Schedule for Children and Adolescents (Herjanic & Reich, 1982; Reich et al., 1982), the Kiddie Schedule for Affective Disorders and Schizophrenia-E (Orvaschel et al., 1982), the National Institute of Mental Health Diagnostic Interview Schedule for Children (J. Costello, Edelbrock, & A. Costello, 1984, 1985; Robins et al., 1981), and the Child Assessment Schedule (Hodges et al., 1982).

Concluding the Assessment. A substance abuse assessment ends with providing adolescents and their parents with feedback about the results. The clinician should keep in mind that personalized feedback can be potentially persuasive input for convincing substance-abusing teens and their significant others of the need for treatment (see Miller & Rollnick, 1991). Initially, important findings from the assessment should be described to the adolescents and their parents, along with the information necessary to understand what each finding means. In order to avoid eliciting resistance and defensiveness, results can be presented in a manner that emphasizes freedom of choice (e.g., "I don't know what you will make of this result, but. . . ."). The clinician should expressly avoid an accusatory or scare tactic tone, especially with adolescents, and empathize instead with common social pressures for drug use.

Once the results from each of the assessment domains have been presented, the adolescents' and their parents' reactions to this information should be solicited and reflected. Because assessment feedback will occasionally arouse strong emotions from adolescents and/or their parents, the clinician should be prepared to deal with such reactions. The feedback session should conclude with a summary of what has transpired including the risks and problems that have been identified during the evaluation, the adolescents' and their parents' reactions to the evaluation (with particular attention to any self-motivational statements that have been made), and an invitation for the adolescents or their parents to append or correct the summary.

TREATMENT OF ADOLESCENT SUBSTANCE ABUSE

OVERVIEW

Adolescent substance abuse treatment is delivered in a variety of modalities and with differing levels of intensity of intervention. Before presenting a treatment outline, this section begins with a brief summary of the theoretical and empirical foundations of the program contained herein, a discussion of important developmental considerations when treating adolescents, and guidelines for matching the intervention to the needs of the individual teen. Although it is beyond the scope of this contribution to provide an exhaustive description for all possible components of treatment, we outline in detail a cognitive-behavioral coping skills approach to adolescent substance abuse treatment. This cognitive behavioral treatment can be administered as a free-standing intervention or incorporated as part of a more comprehensive program, and is applicable within a variety of settings (e.g., inpatient, partial hospital, or outpatient). We present an individual focused intervention, but this approach is easily adapted for group therapy. The cognitive-behavioral intervention outlined here focuses on skills training relevant to deficits commonly experienced by teen substance abusers. Because this approach may comprise just one part of a more comprehensive treatment, additional components must be determined by the particular needs of each individual teen.

BACKGROUND AND RATIONALE

A cognitive-behavioral approach to treatment has at its roots a social learning theory conceptualization of the development of substance abuse (e.g., Abrams & Niaura, 1987). Simply put, this perspective recognizes the contribution of many domains to the emergence of alcohol and

TABLE 1: SELF-REPORT ADOLESCENT SUBSTANCE ABUSE MEASURES

Screening Measures

Measure and Source	Description
The Adolescent Alcohol Involvement Scale (Mayer & Filstead, 1979; Robertson, 1989)	14 items; evaluates the degree to which drinking interferes with psychological functioning, social relations, and family living; designed to identify adolescents who are misusing alcohol, but does not provide for discrimination between different problem types and configurations.
The Adolescent Drinking Inventory: Drinking and You (Harrell, Sowder, & Kapsak, 1988; Harrell & Wirtz, 1989)	24 items; designed for use by clinicians without specialized training in substance abuse assessment; utilizes multidimensional conceptualization of adolescent drinking; possesses good psychometric properties.
The Rutgers Alcohol Problem Index (White & Labouvie, 1989)	23 items; covers all the criteria required for a *DSM-III-R* alcohol abuse diagnosis with the exception of reasons for use; possesses good psychometric properties, however data have not yet been published on clinical samples and clinical versus nonclinical sample comparisons.
The Perceived-Benefit-of-Drinking Scale (Petchers & Singer, 1987; Petchers et al., 1988)	Five items; developed to address the need for a quick, easy-to-administer instrument to be used in health care settings; a potential advantage is that it is not dependent upon directly eliciting information about substance use patterns or negative consequences; good reliability and validity in high school samples, but no data have been published on clinical samples.
The Drug and Alcohol Problem Quick Screen (Schwartz & Wirtz, 1990)	30 items; designed to detect adolescent substance misuse; a 14-item short form has also been developed; designed to be used in primary care settings; has not been independently validated and data have not been published on clinical samples.
The Personal Experience Screening Questionnaire (Winters, 1991)	40 items; designed to identify adolescents in need of a drug abuse assessment referral; includes a problem severity scale, two response distortion scales, and a supplemental information section on psychosocial status and drug use history; shares many items in common with the more comprehensive Personal Experience Inventory; excellent psychometric properties with both nonclinical and clinical populations.
The Personal Experience Inventory (Winters & Henly, 1989)	Includes 15 clinical scales measuring the severity of drug use and 17 additional scales measuring psychosocial functioning; attempts to (a) measure the adolescent's behavioral involvement with substances; (b) assess the frequency, style, duration, and sequelae of drug use; (c) evaluate personality characteristics and environmental circumstances of the user; (d) assist in the formulation of *DSM-III-R* diagnoses; (e) identify psychosocial stressors; and (f) examine for the presence of other disorders; excellent psychometric properties.

Multidimensional Measures

Measure and Source	Description
The Drug Use Screening Inventory (Tarter, 1990)	Profiles substance use involvement in conjunction with the severity of disturbance in nine spheres of everyday functioning; produces a needs assessment and diagnostic summary intended to lead directly to the development of a treatment plan; good psychometric properties.

TABLE 2: INTERVIEW-BASED ADOLESCENT SUBSTANCE ABUSE MEASURES

Measure and Source	Description
The Guided Rational Adolescent Substance Abuse Profile (Addiction Recovery Corporation, 1986)	Collects information regarding family interactional patterns, drug and alcohol involvement, behavior, and personality disorder, which can be used to yield a *DSM-III* diagnosis; supporting psychometric studies have not been published.
The Adolescent Drug Abuse Diagnosis (Friedman, 1987)	Evaluates substance use patterns, medical and legal status, family problems and background, school or employment record, psychological well-being, and social as well as peer relationships; intended for use in clinical settings to aid treatment planning; supporting psychometric studies have not been published.
The Teen Addiction Severity Index (Kaminer et al., 1991; Kaminer et al., 1993)	An adaptation of the Addiction Severity Index (McLellan et al., 1980), this interview evaluates seven domains, including substance use, school, employment, family, peer/social, legal, and psychiatric disturbance; adequate psychometric properties.
Home, Education, Activities, Drug use and abuse, Sexual behavior, and Suicidality and depression (HEADSS; E. Cohen et al., 1991)	A screening interview intended to provide a psychosocial database from which to draw information in a clinical setting; supporting psychometric studies have not been published.
The Drug Taking Evaluation Scale (Holsten & Waal, 1980; Waal & Holsten, 1980)	Evaluates older adolescents and young adults on four dimensions: (a) drug use behavior; (b) social functioning and adjustment; (c) social role identification, particularly as it relates to family relationships; and (d) maturity, psychopathology, personality disorder, and treatment needs; this measure was developed on a Norwegian sample; data from an American sample have not been published.

drug use problems (i.e., the biobehavioral model), but focuses on the role of environmental influences and learned beliefs and behaviors.

Behaviors related to alcohol and drug use are believed to emerge as a result of modeling by family members, peers, and society. In the process of observing the use of alcohol and drugs within the context of family, peers, and society/culture, beginning in childhood, individuals develop beliefs regarding the influence or effects of substances (Christiansen, Goldman, & Inn, 1982; Goldman, Brown, & Christiansen, 1987). It is these beliefs about the anticipated effects of alcohol and drug use that are often found to predict later involvement (Christiansen et al., 1989). So, to the extent that teens anticipate that use of alcohol or drugs will provide them with stress relief, facilitate social interactions (e.g., allow them to be seen as "cool" and accepted into a peer group), or make them feel good (i.e., "high"), they may begin to engage in alcohol and drug use. Although some experimentation with alcohol and drugs is normative during adolescence (Shedler & Block, 1990), teens who lack or are deficient in skills or abilities to manage negative moods, to engage in comfortable social interactions, to generate positive feelings in the absence of alcohol and drug use, or to effectively manage social pressures for substance involvement are at greater risk for developing problems (e.g., Bentler, 1992; Pandina & Schuele, 1983). It is from this perspective that skills-based approaches to substance abuse treatment have emerged (e.g., Monti et al., 1989). The notion is that effective treatment for substance abuse must provide skills for altering the situations and conditions that give rise to substance use and teach alternate means to achieve reinforcing experiences other than the effects obtained from alcohol and drug use. Additionally, coping skills for managing social pressures to use alcohol and/or drugs have been found to play an important role in successful outcome following treatment for teen substance abuse (e.g., Myers & Brown, 1990a, 1990b; Myers, Brown, & Mott, 1993). In particular, concern with the negative consequences of substance use and strategies that provide specific means for maintaining abstinence in the face of pressure to use are found associated with better outcome following treatment for teen substance abuse (Myers & Brown, 1993). The approach presented herein focuses on identifying the functions served by alcohol and drug use and providing appropriate strategies for changing substance use behavior.

GENERAL CONSIDERATIONS FOR TREATMENT

Adolescent Development. Two of the key developmental issues that must be considered when treating adolescent substance abusers are peer groups and identity formation.

Peer Issues. During adolescence, the peer group influences behaviors and plays an important role in the development and maintenance of drug use. Teens with less self-confidence and esteem tend to be more dependent on peer influences. In particular, teens exhibiting problem behaviors tend to be influenced more by peers than by parents. The social resources of teens are clearly prognostic of clinical course once abusive patterns have developed (Vik, Grizzle, & Brown, 1992).

Identity Development. Much of the identity development in adolescence occurs in the context of friendships. Close friendships play a crucial role in helping teens develop a sense of their own identity. The perceived acceptance of teens by their friends functions to bolster self-confidence and self-esteem, which are factors related to treatment success (Richter, Mott, & Brown, 1991).

Client Treatment Matching. As noted in the assessment section previously, the heterogeneity of presenting problems found with teen substance abusers demands that treatment be carefully tailored to each adolescent. Following are some suggestions for developing a comprehensive and effective treatment plan based on a broad assessment of teen functioning and needs.

General Guidelines for Matching (Hester & Miller, 1988). In general, clients show greater improvement with interventions matched to their cognitive style. This is an important consideration for adolescents because they will vary in their level of cognitive development.

Providing choices is also important; allowing teens to play a role in selecting their treatment may be effective in increasing motivation, commitment, and compliance. Additionally, this approach may help reduce resistance. Although we recommend that the skills training form the core of treatment, choice can be provided in offering other elements of treatment (e.g., family therapy, therapy focused on other problem areas, etc.).

Clients with more severe problems benefit differentially from more intense treatment, while those with less severe problems may benefit at least as much from a minimal intervention.

Client Matching Factors to Consider:

1. Severity of the substance use problem.
2. Concurrent psychopathology.
3. Adequacy of available support systems: home environment, family relationships, community resources, involvement in school, and peer relationships.
4. Severity of problem behaviors.
5. Intrapersonal characteristics: aggression, impulsivity, and self-esteem.
6. Interpersonal skills and functioning.
7. Physical health of the teen.
8. Academic functioning.

Following a comprehensive assessment, the process of client-treatment matching begins. Several sequential components are incorporated into this process: negotiation of treatment goals with the teen, selection of level of intervention, choice of type of intervention, maintenance arrangements (i.e., plans for how teens will maintain their recovery), and follow-up assessment (Miller, 1989).

Goals must be developed for each of the various areas of deficit or difficulty identified, rather than focusing solely on substance abuse. Goals of teens may not be consistent with the results of assessment, that is, they may resist change in areas where problems are identified because their perception of problems differs from that of parents and clinical staff. If so, the challenge becomes one of motivating the teen to change. "Rolling" with the resistance can help to reduce opposition. This consists of offering a fair trial of the client's goal. If it succeeds, teens may be more amenable to continuing the intervention process. If efforts fail, the failure is a persuasive diagnostic experience for the adolescent.

Of the domains to be considered for intervention, family relations are often an important area to be addressed. Recent research finds that following treatment, family relations improve with decreased teen substance use (M. A. Stewart & Brown, 1994), and family reintegration is one avenue to successful resolution of teen substance abuse, particularly for younger adolescents (Brown, 1993). Therefore, family interventions are often an important component of treatment, and the need for this approach can be determined following assessment of family functioning and discussion with family members. Although family treatment approaches are not described in this contribution, family-based interventions have been found effective in treating teen substance abuse (e.g., Szapocznik, Kurtines, et al., 1986; Szapocznik, Perez-Vidal, et al., 1988).

Level of Intervention. A range of intensity is available for teen substance abuse treatment. At the low-intensity end of the continuum there are brief interventions and school-based programs. These programs are typically considered secondary prevention, that is, preventing teens with early problem signs from progressing further. Moderate-intensity interventions include self-help groups (e.g., AA, NA) and outpatient treatment. On the high-intensity end of the intervention spectrum are day/partial hospital programs, inpatient treatment, and long-term residential settings. Basic guidelines for level of intervention decisions include:

1. Choose the least intensive intervention likely to be sufficient. If it fails, move to the next level.

2. More supervised care may be warranted by special conditions such as psychiatric comorbidity, medical complications, suicidality, or violence, which may require inpatient treatment.
3. Severity of abuse must be considered in combination with social stability/environmental resources supportive of change efforts.

Selection of the type of intervention also depends on identified deficits. For example, presence of concurrent psychiatric problems are an important matching consideration. Noncompliance, teen dissatisfaction, or poor early response may signal the need to change intervention modalities.

COGNITIVE-BEHAVIORAL COPING SKILLS TRAINING: TECHNIQUES

Several common tools and techniques comprise the treatment approach to coping skills training. The core techniques frequently used in this intervention are functional analysis and role plays.

Functional Analysis (McCrady et al., 1985). Functional analysis refers to examining the role of substance use in the teen's life: What do they get from drinking and drug use? The tool used in the functional analysis is called the behavior chain.

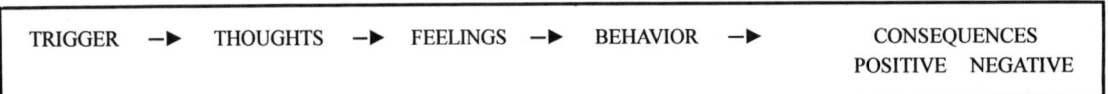

Trigger. The "trigger" refers to something that happens before the alcohol and drug use. A trigger can be an event, a person, a place, or a combination of these things (e.g., argument with parents, being offered beer by a friend, being under pressure to get something done). A trigger does not cause, but increases the likelihood of, substance use.

Thoughts. Thoughts in reaction to a trigger can be positive or negative. This reflects the individual's perception and interpretation of what is going on in the trigger situation. For example, when a teen is offered a beer by a friend, the thoughts in response might be: "What will they think if I say no?" "I'll look like a wimp if I don't drink it."

Feelings. Feelings are another type of internal reaction to a trigger. The cognitive-behavioral perspective focuses on the importance of thoughts in leading to feelings: How you think about a trigger has a lot to do with how you will feel in response. Here, too, feelings can be positive or negative. To follow from the preceding example, in response to being offered a beer, a thought of "What will they think if I say no?" may lead to feeling anxious, uncertain, or pressured in the situation.

Behavior. The behavior is the action or response to the trigger and resulting thoughts and feelings. In the current context the focus will usually be on the behavior of substance use.

Consequences. In this part the positive and negative consequences of alcohol and drug use are examined. It is important to acknowledge that teens use alcohol and drugs because of positive consequences. Likewise, examining negative consequences is important to identifying and understanding the personal costs of alcohol and drug use.

The behavior chain provides a concrete means for examining and understanding the substance use behavior. The first links in the behavior chain are called the antecedents which refer to the trigger, thoughts, and feelings portion of the chain (i.e., what occurs prior to the behavior). The notion is that behaviors (here, alcohol and drug use) occur as a result of the thoughts and feelings that arise in response to a trigger. The consequences part of the chain examines:

1. Positive consequences follow on the heels of the behavior (or substance use), thus reinforcing the behavioral response and making it more likely to occur again (e.g., feeling high, escaping from unpleasant feelings or thoughts).
2. Negative consequences usually occur later in time (e.g., having a hangover after the alcohol and drugs have worn off, having an accident while under the influence, getting in trouble with family or at school) and thus are often ignored or minimized.

An advantage of the behavior chain as an intervention tool is that it clearly specifies the points of intervention for behavior change. Strategies can be aimed at altering the antecedents (trigger, thoughts, and feelings) and the behavior itself. Thus, by acting on the antecedents, the conditions that set the stage for alcohol and drug use may be avoided or diminished. In addition, because situations that present opportunity or temptation for substance use are sometimes unavoidable, it is important to provide teens with alternative behaviors or responses other than substance use.

Guidelines for Role Plays (Kadden et al., 1992). Rehearsal of behavioral skills by role play is an essential part of skills acquisition. Practice in session is necessary prior to skills being attempted in the real world. The focus should be on working through role plays rather than engaging in discussion of problem situations and strategies.

Although this may be a particularly useful strategy, teens normally express discomfort when asked to role play. It is important to acknowledge that this discomfort is normal and inform them that this improves with time and practice. Start by having teens describe relevant situations from their own personal experience. It is important that initial role plays for a given skill area revolve around situations identified as moderately difficult and, with practice and improvement, move on to more difficult scenes. In setting up a scene, it is important to generate details as to where it occurs, who is present, what the problem is, who is the other person in the role play, how the individual being played would behave, and a description of the goal or purpose of the interaction. Such role plays can be conducted in individual sessions or in group sessions with other teens.

To help adolescents generate scenes:

1. Ask for a recent situation in which the skill being rehearsed would have been helpful but was not utilized.
2. Ask for a situation that might occur in the future where the skill would be helpful.
3. Suggest situations based on your knowledge of the teen.

Following each role play, the adolescent must be reinforced for participating, and both therapist and teen discuss reactions to the performance. Next, feedback is provided by the therapist on role-play performance, including praise for improvement and participation along with constructive criticism about areas that need improvement. This is where the therapist must identify weaknesses and work to improve teen communication skills. Select only one or two areas for attention each time so as not to discourage or overwhelm the adolescent. If the teen is having particular difficulty with a certain skill, one useful approach is role reversal, whereby the therapist models the use of the desired skill.

Structure of Sessions. Skills-training sessions are designed to be structured. Sessions begin with a review of material discussed in the previous session. When introducing new material, it is always prefaced with a rationale, and is explained in context of the adolescent's personal behavior chain. Thus, the skills to be taught are presented with respect to how they can help change alcohol and drug use for this teen. We recommend the use of a behavior chain handout (see p. 116), or a chalkboard on which the behavior chain is outlined, when discussing skills and alternative behaviors. This helps make the intervention concrete and provides a visual image of the material. Handouts with outlines of the skills, examples, and materials are also useful. Lecturing for extended periods is to be avoided; it is important to involve the teens and solicit their input and ideas constantly so as to maintain their attention and enhance their self-esteem, so that they develop a sense of personally directing their efforts at behavior change. When appropriate, the therapist first models skill performance and then engages the teen in a role play. Role plays are integral to acquiring new skills, and a significant proportion of each session should be devoted to them.

It is important to deemphasize the structure of the sessions so that teens feel that they have input and are not merely following the therapist's agenda. This generally is not difficult because the sessions focus on issues and problems identified by the teens during the functional analysis of different aspects of their substance use.

Homework. Homework assignments are important for practicing and acquiring skills and should be part of each session. Provide a rationale for homework, for example: "Using the behavior chain and other skills we'll learn often doesn't come naturally and requires practice. The assignments we develop will help you learn and become comfortable with these ideas and behaviors. How much you learn and change your behaviors is directly related to how much effort you put into practice." Note that it is important to negotiate homework with teens, let them decide how much they want to do, and ask them for a commitment to what has been agreed upon. Identify barriers and suggest strategies to help assure they do homework (e.g., time management, scheduling work time). For behavior rehearsal practice, use an approach that gradually introduces more difficult challenges: Success experiences are very important, while failure is to be avoided.

Alternative Activities. Extracurricular activities are found to play an important role in recovery from adolescent substance abuse. Such activities provide teens with an opportunity to build self-esteem and form healthy peer networks. To this end, it is important to work with the teens to identify potential alternative activities and facilitate participation. In collaboration with the teens, identify potential activities such as hobbies, sports, and organized groups, and then formulate a plan. Planning alternative activities will involve identifying potential barriers to participation (concerns, doubts, practical obstacles such as transportation and money), problem solving to remove or diminish obstacles, and setting up a schedule for following through. The teens should be encouraged to provide most of the input in this process. The therapist will need to be familiar with a range of available activities and organizations within the community to help in identifying appropriate activities. The discussion and planning of alternative activities can play a role in several of the skills-training components. Such activities provide opportunities for practicing and utilizing social skills as well as provide means for combating negative feelings (in particular, depression).

COGNITIVE-BEHAVIORAL COPING SKILLS TRAINING: TREATMENT OUTLINE

Following is an outline of a sample skills-training program for adolescent substance abusers. Each topic does not correspond to a single session; the amount of time devoted to each will depend on the individual needs and abilities of each teen.

1. Introduction/Rationale for skills training and functional analysis.
2. Interpersonal skills: assertiveness.
3. Interpersonal skills: dealing with conflict (anger and frustration).
4. Interpersonal skills: giving and receiving criticism, expressing feelings.
5. Intrapersonal skills: managing emotions.
6. Relapse prevention: identifying and coping with high-risk situations.
7. Personal risks: alternative activities.

Introduction to Functional Analysis. Begin by presenting the rationale for a skills-training approach as described in the functional analysis section previously. Introduce the behavior chain, emphasizing the function of the behavior of substance use, and show how each element can lead to the other; emphasize that this does not mean each necessarily causes the next. Explain that using the behavior chain takes time and practice, and there will be many opportunities for practice during the sessions and as part of homework assignments. The idea is for teens to ultimately learn to use the behavior chain on their own.

Next, introduce each element of the behavior chain as described previously, beginning with the antecedents. Use a sample trigger to illustrate each of the elements. (*Note:* This initial example need not involve substance use as the behavior of focus; this allows for a broader understanding of the applicability of the behavior chain.) This example is used to illustrate how one can have very different reactions to the same trigger. As you proceed through each element, check with teens to see if the ideas are understood.

Trigger	*Thoughts*
A new student starts school in one of your classes, and is very quiet and stays to herself.	a. "She must be a snob." "Maybe she thinks she's too good for us." "She seems like a boring person." b. "It must be tough starting in new school." "She must be shy, she probably doesn't have any friends here."

Before proceeding to "feelings," ask teen to suggest feelings that might result from the different thoughts.

Feelings

a. Put-off, hostile, uninterested.
b. Sympathetic, curious.

At this point define antecedents, and the idea that these are what occur prior to a behavior. Focus attention on how different thoughts in response to the same trigger can lead to a very different reaction. Explain that how we react to triggers happens so quickly that we usually are not aware of the thoughts going on, but are more likely to notice the feelings. Stopping to figure out what the thoughts are can help understand and change feelings. Move on to behavior: What behaviors might you expect in response to the feelings?

Behavior

a. Ignore or avoid her in the future, criticize her to others.
b. Make an effort to be friendly, introduce her to friends, invite her to join group activities.

Point out how negative thoughts and feelings lead to negative behaviors, while positive thoughts and feelings lead to positive behaviors. Move on to the last part of the chain, "consequences."

Consequences

a. The new student feels alienated, isolated; you miss chance to make a new friend; you end up disliking someone you don't even know.
b. You make a new friend; she feels accepted and more comfortable in her new school; you feel good for having been friendly and helpful.

Now elicit questions regarding the behavior chain, making sure the concepts are understood. Emphasize that behavior can be analyzed starting anywhere on the chain, and can be understood working backwards or forward. Importantly, behavior can be changed by making a change in the chain, either by changing one or all of the antecedents, or by stopping and thinking of the negative consequences and choosing an alternative behavior. Solicit a trigger from teens, ask for an interpersonal situation where they ended up feeling uncomfortable or unhappy, and work through it together.

Once the teens understand the behavior chain and how it suggests ways to change behavior, relate it to substance use: Focus on substance use as the behavior of interest, and find out what kind of triggers surround their substance use. Ask the teens specifically for social/interpersonal triggers, because these are very common situations for adolescent substance use. Again, use the behavior chain and focus on the thoughts and feelings that occur between the trigger and behavior.

After identifying an appropriate trigger and working through the antecedents, elicit the consequences of substance use (positive and negative). Next, focus on alternatives: What are other behaviors that could achieve the same positive consequences without having the negatives?

Next, orient the teens to the components of treatment and discuss their specific triggers. It is important to acknowledge that individuals differ in their particular triggers, but that the components discussed are commonly important for teens. Allow them to prioritize those elements they perceive as most important. It is important to emphasize and explain how the various components of treatment might be helpful in improving the teens' ability to communicate effectively with others, cope better with negative feelings, and consequently change their substance use behavior.

Homework. For the next session, ask the teens to work on behavior chains for triggers related to interpersonal situations. These don't necessarily need to be substance use situations, but can also be situations that result in negative feelings (angry, anxious, uncomfortable, sad, lonely, etc.).

Interpersonal Skills: Assertiveness. *Note:* assertiveness training should progress at a pace dictated by each teen's level of ability. Don't overload with information. Practice concepts and skills frequently to assess progress.

Rationale. Assertiveness improves our relationships with others. Good relationships decrease the likelihood of negative feelings. Good relationships decrease the likelihood of drug use.

Elicit and help teen list and elaborate upon rights we all have as human beings:

1. To decide things and make our own decisions.
2. To have our own feelings.
3. To have our own thoughts and opinions.
4. To express our own thoughts and opinions.
5. To say no or yes to requests.
6. To be healthy and safe and not be abused physically, emotionally, or sexually.

Elicit, define, and discuss different patterns of behavior:

1. Assertive: respects own rights and rights of others.
2. Passive: respects others rights but not own.
3. Aggressive: respects own rights but not others.

At this point, refer to the triggers homework and ask teens for personal examples involving passive and/or aggressive behavior. Use the behavior chain to work through examples of passive and aggressive behavior.

Next, define and discuss assertiveness guidelines (*note:* these can be divided according to the appropriate topics - it is generally too much to get through in one session):

1. We can only control our own, not others', behavior. You can ask others to change, but they can say no.
2. Do now what you want in a situation.
3. Be specific about what you want.
4. Pay attention to body language consistent with what you want.
5. Timing is important (e.g., if you're mad, take some time to calm down before confronting someone).
6. Use "I" statements; avoid words like "should" and "never."
7. Criticize the behavior, not the person.
8. When criticizing, use the "sandwich" technique: first say something positive about the issue/person, then give criticism, then end with something positive.
9. Be prepared to negotiate (plan what you are willing and unwilling to compromise).

Return to triggers involving passive and aggressive behavior, and engage in role play using the preceding guidelines for assertive behavior. Try to work through two examples to the point where the teens demonstrate comprehension and improvement.

Homework. Have teens initially select a relatively nonthreatening situation in which to practice assertiveness skills. Work on behavior chains for triggers relevant to current or upcoming topic (examples from their daily experiences are good for providing concrete examples and increasing awareness of their own behavior).

Interpersonal Skills: Dealing With Conflict (Anger and Frustration). Have teens generate situations in which they have had difficulty dealing with conflict (arguments, fights), particularly, but not necessarily, related to substance use. Go through the behavior chain for selected triggers; focus on ways of changing the behavior by altering the antecedents and generating alternative behaviors to achieve the desired consequences. Role play the selected examples.

Homework. Have teens select a relatively nonthreatening situation in which to practice assertiveness skills. Work on behavior chains for triggers relevant to current or upcoming topic.

Interpersonal Skills: Criticism, Expressing Feelings. Have teens generate situations in which they have had difficulty giving or accepting criticism or expressing their feelings (positive or negative), particularly, but not necessarily, related to substance use. Go through the behavior chain for selected triggers; focus on ways of changing the behavior by altering the antecedents and generating alternative behaviors to achieve the desired consequences. Role play the selected examples.

Homework. Have teens select a relatively nonthreatening situation in which to practice these skills. Assign identification of behavior chains for triggers relevant to current or upcoming topic.

Intrapersonal Skills: Managing Emotions. This section is designed to address coping with negative feelings such as depression, anxiety, and anger. It is best to discuss a variety of strategies so as to allow teens to match the skills with their particular circumstances and style. In addition to the interpersonal skills previously described, methods for managing mood include relaxation training or meditation (for anxiety and tension, anger management), involvement in pleasant activities (for depression, boredom), and cognitive strategies focused on identifying and changing negative or "irrational" thoughts.

Initially, it is helpful to elicit from teens their own experiences with negative feelings and, using the behavior chain, work through the elements of these experiences. With the teens, identify and select which types of negative feelings are most problematic. Once a particular feeling has been chosen, provide a description of strategies for managing feelings and how they fit into the behavior chain (e.g., relaxation is a behavioral response to feeling tense or anxious that will change the feeling; pleasant activities are alternative behaviors that provide a way of feeling good without using drugs; doing fun things helps you feel better when you're down; cognitive strategies to change irrational thinking will help change negative feelings by having a more positive and realistic attitude). It is important that the teens understand how the skills or strategies discussed will work to influence feelings.

Although a detailed description of each of these strategies is beyond the scope of this contribution, selection of the strategies should proceed in collaboration with the teens. A variety of references are available to describe simple relaxation techniques. Likewise, many references are available which provide detailed effective cognitive-behavioral approaches to mood management. For example, an easy-to-understand description of changing irrational thinking can be found in *Feeling Good: The New Mood Therapy* (Burns, 1981). Similarly, the *Coping With Depression Course for Adolescents* (Clarke, Lewinsohn, & Hops, 1990) provides a variety of mood-management techniques for depression, including descriptions of how to implement interventions focused on pleasant activities and positive and negative thinking.

As in previous sessions, rehearsal and practice are important elements of successful mood management training. It is also important to point out how the interpersonal skills previously learned can function to manage negative feelings (e.g., assertiveness, expressing feelings, etc.).

Homework. Assignments will depend upon the specific strategies selected for mood management. Here there will be less focus on behavior chains, but identifying potential triggers related to negative feelings remains an important focus.

Relapse Prevention I: Identifying High Risk for Relapse Situations

Rationale and Background. The cognitive behavior model of relapse (Marlatt & Gordon, 1985) suggests several important elements of relapse prevention.

1. Relapse (a return to a problematic pattern of alcohol and drug use) is not an all-or-none occurrence; a slip or lapse is seen as an opportunity for learning rather than a failure and violation of an absolute rule of abstinence. It is important to prepare teens for feeling guilty and defeated if a lapse occurs. It is important to communicate that a slip is not a total failure, but rather a signal to examine what is going on and redouble efforts to avoid the next slip. Emphasize that discussing the possibility of a lapse is not permission to use again, but rather a lapse is seen as an important learning experience that can be used to improve skills for avoiding substance use.
2. High-risk situations are situations previously associated with substance use or that pose a risk for substance use, and must be identified for each individual. The triggers discussed throughout previous session will provide many examples of high-risk situations.
3. The availability of appropriate/adequate coping skills will reduce the likelihood of relapse.
4. Self-efficacy enhancement is crucial to the successful performance of coping strategies (self efficacy = one's perceived ability to successfully carry out a given behavior). It is important to draw on the teens' success experiences to date in practicing and using the skills and to reinforce their sense of ability to cope successfully in high-risk situations.

After discussing the idea of relapse prevention with teens, work on identifying high-risk-for-relapse situations. First, describe the types of situations/circumstances found related to relapse. For teens, high-risk situations typically involve the presence of peers: Social pressure to use is the most common relapse situation. Teens often underestimate the difficulty of coping with these situations and may fail to label them as "high risk," therefore it is important to pay particular attention to this issue.

Have the teens identify personal high-risk situations. Assess the perceived risk of using for the various situations identified and the teens' sense of confidence for coping with these triggers. If they do not generate many situations, remind them of previously discussed triggers and return to the functional analysis in suggesting high-risk situations.

Homework. Have the teens make a list of high-risk-for-relapse situations for the present, the next 2 weeks, and the next month. Have them start work on behavior chains for one or two situations, coming up with alternative behaviors and other strategies for avoiding relapse.

Relapse Prevention II: Coping With High-Risk Situations. Having previously identified high-risk situations, focus attention on situations likely to be particularly problematic. Examine such situations using the behavior chain. As before, generate alternatives that accomplish the same result as substance use. In addition to alternative behaviors, coping strategies can focus on changing the feelings and thoughts in response to a trigger.

Discussion of refusal skills is particularly important; review assertiveness skills and role play situations in which the teens might be pressured to use.

Assignments focused on having fun are very important. To the extent that substance use served to facilitate social interactions and fight boredom, it is essential that teens perceive that they can have fun and enjoy themselves without using. Coming up with good alternative activities and helping anticipate barriers to following through on these are particularly important.

1. *Plan and Rehearse Coping Responses.* Have teens plan, role play, and rehearse a number of possible coping alternatives for identified high-risk situations. For each plan, discuss execution, consequences, possible reactions, and confidence.
2. *Anticipate Problem Situations.* It is important to preplan a coping response before being confronted with the situation. Work on anticipation and accurate appraisal of risky situations: Teens who return to heavy use following treatment often display limited forethought prior to relapse and tend to underestimate the difficulty of high-risk situations. For each major problem area, review upcoming events and identify potentially difficult situations. Make plans for coping with a potential slip, framing this as a learning experience.
3. *Build Self-Efficacy.* Practice new coping skills in increasingly more difficult situations. Avoidance of high-risk situations is useful early in treatment, but will not provide for lasting effects on confidence and preventing relapse. Use external aids (accompaniment by reliable others or the therapist if appropriate) to help insure success in homework assignments. It is important that teens make self-attributions with respect to improvement in treatment. Fade out (i.e., gradually decrease) avoidance (within reason) and external supports as the end of treatment nears.

Homework. Work on plans for coping with high-risk situations. Practice skills, initially in easy, safe settings, and progress gradually to more difficult situations.

Personal Risks: Alternative Activities. In addition to focusing on specific relapse prevention skills and strategies, a more global focus on developing activities that will provide reinforcement and nonsubstance-abusing environments is important. This task can be conceptualized as goal setting, and time set aside to discuss what types of activities or pursuits the teens might enjoy. Because substance-abusing teens often present with impoverished interests, it is helpful to find out what activities were important before the onset of substance use and what types of other pursuits the teens might be interested in developing. A variety of domains should be considered, including hobbies, recreational activities (e.g., sports), social activities, employment opportunities, and so on. These types of pursuits will assist in enhancing self-esteem and developing an autonomous identity, and are found to provide an avenue for successful resolution of substance abuse problems for some teens (Brown, 1993).

This portion of the intervention involves several steps:

1. Identify domains for increased involvement in activities, for example, by providing menus or lists of potential activities.
2. Have the teens prioritize which domains are more or less important.
3. Help the teens generate ideas for involvement within each domain.
4. Discuss how the teens plan to get involved in activities; it is important to be concrete and anticipate potential barriers to following through on plans. It may require coming up with concrete steps to follow through on a specific goal.
5. Help the teens select realistic and attainable activities and set goals for taking action (when, how, etc.).

MAINTENANCE OF BEHAVIOR CHANGE

Decades of research on addictive disorders have demonstrated that it is less difficult for interventions to produce abstinence than to sustain the nondrug-use states over extended periods of time. Several recent studies of clinical courses of adolescents following treatment for alcohol and drug abuse support this conclusion (e.g., Brown, 1993; Brown et al., 1989). Just as with adult addictive disorders, relapse is a common problem in the early months after treatment (Brown, Mott, & Myers, 1990), with the first 6 months constituting the greatest risk period (Brown, 1993). In contrast to findings from adult studies, adolescents often demonstrate resiliency after post-treatment use episodes. For example, approximately one-third of teens who fall prey to heavy substance involvement in the first 6 months post-treatment are able to abstain or engage in limited or sporadic nonproblematic substance involvement by 1 year post-treatment.

In light of these findings, there are several practical ways to enhance the likelihood of adolescent success following the initial phase of treatment. First, maintain contact with the adolescent during the highest risk period for relapse. Risk for adolescent alcohol or other drug relapse is greatest during the 1st month after treatment completion, with diminished but sustained risk over the subsequent 5 months. Face-to-face or phone contact with a goal of preventing and minimizing relapse may significantly improve treatment outcome during the highest risk periods. These contacts provide opportunities for resolving problems that arise in the behavior change program as well as for assessing the clinical significance of new symptoms which may emerge (e.g., anxiety, depression).

A second clinical technique that may enhance adolescent success is rapid response to new drug use and to relapse episodes. Adolescent post-treatment substance involvement differs from adult involvement in two ways: Adolescents often experiment with alternative drugs to those originally provoking problems, and a significant proportion (approximately 25%) of use episodes do not result in a return to abusive patterns of alcohol or other drug involvement. Consequently, rapid response by the clinician may disrupt the progression to greater or alternative drug involvement. Nonjudgmental discussion of use episodes provides an opportunity for the adolescent to assimilate post-treatment drug use experiences into the broader framework of how a psychoactive substance impacts them and the nature of their personal relapse risks. Because guilt and the perception of failure are common for those relapsing, early intervention can facilitate more realistic self-appraisal and provide hope for more effective responding in future relapse risk situations. With regard to the latter, relapse prevention strategies of improved risk identification and coping skill rehearsal may be particularly helpful.

A third way to enhance success following treatment of adolescent substance abuse is to support nontraditional abstinence efforts of teens. Although participation in 12-step and other support-oriented groups is most predictive of longer term abstinence among adolescents, teens have been found to successfully utilize alternative efforts which result in positive outcomes (Brown, 1993). For example, among younger teens not active in self-help activity, increased involvement within the family has been shown to provide an alternative means whereby youth have been able to sustain addictive behavior change. Thus, to the extent that family resources permit, therapeutic encouragement of family recreational and social activities, as well as routine structured communication opportunities, may provide sufficient environmental structure and emotional support to sustain abstinence efforts. Alternatively, encouragement of early individuation in the family and reduced family contact has proved a viable means to sustain abstinence for some older teens who have not been able to develop a commitment to support-group efforts. Such individuals often come from families with a history of alcohol or other drug abuse among the parents, and they can participate in structured activities outside the family (e.g., work, extracurricular activities, hobbies) which provide drug-free environments and direct rewards for self-esteem-enhancing activities. Although these approaches are used by only a small proportion of teens who abstain for extended periods after treatment, they do offer clinicians alternative strategies for teens who, for whatever reason, will not regularly participate in abstinence-focused support groups.

In closing, clinical efforts following the primary intervention phase appear critical to extended success for adolescent substance abusers. Continued contact during periods of greatest risk for relapse and rapid response in use situations may markedly enhance success rates when working with adolescent substance abusers. Additionally, given the resiliency demonstrated by youth who have relapsed to alcohol or other drug use, and the variety of means through which teens have been found to maintain their abstinence, clinical work with adolescents following substance abuse treatment requires considerable flexibility to maximize treatment success. Support for adolescent efforts to sustain abstinence is critical, as teens have been found to develop successful outcomes by using efforts not traditionally encouraged in treatment programs.

BEHAVIOR CHAIN WORKSHEET

TRIGGER → THOUGHTS → FEELINGS → BEHAVIOR → CONSEQUENCES
POSITIVE   NEGATIVE

ALTERNATIVES

Eric F. Wagner, PhD, is currently Senior Fellow in the Post-Doctoral Training Program in Research on Alcohol Treatment and Intervention at the Center for Alcohol and Addiction Studies at Brown University. His training is in clinical psychology with special interests in the areas of adolescent substance abuse and adolescent risk-taking behavior. He has published several articles on these topics. In 1993, he was the recipient of the New Investigator Award at the Sixth International Conference on Treatment of Addictive Behaviors for his work on the relations among delay of gratification, stress-coping, and substance use in adolescence. Dr. Wagner may be contacted at the Center for Alcohol and Addiction Studies, Brown University Box G-BH, Providence, RI 02912.

Mark G. Myers, PhD, is Assistant Professor of Psychiatry at the University of California, San Diego. Previously, he completed a post-doctoral fellowship at the Brown University Center for Alcohol and Addiction Studies. Dr. Myers is a clinical psychologist whose interests center on adolescent substance abuse and relapse. He has published numerous articles in this area, and recently received a grant from the National Institute on Drug Abuse to study conduct disorder and outcome following adolescent substance abuse treatment. Dr. Myers can be contacted at Psychology 116B, VA Medical Center, 3350 La Jolla Village Drive, San Diego, CA 92161.

Sandra A. Brown, PhD, is Professor of Psychiatry at the University of California, San Diego, and Chief, Psychology Service, Department of Veterans Affairs Medical Center, San Diego. She has conducted extensive research on reinforcement characteristics of various drugs, most notably alcohol, cocaine, and marijuana, and factors affecting the clinical course of addictive disorders for both adolescent and adult substance abusers. Dr. Brown is known nationally for her training workshops on assessment and interventions for addictive disorders. Dr. Brown may be contacted at Psychology Service (116B), VA Medical Center, 3350 La Jolla Village Drive, San Diego, CA 92161.

RESOURCES

Abrams, D. B., & Niaura, R. S. (1987). Social learning theory. In H. T. Blane & K. E. Leonard (Eds.), *Psychological Theories of Drinking and Alcoholism* (pp. 131-172). New York: Guilford.

Addiction Recovery Corporation. (1986). *Guided Rational Adolescent Substance Abuse Profile.* Waltham, MA: Author.

American Psychiatric Association. (1987). *Diagnostic and Statistical Manual of Mental Disorders* (3rd ed. rev.). Washington, DC: Author.

American Psychiatric Association. (1994). *Diagnostic and Statistical Manual of Mental Disorders* (4th ed.). Washington, DC: Author.

Bentler, P. M. (1992). Etiologies and consequences of adolescent drug use: Implications for prevention. *Journal of Addictive Diseases, 11,* 47-61.

Blum, R. W. (1987). Adolescent substance abuse: Diagnostic and treatment issues. *Pediatric Clinics of North America, 34,* 523-537.

Brown, S. A. (1993). Recovery patterns in adolescent substance abuse. In J. S. Baer, G. A. Marlatt, & R. J. McMahon (Eds.), *Addictive Behaviors Across the Lifespan: Prevention, Treatment and Policy Issues* (pp. 161-183). Beverly Hills, CA: Sage.

Brown, S. A., Mott, M. A., & Myers, M. G. (1990). Adolescent drug and alcohol treatment outcome. In R. R. Watson (Ed.), *Prevention and Treatment of Drug and Alcohol Abuse* (pp. 373-403). Clifton, NJ: Humana.

Brown, S. A., Mott, M. A., & Stewart, M. A. (1992). Adolescent alcohol and drug abuse. In C. E. Walker & M. C. Roberts (Eds.), *Handbook of Clinical Child Psychology* (2nd ed., pp. 677-693). New York: John Wiley & Sons.

Brown, S. A., Vik, P. W., & Creamer, V. A. (1989). Characteristics of relapse following adolescent substance abuse treatment. *Addictive Behaviors, 14,* 291-300.

Burns, D. (1981). *Feeling Good: The New Mood Therapy.* New York: Signet.

Christiansen, B. A., Goldman, M. S., & Inn, A. (1982). Development of alcohol-related expectancies in adolescents: Separating pharmacological from social-learning influences. *Journal of Consulting and Clinical Psychology, 50,* 336-344.

Christiansen, B. A., Roehling, P. V., Smith, G. T., & Goldman, M. S. (1989). Using alcohol expectancies to predict adolescent drinking behavior after one year. *Journal of Consulting and Clinical Psychology, 57,* 93-99.

Clarke, G., Lewinsohn, P., & Hops, H. (1990). *Leader's Manual for Adolescent Groups: Adolescent Coping With Depression Course.* Eugene, OR: Castalia.

Cohen, E., MacKenzie, R. G., & Yates, G. L. (1991). HEADDS, a psychosocial risk assessment instrument: Implications for designing effective intervention programs for runaway youth. *Journal of Adolescent Health, 12,* 539-544.

Cohen, M., Karras, A., & Hughes, R. (1977). The usefulness and reliability of a drug severity scale. *International Journal of the Addictions, 12,* 417-422.

Costello, J., Edelbrock, C., & Costello, A. (1984). *The Reliability of the NIMH Diagnostic Interview for Children: A Comparison Between Pediatric and Psychiatric Referrals.* Pittsburgh, PA: Western Psychiatric Institute and Clinic.

Costello, J., Edelbrock, C., & Costello, A. (1985). Validity of the NIMH Diagnostic Interview for Children: A comparison between psychiatric and pediatric referrals. *Journal of Abnormal Child Psychology and Psychiatry, 13,* 579-595.

Donovan, D. M. (1988). Assessment of addictive behaviors: Implications of an emerging biopsychosocial model. In D. M. Donovan & G. A. Marlatt (Eds.), *Assessment of Addictive Behaviors* (pp. 3-50). New York: Guilford.

Donovan, D. M., & Marlatt, G. A. (Eds.). (1988). *Assessment of Addictive Behaviors.* New York: Guilford.

Dunnette, M. D., Peterson, N. G., Houston, J. S., Rosse, R. L., Bosshardt, M. J., & Lammlein, S. E. (1980). *Causes and Consequences of Adolescent Drug Experiences: A Final Report* (Technical Report 58). Minneapolis, MN: Personnel Decisions Research Institute.

Farrell, M., & Strang, J. (1991). Substance use and misuse in childhood and adolescence. *Journal of Child Psychology, Psychiatry, and Allied Disciplines, 32,* 109-128.

Friedman, A. S. (1987). *Adolescent Drug Abuse Diagnosis.* Unpublished manuscript, Philadelphia Psychiatric Center.

Goldman, M. S., Brown, S. A., & Christiansen, B. A. (1987). Expectancy theory: Thinking about drinking. In H. T. Blane & K. E. Leonard (Eds.), *Psychological Theories of Drinking and Alcoholism* (pp. 173-220). New York: Guilford.

Harrell, A. V., Sowder, B., & Kapsak, K. (1988). *Field Validation of Drinking and You: A Screening Instrument for Adolescent Problem Drinking* (Contract No. ADM 281-85-0007). Rockville, MD: National Institute on Alcohol Abuse and Alcoholism.

Harrell, A. V., & Wirtz, P. W. (1989). Screening for adolescent problem drinking: Validation of a multidimensional instrument for case identification. *Psychological Assessment: A Journal of Consulting and Clinical Psychology, 1,* 61-63.

Henly, G. A., & Winters, K. C. (1989). Development of psychosocial scales for the assessment of adolescents involved with alcohol and drugs. *The International Journal of the Addictions, 24,* 973-1001.

Herjanic, B., & Reich, W. (1982). Development of a structured interview for children: Agreement between child and parent on individual symptoms. *Journal of Abnormal Psychology, 10,* 307-324.

Hester, R. K., & Miller, W. R. (1988). Empirical guidelines for optimal client-treatment matching. In E. R. Rahdert & J. Grabowski (Eds.), *Adolescent Drug Abuse: Analyses of Treatment Research* (National Institute on Drug Abuse Research Monograph 77, DHHS Publication No. ADM 88-1523, pp. 27-38). Washington, DC: U.S. Government Printing Office.

Hodges, K. K., Kline, J., Stern, L., Cytryn, L., & McKnew, D. (1982). The development of a child assessment interview for research and clinical use. *Journal of Abnormal Child Psychology, 10,* 173-189.

Holsten, F., & Waal, H. (1980). The DTES -- Drug Taking Evaluation Scale: A simple scale for the evaluation of drug taking behaviour. *Acta Psychiatrica Scandanavica, 61,* 275-305.

Johnston, L. D., O'Malley, P. M., & Bachman, J. G. (1991). *Drug Use Among American High School Seniors, College Students and Young Adults, 1975-1990* (National Institute of Drug Abuse, DHHS Publication No. ADM 91-1813). Washington, DC: U.S. Government Printing Office.

Kadden, R., Carroll, K., Donovan, D., Cooney, N., Monti, P., Abrams, D., Litt, M., & Hester, R. K. (1992). *Cognitive-Behavioral Coping Skills Therapy Manual* (National Institute on Alcohol Abuse and Alcoholism Project MATCH Monograph Series, Vol. 3, DHHS Publication No. ADM 92-1895). Washington, DC: U.S. Government Printing Office.

Kaminer, Y. (1991). Adolescent substance abuse. In R. J. Frances & S. I. Miller (Eds.), *Clinical Textbook of Addictive Disorders* (pp. 320-346). New York: Guilford.

Kaminer, Y., Bukstein, O. G., & Tarter, R. E. (1991). The Teen Addiction Severity Index: Rationale and reliability. *International Journal of the Addictions, 26,* 219-226.

Kaminer, Y., Wagner, E. F., Plummer, B. A., & Seifer, R. (1993). Validation of the Teen Addiction Severity Index (T-ASI): Preliminary findings. *The American Journal on Addictions, 2,* 250-254.

Marlatt, G. A., & Gordon, J. R. (1985). *Relapse Prevention: Maintenance Strategies in the Treatment of Addictive Behaviors.* New York: Guilford.

Mayer, J., & Filstead, W. J. (1979). The Adolescent Alcohol Involvement Scale: An instrument for measuring adolescents' use and misuse of alcohol. *Journal of Studies on Alcohol, 3,* 291-299.

McCrady, B. S., Dean, L., Dubreuil, E., & Swanson, S. (1985). The problem drinkers' project: A programmatic application of social-learning based treatment. In G. A. Marlatt & J. R. Gordon (Eds.), *Relapse Prevention: Maintenance Strategies in the Treatment of Addictive Behaviors* (pp. 417-471). New York: Guilford.

McLellan, A. T., Luborsky, L., Woody, G. E., & O'Brien, C. P. (1980). An improved diagnostic evaluation instrument for substance abuse patients. *Journal of Nervous and Mental Disease, 40,* 620-625.

Miller, W. R. (1989). Matching individuals with interventions. In R. K. Hester & W. R. Miller (Eds.), *Handbook of Alcoholism Treatment Approaches* (pp. 261-272). New York: Pergamon.

Miller, W. R., & Rollnick, S. (Eds.). (1991). *Motivational Interviewing: Preparing People to Change Addictive Behavior.* New York: Guilford.

Monti, P. M., Abrams, D. B., Kadden, R. M., & Cooney, N. L. (1989). *Treating Alcohol Dependence.* New York: Guilford.

Moore, D. (1980). *Client Substance Abuse Index.* Unpublished manuscript, Olympic Counseling Services, Tacoma, WA.

Myers, M. G., & Brown, S. A. (1990a). Coping and appraisal in relapse risk situations among substance abusing adolescents following treatment. *Journal of Adolescent Chemical Dependency, 1,* 95-116.

Myers, M. G., & Brown, S. A. (1990b). Coping responses and relapse among adolescent substance abusers. *Journal of Substance Abuse, 2,* 177-190.

Myers, M. G., & Brown, S. A. (1993, November). *Factor Analysis of an Instrument to Assess Coping in Drug and Alcohol High Risk for Relapse Situations.* Paper presented at the Association for Advancement of Behavior Therapy Annual Meeting, Atlanta, GA.

Myers, M. G., Brown, S. A., & Mott, M. A. (1993). Coping as a predictor of adolescent substance abuse treatment outcome. *Journal of Substance Abuse, 5,* 15-29.

National Institute of Drug Abuse. (1990). *National Household Survey on Drug Abuse: Main Findings 1988* (NIDA, DHHS Publication No. ADM 91-1813). Washington, DC: U.S. Government Printing Office.

Newcomb, M. D., & Bentler, P. M. (1988). *Consequences of Adolescent Drug Use: Impact on the Lives of Young Adults*. Newbury Park, CA: Sage.

Oetting, E. R., & Beauvais, F. (1986). *The American Drug and Alcohol Survey*. Fort Collins, CO: Rocky Mountain Behavioral Sciences Institute.

Orvaschel, H., Puig-Antich, J., Chambers, W., Tabrizi, M. A., & Johnson, R. (1982). Retrospective assessment of prepubertal major depression with the Kiddie-SADS-E. *Journal of the American Academy of Child Psychiatry, 21,* 392-397.

Owen, P., & Nyberg, L. (1983). Assessing alcohol and drug problems among adolescents: Current practice. *Journal of Drug Addiction, 13,* 249-254.

Pandina, R. J., & Schuele, J. A. (1983). Psychosocial correlates of alcohol and drug use of adolescent students and adolescents in treatment. *Journal of Studies on Alcohol, 44,* 950-973.

Petchers, M. K., & Singer, M. I. (1987). Perceived-benefit-of-drinking: An approach to screening for adolescent alcohol abuse. *Journal of Pediatrics, 110,* 977-981.

Petchers, M. K., Singer, M. I., Angelotta, J. W., & Chow, J. (1988). Revalidation and expansion of an adolescent substance abuse screening measure. *Journal of Developmental and Behavioral Pediatrics, 9,* 25-29.

Reich, W., Herjanic, B., Welner, Z., & Gandhy, P. R. (1982). Development of a structured psychiatric interview for children: Agreement on diagnosis comparing child and parent interviews. *Journal of Abnormal Child Psychology, 10,* 325-336.

Richter, S. S., Mott, M. A., & Brown, S. A. (1991). The impact of social support and self-esteem on adolescent substance abuse treatment outcome. *Journal of Substance Abuse, 3,* 371-386.

Robertson, J. F. (1989). A tool for assessing alcohol misuse in adolescence. *Social Work, 34,* 39-44.

Robins, L. N., Helzer, J. E., Croughan, J., & Ratcliff, K. (1981). National Institute of Mental Health Diagnostic Schedule: Its history, characteristics and validity. *Archives of General Psychiatry, 38,* 381-389.

Schwartz, R. H., & Wirtz, P. W. (1990). Potential substance abuse: Detection among adolescent patients: Using the Drug and Alcohol Problem (DAP) Quick Screen, a 30-item questionnaire. *Clinical Pediatrics, 29,* 38-43.

Shedler, J., & Block, J. (1990). Adolescent drug use and psychological health: A longitudinal inquiry. *American Psychologist, 45,* 612-630.

Smart, R., & Jones, D. (1970). Illicit LSD users: Their personality characteristics and psychopathology. *Journal of Abnormal Psychology, 75,* 286-292.

Stewart, D. G., & Brown, S. A. (1993, March). *Withdrawal and Dependency Symptoms Among Adolescent Substance Abusers*. Poster presented at The Society for Behavioral Medicine Annual Meeting, San Francisco, CA.

Stewart, M. A., & Brown, S. A. (1994). Family functioning following adolescent substance abuse treatment. *Journal of Substance Abuse, 5,* 327-339.

Szapocznik, J., Kurtines, W. M., Foote, F. H., Perez-Vidal, A., & Hervis, O. (1986). Conjoint versus one-person family therapy: Further evidence for the effectiveness of conducting family therapy through one person with drug abusing adolescents. *Journal of Consulting and Clinical Psychology, 54,* 395-397.

Szapocznik, J., Perez-Vidal, A., Brickman, A. L., Foote, F. H., Santisteban, D., & Hervis, O. (1988). Engaging adolescent drug abusers and their families in treatment: A strategic structural systems approach. *Journal of Consulting and Clinical Psychology, 56,* 552-557.

Tarter, R. E. (1990). Evaluation and treatment of adolescent substance abuse: A decision tree method. *American Journal of Drug and Alcohol Abuse, 16,* 1-46.

Tarter, R. E., Ott, P. J., & Mezzich, A. C. (1991). Psychometric assessment. In R. J. Frances & S. I. Miller (Eds.), *Clinical Textbook of Addictive Disorders* (pp. 237-267). New York: Guilford.

Vik, P. W., Grizzle, K., & Brown, S. A. (1992). Social resource characteristics and adolescent substance abuse relapse. *Journal of Adolescent Chemical Dependency, 2,* 59-74.

Waal, H., & Holsten, F. (1980). Evaluation of drug taking behaviour. *Acta Psychiatrica Scandanavica, 61,* 127-134.

White, H. R., & Labouvie, E. W. (1989). Towards the assessment of adolescent problem drinking. *Journal of Studies on Alcohol, 50,* 30-37.

Winters, K. C. (1990). The need for improved assessment of adolescent substance use involvement. *Journal of Drug Issues, 20,* 487-502.

Winters, K. C. (1991). *The Personal Experience Screening Questionnaire.* Los Angeles: Western Psychological Services.

Winters, K. C., & Henly, G. A. (1989). *Personal Experience Inventory.* Los Angeles, CA: Western Psychological Services.

ASSESSMENT AND TREATMENT OF ATTENTION-DEFICIT/ HYPERACTIVITY DISORDER IN CHILDREN

Gerald McMullen, David T. Painter, and Thomas J. Casey

All therapists dealing with children should have a solid working knowledge of diagnostic and treatment issues regarding Attention-Deficit/Hyperactivity Disorder (ADHD). ADHD is one of the most common reasons for referring children to mental health practitioners (Barkley, 1990). The disorder is estimated to exist for 3% to 5% of school-aged children, and is found in a much higher percentage among those who are referred to clinics. ADHD children experience a great deal of social and emotional stress and frustration because of problems imposed by this condition. Performance problems associated with ADHD manifest themselves in family, school, and other social or work-related situations.

This contribution will provide an overview of ADHD for practitioners. Those interested in more detailed analyses are encouraged to read Barkley (1990), S. Goldstein and M. Goldstein (1990), Fowler (1992), Parker (1992), or recent issues of professional journals (e.g., "Council for Exceptional Children," 1993; "National Association of School Psychologists," 1991) that have focused on ADHD.

Despite abundant literature regarding ADHD, the disorder's definition, prevalence, and presumed neurological underpinnings still are debated. Reid, Maag, and Vasa (1993) assert that ADHD diagnosis is societally driven. They state, "Medical classifications appease everyone because they exculpate physicians, parents, teachers, and administrators of responsibility. Medical classifications are, in essence, 'no fault' labels. Even the child cannot be culpable because his or her academic failures now can be attributed to some organic etiology rather than lack of effort or motivation" (p. 208). To support their perspective, they cite Rutter's (1983) finding that children in the United States are 50 times more likely to be diagnosed ADHD than children in England and France. From a more moderate perspective, Achenbach (1980) cautions that our efforts to define childhood psychiatric disorders "represent provisional, state-of-the-art compromises with ignorance rather than definitive achievements" (p. 396). This caution holds true for ADHD.

DEFINITION

The diagnosis of overactivity, impulsivity, and inattention among children can be traced through definitional changes in the *Diagnostic and Statistical Manual of Mental Disorders* (*DSM*) published by the American Psychiatric Association. Definitional changes in the various *DSM* editions were, of course, influenced by research findings and hypotheses generated by clinical experience. *DSM-II* (American Psychiatric Association [APA], 1968) included the diagnostic classification Hyperkinetic Reaction of Childhood Disorder. This brief and simplistic definition emphasized the excessive activity level of these children. The only diagnostic decision to be made was whether or not the general syndrome was present.

Among influential research conducted after the publication of *DSM-II* was that of Douglas and her colleagues at McGill University. By 1979, Douglas and Peters suggested that the four most important characteristics of attention-disordered children were (a) inattention and distractibility, (b) overarousal, (c) impulsivity, and (d) difficulty delaying gratification. The diagnostic and treatment implications of this research were reflected in *DSM-III* (APA, 1980).

DSM-III contained the diagnostic category Attention Deficit Disorder (ADD). The features essential for ADD diagnosis were developmentally inappropriate levels of inattention and impulsivity. Two major subtypes were identified: Attention Deficit Disorder With Hyperactivity (ADD/+H) and Attention Deficit Disorder Without Hyperactivity (ADD/-H). ADD/+H was diagnosed when there were developmentally inappropriate levels of inattention, impulsivity, and hyperactivity. Hyperactivity was manifested by difficulty sitting still and "running like a motor," although the latter trait could diminish with maturation. Symptoms were clearly outlined and numerical cutoff scores were established in the areas of inattention (exhibiting at least three of five symptoms), impulsivity (exhibiting at least three of six symptoms), and hyperactivity (exhibiting at least two of five symptoms). Onset of symptoms must have occurred before age 7, and duration of symptoms had to be at least 6 months. ADD/-H required the same diagnostic criteria as ADD/+H, with the exception of meeting the cutoff criterion for hyperactivity. This system of identification shifted clinical decision making from the syndrome level to the symptom level, with specified scores required to determine classification.

Substantial changes in diagnostic criteria for ADD were made when *DSM-III* was revised (*DSM-III-R*, APA, 1987). The disorder was renamed Attention Deficit Hyperactivity Disorder (ADHD). The ADD/-H subcategory was eliminated; children formerly classified ADD/-H could be diagnosed as Undifferentiated Attention-Deficit Disorder (UADD). The three lists of symptoms for inattention, impulsivity, and hyperactivity were replaced with a single list on which 8 of 14 symptoms, or behavioral characteristics, must be present for at least 6 months, with onset before age 7 for diagnostic classification. Criteria are delineated for mild, moderate, and severe levels of the disorder based upon the pervasiveness and number of symptoms.

Upon publication, *DSM-III-R* quickly received criticism. Werry (1988) claimed that the new criteria were "hastily derived" and "largely untested." The single list of 14 symptoms was seen as heavily weighted toward impulsivity and hyperactivity, with 10 of the 14 symptoms related to impulsivity, hyperactivity, or behavior problems. Failure to include ADD/+H and ADD/-H as separate categories was viewed by many as a serious mistake, because several studies indicated that these are distinctly different disorders in children (Edelbrock, Costello, & Kessler, 1984; Lahey et al., 1987).

DSM-IV (American Psychiatric Association, 1994) maintains the label Attention Deficit Hyperactivity Disorder (ADHD) and many of the symptoms (behavioral characteristics) that appeared in *DSM-III-R*; however, the symptoms are divided into two lists.

The first list, *Inattention*, includes the following nine symptoms (abbreviated): (a) fails to give close attention to details or makes careless mistakes; (b) has difficulty sustaining attention; (c) does not seem to listen when spoken to directly; (d) does not follow through on instructions and fails to finish duties; (e) has difficulty organizing tasks and activities; (f) avoids, dislikes, or is reluctant to engage in tasks that require sustained mental effort; (g) loses things necessary for tasks or activities; (h) is often easily distracted by extraneous stimuli; and (i) is often forgetful.

The second symptom list, *Hyperactivity-Impulsivity*, contains the following behavioral characteristics (abbreviated): (a) fidgets or squirms, (b) leaves seat in situations in which remaining seated is expected; (c) runs about or climbs excessively; (d) has difficulty playing or engaging in leisure activities quietly; (e) acts as if "driven by a motor"; talks excessively; (g) blurts out answers before questions have been completed; (h) has difficulty awaiting turn; and (i) interrupts or intrudes on others. The first six items relate primarily to hyperactivity, and the last three relate primarily to impulsivity.

For diagnostic purposes, six (or more) symptoms from the Inattention and/or Hyperactivity-Impulsivity lists must persist for at least 6 months to a degree that is maladaptive and inconsistent with developmental level. In addition, some of the symptoms causing impairment must be present before age 7 years; some impairment must be present in two or more settings (e.g., home and school); and there must be clear evidence of impairment in social, academic, or occupational functioning. ADHD is not diagnosed if symptoms occur exclusively during the course of a Pervasive Developmental Disorder, Psychotic Disorder, other mental disorders, or in relation to the use of medications (e.g., bronchodilators).

According to the number of symptoms manifested, individuals can be diagnosed as one of three ADHD types. Those exhibiting six of the nine symptoms on both Inattentive and Hyperactivity-Impulsivity lists are classified *ADHD, Combined Type* (similar to ADHD under the *DSM-III-R* classification). Those meeting six of nine symptoms on the Inattention list are classified *ADHD, Predominantly Inattentive Type* (similar to ADD/-H). Those meeting six of nine symptoms on the Hyperactivity-Impulsivity list are classified *ADHD, Predominantly Hyperactive-Impulsive Type*. There also is a category of *ADHD, Not Otherwise Specified*, for individuals with prominent symptoms of inattention or hyperactivity-impulsivity who do not fully meet criteria for the three major ADHD types.

PREVALENCE

DSM-IV states that ADHD occurs in 3% to 5% of school-age children; furthermore, the disorder is estimated to be four times more common among males than females in community samples, and nine times more common in males in clinic samples.

ETIOLOGY

The primary cause of ADHD appears to be heredity. Goodman and Stevenson (1989) estimate that heritability for ADHD traits accounts for 30% to 50% of variance, while common environmental factors account for up to 30%. Fewer than 5% of ADHD children have hard evidence of neurological impairment (Ferguson & Rapoport, 1983). Large-scale studies indicate that difficulties during pregnancy, labor, or delivery, or factors such as birth weight or low Apgar score do not place children at significant risk for ADHD (Parker, 1992). Environmental toxins (e.g., lead poisoning) and maternal alcohol consumption or cigarette smoking during pregnancy may be the cause of ADHD for a small percentage of children. There is no research evidence to suggest that dietary intake of refined sugar or food additives (as per Feingold, 1975) are significant contributors to attentional deficits (S. Goldstein & M. Goldstein, 1990). Inattention and hyperactivity can be side-effects of antiseizure medications, especially phenobarbital and diphenylhydantoin (Dilantin; Committee on Drugs, 1985).

NEUROLOGICALLY BASED CAUSATIVE HYPOTHESES

Throughout this century it has been suspected that atypically high levels of inattention, impulsivity, and hyperactivity in children have a neurological basis. Riccio et al. (1993) summarized findings from three perspectives regarding the neurological bases of ADHD: neuroanatomical, neurochemical, and neurophysiological.

The neuroanatomical approach emphasizes the importance of specific areas of the brain (frontal lobe, caudate nucleus in the basal ganglia, and right hemisphere) associated with the regulation of attention, impulsivity, and hyperactivity.

The neurochemical approach explores the role of neurochemistry in facilitating communication among neuronal circuits. Neurochemical research has pointed to the importance of dopamine and norepinephrine (e.g., Zametkin & Rapoport, 1987). These catecholamine neurotransmitters serve an inhibitory function that can influence attention, behavioral inhibition, and motor activity.

Those espousing a neurophysiological approach feel that neurological explanations of ADHD must consider the interaction of neuroanatomy and neurochemistry. Riccio et al. (1993) discuss the hypothesis that "certain ascending/arousal and descending/inhibitory pathways (e.g., the loops that connect the frontal lobes, basal ganglia, and thalamus) constitute a system that activates/inactivates other brain regions" (p. 121). Disruption of function along the ascending/arousal loop could interfere with the level of arousal to specific regions of the cerebral cortex. Interruption along the descending/inhibitory loop could diminish inhibition or selective attention.

IDENTIFICATION

According to Connors (1975) there are no critical tests, few exclusionary developmental criteria, and no unequivocal positive developmental markers for ADHD. The "symptoms" of ADHD are behavioral characteristics, many of which are natural for children, especially young children. ADHD presents a major diagnostic challenge because key symptoms (inattentiveness, impulsivity, and high activity levels) can result from disparate factors including maturation, poor behavior management, inappropriate environmental demands, lack of motivation, oppositionality, intolerance of those reporting the behaviors, or actual ADHD.

Because of the complexity of ADHD and its identification, a multifaceted approach to diagnosis should be used. D. M. Ross and S. A. Ross (1982) suggest that intensity, persistence, and clustering of symptoms should form the basis for diagnosis. Techniques useful for ADHD diagnosis are behavioral observations, parent interviews, teacher interviews, behavior rating scales, situational questionnaires, psychoeducational testing, and medical evaluation. Barkley (1991) provides a compendium of evaluative techniques, approaches to rating behaviors, and interview and observation forms in his clinical workbook.

DIRECT OBSERVATIONS

Practitioners usually see patients in their offices, not in the settings where ADHD symptoms typically occur. Some children who are very hyperactive exhibit ADHD behavioral characteristics in office settings. Children classified ADHD, Predominantly Inattentive Type, often do not manifest symptoms in office settings where they encounter a relatively high level of individual attention, few competing distractions, and a narrow range of task demands. Observing the child in school or at home can provide a great deal of understanding and insight; however, on-site observations are time-consuming, and the observer is an intervening variable whose presence may alter behaviors.

PARENT INTERVIEWS

Parent interviews are essential to the ADHD diagnostic process. Whenever possible, it is beneficial to interview both parents to obtain their individual perspectives and to explore differences that may exist between them. This interview should determine if the child exhibits behavioral characteristics associated with ADHD and the cross-situational persistence or variability of these characteristics. Age of onset and duration of ADHD symptoms also must be established. Medical, developmental, social, and educational background should be obtained. Because heredity is believed to be a primary causative factor, background history must include whether ADHD symptoms are present in other family members.

TEACHER INTERVIEWS

It is not until confronted with demands imposed by formal education that behavioral characteristics of many children are perceived as problematic. The high incidence of school referrals for ADHD screening underscores the fact that ADHD is a disorder manifested in reciprocal interaction between the child and environmental demands. Teachers are valuable informants about the interaction of the child and the school environment where problems have occurred. The perspectives of several teachers who deal with the child can be helpful, but it must be kept in mind that teachers' tolerance for behaviors associated with ADHD vary tremendously. Areas to be explored with teachers include the child's academic, social, and emotional adjustment, and the persistence or situational variability of symptoms.

BEHAVIOR RATING SCALES

There is a growing number of rating scales to assess children's behavior; many are available in parent and teacher versions. Use of these scales is enticing because they are time-effective and inexpensive; furthermore, they yield standardized scores with interpretive guidelines. It is good practice to administer a broad-banded behavior rating scale such as the Child Behavior Checklist (Achenbach & Edelbrock, 1991) or the Devereux Behavior Rating Scale (Naglieri, LeBuffe, & Pfeiffer, 1993) as a first step in differential diagnosis. If ADHD is suspected, administration of a rating scale specifically designed to investigate ADHD characteristics, such as the Connors' Rating Scales (Connors, 1990) or the Attention Deficit Disorders Evaluation Scale (McCarney, 1989), is warranted.

Research supports a cautious approach in the interpretation of scores from behavior rating scales. Morriss (1992) emphatically states that rating scales should never be used as "tests" for ADHD because they lead to overidentification (false positives). Barkley (1989) found that even the best ADHD rating scales had only a moderate correlation (.30 to .50) with actual behavioral observations of ADHD symptoms in home or school settings. Interrater agreement is unacceptably low for diagnostic purposes. For example, rating scale reliability coefficients between parents and teachers are less than .50, and those between mothers and fathers are in the .60 to .70 range (Achenbach, McConaughy, & Howell, 1987). These findings suggest that variability among informants' ratings should be anticipated. Differences may result from situational demands such as setting, task requirements, and interpersonal dynamics. Comparison of individual item ratings obtained from different informants provides valuable understanding of how the child is perceived by significant adults in his or her life and reveals information about the dynamics of the relationship with each informant. Item level analysis also is useful for designing treatment/intervention plans. Rating scales should be just one of multiple information sources considered for ADHD identification.

SITUATION QUESTIONNAIRES

Refinement of a treatment plan sometimes requires delineation of where and/or under what circumstances symptoms arise. Barkley's clinical workbook (Barkley, 1991) provides copies of his Home Situations Questionnaire and School Situations Questionnaire, which originally were designed to obtain information about oppositional, defiant, or aggressive behavior. Also included in the workbook are revised questionnaires that specifically target Attention Deficit Disorder With and Without Hyperactivity. These revisions by DuPaul (1991) yield four scores: (a) number of problem settings, (b) mean severity, (c) compliance situations, and (d) leisure situations. These scores can provide useful information with regard to number and pervasiveness of symptoms.

PSYCHOEDUCATIONAL TESTING

Cognitive, academic, and affective abilities will directly impact a child's behavior, particularly when dealing with school and school-related work. Psychoeducational assessment can provide valuable information about these abilities; however, there is no unique test scoring pattern for the differential diagnosis of ADHD. To associate ADHD with depressed scores on an ability dimension such as the freedom from distractibility factor on the Wechsler Intelligence Scale for Children-III (WISC-III) has intuitive appeal; however, a review of research involving earlier versions of the WISC (McMullen, 1989) found this factor typically was depressed for samples of children with learning disabilities, social/emotional disturbance, and mental retardation. Although

ADHD may have coexisted with other disabilities among subjects in these samples, the prevalence of depressed freedom-from-distractibility-factor scores across educational exceptionalities precludes its presence as a means of differential diagnosis. Psychoeducational test results must be carefully integrated with information obtained through other sources.

MEDICAL EVALUATION

Physicians are important members of the diagnostic and treatment team for children with ADHD. As with other specialists involved in the process of identifying ADHD, physicians are constrained by the necessity of determining the presence or absence of symptoms that are behavioral characteristics. There is no definitive medical test for ADHD. Electroencephalogram (EEG), computerized axial tomography (CT) scans, and magnetic resonance imaging (MRI) are inconclusive for identification of ADHD; furthermore, only about 5% of ADHD children have hard evidence of neurological dysfunction (Parker, 1992). Physicians must not only examine the patient, but also spend time gathering information from parents and others having pertinent involvement. Adequate diagnosis and treatment of ADHD demands collaborative effort.

SPECIAL EDUCATION ELIGIBILITY

Public Law 94-142 (the Education for all Handicapped Children Act; EHA, 1975) did not include ADHD as a special education classification. During 1990 when Congress accepted input for amendments as part of the reauthorization of EHA, there was impetus to designate ADHD as a separate special education classification; however, PL 94-142's revision, Part B of the Individuals With Disabilities Act (IDEA), did not introduce ADHD as a special education classification.

In September 1991, the U.S. Department of Education issued a policy memorandum (Davila, Williams, & MacDonald, 1991) to clarify services available to address the needs of ADHD children within general or special education programs. In summary, this memorandum states that ADHD children may qualify for special assistance or accommodations in general education under Section 504 of the Rehabilitation Act of 1973 if they are considered "handicapped persons." The Section 504 regulation defines a "handicapped person" as anyone who has a physical or mental impairment which substantially limits a major life activity (e.g., learning). Furthermore, the memorandum specifies that under IDEA, ADHD children who meet criteria for an established special education classification (e.g., learning disability, serious emotional disturbance) are eligible for special education and related services. ADHD children also can be classified under the special education category "other health impaired" if the condition is a chronic or acute health problem that results in limited alertness, which adversely affects educational performance.

This memorandum has significant implications for educational programming. Schools must be sensitive to meeting the needs of ADHD students under both special education regulations and the antidiscrimination requirements assured in Section 504. This does not mean that all students identified as ADHD are automatically eligible for special services; it means that school districts are obliged to systematically determine needs and eligibility.

SCHOOL-BASED INTERVENTIONS AND SERVICES

GENERAL PRACTICES

Inclusive. The current trend in education is to provide all children the opportunity to receive instruction in the least restrictive classroom environment. Children with special needs, including those with attention problems, should be provided with assessment, intervention, and support services with the goal of maintaining their placement in regular education classes with their peers.

Team Approach. Because children with attention disorders are a heterogenous group with potential for multiple comorbid conditions, a collaborative multidisciplinary team approach best provides the basis for comprehensive strategies and services. Most schools are familiar with a child study team, instructional support team, or individualized educational plan (IEP) team approach to assessment, consultation, and intervention. Typically these teams include personnel such as a school psychologist, guidance counselor, teacher, principal, special education teacher, school nurse, speech and language clinician, and reading specialist. Parents can actively participate in team meetings and request involvement of child advocates and/or private clinicians.

Service Plans. When children with attention disorders are also eligible for special education services, an IEP with specific goals and objectives must be developed and implemented by the school. Conditions relevant to attention and school performance problems should be addressed in the IEP. When children with attention disorders are considered handicapped through Section 504 of the Rehabilitation Act of 1973, a service delivery plan with specific goals and objectives designed to prevent discrimination on the basis of the child's handicap must be developed. When children attending school are identified as having an attention disorder that interferes with school performance, a team assessment and team-derived service plan are considered essential elements of best practice. Private practitioners can make significant contributions to this process by providing practical recommendations relevant to the individual child.

Family Involvement. Families play a vital role in the identification and management of ADHD. By definition, children with ADHD have an early onset of problems that are chronic in nature. Their parents and families have the most complete developmental perspective of the manner in which the attention disorder is expressed. When service plans are developed, families are in a unique position to identify salient features of motivation and performance. Children with attention problems benefit most from ordered and consistent environments. When parents are actively involved with the specification of school-based interventions, behavioral expectations and contingencies between school and home can be made more consistent, and options for positive reinforcement of goals accomplished at school can be maximized.

Continuous Assessment. It has been said that children with attention problems are consistent only in their inconsistency. For long-term effectiveness, intervention plans must be continually monitored and modified. There should be some mechanism by which all stakeholders (including the child) are informed of progress and the need to modify plans.

Promising Programs. Burcham, Carlson, and Milich (1993) reported eight themes in promising field-based practices that should be considered when developing educational plans for students with ADHD.

1. Before implementing a program or practice, one should determine whether implementing a change in the educational design is likely to have a positive effect. Further, one should begin to evaluate how one knows that change has occurred and account for maintenance and generalization.
2. It is important to note if the strategy has practical value in school or home situations. Experimental interventions that are conducted in controlled laboratory settings may effect positive change; however, the reality of school life may prohibit the use of such practice. Issues such as enhanced academic and/or behavioral performance as well as acquisition, maintenance, and generalization of skills should be considered when determining if an intervention has practical meaning.

3. At least one of the three major components of ADHD (inattention, impulsivity, and overactivity) must be addressed. These factors influence children's academic performance as well as their behavior. Ideally, there should be an attempt to address these issues early in a child's educational career.
4. Many practices concentrate on the child's, the parent's, the school's, or the community's weaknesses, without appropriate consideration of assets. Practices that show promise focus also on the strengths of individuals or groups involved.
5. The work of identifying and intervening with students with ADHD should be a team accomplishment. To achieve positive educational outcomes for children with ADHD, school personnel, families, and community service providers must work together.
6. Better outcomes for students with ADHD can be achieved from practices that proactively plan for continuous, positive parental involvement in the assessment and intervention process.
7. Evaluations and interventions used with students with ADHD from diverse cultures should address potential bias in assessment procedures, tease out language issues that may be contributing to inattention, and develop interventions that are sensitive to the child's background.
8. Pharmacological intervention is the most common form of treatment for children with ADHD, and schools play a critical role in monitoring its use. Physicians often need behavioral data to assist in determining the need for the medication as well as school-based data to adjust dosages. In addition, schools often provide the best vantage point for observing and reporting side-effects of medication.

CLASSROOM METHODS

Behavior Management. Stimulant medication is the most frequent form of treatment for children with attention disorders, and reportedly it is effective in 80% to 90% of cases (DuPaul & Barkley, 1990; Pelham et al., 1993). Research indicates that stimulant medication is even more effective when combined with behavior management techniques (Gittelman-Klein et al., 1980). Pelham et al. (1993) found that behavioral interventions added to the utility of medication in 41% of cases.

Behavior management techniques are the second most consistently effective form of treatment for attention deficit disorders (Barkley, 1990; S. Goldstein & Ingersoll, 1993). Off-task behaviors are probably the most frequent targets for behavior intervention. Barkley (1990) cautions that targeting off-task behaviors does not guarantee improvement in academic performance. A comprehensive plan, which is generally the recommended approach for behavior change, should consider the child's classroom conduct, academic performance, and social skills. When making specific recommendations for behavior management programs, clinicians need to be sensitive to ease of implementation and time demands imposed on teachers or other school personnel.

Behavior management approaches for children with attention problems generally have focused on characteristics of the classroom environment and learning tasks (antecedents; Abramowitz & O'Leary, 1991). Early work in modifying classroom environments for ADHD children attempted to reduce stimulation through the use of study carrels and barren, muted classrooms. These practices, which were largely ineffective, have been abandoned because of their unfairness to non-ADHD classmates and their stigmatizing effect on ADHD children. Abramowitz and O'Leary (1991) concluded that no studies have specifically examined the effect of classroom seating arrangements for ADHD children. Generally, clustered seating increases social interaction but interferes with on-task behavior during independent work for all children. Circle seating can increase participation in teacher-led discussions, while sitting in rows can improve productivity for independent work. Common sense dictates that preferred seating near the teacher for the ADHD child provides more opportunities for teacher monitoring and one-to-one intervention.

The impact of task characteristics on the behavior of ADHD children also has been examined. Classroom noise, difficult tasks, and tasks paced by others (as opposed to self-paced) have been found to detract from on-task behavior (Whalen et al., 1979). Zentall (1993) argues that children with attention problems are more accurately described as having an "attentional bias" as opposed to an attention disorder. Using her "optimal stimulation theory," Zentall has shown that novelty and stimulation using color, shape, and texture enhancers can improve performance on easy and repetitive tasks, but not for new or difficult tasks for ADHD children.

Barkley (1993) investigated the effect of consequences or contingencies on the behavior of ADHD children and found that ADHD children generally require consequences that are more immediate, more powerful or tangible, and more frequent than those for other children. An exhaustive review of contingency management literature pertaining to ADHD children is beyond the scope of this contribution. Major approaches to consequences or contingencies that clinicians should consider include positive reinforcement, response cost, reprimands, token systems, home and school communication, and self-management.

Teacher attention often is presumed to be the most commonly dispensed positive reinforcer in the classroom. Verbal praise alone is unlikely to significantly alter or effectively manage the behavior of ADHD children. Abramowitz and O'Leary (1991) found that prudent reprimands for off-task behaviors combined with positive attention for desirable behaviors is more effective than positive attention techniques alone.

Token, check mark, or point systems have appeal for classroom application because of their relative ease of use and possible inclusion of a response cost component. Token systems can be applied to the entire class, involve individual or group contingencies, be implemented during portions of the day, and utilize a variety of back-up reinforcers administered at school and at home. The challenge is to design a program that targets relevant behaviors and consistently results in the child's earning more points than are lost. If a deficit economy results, the token system should be revised immediately to include more salient back-up reinforcers, lower criteria for reward, or shorter intervals for reward. Token systems often have problems associated with generalization and transfer. There is very little evidence of spontaneous generalization or transfer to settings where the system is not being employed. Sending daily or weekly report cards to parents provides useful feedback and facilitates dispensing of back-up reinforcers. These reports should include only a few target behaviors that are defined in specific, positive terms (e.g., "raises hand before talking" instead of "does not call out").

Self-management approaches appeal to teachers, families, and clinicians because ADHD children are trained to assume responsibility for monitoring and reinforcing their own behavior. These approaches can be regarded as cognitive-behavioral and contingency management because elements of both are combined when ADHD children participate in measurement of behaviors, determination of reaching criteria, and delivery of rewards. Fantuzzo and Polite (1990) reviewed 30 studies of self-management procedures and discovered that a majority were primarily teacher managed. Teachers and practitioners need to understand that students, especially younger ones, need a great deal of assistance to establish realistic goals and criteria and learn techniques of observation and recording. Similar to token systems, self-management strategies must include mechanisms for transfer and generalization of behaviors between settings.

A relatively simple self-management approach requires that the ADHD child rate himself or herself on a 3-point scale for one, two, or three target behaviors. The teacher also rates the target behaviors on the same 3-point scale. Bonus points may be awarded for agreement of student and teacher ratings, and penalty points may be deducted when student ratings are inflated. When appropriate, teacher ratings are faded to a random or intermittent schedule.

Self-management strategies and behavior contracting are approaches that may be more applicable to older children and adolescents. Very few educational interventions for ADHD adolescents in regular education programs have been researched. Generally, it is agreed that adolescents should be included in the planning and implementation of strategies in order to avoid countercontrol behaviors.

Self-Instruction. Cognitive-behavioral strategies employ variations of the well-known "Stop-Look-Think" sequence pioneered for impulsive, acting-out children. These strategies have fallen short of expectations when implemented with ADHD children, perhaps because original expectations were unrealistic. To promote success, cognitive-behavioral strategies must be tightly focused on specific tasks in specific settings. For example, it is much more realistic to expect a child to learn a self-instruction strategy for checking the operation sign of a math problem before solving it (a specific task in a specific setting) than it is to expect a child to learn a self-instruction strategy for responding to teasing (a subjective, interpretive task across social settings). Generally, in order to anticipate success, practitioners should consider the following: self-instruction must be designed to increase a specific skill, self-instruction should be in the child's own words, and self-instruction must be modeled, monitored, and reinforced.

Social Skills Training. These highly structured programs usually are taught in small groups by specially trained facilitators. Their underlying theory is that certain children do not have an adequate repertoire of pro-social behaviors for effective interpersonal relations. This is not a safe assumption for all children with attention disorders; ADHD is primarily a disorder of performance, not of skill deficit. Many ADHD children can state appropriate responses to social situations, but have severe difficulty applying their knowledge. To maximize effectiveness, social skills training for ADHD children should be close to the point of performance. Group social skills training in clinic settings may help ADHD children by providing a positive social experience, but transfer of skills to more naturalistic settings cannot be expected without specific mechanisms designed to promote it.

Peer-Mediated Approaches. Attention to tasks is enhanced for ADHD children when active responses are required, when performance feedback is immediate and individualized, when tasks are matched to students' abilities, and when instruction is self-paced. Cooperative learning activities potentially meet all of the preceding criteria. DuPaul and Henningson (1993) report successful use of peer tutoring with ADHD children. They list the following components for effective peer tutoring: contains a high degree of structure; provides immediate feedback; offers error correction procedures; tallies points and charts progress; and includes monitoring by the classroom teacher.

Parent Training. Many parents of ADHD children do not have extensive knowledge of behavior management or behavior problem-solving techniques. It can be beneficial to provide training designed to develop and refine attitudes and parenting skills with regard to ADHD behavioral characteristics. A comprehensive rationale, theoretical considerations, and parent training prototypes are presented in Barkley's (1990) text. Parent training programs should be customized to the age (or developmental level) of the ADHD child, the severity of ADHD symptoms (and comorbid conditions), and, to some extent, the experiences and needs of the families involved. Parent training programs usually involve an overview of the disorder, behavior management concepts, opportunities for application of skills and critical feedback, opportunities for parents to express feelings and attitudes, communication skills, and problem-solving approaches.

COMORBIDITY AND MEDICAL INTERVENTION

The processes of attention, behavioral inhibition, and motoric regulation are complex; determination of when these normally occurring processes reach levels of significance for ADHD diagnosis provides considerable challenge. The fact that ADHD often coexists with other disorders increases this challenge. Szatmari, Offord, and Boyle (1989) estimate that ADHD occurs with at least one other psychiatric disorder in up to 44% of cases; therefore, practitioners must be sensitive to the unique array of symptoms for each patient. Because of the complexity of ADHD, a physician's involvement is often vital for identification and treatment. This section, written from a physician's perspective, provides an overview of important coexisting conditions that form the basis for ADHD subclassifications and suggests psychopharmacological interventions to treat them.

ATTENTION-DEFICIT/HYPERACTIVITY DISORDER SUBCLASSIFICATIONS

Children with attention deficit disorders may exhibit multiple symptoms. When symptoms cluster distinctly, different subtypes of ADHD classification are suggested. As with any classification scheme, distinctions may be somewhat artificial because there are areas where one subtype blends into another.

Subclassification of children with ADHD has implications for diagnostic interviewing, diagnosis, and treatment. Standard procedure for recording medical history of a child suspected of having attention deficit disorder should include questioning parents about a variety of behavioral symptoms and problems. If parents report one symptom, it should be determined if the child has related symptoms. This additional information helps to develop a complete diagnostic picture of the child. The grouping of symptoms influences treatment with medication and other modalities. Subclassification also helps parents understand where their child fits into the complex of all children with attention deficit disorders.

Attention-Deficit/Hyperactivity Disorder-Uncomplicated. This condition is clearly genetic. There is often a history of symptoms in male relatives on one or both sides of the family; symptoms are found less often among female relatives. The reported ratio of affected males to females is approximately 4 to 1. In families of children with ADHD, mothers and fathers seem to be more equally affected than the reported male preponderance suggests. Fathers are more often described by other family members as hyperactive or as having been hyperactive in childhood, while mothers may report difficulties with organization and focus.

In ADHD-Uncomplicated, significant problems usually involve short attention span, distractibility, and impulsivity - traits that interfere with school performance. Parents may not view their child as having problems before entering elementary school. In many cases where hyperactivity is not extreme, families have learned to adapt to a child's activity level. Problems may not be pronounced in social, family, or sports activities outside of school.

Even without treatment, hyperactivity improves with age. Physical restlessness may diminish or disappear during adolescence. Distractibility and short attention span also may improve without treatment, but to a lesser degree. Even though attention span has improved, increased attentional demands at higher grade levels present a continuing challenge to ADHD students; therefore, academic achievement may suffer. Impulsivity also remains a problem. Frequency of disciplinary problems may increase in middle school and high school for some ADHD students.

Children with ADHD-Uncomplicated are very likely to respond well to stimulant medications such as methylphenidate (Ritalin), pemoline (Cylert), or dextroamphetamine (Dexedrine). Clonidine (an antihypertensive medication) is often a useful addition to the pharmacological regimen for children with marked hyperactivity that is only partly responsive to stimulants.

Attention-Deficit/Hyperactivity Disorder, Predominantly Inattentive Type. Parker (1992) claims that 30% of ADD children fall into *DSM-III-R*'s UADD category (ergo ADD/-H or ADHD, Predominantly Inattentive Type). *DSM-IV*'s inclusion of ADHD, Predominantly Inattentive Type suggests that the view of ADD without hyperactivity as a distinct subtype of attention deficit disorder has validity.

As a group, ADHD, Predominantly Inattentive Type children are less impulsive, less active, and less aggressive than ADHD children with hyperactivity. Because of this, they may experience less overt social antagonism and conflict than ADHD, Predominantly Hyperactive-Impulsive Type children; however, their social interactions may be passive and awkward. Other problems may include disorganization, inability to finish tasks, need for external structure and guidance, clumsiness, and learning problems. Differential diagnosis in these cases should attempt to rule out the presence of depression and nonverbal (perceptually based) learning disabilities.

Stimulant medication can be useful for treating ADHD, Predominantly Inattentive Type children. Necessary educational and social supports should be provided to assure needs in these areas are addressed.

Attention-Deficit/Hyperactivity Disorder With Oppositionality. ADHD With Oppositionality is another subgroup of children frequently seen in clinical practice. In addition to difficulty with inattention, impulsivity, and hyperactivity, these children exhibit negative, hostile, and/or defiant behaviors.

These children often present oppositionality during preschool years; however, it is typically during the early elementary grades that they are referred for medical evaluation. Although they may have few or no academic difficulties, social interactions frequently are problematic. These children have difficulty perceiving other points of view and fail to see why their own behavior is unreasonable. Such weaknesses limit effectiveness for developing strategies to reduce or curb negative social interactions. Considerable effort must be dedicated to teaching them what is and what is not socially acceptable. ADHD With Oppositionality children tend to elicit negative or punitive responses from authority figures at home and in school.

Although symptoms of distractibility and hyperactivity generally respond well to the use of methylphenidate or other stimulant medications, this group's impulsivity and oppositional behaviors respond less consistently. In many cases, other kinds of medication are needed to address these symptoms.

Attention-Deficit/Hyperactivity Disorder and the Angry Child With Symptoms of Depression. This group of children blends into the previous classification of ADHD With Oppositionality; the distinction, in fact, may be artificial. Complaints bringing these children to medical attention typically are related to ADHD symptoms, but problems in social relationships with adults and peers also are salient. They often verbally or physically abuse their parents, particularly their mothers. They habitually complain of unfairness or favoritism displayed to siblings. They may seem insatiable in their demand for attention and material possessions. Episodes of aggressive behavior and destruction of property may occur beyond the age at which tantrums are common.

These children have an increased likelihood of family histories of depression in parents, grandparents, aunts, or uncles. It seems possible that this complex of ADHD and angry, oppositional behavior might represent a precursor to what will appear as depression in adolescence and adulthood. Although behavioral symptoms have been present a long time, feelings of worthlessness and other symptoms more typical of depression are not expressed until later in childhood after social isolation has occurred. This group seems different from children who are primarily depressed in that their social isolation is involuntary. They have not withdrawn from peers, their peers have withdrawn from them.

ADHD symptoms in this group respond well to stimulant medication, whereas behavioral difficulties and mood disorder do not; in fact, they may worsen when a stimulant is taken. Antidepressant medication may help behavioral difficulties and mood disorder, but does little for ADHD symptoms. Careful monitoring and regulation of medications is necessary. Typically, these children respond to lower doses of antidepressants than are used to treat overt depression.

Attention-Deficit/Hyperactivity Disorder and Language-Based Learning Disabilities. Difficulty understanding and using language is a common learning disability. Children with this type of learning disability often have delayed speech and problems in the following areas: understanding and using abstract words and grammatical forms such as prepositions, tenses, and pronouns; expressing or understanding sequences of events; and following verbal directions. Reading problems also are common with this group. When ADHD and a language-based learning disability coexist, problems are compounded because listening and completing assignments place high demands on language skills and concentration. Exertion and frustration in the classroom produce exhaustion, which leads to higher levels of restlessness, inattention, and impulsivity. These children do not tend to demonstrate excessive hyperactivity or impulsivity outside of school. Diagnosis of these children should be multidisciplinary, including medical, psychoeducational, speech and language, and audiological evaluations.

At times, the question of whether a child with language problems also has attention deficit disorder can only be answered by a trial of medication. Children who have ADHD and language-based learning disabilities generally respond to medications similarly to children with other varieties of ADHD. In addition, it is essential that appropriate support be provided at home and in school. It is vital that parents have a good understanding of their child's disabilities (both ADHD characteristics and the specific nature of problems imposed by the learning disability) so that necessary adjustments in expectations and parenting can be made. Appropriate educational programming with adequate support services also must be provided for ADHD children with language-based learning disabilities.

Attention-Deficit/Hyperactivity Disorder and Tourette's Syndrome. A very small percentage of children with ADHD have Gilles de la Tourette's syndrome; however, over 70% of children with Tourette's syndrome are likely to have ADHD (Barkley, 1990). Practitioners treating children with attention disorders should be familiar with Tourette's syndrome.

Tourette's syndrome is a long-term waxing and waning of motor and vocal tics that begin in childhood. It has been described as an autosomal dominant disorder with variable penetrance, meaning that it may be expressed severely, mildly, or not at all. The disorder often begins during the early elementary school years in the form of facial tics. Although every case is different, motor tics can follow a cephalocaudal progression involving the neck, shoulders, arms, trunk, and legs. Vocal tics may include repetitive throat clearing, coughing, or inappropriate vocalizations. Other traits associated with Tourette's syndrome are insatiability, thrill seeking, compulsion to use unacceptable language, and unusual fears. Symptoms can be exacerbated by stress, excitement, or ingestion of stimulants such as caffeine.

Some controversy exists regarding the relationship of stimulant medication and the onset of Tourette symptoms. Specifically, children treated with stimulant medication sometimes develop tics. In their examination of 1,520 children treated with methylphenidate, Denckla, Bemporad, and MacKay (1976) found tics in 20 cases (1.3%). In 19 of these 20 cases, tics resolved entirely when medication was withdrawn. Erenberg, Cruse, and Rothner (1985) concluded that stimulant medication can prompt premature onset of Tourette symptoms in some patients for whom these symptoms might emerge spontaneously at a later age.

The current consensus is that stimulant medication rarely, if ever, is a primary cause of Tourette's syndrome. Stimulant medication is beneficial for many children with Tourette's syndrome; however, if tics increase to an intolerable level, use of stimulants should be discontinued. Depending on the specific nature of the symptoms, other psychotropic medications, including clonidine (Catapres), fluoxetine (Prozac), haloperidol (Haldol), and pimozide (Orap) may be beneficial.

CONCLUSION

The condition known as Attention-Deficit/Hyperactivity Disorder is complex; its diagnosis and treatment are fraught with controversy. There is no definitive medical or psychometric test for diagnosis of ADHD. The definition of ADHD has evolved, with much debate regarding whether the condition is best characterized as having two major subcategories: attention deficit disorder with hyperactivity and attention deficit disorder without hyperactivity. Prevalence also is questioned, with critics such as Reid et al. (1993) suggesting that ADHD is a societally driven diagnosis that is grossly overused in the United States.

Practitioners should be thoroughly familiar with the research and literature on ADHD. It is essential to remember that ADHD is a disorder manifested in reciprocal interaction between the child and environmental demands. To be sensitive to situational variables, diagnosis should be made through a "team" approach that includes the child, the child's parents and teachers, psychologists, physicians, and others as appropriate. Interventions to address ADHD symptoms should start with behavioral, educational, and psychotherapeutic methods, and move to the use of medication only when necessary.

Gerald McMullen, PhD, is currently Supervisor of Diagnostic Services for Chester County Intermediate Unit in Exton, Pennsylvania. In addition, he is a licensed private practitioner who provides psychoeducational evaluations and psychotherapy. His professional background includes 20 years experience as a school psychologist working with a wide range of students from preschool through high school. He earned his doctorate in Human Development from Bryn Mawr College. Dr. McMullen may be contacted at Chester County Intermediate Unit, 150 James Hance Court, Exton, PA 19341.

David T. Painter, PhD, is currently on the psychology staff of the Chester County Intermediate Unit in Exton, Pennsylvania. He has held school psychologist positions in special education centers and in public school districts. Presently Dr. Painter provides a full range of school psychological services at Conestoga High School in Berwyn, Pennsylvania. He also maintains a private practice with a special interest in developmental, affective, and behavior disorders of children and adolescence. Dr. Painter is an allied health professional with attending privileges at Belmont Comprehensive Treatment Center, Philadelphia, Pennsylvania. He is president-elect of the School Division of the Pennsylvania Psychological Association for 1994-1995. Dr. Painter can be contacted at 47 Marchwood Road, Suite 1-J, Exton, PA 19341.

Thomas J. Casey, MD, is a Developmental Pediatrician in private practice in Bryn Mawr, Pennsylvania. He is an attending physician at the Bryn Mawr Hospital. He is a Fellow of the American Academy of Pediatrics and the American Academy for Cerebral Palsy and Developmental Medicine. He is past president of the Philadelphia Pediatrics Society and the Greater Philadelphia Branch of the Oton Dyslexia Society. His clinical interests are in children with learning disabilities, attention deficit disorder, mental retardation, pervasive developmental disorder, and cerebral palsy. Dr. Casey may be contacted at 830 Old Lancaster Road, Bryn Mawr, PA 19010.

RESOURCES

Abramowitz, A. J., & O'Leary, S. G. (1991). Behavioral interventions for the classroom: Implications for students with ADHD. *School Psychology Review, 20,* 220-234.

Achenbach, T. M. (1980). DSM-III in light of empirical research on the classification of child psychopathology. *Journal of the American Academy of Child Psychiatry, 19,* 395-412.

Achenbach, T. M., & Edelbrock, C. S. (1991). *Manual for the Child Behavior Checklist and Revised Child Behavior Profile.* Burlington, VT: T. M. Achenbach.

Achenbach, T. M., McConaughy, S. H., & Howell, C. T. (1987). Child/adolescent behavioral and emotional problems: Implications of cross-informant correlations for situational specificity. *Psychological Bulletin, 101,* 213-232.

American Psychiatric Association. (1968). *Diagnostic and Statistical Manual of Mental Disorders* (2nd ed.). Washington, DC: Author.

American Psychiatric Association. (1980). *Diagnostic and Statistical Manual of Mental Disorders* (3rd ed.). Washington, DC: Author.

American Psychiatric Association. (1987). *Diagnostic and Statistical Manual of Mental Disorders* (3rd ed. rev.). Washington, DC: Author.

American Psychiatric Association. (1994). *Diagnostic and Statistical Manual of Mental Disorders* (4th ed.). Washington, DC: Author.

Barkley, R. A. (1989). The ecological validity of laboratory and analogue assessments of ADHD symptoms. In J. Sargeant & A. Kalverboer (Eds.), *Proceedings of the Second International Symposium on ADHD.* Oxford: Pergamon.

Barkley, R. A. (1990). *Attention-Deficit Hyperactivity Disorder: A Handbook for Diagnosis and Treatment.* New York: Guilford.

Barkley, R. A. (1991). *Attention-Deficit Hyperactivity Disorder: A Clinical Workbook.* New York: Guilford.

Barkley, R. A. (1993). Eight principles to guide ADHD children. *ADHD Report, 1*(2), 1-4.

Burcham, B., Carlson, L., & Milich, R. (1993). Promising school-based practices for students with Attention Deficit Disorder. *Exceptional Children, 60,* 174-180.

Committee on Drugs, American Academy of Pediatrics. (1985). Behavioral and cognitive effects of anticonvulsant therapy. *Pediatrics, 76,* 644-647.

Connors, C. K. (1975). Minimal brain dysfunction and psychopathology in children. In A. Davids (Ed.), *Child Personality and Psychopathology: Volume 2. Current Topics.* New York: Wiley Interscience.

Connors, C. K. (1990). *Connors' Rating Scales Manual.* North Tonawanda, NY: Multi-Health Systems.

Council for Exceptional Children. (1993). *Exceptional Children, 60*(2).

Davila, R. R., Williams, M. L., & MacDonald, J. T. (1991). *Memorandum to Chief State School Officers Re: Clarification of Policy to Address the Needs of Children With Attention Deficit Disorders With General and/or Special Education.* Washington, DC: U.S. Department of Education.

Denckla, M. B., Bemporad, J. R., & MacKay, M. C. (1976). Tics following methylphenidate administration. *Journal of American Medical Association, 235,* 1349-1351.

Douglas, V. I., & Peters, K. G. (1979). Toward a clearer definition of the attentional deficit of hyperactive children. In G. A. Hale & M. Lewis (Eds.), *Attention and the Development of Cognitive Skills* (pp. 173-248). New York: Plenum.

DuPaul, G. J. (1991). The Home and School Situations Questionnaires - Revised. In R. A. Barkley (Ed.), *Attention-Deficit Hyperactivity Disorder: A Clinical Workbook.* New York: Guilford.

DuPaul, G. J., & Barkley, R. A. (1990). Medication therapy. In R. A. Barkley (Ed.), *Attention-Deficit Hyperactivity Disorder: A Handbook for Diagnosis and Treatment* (pp. 573-612). New York: Guilford.

DuPaul, G. J., & Henningson, P. N. (1993). Peer tutoring effects on the classroom performance of children with Attention Deficit Hyperactivity Disorder. *School Psychology Review, 22,* 134-143.

Edelbrock, C. S., Costello, A., & Kessler, M. D. (1984). Childhood hyperactivity: An overview of rating scales and their applications. *Clinical Psychology Review, 5,* 429-445.

Erenberg, G., Cruse, R. P., & Rothmer, A. D. (1985). Gilles de la Tourette's syndrome: Effect of stimulant drugs. *Neurology, 35,* 1346-1348.

Fantuzzo, J. W., & Polite, K. (1990). School-based, behavioral self-management: A review and analysis. *School Psychology Quarterly, 5,* 180-198.

Feingold, B. (1975). *Why Your Child Is Hyperactive.* New York: Random House.

Ferguson, H. B., & Rapoport, J. L. (1983). Nosological issues and biological variation. In M. Rutter (Ed.), *Developmental Neuropsychiatry* (pp. 369-384). New York: Guilford.

Fowler, M. (1992). *CH.A.D.D. Educators Manual.* Plantation, FL: CH.A.D.D.

Gittelman-Klein, R., Abikoff, H., Pollack, E., Klein, D., Katz, S., & Mattes, J. (1980). A controlled trial of behavior modification and methylphenidate in hyperactive children. In C. Whalen & B. Henker (Eds.), *Hyperactive Children: The Social Ecology of Identification and Treatment* (pp. 221-246). New York: Academic.

Goldstein, S., & Goldstein, M. (1990). *Managing Attention Disorders in Children.* New York: John Wiley & Sons.

Goldstein, S., & Ingersoll, B. (1993). Controversial treatments for ADHD: Essential information for clinicians. *ADHD Report, 1,* 4-5.

Goodman, R., & Stevenson, J. (1989). A twin study of hyperactivity: II. The aetiological role of genes, family relationships, and perinatal adversity. *Journal of Child Psychology and Psychiatry, 30,* 691-709.

Lahey, B. B., Schaughency, E. A., Hynd, G. W., Carlson, C. L., & Nieves, N. (1987). Attention deficit disorder with and without hyperactivity: See comparison of behavioral characteristics of clinic-referred children. *Journal of the American Academy of Child and Adolescent Child Psychiatry, 26,* 718-723.

McBurnett, K., Lahey, B. B., & Pfiffner, L. (1993). Diagnosis of attention deficit disorders in DSM-IV: Scientific basis and implications for education. *Exceptional Children, 60,* 108-117.

McCarney, S. B. (1989). *Manual for the Attention Deficit Disorders Evaluation Scale.* Columbia, MO: Hawthorne Educational Services.

McMullen, G. M. (1989). *The Contribution of WISC-R Factors to Psychoeducational Evaluation: A Developmental Study.* Ann Arbor, MI: University Microfilms International.

Morriss, R. (1992). The use and abuse of rating scales in the assessment of attention disorders. *NASP Communique, Nov. 92,* 11-13.

Naglieri, J. A., LeBuffe, P. A., & Pfeiffer, S. I. (1993). *Manual for the Devereux Behavior Rating Scale.* San Antonio: The Psychological Corporation.

National Association of School Psychologists. (1991). *School Psychology Review, 20*(2).

Parker, H. C. (1992). *The ADD Hyperactivity Handbook for Schools.* Plantation, FL: Impact Publications.

Pelham, W. E., Carlson, C., Sams, S. E., Vallano, G., Dixon, M. J., & Hoza, B. (1993). Separate and combined effects of methylphenidate and behavior modification on the classroom behavior and academic performance of ADHD boys: Group effects and individual differences. *Journal of Consulting and Clinical Psychology, 61,* 506-515.

Reid, R., Maag, J. W., & Vasa, S. F. (1993). Attention deficit hyperactivity disorder as a disability category: A critique. *Exceptional Children, 60,* 198-214.

Riccio, C. A., Hynd, G. W., Cohen, M. J., & Gonzalez, J. J. (1993). Neurological basis of attention deficit hyperactivity disorder. *Exceptional Children, 60,* 118-124.

Ross, D. M., & Ross, S. A. (1982). *Hyperactivity: Current Issues, Research and Theory* (2nd ed.). New York: John Wiley & Sons.

Rutter, M. (1983). Behavioral studies: Questions of findings on the concept of a distinctive syndrome. In M. Rutter, A. H. Tuma, & I. S. Lann (Eds.), *Assessment and Diagnosis in Child Psychopathology* (pp. 437-452). New York: Guilford.

Szatmari, P., Offord, D. R., & Boyle, M. H. (1989). Ontario child health study: Prevalence of attention deficit disorder with hyperactivity. *Journal of Child Psychology and Psychiatry, 30,* 219-230.

Werry, J. S. (1988). In memorium - DSM-III [Letter to the editor]. *Journal of the American Academy of Child and Adolescent Psychiatry, 27,* 138-139.

Whalen, C. K., Henker, B., Collins, B. E., Finck, D., & Dotemoto, S. (1979). A social ecology of hyperactive boys: Medication effects in systematically structured classroom environments. *Journal of Applied Behavioral Analysis, 12,* 65-81.

Zametkin, A. J., & Rapoport, J. L. (1987). Neurobiology of attention deficit disorder with hyperactivity: Where have we come in 50 years? *American Academy of Child and Adolescent Psychiatry, 26,* 676-686.

Zentall, S. S. (1993). Research on the educational implications of Attention Deficit Hyperactivity Disorder. *Exceptional Children, 60,* 143-153.

DEPENDENCY IN PSYCHOTHERAPY: EFFECTIVE THERAPEUTIC WORK WITH DEPENDENT PATIENTS

Robert F. Bornstein

Dependency is a natural part of the psychotherapeutic process. Given that patients typically initiate therapy because they are unable to deal effectively with some problematic aspect of their lives, it is only natural that most patients will, at least to some degree, become dependent upon the therapist for guidance, support, and reassurance. In fact, as Goldfarb (1969) observed, patient dependency is in some respects a prerequisite for successful psychotherapy. As Goldfarb pointed out, the patient's dependent, help-seeking stance during the early stages of therapy can motivate him or her to engage in productive therapeutic work in order to please the therapist and strengthen the patient-therapist relationship.

Although a certain degree of patient dependency is to be expected during the course of psychotherapy, some patients are more dependent than others. Some patients show exaggerated dependency needs which are so pronounced that they interfere with the patient's functioning, both within and outside of therapy. The purpose of this contribution is to (a) familiarize therapists with the clinical features of patients who show exaggerated dependency needs, (b) describe the ways that these exaggerated dependency needs may affect therapeutic process and outcome, and (c) present strategies for working with dependent patients in such a way that the patient receives maximum benefit from therapy.

BACKGROUND

Psychiatrists, psychologists, counselors, and other mental health professionals have long recognized that certain patients show exaggerated dependency needs. Not surprisingly, early clinical descriptions of such patients were generally quite negative. For example, Emil Kraeplin, one of the founders of modern psychiatry, referred to overly dependent patients as "shiftless" and "weak-willed." Early psychoanalytic theorists such as Freud, Abraham, and Fenichel gave similar negative descriptions of dependent psychotherapy patients. Fromm (1947) subsequently provided one of the more articulate descriptions of the personality characteristics of dependent patients, noting that such persons "are dependent not only on authorities for knowledge and help, but on people in general for any kind of support. They feel lost when alone because they feel that they cannot do anything without help. It is characteristic of these people that their first thought is to find somebody else to give them needed information rather than to make even the slightest effort on their own" (p. 62). Recent clinical descriptions of dependent psychotherapy patients (e.g., Millon, 1981) are very similar to these early descriptions.

Broadly speaking, the overly dependent patient brings two unique sets of problems to therapy. These problems may or may not be a part of the patient's presenting complaint, but nonetheless, they are difficulties that are frequently - if not invariably - encountered in clinical work with dependent individuals.

First, the patient's dependency is likely to be causing difficulties in his or her interpersonal relationships outside of therapy. For example, the dependent patient may have developed a submissive, clinging relationship with his or her spouse, which can result in marital conflict (Birtchnell, 1988). Alternatively, the dependent patient may be so fearful of damaging a romantic relationship that he or she tolerates psychological and/or physical abuse from the romantic partner (Bornstein, 1993). Along different lines, the patient's dependency can cause him or her to experience problems at work or school due to a lack of assertiveness and an inability to function independently (Millon, 1981).

Second, the patient's exaggerated dependency needs can cause difficulty within therapy. In this case, the therapist may find that the patient quickly becomes overly dependent upon the therapist, and that this dependency hinders therapeutic progress. For example, an overly dependent transference can produce a strong negative countertransference reaction on the part of the therapist (Emery & Lesher, 1982). Patient dependency can also interfere with termination of therapy insofar as the dependent patient is unwilling to relinquish a relationship with an important caretaking figure (Greenberg & Bornstein, 1989). These and other dependency-related difficulties can adversely affect therapeutic process and outcome.

IDENTIFYING THE DEPENDENT PATIENT

The first step in working effectively with dependent psychotherapy patients is identifying patient dependency and understanding the particular ways in which a patient expresses his or her dependency needs. There are numerous measures available to assess and quantify level of dependency in children, adolescents, and adults. These are described in detail by Bornstein (1993). The therapist who wants to become familiar with the various measures that have been used to assess and quantify psychiatric patients' dependency needs can easily obtain whatever objective or projective dependency measures seem most appropriate for his or her practice. Over 35 different measures of patient dependency have been developed and validated during the past several decades.

Examples of widely used dependency measures include Blatt, D'Afflitti, and Quinlan's (1976) Depressive Experiences Questionnaire (DEQ) Dependency Scale, the Millon Clinical Multiaxial Inventory (MCMI) Dependency Scale (Millon, 1987), and the Hirschfeld et al. (1977) Interpersonal Dependency Inventory (IDI). These are all paper-and-pencil measures that can be administered to the patient during (or after) the intake process. Although these measures are all widely available, some of these scales (e.g., the MCMI Dependency Scale) must be purchased from national distributors. Other dependency scales (e.g., the IDI) can be obtained free of charge. A detailed description of objective, projective, interview, and observational measures of dependency is provided by Bornstein (1993).

For many therapists, the most appropriate way to assess patient dependency is through the *DSM-IV* (American Psychiatric Association [APA], 1994) diagnostic criteria for Dependent Personality Disorder (DPD). The *DSM-IV* provides a great deal of information regarding the clinical characteristics of patients with exaggerated dependency needs, although the general thrust of this information can be summarized simply. According to the *DSM-IV*, the essential feature of DPD is "a pervasive and excessive need to be taken care of that leads to submissive and clinging behavior and fears of separation" (APA, 1994, p. 665). The *DSM-IV* goes on to note that people with this disorder are unable to make everyday decisions without an excessive amount of advice and reassurance from others, and will even allow others to make most of their important decisions. This excessive dependence on others leads to difficulties in initiating projects or doing things on one's own. People with this disorder tend to feel uncomfortable or helpless when alone. They are devastated when close relationships end, and tend to be preoccupied with fears of being abandoned. These people are easily hurt by criticism or disapproval, and tend to subordinate themselves to others for fear of being rejected. They will volunteer to do things that are unpleasant or demeaning in order to get others to like them (APA, 1994, pp. 665-666).

In addition to describing the clinical features of DPD, the *DSM-IV* also describes the specific symptoms that characterize this disorder. A total of eight DPD symptoms are included in the *DSM-IV*. The individual must show five or more of these symptoms in order to receive the DPD diagnosis. According to the *DSM-IV*, the individuals suffering from DPD (a) are unable to make independent decisions; (b) allow others to make important decisions for them; (c) have excessive fear of rejection; (d) have difficulty initiating projects or activities; (e) volunteer to perform unpleasant tasks in order to please others; (f) feel helpless when alone; (g) feel devastated when important relationships end; and (h) are preoccupied with fears of being abandoned (APA, 1994, pp. 668-669).

Three things are noteworthy about the *DSM-IV* criteria for DPD. First, it is important to keep in mind that a patient need not have all (or even most) of these symptoms in order to be overly dependent (Bornstein, 1993; Overholser, 1987). Although a patient must show at least five DPD symptoms to receive the DPD diagnosis, patients who show three or four of these symptoms can - depending upon the intensity of the symptoms and the way that they are expressed - also show high levels of dependency. Millon (1981) provides a thorough discussion of this issue.

Second, it is worth noting that the eight *DSM-IV* DPD symptoms can be divided into two broad areas. Four of these symptoms (listed previously as a, b, d, and e) reflect behavioral difficulties, while the remaining four symptoms (c, f, g, and h) represent problematic emotional responses. There are no DPD symptoms reflecting the cognitive features of dependency (i.e., a view of oneself as powerless and ineffectual, along with a perception of other people as being powerful and in control), despite the fact that research on dependent persons suggests that such cognitive features are central to a dependent personality orientation (see Bornstein, 1992, 1993 for detailed reviews of the empirical literature on this topic).

Third, the therapist should keep in mind that there is some degree of overlap between the DPD symptom criteria and the diagnostic criteria for several other psychological disorders. In particular, the DPD symptom criteria show substantial overlap with the diagnostic criteria for avoidant and passive-aggressive personality disorders, as well as having moderate overlap with the diagnostic criteria for depression and certain anxiety disorders (e.g., agoraphobia, panic disorder). Several recent investigations have examined the covariation of DPD symptoms with symptoms of other psychological disorders (e.g., Alnaes & Torgerson, 1988; Widiger & Sanderson, 1987). Detailed information regarding the overlap of DPD symptoms with symptoms of other psychopathologies can be found in these studies.

RECENT CLINICAL AND EMPIRICAL FINDINGS

During the past several decades there has been an enormous amount of research on dependency. In this section two areas of research that are of particular interest to the practicing clinician will be summarized: (a) investigations of dependency as a risk factor for other psychological disorders and (b) studies of dependency and various patient-related behaviors.

DEPENDENCY AS A RISK FACTOR FOR OTHER PSYCHOLOGICAL DISORDERS

Clinicians and researchers have long speculated that dependent personality traits can place individuals at risk for a wide variety of psychological disorders, including depression, anxiety disorders, dissociative disorders, schizophrenia, substance use disorders, psychosomatic disorders, and eating disorders. Masling and Schwartz (1979) summarized much of the early work in this area.

Although anecdotal accounts of dependent psychotherapy patients suggested that these individuals are at risk for a variety of psychopathologies, recent research indicates that dependency is in fact an established risk factor for only three psychological disorders: depression, substance use disorders, and eating disorders (i.e., anorexia and bulimia).

Depression. There have been dozens of studies assessing the relationship between level of dependency and presence of (or level of) depression in psychiatric inpatients, psychiatric outpatients, medical patients, and nonclinical subjects (e.g., college students). Many of these studies are summarized in a recent review of the dependency-depression literature by Nietzel and Harris (1990). The general conclusion that may be drawn from these investigations is clear: Exaggerated dependency needs do in fact place individuals at increased risk for depression. However, the onset of depression in a dependent person is generally precipitated by a stressful life event - in particular, a stressful life event involving interpersonal loss or interpersonal conflict.

A recent study by Hammen et al. (1985) illustrates the dependency-life stress-depression relationship. Hammen et al. divided a mixed-sex sample of college students into dependent and nondependent groups based on the students' responses to Blatt et al.'s (1976) DEQ Dependency Scale (described earlier). Four months later, Hammen et al.'s subjects reported the number of stressful interpersonal events (e.g., rejection by a friend) and stressful achievement-related events (e.g., failure on a test) that they had experienced since the first session. Level of depression at follow-up was assessed via the Beck Depression Inventory (BDI). Hammen et al. found that dependent subjects of both sexes reported elevated levels of depression at follow-up only when they had experienced high levels of interpersonal stressors. As expected, there was no relationship between BDI depression scores and level of achievement-related stressors in the dependent subjects. Subsequent studies have confirmed Hammen et al.'s findings in samples of psychiatric inpatients and outpatients (see Bornstein, 1993, for a review of these investigations).

The implications of these studies are straightforward: A dependent patient is likely to develop depression when confronted with stressful interpersonal events. Thus, the therapist working with a dependent patient should monitor the patient's level of interpersonal stressors periodically in order to assess the patient's risk for developing clinically significant depression. This can be done either informally (i.e., during therapy sessions) or formally (i.e., via questionnaire or structured interview). There are a number of procedures available for assessing a client's level of interpersonal stressors; several of these methods are discussed by Hammen et al. (1985).

Substance Use Disorders. There is some indication that dependent persons are at increased risk for the development of substance use disorders, especially alcohol and tobacco addiction. In addition, a few studies have found that dependent psychiatric patients show higher-than-expected rates of other substance use disorders (e.g., opiate, cocaine, and poly-drug abuse), but these findings must be regarded as preliminary, as they have not been replicated on independent subject samples.

The therapist who seeks to explore the dependency-substance use disorder relationship in a particular patient would do well to keep in mind one important caveat: Although dependency appears to represent a risk factor for the onset of certain substance use disorders, it also seems that the onset of a substance use disorder produces increases in dependent thoughts, feelings, and behaviors (see Bornstein, 1992). Thus, obtaining information regarding the onset of a patient's exaggerated dependency needs and the onset of his or her substance use is critical. In one case (i.e., when dependency preceded the onset of substance use), the patient has a substance use disorder that is secondary to the dependency. In the other case (i.e., when increases in dependency follow, rather than precede, substance abuse), the substance abuse diagnosis is primary, and the patient may be said to show a secondary dependency-related disorder. Unfortunately, there are no data available that address the question of whether these two situations require different treatment approaches. Nonetheless, understanding the temporal relationship between a patient's exaggerated dependency needs and his or her substance abuse may be important in formulating and implementing a treatment plan for that patient.

Eating Disorders. In a sense, findings regarding the relationship of dependency to eating disorders parallel the findings obtained regarding the dependency-depression relationship. Again, dependency seems to place patients at increased risk for eating disorders (i.e., anorexia and bulimia). However, like depression, eating disorders tend to appear following some significant interpersonal stressor in the dependent person's life. Several studies (e.g., Lacey, Coker, & Birtchnell, 1986; Pyle, Mitchell, & Eckert, 1981) have suggested that underlying dependency needs and interpersonal stressors combine to predict the onset of eating disorder symptomatology in both clinical and nonclinical subjects. Thus, the therapist working with a dependent patient must be sensitive to the occurrence of interpersonal stressors in the patient's life, in that these stressors not only place the patient at increased risk for depression, but may place him or her at increased risk for eating disorders as well.

DEPENDENCY AND PATIENT-RELATED BEHAVIORS

There are three areas in which laboratory and clinical studies have produced highly consistent results that allow strong conclusions to be drawn regarding the relationship of dependency to various patient-related behaviors. In this section, I review research on the relationship of dependency to (a) compliance with medical and psychotherapeutic regimens, (b) sensitivity to interpersonal cues, and (c) need for feedback and support.

Compliance With Medical and Psychotherapeutic Regimens. Because dependent individuals are preoccupied with obtaining nurturance and support from others, they should be more willing than nondependent persons to comply with the demands and expectations of others, especially figures of authority. In this context, it is not surprising that clinical studies have demonstrated that dependent patients comply very well with medical and psychotherapeutic regimens. Two recent investigations illustrate nicely the dependency-compliance relationship in clinical settings.

In one of the first studies of this issue, Nacev (1980) assessed level of dependency in a mixed-sex sample of adult psychotherapy patients, using an MMPI measure of dependency that was administered during the intake process. Records of each patient's attendance in weekly psychotherapy sessions (i.e., the number of sessions missed but not canceled beforehand) were kept by their outpatient therapists. As predicted, there was an inverse relationship between the patients' level of dependency and the number of sessions missed: The more dependent the patient, the fewer sessions missed. Poldrugo and Forti (1988) subsequently obtained similar results in a sample of men undergoing outpatient treatment for alcoholism. In this study, dependent patients showed higher rates of treatment compliance (and treatment follow-through) than did nondependent patients. Specifically, Poldrugo and Forti found that 75% of the dependent patients in their sample completed the 1-year course of prescribed outpatient treatment, while only 33% of the nondependent patients completed the 1-year course of treatment.

These two investigations suggest that dependency is associated with a willingness to follow through on outpatient treatment. Thus, these results point to the possibility that patient dependency is not always a deficit, but in certain contexts can be a strength as well: To the extent that dependent patients are more willing than nondependent patients to become actively engaged in treatment, the likelihood of a positive treatment outcome should increase.

Sensitivity to Interpersonal Cues. One would expect that dependent persons should be particularly sensitive to interpersonal (i.e., verbal and nonverbal) cues, for two reasons. First, the dependent person is highly motivated to understand the behaviors, thoughts, and feelings of other people. Second, the dependent person is likely to have developed considerable skill in this area, because sensitivity to interpersonal cues will allow the dependent person to develop and maintain good relationships with potential caretakers and protectors (e.g., physicians, therapists, supervisors, teachers, romantic partners). In this context, several laboratory and clinical studies have assessed the dependency-interpersonal sensitivity relationship.

The best-designed study of this issue was conducted by Masling, Shiffner, and Shenfeld (1980). In this investigation, the researchers first assessed level of dependency in members of a mixed-sex sample of adult patients undergoing outpatient psychotherapy at a University Counseling Center. Following the third therapy session, and again immediately following termination of therapy, each patient completed a questionnaire that asked them to make a series of judgments about their therapist's political beliefs, personal interests, and attitudes regarding various social issues (e.g., abortion, capital punishment). Each therapist had previously completed a questionnaire on which they had indicated their actual attitudes and beliefs in these areas. Masling et al. found that dependent patients gave very accurate responses when attempting to infer their therapist's attitudes and personal beliefs. In contrast, the responses provided by the nondependent patients were inaccurate and generally were unrelated to the therapist's actual attitudes and beliefs.

These findings are noteworthy in two respects. First, they demonstrate that dependent subjects are accurate perceivers of subtle interpersonal cues. Second, these findings are made even more compelling by virtue of the fact that therapists typically go to great lengths to avoid revealing personal information that might bias or adversely affect the therapist-patient relationship. Thus, even though the therapists in Masling et al.'s (1980) study presumably were motivated to maintain a neutral stance and not reveal personal information, dependent patients in this study were able to infer accurately some important aspects of their therapist's attitudes and personal beliefs. This finding - which has now been replicated several times in different contexts - has important implications for working with the dependent patient. At the very least, the dependent patient's ability to make accurate inferences regarding the therapist's attitudes and personal beliefs might have a significant effect on the kinds of transference (and countertransference) reactions that occur in therapeutic work with such patients. These dependency-related transference and countertransference effects will be discussed in detail in a later section of this contribution.

Need for Feedback and Support. Several studies indicate that dependent persons ask for feedback regarding psychological test data more frequently than do nondependent persons. Other studies indicate that dependent psychiatric patients show a help-seeking response set on psychological tests such as the MMPI and show greater apprehension regarding testing than do nondependent patients. The findings are discussed in detail by Bornstein (1993).

The results of these investigations converge to indicate that in general, the dependent person is particularly anxious about psychological testing and evaluation, and responds to this anxiety by actively seeking feedback regarding his or her test performance. These findings therefore suggest that the therapist must be sensitive to the concerns and apprehensions that dependent patients may have regarding psychological testing and evaluation. Discussing openly the ways in which testing can assist the therapy process (and strengthen the therapist-patient relationship) will be important in this context. Moreover, in light of the fact that dependent patients tend to adopt a help-seeking response set on psychological tests, it will be necessary for the therapist to emphasize the importance of the patient's responding honestly and accurately to test items.

Along somewhat different lines, the dependent person's need for guidance and support is often expressed in concerns regarding treatment termination. Perhaps this is not surprising, given the dependent person's general desire to obtain support and guidance from others in a variety of situations and settings. In any case, research indicates that dependent psychotherapy patients (a) remain in treatment significantly longer than do nondependent patients and (b) express greater concern regarding treatment termination than do nondependent patients. In fact, some studies suggest that dependent patients remain in treatment nearly twice as long as do nondependent patients with comparable psychological disorders (see Greenberg & Bornstein, 1989, for an example of recent findings regarding this issue). These studies suggest that treatment termination is likely to be particularly problematic for the dependent patient.

EFFECTIVE PSYCHOTHERAPY WITH THE DEPENDENT PATIENT: A PRACTICAL GUIDE

With the aforementioned clinical and research findings in mind, it is possible to describe some of the specific problems and issues that are likely to arise in psychotherapeutic work with dependent patients. In this section I discuss some of the most important of these issues and provide recommendations regarding strategies that the therapist can use to minimize the adverse effects of patient dependency on the therapeutic process.

1. *Assess Dependency Early.* As noted earlier, there are numerous formal and informal measures available for assessing patient dependency. The only way that a therapist can effectively minimize the negative effects of dependency is to become aware of the patient's dependency needs early in therapy. If possible, the therapist should routinely screen patients for level of dependency during the intake process, either formally (i.e., via questionnaire or structured interview) or informally (i.e., via discussion of life-history information that typically occurs during the first few therapy sessions). Once the therapist is aware of a patient's level of dependency, treatment can be structured so as to deal with the patient's dependency needs in as constructive a way as possible.

   As Bornstein et al. (1993) noted, although there are many objective and projective measures available to the clinician who wants to assess level of dependency in a patient, the choice of which type of measure to use in a given testing situation depends upon the goals of that testing procedure. If assessing a person's underlying dependency needs is the central goal of testing, then a projective dependency measure may be superior to an objective dependency scale. However, if one is interested primarily in assessing a person's overt expression of dependent traits and behaviors, then an objective dependency scale will likely be superior to a projective dependency measure. In this context, an interesting strategy would be to administer objective and projective dependency measures to the same patient. The tester would then be in a position to assess directly any inconsistencies that exist between that patient's underlying and expressed dependency needs.

2. *Set Limits on the Patient's Dependent Behavior.* Emery and Lesher (1982) discussed in detail the kinds of strategies that are used by dependent psychiatric patients to shift responsibility for therapeutic progress from themselves to the therapist. These strategies include (but are not limited to) requesting extra therapy sessions; adopting a passive, helpless stance during sessions; seeking a great deal of guidance and structure from the therapist; and making after-hours phone calls to the therapist to report "pseudo-emergencies" that, upon scrutiny, turn out to be relatively mundane events. Of course, different dependent patients will adopt somewhat different strategies for externalizing responsibility in the clinical setting.

   In any case, it is critical that the therapist set appropriate limits on the patient's dependent behavior. Communicating these limits to the patient firmly and consistently is of primary importance. In addition, it is clear that one important therapeutic strategy that is useful in limiting the patient's dependent behaviors is to not reinforce the patient's attempts to become overly dependent on the therapist (Overholser, 1987). In general, requests for extra sessions should be refused, and strict guidelines regarding when - if ever - the patient may initiate after-hours contact with the therapist should be discussed early in therapy.

3. *Be Nonjudgmental.* Although it is important to set limits on the patient's dependent behavior early in therapy, it is almost always a mistake to confront the patient directly regarding his or her exaggerated dependency needs or inappropriate dependent behaviors until after the therapist-patient relationship has been firmly established. The patient may well be largely (or completely) unaware of his or her underlying dependency needs, and

he or she will likely feel hurt and rejected if confronted with this information early in therapy. This is particularly true for dependent male patients, for as most of us are well aware, it is generally not acceptable for men in our society to express dependent feelings and needs directly. Open discussion of a patient's dependency needs can be particularly sensitive when the situation involves a male patient working with a male therapist (see Gilbert, 1987, for a detailed discussion of this issue).

After the therapist-patient relationship has become firmly established, there might come a time when giving the patient feedback regarding his or her dependency needs is appropriate and therapeutic. However, this must be done cautiously, and above all, the feedback should be given to the patient in a nonjudgmental manner. In this context, it is important that the therapist avoid using terms like "dependent" or "passive," and instead describe the patient's dependency needs in a way that is less likely to be perceived as criticism by the patient. Terms like "sensitive to others' wishes," "inclined to seek other people's help," and "tend to rely on others" are likely to elicit a more positive response from the patient than terms like "dependent," "submissive," or "passive."

4. *Include in the Treatment Plan Some Goals Related to Increasing the Patient's Independent Behavior.* Even if dependency is not part of the patient's presenting complaint, it is useful to include in the treatment plan some goals related to increasing the patient's independent, autonomous functioning. Whether these goals are to be communicated directly to the patient or are simply made a part of the therapists's unspoken agenda depends upon the particular patient and upon the circumstances surrounding the patient's therapy experience. In general, if the patient's presenting complaint involves a pressing problem that must be dealt with immediately, it is not helpful to confuse the situation by bringing in issues regarding the patient's exaggerated dependency needs. However, if the presenting complaint involves a matter that is less pressing, then bringing in issues regarding the patient's dependency can be useful, especially if the patient's presenting complaint is in some way related to his or her dependency needs or dependent behaviors.

A useful way to help the patient feel (and act) more independent is to explore the patient's dependency-related cognitions and self-statements. As noted earlier, several kinds of dependency-related cognitions are characteristic of patients who show exaggerated dependency needs. The kinds of cognitions that are characteristic of such patients include a perception of himself or herself as powerless and ineffectual, and a belief that others are powerful and in control of situations (Bornstein, 1992, 1993). In addition, dependent patients tend to perceive themselves as shy, unattractive, and socially awkward (Millon, 1981). Although helping the patient recognize his or her dependency-related behaviors and emotional responses can be very useful, it appears that helping the patient to understand his or her dependency-related cognitions and self-statements is a particularly effective way of altering problematic dependent behavior (Bornstein, 1993; Overholser, 1987).

5. *Make Aspects of the Patient's Dependent Transference Explicit to the Patient.* Although open discussion of the patient's dependency needs may not always be useful, especially early in therapy, some explicit interpretation of the patient's dependent transference can be an important therapeutic tool when working with highly dependent patients. As with all transference interpretations, the timing of this feedback is critical. Ideally, such feedback should be communicated to the patient in the context of a situation that has arisen (either within or outside of therapy) wherein the patient's dependent feelings or behaviors have caused some sort of difficulty. In this context, Crowder (1972) pointed out that the therapist should not interfere with a dependent transference reaction early in therapy, since such a transference reaction can strengthen the therapist-patient relationship and can also be useful in encouraging the patient to become emotionally invested in therapy and adhere to the therapeutic regimen. Crowder further suggested that once the therapist-patient relationship has become firmly established and the dependent transference has emerged full-blown, then (and only then) it may be useful to discuss openly the positive and negative aspects of the patient's dependency.

6. *Be Aware of Dependency-Related Countertransference Reactions That May Impede Therapeutic Progress.* The dependent patient looks up to - and may even idolize - the therapist. This can produce a countertransference reaction on the part of the therapist that impedes therapeutic progress. In fact, two general forms of problematic countertransference reactions can result from the patient's dependent transference. First, the therapist might find such a transference reaction very gratifying. In this situation, the therapist may, consciously or unconsciously, subvert therapeutic progress and foster the patient's dependency in order to avoid losing the adulation and adoration that accompanies the patient's dependent transference (Bornstein, 1993).

    Alternatively, the therapist might become angry or frustrated at the patient's dependency (Overholser, 1987). In this situation, the therapist's ability to maintain positive regard for the patient may diminish, and the possibility that the therapist will act in ways that serve to distance himself or herself from the patient will increase. The dependent patient is particularly likely to experience such distancing as abandonment or rejection, which will (a) raise concerns on the part of the patient that he or she will be abandoned by the therapist, (b) cause the patient to feel anxious and threatened, and therefore (c) produce even stronger efforts on the part of the patient to strengthen the therapist-patient relationship via increases in dependent, help-seeking behavior.

7. *Assume That the Patient's Dependent Relationship With the Therapist Is Characteristic of the Patient's Other Relationships.* To some degree, all transference reactions provide information regarding other important relationships in a patient's life. In the case of the dependent patient, the therapist-patient relationship can provide two types of useful information in this area. First, by carefully monitoring his or her feelings regarding the patient, the therapist can get a good sense of how other people in the patient's life must perceive the patient. In other words, if the therapist feels overwhelmed by the patient's demands for nurturance and support, it is likely that the patient's spouse, friends, co-workers, and others feel much the same way in their relationships with the patient. Second, the kinds of fears and feelings that the patient expresses toward the therapist (e.g., fears of abandonment or rejection) are often a reflection of the kinds of feelings that the patient experiences in other important relationships. Thus, the dependency-related concerns that are expressed during the therapy session are likely to be expressed outside the therapy session as well. By being sensitive to these concerns as they arise during therapy, the therapist can anticipate the kinds of interpersonal problems that the patient is likely to experience in other important relationships.

8. *Be Aware That the Patient's Dependency May Adversely Affect His or Her Romantic Relationships.* Birtchnell (1988) conducted an extensive study examining the marital relationships of dependent persons. He found that high levels of dependency needs in either spouse were associated with decreased marital satisfaction and increased marital conflict. When both spouses showed high levels of underlying dependency needs, marital problems were particularly likely to result. Although there are no data available that indicate what proportion of dependent individuals experience marital problems that are severe enough to warrant treatment, the therapist should be aware that a dependent patient is likely to be experiencing some dependency-related difficulties in his or her romantic relationships.

9. *Be Aware of the Various Risk Factors Associated With Dependency.* As discussed earlier, dependency is associated with increased risk for depression, substance use disorders, and eating disorders, especially in patients who are undergoing high levels of interpersonal stress. The therapist should periodically monitor the patient's behaviors in each of these areas in order to identify the onset of related psychopathologies as early as possible. In addition, evidence is beginning to accumulate that suggests that dependent persons may be at increased risk for engaging in child abuse. Bornstein (1993) summarized many of the findings in this area, and concluded that dependent persons' strong need for nurturance and support may cause them to become frustrated with the demands of parenting and

caregiving, and lash out at those who are dependent upon them (e.g., children, frail elders). The therapist working with a dependent patient should gather information regarding the patient's family dynamics, frustration tolerance, and parenting/caretaking skills in order to assess the likelihood that the patient may engage in abusive behavior.

10. *Plan Termination With Care.* Termination of therapy can be very difficult for the dependent patient, because termination involves relinquishing an important relationship with a nurturing, caretaking figure. Thus, termination is likely to be particularly anxiety-producing for the dependent patient. Consequently, the therapist can (and should) take steps to minimize the negative effects of termination, and try, as much as possible, to turn termination into a therapeutic intervention in and of itself. Two therapeutic strategies can facilitate treatment termination with the dependent patient. First, termination will be made easier if the therapist makes it clear that termination does not require a permanent break in the therapist-patient relationship. Clearly, the therapist does not want to send the patient a mixed message, indicating that the patient is ready to terminate but that they are not "really" terminating. Rather, the therapist must frame termination in terms that emphasize the patient's successful work during therapy.

Second, the therapist should make explicit his or her belief that the patient's dependency needs may make termination difficult. If this information is conveyed to the patient in a nonjudgmental manner, it can simultaneously (a) preempt the patient's (conscious or unconscious) desire to subvert termination and continue therapy indefinitely and (b) provide the patient with useful feedback regarding the ways in which his or her dependency strivings can adversely affect other important interpersonal relationships.

CONCLUSION

Clearly, patient dependency can have both positive and negative effects on psychotherapeutic process and outcome. On the negative side, the dependent patient's passive, help-seeking stance may impede therapeutic progress and may even provoke a countertherapeutic response from the frustrated therapist. However, on the positive side, the patient's dependency can, if identified accurately and nurtured carefully, be utilized by the therapist to increase the patient's investment in therapy and to motivate the patient to engage in productive therapeutic work. Like many personality traits that seem at first glance to represent flaws or deficits in functioning (e.g., introversion, narcissism), dependency is neither "all good" or "all bad." Rather, dependency is a weakness in certain contexts and an asset in others.

In any case, clinical and empirical findings indicate that the therapist can play a key role in maximizing the positive aspects of patient dependency and minimizing the negative effects of patient dependency on therapeutic progress. To the extent that the therapist becomes familiar with the various strategies that have proved useful in working with dependent psychotherapy patients, his or her ability to work effectively with these patients in the clinical setting will be enhanced.

Robert F. Bornstein, PhD, is Associate Professor of Psychology at Gettysburg College. He received his PhD in clinical Psychology from the State University of New York at Buffalo in 1986. Dr. Bornstein has published numerous articles on the antecedents, correlates, and consequences of dependent personality traits in children, adolescents, and adults. In 1993, he published *The Dependent Personality*, a comprehensive review of the clinical and empirical literature on dependency. Dr. Bornstein may be contacted at the Department of Psychology, Gettysburg College, Gettysburg, PA 17325.

RESOURCES

Alnaes, R., & Torgerson, S. (1988). The relationship between DSM-III symptom disorders (Axis I) and personality disorders (Axis II) in an outpatient population. *Acta Psychiatrica Scandinavica, 78,* 485-492.

American Psychiatric Association. (1994). *Diagnostic and Statistical Manual of Mental Disorders* (4th ed.). Washington, DC: Author.

Birtchnell, J. (1988). The assessment of the marital relationship by questionnaire. *Sexual and Marital Therapy, 3,* 57-70.

Blatt, S. J., D'Afflitti, J. P., & Quinlan, D. M. (1976). Experiences of depression in normal young adults. *Journal of Abnormal Psychology, 85,* 383-389.

Bornstein, R. F. (1992). The dependent personality: Developmental, social and clinical perspectives. *Psychological Bulletin, 112,* 3-23.

Bornstein, R. F. (1993). *The Dependent Personality.* New York: Guilford.

Bornstein, R. F., Manning, K. A., Krukonis, A. B., Rossner, S. C., & Mastrosimone, C. C. (1993). Sex differences in dependency: A comparison of objective and projective measures. *Journal of Personality Assessment, 61,* 169-181.

Crowder, J. E. (1972). Relationship between therapist and client interpersonal behaviors and psychotherapy outcome. *Journal of Counseling Psychology, 19,* 68-75.

Emery, G., & Lesher, E. (1982). Treatment of depression in older adults: Personality considerations. *Psychotherapy, 19,* 500-505.

Fromm, E. (1947). *Man for Himself.* New York: Rinehart.

Gilbert, L. A. (1987). Male and female emotional dependency and its implications for the therapist-client relationship. *Professional Psychology, 18,* 555-561.

Goldfarb, A. I. (1969). The psychodynamics of dependency and the search for aid. In R. A. Kalish (Ed.), *The Dependencies of Old People* (pp. 1-15). Ann Arbor, MI: University of Michigan Institute of Gerontology.

Greenberg, R. P., & Bornstein, R. F. (1989). Length of psychiatric hospitalization and oral dependency. *Journal of Personality Disorders, 3,* 199-204.

Hammen, C. L., Marks, T., Mayol, A., & DeMayo, R. (1985). Depressive self-schemas, life stress, and vulnerability to depression. *Journal of Abnormal Psychology, 94,* 308-319.

Hirschfeld, R. M. A., Klerman, G. L., Gough, H. G., Barrett, J., Korchin, S. J., & Chodoff, P. (1977). A measure of interpersonal dependency. *Journal of Personality Assessment, 41,* 610-618.

Lacey, J. H., Coker, S., & Birtchnell, S. A. (1986). Bulimia: Factors associated with its etiology and maintenance. *International Journal of Eating Disorders, 5,* 475-487.

Masling, J. M., & Schwartz, M. A. (1979). A critique of research in psychoanalytic theory. *Genetic Psychology Monographs, 100,* 257-307.

Masling, J. M., Shiffner, J., & Shenfeld, M. (1980). Client perception of the therapist, orality, and sex of client and therapist. *Journal of Counseling Psychology, 27,* 294-298.

Millon, T. (1981). *Disorders of Personality.* New York: Wiley.

Millon, T. (1987). *Millon Clinical Multiaxial Inventory--II Manual.* Minneapolis, MN: National Computer Systems.

Nacev, V. (1980). Dependency and ego strength as indicators of patients' attendance in psychotherapy. *Journal of Clinical Psychology, 36,* 691-695.

Nietzel, M. T., & Harris, M. J. (1990). Relationship of dependency and achievement/autonomy to depression. *Clinical Psychology Review, 10,* 279-297.

Overholser, J. C. (1987). Facilitating autonomy in passive-dependent persons: An integrative model. *Journal of Contemporary Psychotherapy, 17,* 250-269.

Poldrugo, F., & Forti, B. (1988). Personality disorders and alcoholism treatment outcome. *Drug and Alcohol Dependence, 21,* 171-176.

Pyle, R. L., Mitchell, J. E., & Eckert, E. D. (1981). Bulimia: A report of 34 cases. *Journal of Clinical Psychiatry, 42,* 60-64.

Widiger, T. A., & Sanderson, C. (1987). The convergent and discriminant validity of the MCMI as a measure of DSM-III personality disorders. *Journal of Personality Assessment, 51,* 228-242.

ASSESSMENT AND TREATMENT OF DEPRESSION AND LOSS IN THE ELDERLY*

Ruby Takushi Chinen and Linda Berg-Cross

The elderly are by far the fastest growing segment of the U.S. population. It has been estimated that approximately 12% of the United States population is over the age of 65, and by the year 2025 this will increase to 20%. Waxman and Carner (1984) point out that although the elderly comprise a substantial segment of the population, and are at particular risk for mental disorders, their utilization of mental health services is relatively low. He argues that this underutilization of available services is related to inadequate recognition, diagnosis, and treatment of mental health disorders in the elderly. In an analysis of the cost implications of mental disorders, Gottlieb (1988) also reported disproportionately low utilization of psychiatric services. However, he also noted that, overall, the elderly account for nearly 30% of all health care resources. These research clinicians suggest that these figures are related in part to the tendency of elderly patients to offer complaints of physical problems that are related to a depressive syndrome, but present them in the absence of depressed mood.

Recently, the American Psychological Society, in cooperation with several other organizations, sought to address the specific needs of the elderly (American Psychological Society [APS], 1993). This group has prepared a document which outlines specific priorities to "sustain human vitality across the adult life span into old age and ensure quality of life" (p. 2). These priorities are:

1. To develop health-promoting behaviors such as exercise and good nutrition.
2. To develop strategies that maximize adjustment to aging and independent living (e.g., improved vision via eye examinations or use of electronic mail as reminders of daily routine).
3. To develop home and work environments that are sensitive to the changing needs of the older adult (e.g., driving simulators, architectural changes such as ramps).
4. To improve our ability to assess and treat mental disorders in this age group.

In light of these suggestions, and with a recognition that depression is the most frequently seen psychiatric disorder in a general practice (Avant, 1987), this contribution will discuss the assessment/diagnosis of depression and treatment implications for the elderly. This discussion is specifically geared towards the depressed elderly population that lives independently in the community. Although much of the material is applicable to people in assisted care living arrangements or nursing homes, these situations pose additional challenges to the therapist which

---

*The authors wish to thank their research assistant, Rhonda Harrell, for all the help she gave in the preparation of this manuscript.

are beyond the scope of this contribution. However, the "Additional Resources" at the end of the contribution contain information on these other situations.

ASSESSMENT AND DIAGNOSIS OF DEPRESSION IN THE ELDERLY

DIAGNOSTIC CRITERIA

For now, depression criteria are the same for all age groups. Researchers feel this may soon need to change. The Fourth Edition of the *Diagnostic and Statistical Manual of Mental Disorders* (American Psychiatric Association, 1994) provides a system for classification of mental disorders based on behavioral or psychological syndromes. There are two categories of depressive mood disorder: the Major Depressive Disorder and Dysthymic Disorder. There are two additional diagnostic categories for mood disorders due to medical conditions or use of substances such as drugs of abuse.

A diagnosis of Major Depression is made if symptoms include at least 2 weeks of depressed mood, and/or at least 1 week of loss of interest or pleasure in previously pleasurable activities. Symptoms must be present for at least 2 weeks and must represent a change from a previous level of functioning. In addition to depressed mood or loss of interest, at least three or four of the following symptoms must be present so that a total of five symptoms are identified. They are:

1. Significant unintentional weight change (e.g., more than 5% of body weight in a month), or loss of appetite almost daily.
2. Insomnia or hypersomnia nearly every day.
3. Psychomotor agitation or retardation.
4. Fatigue or loss of energy nearly every day.
5. Feelings of worthlessness or excessive or inappropriate guilt.
6. Diminished ability to think or concentrate.
7. Recurrent thoughts of death, recurrent suicidal ideation or intention.

Before the diagnosis can be made, it must be established that organic factors cannot account for the change in mood. This is particularly important when assessing elderly patients, because complicating physical conditions such as endocrine disorders, viral illness, cardiovascular disorders, or medication side effects may present with depressive symptoms. Normal changes in sleep patterns also may occur in the elderly, and changes in taste sensation may result in loss of appetite (Thompson & Gallagher, 1985).

Also, an Uncomplicated Bereavement must be ruled out. Because the elderly are in an age cohort that is apt to experience significant relationship losses, the clinician must be especially careful to discern when a depressive syndrome is a normal response to some real loss. The *DSM-III-R* describes the Uncomplicated Bereavement as similar to a Major Depression, but typically the patient does not present with morbid preoccupations and feelings of worthlessness. In bereavement, the individual tends to regard the feelings of depression as a somewhat "normal" response.

The Major Depressive episode is classified as mild, moderate, severe with or without psychotic features, in partial remission, in full remission, or unspecified. The *DSM-III-R* also includes criteria for distinguishing a chronic versus melancholic type, and for a seasonal pattern of the depressive disorder. A diagnosis of Dysthymia is made using similar criteria for the Major Depression. The two diagnoses differ primarily in severity and duration. The essential feature of Dysthymia is chronic depressed mood for at least 2 years duration with the presence of appetite or sleep changes, low energy, low self-esteem, poor concentration, or feelings of helplessness.

MEDICATION COMPLICATIONS

Depressive complications associated with medications and medical conditions that have depressive symptomatology should be checked. Avant (1987) has summarized medications that may be associated with symptoms of depression, and cautions the clinician to ask patients to name any medications they are currently taking. He reports that analgesics, antibiotics, anticonvulsants, antihistamines, antihypertensives, cardiac drugs, and immunosuppressive drugs, to name a few, may affect mood. The diagnostic task is further complicated when we consider that the underlying physical condition that led to the prescribed medication may be contributing to the depressive symptomatology (e.g., fatigue, insomnia, poor appetite).

PREVALENCE OF DEPRESSION

The prevalence of depression in the elderly is probably in the vicinity of 10% to 15% (Nakra & Grossberg, 1990). However, estimates are difficult to obtain given the tendency of both researchers and clinicians to "accept depressive symptoms in elderly subjects as not indicative of depressive illness" (Blazer & Williams, 1980, p. 439) or to focus primarily on physical concerns. Also, the elderly are in an age cohort likely to view mental disorders as stigmatizing, and therefore are less likely to seek mental health care (German et al., 1987).

There appears to be a greater tendency for women to describe depressive symptoms than men, but by age 55, men begin to report depression as often as women (Nakra & Grossberg, 1990). In general, adults over the age of 75 (the old-old) are significantly more likely to be depressed when compared to a 65 to 74 (young-old) age group. Household income and level of education also produces differences in level of measured depression, with lower income persons and those with fewer number of years of education scoring higher on a measure of depression (L. F. Berkman et al., 1986).

ASSESSMENT INSTRUMENTS

There are several commonly used, relatively easy to administer tools for the assessment of depression. The Beck Depression Inventory (Beck et al., 1961) is a 21-item questionnaire that can be administered via a trained interviewer who reads the items, or the test can be self-administered. The items focus on the cognitive elements of depression (e.g., guilt, feelings of failure, punishment), as well as the somatic elements commonly associated with depression (e.g., weight change, physical concern).

The Self-Rating Depression Scale (SDS) developed by Zung et al. (1965) is a short, 20-item scale which includes items from affective, biological, and psychological arenas. The subject is required to endorse each item, for example "I feel down-hearted and blue," as characteristic of their mood a little of the time, some of the time, a good part of the time, or most of the time (Zung et al., 1965). Glazer, Clarkin, and Hunt (1981) argue that this instrument is of limited utility because items are easily faked and because it relies heavily on self-reporting of psychological distress.

The Geriatric Depression Scale (GDS) is a 30-item scale developed to specifically screen for those depressive symptoms typically seen in the elderly (Brink et al., 1982). The test authors argue that because the Beck Depression Inventory includes items more relevant to the younger patient, it tends to "under-emphasize those symptoms most characteristic of geriatric depression while giving excessive weight to some factors irrelevant in the senium" (p. 39). This results in both false positives and false negatives when used to diagnose depression in the elderly (Brink et al., 1982).

The GDS was developed to be (a) self-rating in order to be suitable for an office practice, (b) easy to answer and composed of simple yes/no options, and (c) geared toward geriatrics with items generated by clinicians experienced in the field of geriatrics. Items include questions such as, "Do you often get bored?" or "Do you have trouble concentrating?" Brink et al. (1982; see also Yesavage et al., 1983) were concerned that the scale be sensitive to mild depression in the elderly, and thus included fewer items specifically related to physical complaints. Yesavage et al. (1983) report reliability and validity data on the GDS in support of its use with the elderly. The GDS is reproduced on page 162.

SUICIDE IN THE ELDERLY

There is evidence to suggest that the elderly are at particular risk for suicide. Reporting on data from Finland, Achte (1988) notes that although suicide attempts decrease, the rate of successful suicide increases with age. She suggests that the risk of suicide increases in persons who were born in a year with a high birth rate. This is because that individual is thus subject to a greater amount of lifelong competition for resources. Because the proportion of elderly in the population is steadily growing, a corresponding increase in the suicide rate of the elderly can be expected. Similarly, Kirsling (1986) reports a substantially higher incidence of suicide among older adults when compared to younger aged U.S. adults. In the United States, it also appears that the elderly have more suicides and fewer suicide attempts or gestures. Of course, there are an unknown number of suicides among the elderly population that are not due to a clinically identifiable depression. Rather, they are related to a poor medical prognoses or philosophical decisions about the importance of quality of life and the need to live independently.

In clinical practice, look for the following 10 warning signs: Changes in sleep or eating patterns, weight change, a sudden disinterest in activities, or vague physical complaints should be noted. Other risk factors the clinician must be alert to include previous attempts or a family history of suicide, patients who are widowed or divorced, patients who abuse substances, patients who have recently experienced a major loss, or a newly developed rejection of loved ones. The greatest danger of suicide is when the patient is caught in a situation that feels hopeless, and the patient reports feeling helpless, exhausted, and a sense of failure (Achte, 1988).

Possible questions to ask a depressed elderly adult:

1. Do you feel like giving up sometimes?
2. How is this different from how you felt in middle age?
3. Have you been thinking about death and dying more frequently?
4. How often do you find yourself dwelling on lost abilities?
5. Have you ever considered suicide? Do you have a plan for suicide?
6. Do you talk about suicide with your friends?
7. Do you know anyone who has planned or successfully committed suicide?

TAILORING STANDARD THERAPEUTIC STRATEGIES FOR THE TREATMENT OF DEPRESSION IN THE ELDERLY

INDIVIDUAL PSYCHOTHERAPY

One basic guideline for treating the elderly is to "let the treatment suit the patient" (Brink, 1985). The objectives of treatment are typically to remove symptoms of depression, restore psychosocial functioning, improve medical health, and prevent a recurrence of depression (Rush, 1991). The therapist may need to make modifications in a typical treatment approach if the elderly client has difficulty concentrating, is easily fatigued, or perhaps has a communication disorder due to a recent illness. The environment of therapy may vary. For example, sessions may be held in the client's home or in an institutional setting that does not provide for privacy. Flexibility in the frequency and duration of therapy may be necessary. Sessions may be shortened to less than the traditional hour, or the clinician may elect to meet more frequently than once a week if the patient is recently bereaved. Defining who is the actual patient is another necessary professional decision. It may be that, although the patient presents as an individual for therapy, intervention may need to involve family or other available caregivers.

Other issues to consider are those related to socioeconomic status and ethnicity. Sufficient and stable finances in old age afford the elder flexibility and a sense of security that assists in adjusting to retirement or other changes. The clinician must be sensitive to the very real difficulties encountered by the poor, minority, and old person. Demonstrating a sensitivity to these realities and a willingness to openly discuss them can help foster trust in the therapeutic relationship (C. I. Cohen, 1990).

Behavioral/Cognitive-Behavioral Treatment Suggestions. Behavioral approaches with the depressed elderly client are aimed at decreasing the effects of (covert and physiological) aversive stimuli, increasing the level of reinforcement, and fostering a feeling of greater self-control. Several behavioral strategies can be used to achieve these goals. For example, traditional desensitization techniques can assist the elderly patient to overcome fears of using public transportation alone. Or, if the patient is prone to physical pain, the clinician can help the patient differentiate between pain that needs immediate medical attention and pain that can be managed by relaxation techniques or visualization (J. B. Skinner et al., 1990). When using behavioral techniques such as progressive relaxation, be sensitive to physical changes, such as loss of muscle tone or arthritis, that can affect the patient. It may be beneficial to omit certain muscle groups altogether (Cautela, 1981). The clinician can also assist by encouraging the elder to identify (or create) and list new reinforcers to replace those lost due to changes in physical abilities or to the loss of a supportive spousal relationship.

B. F. Skinner (1983) discussed his own experience of aging and wrote, "to develop is not simply to grow older but to unfold a latent structure, to realize an inner potential" (p. 239). He called it "intellectual self-management" and made several suggestions for adjusting to normal changes that occur with aging. A few of his suggestions to pass on to patients include:

1. If you cannot read, listen to book recordings.
2. Flavor food for the aging palate.
3. Seek to make situations as free from aversive consequences as possible. For example, use humor and grace when you forget an acquaintance's name.
4. To compensate for forgetfulness, execute as much of a behavior as possible as soon as possible, that is, place the umbrella near the door as soon as you realize it may rain to minimize the chance you will forget it.
5. Keep a note pad or a tape recorder with you to make notes to yourself, or establish a convenient organizational system which may include a dictating system.

Psychodynamic Psychotherapy. Psychodynamic psychotherapy has also been described as a useful treatment modality with the elderly. Psychodynamic approaches with the older patient may be different from therapy with a younger patient because what constitutes stress may be different for the older adult, or there may be differences in adaptive responses. Goals of psychodynamic psychotherapy with the elderly are:

1. To bring about a change in the functioning of the personality so that the person is more able to have creative and satisfying aging experiences.
2. To assist in the return of the person to a previous, higher level of functioning.
3. To assist the family or caregiver in the home environment in providing support to the patient (Kahana, 1979).

Psychodynamically oriented therapy with the elderly has been characterized as a "mourning-liberation" process (Pollock, 1987, p. 11) in which the elderly patient is able to mourn past states of the self and then move forward. Patients who are unable to mourn the inevitable losses associated with aging, and who have difficulty adapting to change, often present with complaints of loneliness, isolation, fears of loss of basic controls, and helplessness. In particular, patients may need to explore the nature and meaning of changing relationships with spouses, children, and siblings.

GROUP PSYCHOTHERAPY

Group psychotherapy is a particularly useful treatment modality with the elderly. A supportive group setting can be of immense assistance to the isolated elderly adult. Groups help isolated elders make new relationship contacts, they can provide an opportunity for bereaved elders to openly discuss their feelings of loss and loneliness, they can be educational in focus and provide information about the functional consequences of certain physical conditions, they can help the elder develop new hobbies or interests in retirement, or they may be an opportunity for life review and the telling of one's story.

Types of group interventions vary from relatively unstructured social environments where refreshments are served to more formal insight-oriented psychotherapy groups. Two general categories of group psychotherapy that often overlap are (a) insight-oriented, in which emotional conflicts are worked through, and (b) supportive, in which support is provided for current stresses (Gurfein & Stutman, 1993). Short-term group cognitive therapy which provides an opportunity to identify and change irrational beliefs has been effective in treatment of depression in the elderly (Free, Oei, & Sanders, 1991). However, the elderly can also do very well in more open-ended insight-oriented therapy groups. Some typical themes that arise are death and loss, concern about the uncertainty of life, isolation, and loneliness (Solomon & Zinke, 1991). Riley and Carr (1989) suggest that a nonstructured expressive approach allows the development of resources in the group and a sense of mastery that is curative.

Some modifications in the structure of the group or therapy techniques may be helpful with this age group. A partial list includes:

1. Greater structure. Provide a consistent "holding environment" for members by conducting group in the same place at the same time, and by being mindful of boundary management.
2. You may elect to be more active than you typically would be in the group.
3. Gently encourage reminiscence by asking patients to bring in and discuss old photographs of local scenes or personal photographs (Baines, Saxby, & Ehlert, 1987).
4. Encourage extragroup socialization.
5. Vary session length, adapt in other ways to physical limitations of the patients (Gurfein & Stutman, 1993).
6. Make an effort to match the level of functioning, especially cognitive functioning, of group members (Parham et al., 1982).

FAMILY THERAPY

One of the most difficult psychological adjustments for healthy aging is the successful readjustment of family relationships for the final phase of life. David Morgenstern (1992) describes the following seven themes that need to be resolved by the family with aging members. Each of these issues is critical to address with the depressed elderly client.

1. *Dependence-Independence.* With declining abilities, parents and adult children need to decide who will be in control of bills, food, clothes, medicine, and activity schedules. Depressed elderly clients may relinquish responsibilities prematurely, feeling that their lack of energy and ability to complete tasks is permanent. Therapists should educate the family and client about the depression process and help set up temporary or partial supports whenever possible.
2. *Dealing With Loss and Bereavements.* Without the structure and support of a spouse following death, adult children are often expected to "fill the gap." Adult children often be-

come emotional caretakers long before they become physical caretakers. Caregivers often feel "sandwiched" between the demands of their nuclear family and care, and the desire to be a companion to a grieving or depressed parent. Clinicians can offer an additional important source of support during the grieving process. Support groups for widows and widowers are available in most communities, and therapists should be familiar with these groups to make referrals easier. During later stages of the grieving process a family-of-origin session can help the family mourn together and voice concerns and problems they fear in the future.

3. *Relationships, Family Issues, and Interactions.* As parents age and become more dependent upon their children, the angers and resentments of adult children may be rekindled. Once again, children become extremely sensitive to criticism, not living up to expectations, comparisons with siblings, and feelings of not being understood. As these animosities express themselves, depressed elderly parents may feel they have "failed" in their role as parent. The adult children's anger reinforces the parent's sense of worthlessness. Cognitive therapy aimed at uncovering irrational parental beliefs and refuting them and/or testing them can lead to significant improvement in clients.

4. *Physical Concerns.* For many elderly parents, phone calls and visits from adult children are opportunities to discuss every ache and pain that has occurred since their last visit. Children come to feel that the parent is a cranky old person wanting to dwell on the negative. Indeed, happier elderly people do speak less often about symptomatology than the more depressed elderly. Of course, this could be a "chicken and egg" problem. Clearly, the more physical problems people have, the more depressed most people become. Therapists working with the depressed elderly can reduce familial stress by allowing the patient to discuss health concerns in great detail. Asking patients to keep a diary of their health concerns, having them complete a daily mood chart, and noting effective ways of coping in a diary are all useful techniques that allow the client to feel nurtured and able to invest in other topics with their family.

5. *Loss of Power.* When adult children have to deal with sudden illness in a parent, they also need to deal with the idea that this may happen to them in the not-so-distant future. The same is true of memory loss, hearing loss, the fractured hip, stressed or confused communications, or the need to move into a nursing home. On the other hand, depressed elderly parents focus only on the avoidance and rejection they experience from their children. Therapists can help clients reframe the seeming "insensitivity" of their children's behavior. Instead, a more accurate explanation is that the "insensitivity" is a defensive expression of fear based on deep love and identification with the parent.

6. *Finances, the Handling of Money, and Legal Concerns.* Money is often symbolic of how power, control, and independence are distributed in a family. Elderly parents usually are adamant about retaining control over their money; this despite the fact that over 95% of all adults leave their money equitably distributed to all surviving children. Relatives need to be educated about how especially important it is for the depressed elderly to retain control over their finances.

7. *Death and Legacies.* Not surprisingly, most old people have reconciled themselves to the fact that they are going to die. The depressed elderly, however, often want to die. In these situations, family members need help on how to reassure and reinforce the depressed client. Help family members focus on all the different experiences and attitudes they have witnessed in the patient over the years. This often helps place the depression in a less painful context by making it one experience among a lifetime of experiences. Very often a depleted caregiver seeks therapy to deal with stress imposed by their depressed, elderly relative.

ANTIDEPRESSANT MEDICATION AND PSYCHOTHERAPY

Antidepressant medications are often combined with psychotherapy for treatment of depression in the elderly (Reynolds et al., 1992). Generally, the same types of medications are used for the elderly as with other adult groups, but the dosage is usually far lower; typically only 50% of the usual middle-aged adult dosage. An in-depth review of medication issues is beyond the scope of this contribution, but the reader is referred to Jenike (1989), who provides a helpful summary of antidepressant medications. He describes the various medication options available to the clinician, side-effect concerns, and health complications in the elderly, and also comments on the use of electroconvulsive therapy (ECT) with this population (see also Nakra & Grossberg, 1990).

Briefly, some issues the professional must be sensitive to with antidepressant medication are the changing metabolic rates of the elderly, the heightened sensitivity to side effects due to lowered resistances or less resiliency in the elderly, the potential for cardiotoxicity of certain antidepressant medications, or the complications that may arise due to alcohol use or other prescribed medications (Abrams & Alexopoulos, 1987; Salzman, 1991; Sunderland et al., 1990). Medication compliance is often difficult to obtain with the elderly, and the clinician can enhance compliance by carefully explaining any expected side effects, providing clear instructions for when and how the medication is to be taken (at mealtime), or by cautioning elders that they may not experience results immediately. Written explanations of side effects and methods of assuring that the drugs are taken in the proper dosage increases compliance. Therapists working with older depressed patients need to work closely with the primary care physicians to assure that clients are properly medicated.

COUNTERTRANSFERENCE IN THE YOUNGER THERAPIST

As with all patients, the clinician gathers rich therapeutic information by staying attuned to both positive and negative countertransference feelings. Unresolved personal issues of the clinician not only affect the therapy relationship but may determine whether or not an elderly patient even receives care. For instance, in addition to the tendency for clinicians to assume that depressive symptoms in the elderly are "normal" and to therefore underdiagnose depression, a clinician may adhere to the belief that the elder is not a good therapy candidate because of a limited life span (G. D. Cohen, 1981). Or, the clinician may be less attentive to the older client due to feelings related to inadequate reimbursement, or the greater length of time sometimes required to obtain a complete history, or because the clinician has therapeutic goals for the patient that the patient does not necessarily desire (Waxman & Carner, 1984).

There are several other possible countertransference issues that may arise when younger therapists treat older patients. Treating the elderly forces the clinician to confront personal anxieties about physical illness and death. Or, if the therapist has unresolved feelings of hostility toward a parent, these feelings may be stirred by contact with an elderly patient. As noted previously, the clinician may believe that the amount and quality of life left to the patient makes therapy almost a wasted effort. Or, the clinician may fear the patient will die during treatment. It is also possible the clinician is concerned about whether or not professional colleagues will hold work with the elderly in high esteem (Cooper, 1984; Myers, 1986).

TECHNIQUES FOR ADDRESSING LOSS IN THE ELDERLY

Clinicians treating the depressed need to make a thorough assessment of the nature and extent of losses experienced by that patient. A single, relatively simple loss may be difficult for the older adult if it serves as a reminder that future losses are inevitable. In addition, the elderly often encounter several types of loss simultaneously, for example loss of spouse, loss of physical health, loss of siblings, and loss of community or work-related contacts, to name a few. In the following section we will discuss some commonly experienced losses in old age and offer some suggestions for therapeutic intervention.

LOSS OF SPOUSE AND BEREAVEMENT

As noted earlier, an Uncomplicated Bereavement is generally understood as a normal grief reaction to a perceived loss that does not involve a morbid preoccupation with a personal sense of worthlessness. The duration of a "normal" bereavement cannot be predicted because it varies according to the style and timing of the individual. Cultural differences also affect the length and intensity of an Uncomplicated Bereavement. If the older adult is able to utilize supportive social structures and can slowly identify with the new role of widow or widower, the loss of a spouse need not be characterized by social disintegration or health deterioration (Heyman & Gianturco, 1973).

When presented with the bereaved spouse, the clinician has the opportunity to support the patient through the grief and to monitor any changes that may suggest a more serious disorder. Recovery from bereavement can be understood as the return to a level of functioning that had been achieved prior to the loss of the spouse, which may include the formation of new attachments (Conway, 1988).

The loss of a spouse has been cited as significantly related to depression in the elderly, with married men and those never married having the lowest rates of depression when compared to widowers and the divorced or separated elder (Murrell, Himmelfarb, & Wright, 1983). If the individual is unable to resolve feelings of grief or continues to feel dependent upon the lost spouse, recovery from the loss may lead to a depressive disorder. Again, a spouse is often the closest adult attachment one can experience, and, even if the relationship was not always experienced as close or supportive, what is lost is the stability of a relationship and the daily stimulation that even conflict can provide (Sable, 1991).

Some suggestions for helping the bereaved older adult make sense of the loss and thus speed recovery include:

1. Help clients reminisce, to forgive their spouse for certain hurts they inflicted, to forgive themselves when they failed as a spouse, and to rejoice in the couple's triumphs.
2. Have clients bring in photos and mementos to heighten the emotional intensity and clarity of the memories.
3. Have clients develop healing rituals. For example, some clients need permission to "talk" to their dead spouse or visit the cemetery frequently.
4. Help clients reframe the meaning of a new, independent life plan so that it signifies paying tribute to their spouse instead of forgetting the spouse.
5. Emphasize the use of community services such as hospices or educationally oriented bereavement self-help groups, and assist the elder in locating transportation services to these services.
6. If necessary, assist elders in securing financial consultation regarding the economic implications of the loss of their spouse. The clinician may even suggest that elderly couples make financial preparations for the possibility of a major medical illness or death of one of the partners.
7. Consider seeing elders with family members for a session if siblings or children are available.

LOSS OF A SIBLING

The loss of a sibling is also a normative loss experienced by those over the age of 65. S. Z. Moss and M. S. Moss (1989) have pointed out that before the clinician can assess the impact of sibling loss, the nature of that relationship must be determined. Some dimensions of the sibling tie to explore include the nature and degree of the interaction between siblings, the amount of emotional support given to and received from the lost sibling, the nature of sibling rivalry, the importance of the lost sibling as a role model for aging, and the amount of family identity gained from the sibling tie.

It must be noted that in addition to these dimensions, the clinician must be sensitive to the sociocultural differences that bear on the nature of the family tie and the resultant experience of loss. Ethnic minority communities are often highly family oriented and interdependent, and the loss of a sibling may be significantly more devastating than expected, thus placing that person at greater risk for depression. Remember, also, that institutionalized elderly may have reformed their attachments to their new "family" and so the loss of a roommate or friend within the facility may be experienced as a sibling loss (Sanchez, 1992).

However, the loss of a sibling may also serve to strengthen remaining family ties and actually assist the older adult in adjusting to the aging process. The clinician can (a) provide an opportunity for the elder to explore both positive and negative feelings toward the sibling, (b) explore possible feelings of guilt at having survived longer than a sibling, or perhaps guilt at wanting to survive longer, (c) explore the implications for the elder's own sense of mortality in an effort to affirm present vitality, and (d) encourage the elder to maintain or renew other family relationships in an effort to foster a sense of continuity among the generations (S. Z. Moss & M. S. Moss, 1989).

LOSS OF PHYSICAL INTEGRITY OR HEALTH

Many, if not most, older adults suffer from some kind of physical disability. The physical impairment may take the form of a chronic illness, loss of physical mobility, decline in sensory sensitivity, or a loss of mental acuity. As with any change, the individual needs to grieve the lost physical ability; not to do so may increase the likelihood of depression in the elder. In addition to the changes in daily routine or capacity for self-care that may occur with physical illness, the loss of health may contribute to depression if the elder also loses an identification with a valued parent or other figure associated with physical prowess or athletic ability. This may be explored by asking elders to describe what physical ability they have lost and what memories or relationships are associated with that specific ability (Myers, 1989).

Hearing loss or changes in visual acuity are commonly seen in aging and are often associated with psychiatric symptoms of depression. Kalayam et al. (1991) found that 30% of subjects in a speech and hearing clinic could be diagnosed as depressed. They note that paranoid symptoms are also associated with hearing loss, but that patients with paranoid tendencies are not likely to be seen in a speech and hearing clinic.

Some simple but humane interventions that can be used to assist the elderly patient with sensory loss include the following:

1. Touch patients as much as possible to assist in sensory awareness.
2. Be sure that eyeglass prescriptions are correct, and that lenses are clean.
3. If necessary, speak slowly and directly in front of the hearing impaired patient.
4. Recommend frequent assessment of vision and hearing.
5. Assist the patient and caregivers in making changes in the home environment (e.g., recommend the use of large clocks, or a night light to assist in night-time activities; Burnside, 1973).

Tinnitus, or the experience of sound that originates within the hearer, is another hearing disorder seen in the elderly (Sullivan et al., 1988). Most patients with tinnitus do not report significant disability once they are reassured that the disorder does not imply more serious disease (Sullivan et al., 1988). However, those few patients who do report a disruption in their social or work activities due to tinnitus are at significantly higher risk for depression. When presented with a patient who has not habituated to the sound in their ears, the clinician should note that an underlying depression exacerbates the tinnitus, and as depression decreases, so will the symptomatology.

Patients with congestive heart failure and other cardiac conditions are also prone to depressive disorder (Freedland et al., 1991; Morro, 1989). The clinician should encourage older patients to participate in a formal cardiac rehabilitation program in order to maintain a sense of hopefulness by interacting with other recovering cardiac patients. The program may include supportive discussion groups, activity groups designed for the recovering cardiac patient, and education of the patient and the patient's family about the illness.

LOSS OF VOCATIONAL ROLE OR COMMUNITY CONTACTS

Retirement is typically a life change the older adult looks forward to with great anticipation. Plans are made for extended rest and relaxation, but oftentimes, the experienced changes are unexpected. Many retirees are not aware of how closely their social contacts are tied to their work environments. If one partner has taken the traditional homemaker role for a number of years, the adjustments to having a spouse at home full-time may also be experienced as a loss of personal space and time. The elder who is best able to adjust to retirement is one who has interests outside of the workplace or can slowly reduce professional activities; thus it is typically the blue-collar worker who feels the loss of vocation most intensely (Brink, 1985). The loss of vocation in persons who focused their lives around their work may produce a sense of loss of "will to meaning," or the loss of a feeling of life satisfaction (Pintos, 1988).

Life satisfaction, or a sense of one's continued ability to be creative, can be fostered through a program or group that focuses on the cultural arts. The clinician may recommend the patient attend a community program that integrates the enjoyment and performance of music, storytelling, and poetry reading. B. B. Smith (1992) reports that the rewards of such stimulation and opportunity serve her elderly population well. The Independent Living Rehabilitation (ILR) program recognizes the importance of activity and the need to feel effective in the environment. The program is designed to assist the elderly in maximizing self-reliance and the sense of personal control in daily activities (H. Smith, 1986).

SUMMARY

Although the elderly are at risk for numerous physical ailments and experiences of loss, they are often overlooked and underserved. Despite the common societal assumption that old age must be a time of expected decline in all spheres of life, there continues to be much the older adult can celebrate. Aging is a part of the human developmental scheme, and we as clinicians are in a position to offer assistance when an elder is not able to fully experience the positive aspects of aging.

Innovations in Clinical Practice: A Source Book (Vol. 13)

THE GERIATRIC DEPRESSION SCALE*

Choose the best answer for how you felt over the past week (circle "Yes" or "No").

1. Are you basically satisfied with your life? — Yes / No
2. Have you dropped many of your activities and interests? — Yes / No
3. Do you feel that your life is empty? — Yes / No
4. Do you often get bored? — Yes / No
5. Are you hopeful about the future? — Yes / No
6. Are you bothered by thoughts you can't get out of your head? — Yes / No
7. Are you in good spirits most of the time? — Yes / No
8. Are you afraid that something bad is going to happen to you? — Yes / No
9. Do you feel happy most of the time? — Yes / No
10. Do you often feel helpless? — Yes / No
11. Do you often get restless and fidgety? — Yes / No
12. Do you prefer to stay at home, rather than going out and doing new things? — Yes / No
13. Do you frequently worry about the future? — Yes / No
14. Do you feel you have more problems with memory than most? — Yes / No
15. Do you think it is wonderful to be alive now? — Yes / No
16. Do you often feel downhearted and blue? — Yes / No
17. Do you feel pretty worthless the way you are now? — Yes / No
18. Do you worry a lot about the past? — Yes / No
19. Do you find life very exciting? — Yes / No
20. Is it hard for you to get started on new projects? — Yes / No
21. Do you feel full of energy? — Yes / No
22. Do you feel that your situation is hopeless? — Yes / No
23. Do you think that more people are better off than you are? — Yes / No
24. Do you frequently get upset over little things? — Yes / No
25. Do you frequently feel like crying? — Yes / No
26. Do you have trouble concentrating? — Yes / No
27. Do you enjoy getting up in the morning? — Yes / No
28. Do you prefer to avoid social gatherings? — Yes / No
29. Is it easy for you to make decisions? — Yes / No
30. Is your mind as clear as it used to be? — Yes / No

> Items 1, 5, 7, 9, 15, 19, 21, 27, 29, and 30 are scored for depression if the subject responds "No." All other items are scored if the subject responds "Yes." A score of 11 or greater is a possible indicator of depression which needs to be confirmed by clinical evaluation.

*Note. From "Development and Validation of a Geriatric Depression Screening Scale: A Preliminary Report" by J. A. Yesavage, T. L. Brink, T. L. Rose, O. Lum, V. Huang, M. Adey, and V. O. Leirer, 1983, *Journal of Psychiatric Research, 17,* p. 41. Copyright © 1983 by Pergamon Press Ltd. Reprinted by permission.

Ruby Takushi Chinen, PhD, is currently Assistant Professor of Psychology in the Psychology Department at Howard University in Washington, DC. Her training is in clinical psychology with special interests in the areas of group psychotherapy, gerontology, and substance abuse. Dr. Chinen may be contacted at Department of Psychology, Howard University, 525 Bryant Street, N.W., Campus Box 1097, Washington, DC 20059.

Linda Berg-Cross, PhD, ABPP, is currently Director of Clinical Training in the Psychology Department of Howard University. She has special interests in the areas of developmental marital issues and intergenerational interactions. Dr. Berg-Cross is the author of a book on basic concepts in family therapy and a forthcoming book on couples therapy. Dr. Berg-Cross can be contacted at Psychology Department, CB Powell, 525 Bryant Street, N.W., Washington, DC 20059.

RESOURCES

CITED RESOURCES

Abrams, R. C., & Alexopoulos, G. S. (1987). Substance abuse in the elderly: Alcohol and prescription drugs. *Hospital and Community Psychiatry, 38,* 1285-1287.

Achte, K. (1988). Suicidal tendencies in the elderly. *Suicide and Life-Threatening Behavior, 18,* 55-65.

American Psychiatric Association. (1987). *Diagnostic and Statistical Manual of Mental Disorders* (3rd ed. rev.). Washington, DC: Author.

American Psychiatric Association. (1994). *Diagnostic and Statistical Manual of Mental Disorders* (4th ed.). Washington, DC: Author.

American Psychological Society. (1993). Vitality for life: Psychological research for productive aging [Booklet in a series]. *Human Capital Initiative.* Washington, DC: Author.

Avant, R. (1987). Diagnosis and treatment of depression. *Psychopathology, 20,* 13-19.

Baines, S., Saxby, P., & Ehlert, K. (1987). Reality orientation and reminiscence therapy: A controlled cross-overt study of elderly confused people. *British Journal of Psychiatry, 151,* 222-231.

Beck, A. T., Ward, C. H., Mendelson, M., Mock, J., & Erbaugh, J. (1961). An inventory for measuring depression. *Archives of General Psychiatry, 4,* 561-571.

Berkman, L. F., Berkman, C. S., Kasl, S., Freeman, D. H., Leo, L., Ostfeld, A. M., Cornoni-Huntley, J., & Brody, J. A. (1986). Depressive symptoms in relation to physical health and functioning in the elderly. *American Journal of Epidemiology, 124,* 372-388.

Blazer, D., & Williams, C. D. (1980). Epidemiology of dysphoria and depression in an elderly population. *American Journal of Psychiatry, 137,* 439-444.

Brink, T. L. (1985). The grieving patient in later life. *Psychotherapy Patient, 2,* 117-127.

Brink, T. L, Yesavage, J. A., Lum, O., Heersema, P. H., Adey, M., & Rose, T. L. (1982). Screening tests for geriatric depression. *Clinical Gerontologist, 1,* 37-43.

Burnside, I. M. (1973). Multiple losses in the aged: Implications for nursing care. *Gerontologist, 13,* 157-162.

Cautela, J. P. (1981). Behavioral treatments of elderly patients with depression. In J. F. Clarkin & H. I. Glazer (Eds.), *Depression: Behavioral and Directive Intervention Strategies* (pp. 344-365). New York: Garland Publishing.

Cohen, C. I. (1990). Psychotherapy with the elderly in public mental health settings. *New Directions for Mental Health Services, 46,* 81-92.

Cohen, G. D. (1981). Perspectives on psychotherapy with the elderly. *American Journal of Psychiatry, 138,* 347-350.

Conway, P. (1988). Losses and grief in old age. *Social Casework: The Journal of Contemporary Social Work, November,* 541-549.

Cooper, D. E. (1984). Group psychotherapy with the elderly: Dealing with loss and death. *American Journal of Psychotherapy, 38,* 203-213.

Free, M. L., Oei, T. P. S., & Sanders, M. R. (1991). Treatment outcome of a group cognitive therapy program for depression. *International Journal of Group Psychotherapy, 41,* 533-547.

Freedland, K. E., Carney, R. M., Rich, M. W., Caracciolo, A., Krotenberg, J. A., Smith, L. J., & Sperry, J. (1991). Depression in elderly patients with congestive heart failure. *Journal of Geriatric Psychiatry, 24,* 59-71.

German, P. S., Shapiro, S., Skinner, E. A., Von Korff, M., Klein, L. E., Turner, R. W., Teitelbaum, M. L., Burke, J., & Burns, B. J. (1987). Detection and management of mental health problems of older patients by primary care providers. *Journal of the American Medical Association, 257,* 489-493.

Glazer, H. I., Clarkin, J. F., & Hunt, H. F. (1981). Assessment of depression. In J. F. Clarkin & H. I. Glazer (Eds.), *Depression: Behavioral and Directive Intervention Strategies* (pp. 3-30). New York: Garland Publishing.

Gottlieb, G. L. (1988). Cost implications of depression in older adults. *International Journal of Geriatric Psychology, 3,* 191-200.

Gurfein, H. N., & Stutman, G. F. (1993). Group psychotherapy with the elderly. In H. I. Kaplan & B. J. Sadock (Eds.), *Comprehensive Group Psychotherapy* (3rd ed., pp. 584-596). Baltimore: Williams & Wilkins.

Heyman, D. K., & Gianturco, D. T. (1973). Long-term adaptation by the elderly to bereavement. *Journal of Gerontology, 28,* 359-362.

Jenike, M. A. (1989). Treatment of affective illness in the elderly with drugs and electroconvulsive therapy. *Journal of Geriatric Psychiatry, 22,* 77-112.

Kahana, R. J. (1979). Strategies of dynamic psychotherapy with the wide range of older individuals. *Journal of Geriatric Psychiatry, 12,* 71-100.

Kalayam, B., Alexopoulos, G. S., Merrell, H. B., Young, R. C., & Shindledecker, R. (1991). Patterns of hearing loss and psychiatric morbidity in elderly patients attending a hearing clinic. *International Journal of Geriatric Psychiatry, 6,* 131-136.

Kirsling, R. A. (1986). Review of suicide among elderly persons. *Psychological Reports, 59,* 359-366.

Morgenstern, D. (1992). Caregiving interventions with the elderly: Paths, pains, pitfalls, and possibilities. *Psychotherapy in Private Practice, 11,* 63-73.

Morro, B. C. (1989). Post hospital depression and the elderly cardiac patient. *Social Work in Health Care, 14,* 59-66.

Moss, S. Z., & Moss, M. S. (1989). The impact of the death of an elderly sibling. *American Behavioral Scientist, 33,* 94-106.

Murrell, S. A., Himmelfarb, S., & Wright, K. (1983). Prevalence of depression and its correlates in older adults. *American Journal of Epidemiology, 117,* 173-185.

Myers, W. A. (1986). Transference and countertransference issues in treatments involving older patients and younger therapists. *Journal of Geriatric Psychiatry, 19,* 221-239.

Myers, W. A. (1989). I can't play ball anymore. *Journal of Geriatric Psychiatry, 22,* 121-139.

Nakra, B. R. S., & Grossberg, G. T. (1990). Mood disorders. In D. Bienenfeld (Ed.), *Verweordt's Clinical Geropsychiatry* (3rd ed., pp. 107-124). Baltimore: Williams & Wilkins.

Parham, I. A., Priddy, J. M., McGovern, T. V., & Richman, C. M. (1982). Group psychotherapy with the elderly: Problems and prospects. *Psychotherapy: Theory, Research, and Practice, 19,* 437-443.

Pintos, C. C. G. (1988). Depression and the will to meaning: A comparison of the GDS and PIL in an Argentine population. *Clinical Gerontologist, 7,* 3-9.

Pollock, G. H. (1987). The mourning-liberation process: Ideas on the inner life of the older adult. In J. Sadavoy & M. Leszcz (Eds.), *Treating the Elderly With Psychotherapy: The Scope for Change in Later Life* (pp. 3-30). Madison, CT: International Universities Press.

Reynolds, C. F., Frank, E., Perel, J. M., Imber, S. D., Cornes, C., Morycz, R. K., Mazumdar, S., Miller, M. D., Pollock, B. G., Rifai, A. H., Stack, J. A., George, C. J., Houck, P. R., & Kupfer, D. J. (1992). Combined pharmacotherapy and psychotherapy in the acute and continuation treatment of elderly patients with recurrent major depression: A preliminary report. *American Journal of Psychiatry, 149*, 1687-1692.

Riley, K. P., & Carr, M. (1989). Group psychotherapy with older adults: The value of an expressive approach. *Psychotherapy, 26*, 366-371.

Rush, A. J. (1991, November). *Overviewing Treatment Options in the Depressed elderly.* National Institutes of Health Consensus Development Conference, Bethesda, MD.

Sable, P. (1991). Attachment, loss of spouse, and grief in elderly adults. *OMEGA, 23*, 129-142.

Salzman, C. (1991, November). *Pharmacological Treatment of Depression in the Elderly.* National Institutes of Health Consensus Development Conference, Bethesda, MD.

Sanchez, C. D. (1992). Mental health issues: The elderly hispanic. *Journal of Geriatric Psychiatry, 25*, 69-83.

Skinner, B. F. (1983). Intellectual self-management in old age. *American Psychologist, 38*, 239-244.

Skinner, J. B., Erskine, A., Pearce, S., Rubenstein, I., Taylor, M., & Foster, C. (1990). The evaluation of a cognitive behavioral treatment programme in outpatients with chronic pain. *Journal of Psychosomatic Research, 14*, 13-19.

Smith, B. B. (1992). Treatment of dementia: Healing through cultural arts. *Pride-Institute-Journal-of-Long-Term-Home-Health-Care, 3*, 37-45.

Smith, H. (1986). Mastery and achievement: Guidelines using clinical problem solving with depressed elderly clients. *Physical and Occupational Therapy in Geriatrics, 5*, 35-46.

Solomon, K., & Zinke, M. R. (1991). Group psychotherapy with the depressed elderly. *Journal of Gerontological Social Work, 17*, 47-56.

Sullivan, M. D., Katon, W., Dobie, R., Sakai, C., Russo, J., & Harrop-Griffiths, J. (1988). Disabling tinnitus: Association with affective disorder. *General Hospital Psychiatry, 10*, 285-291.

Sunderland, T., Molchan, S. E., Martinez, R. A., & Vitiello, B. (1990). Treatment approaches to atypical depression in the elderly. *Psychiatric Annals, 20*, 474-478.

Thompson, L. W., & Gallagher, D. (1985). Depression and its treatment. *Aging, 348*, 14-18.

Waxman, H. M., & Carner, E. A. (1984). Physicians' recognition, diagnosis, and treatment of mental disorders in elderly medical patients. *Gerontologist, 24*, 593-597.

Yesavage, J. A., Brink, T. L., Rose, T. L., Lum, O., Huang, V., Adey, M., & Leirer, V. O. (1983). Development and validation of a geriatric depression screening scale: A preliminary report. *Journal of Psychiatric Research, 17*, 37-49.

Zung, W. W. M., Richards, C. B., Gables, C., & Short, M. J. (1965). Self-rating depression scale in an outpatient clinic. *Archives of General Psychiatry, 13*, 508-516.

ADDITIONAL RESOURCES

Ben-Sira, Z. (1991). *Regression, Stress, and Readjustment in Aging: A Structured Bio-Psycho-Social Perspective on Coping and Professional Support.* New York: Greenwood Press.

Berezin, M. A. (1987). Reflections on psychotherapy with the elderly. In J. Sadavoy & M. Leszcz (Eds.), *Treating the Elderly With Psychotherapy: The Scope for Change in Later Life* (pp. 45-66). Madison, CT: International Universities Press.

Berland, D. I, & Poggi, R. (1979). Expressive group psychotherapy with the aging. *International Journal of Group Psychotherapy, 29*, 87-108.

Breckenridge, J. N., Gallagher, D., Thompson, L. W., & Peterson, J. (1986). Characteristic depressive symptoms of bereaved elders. *Journal of Gerontology, 41*, 163-168.

Bienenfeld, D. (Ed.). (1990). *Clinical Geropsychiatry.* Baltimore: Williams & Wilkins.

Billig, N. (1986). *To Be Old and Sad: Understanding Depression in the Elderly.* New York: Free Press.

Breslau, L. (1983). *Depression in Aging: Causes, Care and Consequences*. New York: Springer.

Clayton, P. J., Halikas, J. A., & Maurice, W. L. (1972). The depression of widowhood. *British Journal of Psychiatry, 120,* 71-77.

Cohen, C. I, & Sokolovsky, J. (1981). Social networks and the elderly: Clinical techniques. *International Journal of Family Therapy, 3,* 281-294.

Elderly minorities: Mental health issues [Special issue]. (1992). *Journal of Geriatric Psychiatry, 25*.

Foster, J. R., & Martin, C. C. (1990). Dementia. In D. Bienenfeld (Ed.), *Verweordt's Clinical Geropsychiatry* (3rd ed., pp. 66-84). Baltimore: Williams & Wilkins.

Foster, R. P, & Foster, J. R. (1989). Group therapy with geriatric patients. In D. A. Halperin (Ed.), *Group Psychodynamics: New Paradigms and New Perspectives* (pp. 297-310). Chicago: Year Book Medical Publishers.

Garrison, J. E., & Howe, J. (1976). Community intervention with the elderly: A social network approach. *Journal of the American Geriatrics Society, 24,* 329-333.

Goldstein, M. Z. (1990). Evaluation of the elderly patient. In D. Bienenfeld (Ed.), *Verweordt's Clinical Geropsychiatry* (3rd ed., pp. 47-58). Baltimore: Williams & Wilkins.

Grant, I., Patterson, T. L., & Yager, J. (1988). Social supports in relation to physical health and symptoms of depression in the elderly. *American Journal of Psychiatry, 145,* 1254-1258.

Hansson, R. O., Stroebe, M. S., & Stroebe, W. (1988). In conclusion: Current themes in bereavement and widowhood research. *Journal of Social Issues, 44,* 207-216.

Liptzin, B. (1989). Discussion: I can't play ball anymore. *Journal of Geriatric Psychiatry, 22,* 141-144.

Sadavoy, J., & Leszcz, M. (1987). *Treating the Elderly With Psychotherapy: The Scope for Change in Later Life*. Madison, CT: International Universities Press.

Siegel, J. M., & Kuykendall, D. H. (1990). Loss, widowhood, and psychological distress among the elderly. *Journal of Consulting and Clinical Psychology, 58,* 519-524.

Stone, I., & Koonin, M. (1986). A support group in a retirement home. *Aging, 352,* 18-19.

A REVIEW OF SCALES FOR THE BRIEF ASSESSMENT OF ANXIETY

Victoria C. Demos and Maurice F. Prout

The purpose of this contribution is to examine clinical issues related to the self-report assessment of anxiety in adults and children. We begin by outlining the general symptoms of anxiety. Because this is by no means an exhaustive description of the various anxiety disorders, the reader is referred to Prout and Demos (1993) for a more detailed discussion. We present here a survey of the most frequently employed self-report measures to assess the severity of anxiety. The basic psychometric properties of each measure, such as test-retest reliability and validity, are also outlined.

The *DSM-IV* (American Psychiatric Association [APA], 1994) describes many different anxiety disorders: Agoraphobia, Social Phobia, Panic Disorder With Agoraphobia, Panic Disorder Without Agoraphobia, Post-Traumatic Stress Disorder, Acute Stress Disorder, Obsessive-Compulsive Disorder, Specific Phobia, and Generalized Anxiety Disorder. However, most self-report inventories for anxiety assess a variety of anxiety symptoms similar to what might be found in Generalized Anxiety Disorder (GAD).

We have chosen to limit our discussion to brief paper-and-pencil instruments, which can be used as screening devices. Many insurance companies are now questioning the reimbursement of costly psychological testing in this age of managed care. The assessment instruments outlined in this contribution are economical from a cost and time perspective. For these reasons, and because of the greater amount of training required to administer and score such detailed personality inventories as the MMPI (Butcher et al., 1989) and the Rorschach Inkblot Test (Rorschach, 1921/1942), we have eliminated them from our discussion.

ASSESSMENT OF ANXIETY

A number of structured interviews are available for the assessment of anxiety, such as the Anxiety Disorders Interview Schedule-Revised (ADIS-R; Di Nardo et al., 1985). Although these instruments are valid and reliable, most clinicians use them primarily for research or in cases of more difficult diagnostic dilemmas. For a standard intake interview, a detailed assessment interview following the guidelines of the *DSM-IV* (APA, 1994) criteria for Generalized Anxiety Disorder along with one good self-rating scale such as the Beck Anxiety Inventory (Beck et al., 1988) should be sufficient to confirm the presence or absence of anxiety.

CLINICAL INTERVIEW

Anxiety can be defined as "apprehension, tension, or uneasiness that stems from the anticipation of danger, which may be internal or external" (APA, 1980, p. 354). In addition to the general questions that are asked in a thorough interview, and the *DSM-IV* (APA, 1994) criterion-based questions, there are some specific areas which should be addressed:

Appearance and Behavior Within Session. Patients with Generalized Anxiety Disorder may appear anxious in the interview, which may be evident in patients fidgeting, shifting in their seat, constantly playing with something in their hands, or moving their feet in a nervous manner. The symptoms can be classified into three main categories: (a) vigilance - insomnia, irritability, difficulty concentrating, and a heightened startle response; (b) muscle tension - fidgeting, twitching, trembling and restlessness; and (c) autonomic hyperactivity - rapid pulse, dry mouth, sweating, clammy and cold hands, frequent urination, feeling of a lump in the throat or difficulty swallowing, stomach upset, and dizziness (Last & Hersen, 1988).

Mood and Affect. A mood of apprehension or fear suggests anxiety, while a mood of sadness and loss of interest points to depression. Along with anxious mood, a particular characteristic of this disorder is the presence of repetitive thoughts. These thoughts are fearful in content, and are referred to as worries.

Substance Abuse. Alcohol abuse should be ruled out, in particular, as should abuse or use of any other substances that could be used to self-medicate for anxiety. In addition, anxiety can be a symptom of withdrawal from certain substances such as alcohol, caffeine, sedatives, or hypnotics. Daily intake of caffeine should be determined, as well as ingestion of any prescription or over-the-counter medications, such as antihistamines, which can cause symptoms of anxiety in susceptible individuals.

Cognitions. Following from the characteristic feature of Generalized Anxiety Disorder (as defined in the *DSM-IV* of excessive worry about two or more life events), recent research has focused more exclusively on this cognitive aspect of anxiety. In a 1983 study that investigated aspects of worrying, Borkovec et al. found that worrying is dominated by concerns regarding future as opposed to past events, and that these cognitions become uncontrollable once they are underway. This is true for all worrying and anxiety, not just for those persons diagnosed with Generalized Anxiety Disorder. Worry reflects a cognitive aspect of anxiety, which is often focused on one's own behavior. Borkovec et al. defined worry as "a chain of thoughts and images, negatively affect-laden and relatively uncontrollable. The worry process represents an attempt to engage in mental problem-solving on an issue whose outcome is uncertain but contains the possibility of one or more negative outcomes" (p. 10). The most frequent areas of worry for Generalized Anxiety Disorder patients have been reported as family, money, work, and illness, in order of prevalence (Craske et al., 1989).

Based on their research of anxious and nonanxious subjects' worrying activity, Borkovec and Inz (1990) have speculated that for anxious patients, worry may allow them to avoid anxious imagery, its associated emotions, and its physical concomitants. Worry is a purely cognitive function without any associated affect.

Anxiety and Depression. It can be difficult to distinguish between depression and anxiety, because the two conditions can coexist. There is a high incidence of anxiety symptoms in depressed patients (McGlynn & Metcalf, 1989) as well as a high incidence of depression in patients with Panic Disorder (Clayton, 1990). Patients who have mixed symptoms often have more serious psychopathology and poorer outcomes (Clayton, 1990). McGlynn and Metcalf (1989) categorized the symptoms more characteristic of anxiety as difficulty falling asleep, shallow breathing, rapid pulse and general autonomic hyperactivity (tremors, sweating, heart palpitations), feeling faint or lightheaded, and dizziness. In addition, there may be derealization (a feeling that the immediate environment is unreal or unfamiliar), depersonalization (feeling that one is outside one's body and observing oneself), or feelings of dread.

In contrast, McGlynn and Metcalf (1989) describe depression as having more of the following features: sleeping longer hours or awakening in the early morning, feeling much worse in the morning, exhibiting a general slowing of processes (slowed speech, cognition, response time, and body movements), looking and feeling sad, feeling worthless and hopeless, thinking of death or suicide, having less interest in one's usual activities, and experiencing anhedonia (an inability to experience pleasure).

Medical Disorders. The practitioner must be cognizant of various physical disorders that may have anxiety and/or panic as part of the clinical presentation. Areas of consideration include the following four categories of disorders: cardiovascular and respiratory, endocrine, neurological, and substance-related. Table 1 (p. 170) provides a list of specific disorders within each of the four major categories. If there is any suspicion that either a medical disorder or medication might be contributing to or causing the anxiety, the patient should be referred to a physician for a complete physical.

History. Patients should be asked about family history of depression, alcoholism, and anxiety, because these are more common in family members of anxiety-disordered patients (Lipschitz, 1988). The interviewer should also inquire as to previous history of anxiety episodes in the patient's past. Patients may not immediately recognize their previous symptoms as anxiety, so it is often more helpful to ask, "Have you ever felt this way before?" If the answer is yes, it is informative to inquire as to the conditions of the previous occurrence, that is, life circumstances at the time. Anxiety can be related to certain kinds of events in the patient's life, and it can be helpful to the treating clinician to know the trigger events for the onset of anxiety. For example, in some patients, anxiety can follow actual or perceived periods of separation from people they are close to.

In addition, it is useful to determine whether the patient has ever been treated for this problem before, for how long, and what he or she gained from it. It can also be informative to ask what, specifically, the patient found helpful from the previous treatment and what was not helpful. This gives the current therapist some idea of what might be effective with this particular patient.

ANXIETY SEVERITY ASSESSMENT SCALES FOR ADULTS

Using one of the following pencil-and-paper scales can improve on clinical judgment by providing a more objective measure of the presence and level of anxiety. This provides the clinician a way to compare across cases, because the items are identical for all patients and are uniformly scored. They may also be used, as many cognitive-behavioral therapists do, as an ongoing index of level of anxiety during treatment. They can be administered as frequently as before each session. The scales chosen for discussion here have adequate levels of reliability and validity, and are specific to anxiety.

Before describing the specific scales, a brief definition of the different types of reliability and validity to be discussed is in order. Reliability is the "proportion of variance in a set of scores that is due to true and stable differences among the individuals tested for the attribute that is being measured" (Gotlib & Cane, 1989, p. 136). Reliability examines the stability of the test scores, that is, whether the scores are consistent over different parts within the test, and across different administrations of the test over time.

Validity examines whether the test measures what it purports to measure. There are several different kinds of validity which are relevant to examining self-report measures of anxiety. Content validity looks at whether the test gives an adequate sampling of the content area that it was designed to measure. Construct validity is the "extent to which performance on a measure is consistent with the theoretical concepts or constructs it is assumed to measure" (Gotlib & Cane, 1989, p. 136). Convergent validity is examined by measuring the extent to which the test correlates significantly with other tests designed to assess the same domain. For anxiety tests, this would involve investigating the extent of correlation with other established tests that measure anxiety. Finally, discriminant validity is demonstrated when the test has a low correlation with tests that

TABLE 1: MEDICAL DISORDERS ASSOCIATED WITH ANXIETY*

Cardiovascular and Respiratory

Asthma
Cardiac arrhythmias
Chronic obstructive pulmonary disease
Congestive heart failure
Coronary insufficiency
Hypertension
Hyperventilation syndrome
Hyperdynamic beta-adrenergic state
Hypoxia, embolus, infections

Endocrine

Cushing's syndrome
Hyperthyroidism
Hypoglycemia
Menopause
Pheochromocytoma
Premenstrual syndrome
Pregnancy

Neurological

Collagen vascular disease
Epilepsy
Huntington's disease
Multiple sclerosis
Organic brain syndrome: delirium, dementia
Parkinson's disease
Vestibular dysfunction
Wilson's disease

Substance-Related

Anticholinergic drugs
Aspirin
Caffeine
Cocaine
Hallucinogens, including phencyclidine ("angel dust")
Steroids
Sympathomimetics
THC
Withdrawal syndromes: alcohol, narcotics, sedative hypnotics

*Copyright © 1987 by B. A. Raj and D. V. Sheehan, University of South Florida College of Medicine, Department of Psychiatry and Behavioral Medicine, Tampa, FL. Reprinted by permission.

evaluate different, unrelated domains. Essentially, this is to assure that the instrument is assessing the unique concept of anxiety and that it does not overlap significantly with measures of self-esteem or general psychopathology, for example.

Beck Anxiety Inventory (BAI). The BAI (Beck et al., 1988) requires approximately 8 minutes to complete. There are 21 items that are rated on a 4-point scale ranging from 0 to 3. The minimum score is 0, and the maximum score is 63. The 21 items are factored into four clusters assessing the following symptoms: neurophysiological, subjective, panic, and autonomic. However, scores within individual clusters are currently not statistically interpreted with respect to severity. Clinicians use the total BAI score to assess the degree of anxiety. The following guidelines relate to the total score: 0 to 7 = minimal; 8 to 15 = mild; 16 to 25 = moderate; and 26 to 63 = severe anxiety. Gotlib and Cane (1989) reported on the lack of discriminant validity from depression for most of the older self-report measures of anxiety, specifically the Self-Rating Anxiety Scale (SRAS; Zung, 1971), and the State-Trait Anxiety Inventory (STAI; Spielberger, Gorusch, & Lushene, 1970). The BAI was developed specifically in response to this problem and to the need for a scale that would reliably measure anxiety as distinct from depression. Beck et al. (1988) found that the BAI has quite high test-retest reliability ($r = .75$), and high internal consistency ($a = .92$). The BAI was also shown to discriminate validly between nonanxious groups, such as depressed groups, and anxious groups (e.g., Panic Disorder, Generalized Anxiety Disorder). The BAI was also only slightly correlated with the Hamilton Depression Rating Scale (Hamilton, 1960), but was moderately correlated with the Hamilton Anxiety Rating Scale (Hamilton, 1959), providing evidence for concurrent validity. The BAI is published commercially by The Psychological Corporation. Copies may be requested by writing to: 555 Academic Court, San Antonio, TX 78204-2498, or telephoning, (800) 228-0752.

Hamilton Anxiety Rating Scale (HARS). The HARS (Hamilton, 1959) is a clinician rating scale consisting of 14 items with each item rated on a 5-point scale from 0 (not present) to 4 (very severe). The total points range from 0 to 70. Scores of 18 or above have been considered reflective of significant anxiety and constitute patient admission criteria for some antianxiety drug studies (Fankhauser & German, 1987). Cut-off scores used by Fankhauser and German (1987) in their drug studies are: 0 to 5 = no anxiety; 6 to 14 = minor anxiety; and 18 or more = major anxiety. Hamilton has found that the HARS measures two main factors of anxiety: somatic and psychic. The somatic factor includes autonomic activity - cardiovascular and respiratory - while the psychic items assess insomnia, anxious mood, tearfulness, and tension. Maier et al. (1988) found interrater reliabilities for the HARS of between .70 and .74. Riskind et al. (1987) found a discriminant validity for depression of .83, and the HARS has been found to correlate moderately with the BAI (Convergent validity, $r = .51$) (Beck et al., 1988).

A study by Beck and Steer (1991), examining the specific relationship between the BAI and HARS, found that in addition to overlapping in their general measurement of anxiety, the two measures actually assess somewhat different content areas of anxiety. The BAI was found to measure "subjective, neurophysiological, autonomic, and panic symptoms of self-reported anxiety" (Beck & Steer, 1991, p. 220), while the HARS assessed slightly more general "aspects of clinically-rated somatic and psychic anxiety" (p. 220). The authors recommended that, when assessing for anxiety, the clinician use both a self-report scale such as the BAI and a rating scale completed by the examining clinician, such as the HARS. The HARS is included on page 175.

State-Trait Anxiety Inventory (STAI). Spielberger developed the STAI (Spielberger & Krasner, 1988) to measure Freud's concept of neurotic anxiety and Cattell's theory of state and trait anxiety. There are actually two 20-item sections to this self-report test, one measuring state anxiety and the other measuring trait anxiety. Trait anxiety was defined (Spielberger & Krasner, 1988) as a stable individual proneness to anxiety, while state anxiety was conceptualized as a more fluctuating emotional reaction, which would vary according to current life circumstances. The 20-item state anxiety scale is scored along a 4-point intensity scale ranging from "not at all" to "very much so." The 20-item trait anxiety scale is scored along a 4-point frequency scale ranging from "almost never," to "almost always." Scores for both the state and trait can range from a minimum of 20 to a maximum of 80. From a clinical perspective, trait anxiety scores at the 80th percentile or above indicate significant anxiety. Scores below the 20th percentile indicate low anxiety or the use of psychological defenses such as denial or repression. The middle range of trait anxiety scores represent an average, nonclinical status (Spielberger, personal communication, 1994).

Spielberger and Krasner (1988) have found both scales to have high internal consistency (.86 to .95), and the trait form has a good test-retest reliability of .65 to .86. The trait form has also been found to distinguish psychiatric patients from normal controls and to correlate significantly with other measures of anxiety. One criticism levied against the STAI by Beck et al. in 1988 is that it was developed on a nonpsychiatric college population, while it is used largely with psychiatric patients. In addition, there is some question whether the STAI measures only anxiety, or a mixture of anxiety and depression, as Barlow et al. (1986) found the scores on the STAI to be higher in a depressed group than an anxious group. The STAI is published commercially by Western Psychological Services: 12031 Wilshire Boulevard, Los Angeles, CA 90025-1251, telephone (800) 648-8857.

Case Study. A 23-year-old graduate student* was self-referred to the university counseling center. She stated she was depressed, could not sleep, and was frequently tearful. Her local family practitioner had recently prescribed a tricyclic antidepressant (TCA) for the management of her depression.

A history revealed that she had always been an intensely shy person who was sensitive to the criticisms of others. Throughout her education she attained excellent grades, but her fear of criticism precluded her ever having to present a project or paper orally. She became adroit at avoiding her fear by claiming illness, confusion over presentation dates, and so on. Her teachers and professors inadvertently colluded with her by accepting her excuses and basing her grades on superior written work and general enthusiasm. Shortly after entering graduate school, it became clear that her ploys would no longer work. Indeed, numerous presentations in a variety of classes was mandatory.

The patient was clinically assessed with the HARS and attained a total score of 28. She did not exhibit anhedonia or generalized fear. Rather her scores were in the areas of worry, insomnia, and gastrointestinal and autonomic symptoms. She also completed the BAI and attained a total score of 36 with most of the endorsed items falling in the neurophysiological and subjective categories. She endorsed few items related to panic.

The case was conceptualized as one of social phobia of longstanding duration. With her permission, her physician was contacted and the diagnosis and rationale was provided along with a recommendation to discontinue the TCA. She agreed. An intensive cognitive-behavioral approach was instituted over a 4-month period. A BAI was obtained at the beginning of each session. Soon after treatment commenced, the BAI began to drop, only to periodically flair up as the dates of presentation neared. Eventually the patient overcame her terror and was able to present her material.

This case initially was conceptualized as one of depression by both the patient and her physician. Both instruments (HARS, BAI) as well as a clinical interview underscored an anxiety disorder, specifically a social phobia.

ASSESSMENT OF ANXIETY IN CHILDREN AND ADOLESCENTS

To assess child/adolescent anxiety, clinicians need to interview both the child and his or her parents. The interview with the parents should concentrate on the history of the present complaint and the child's developmental milestones. In addition to a standard interview, the history of ma-

---

*Identifying characteristics have been changed to protect the confidentiality of the invidividuals in case examples/studies.

ternal bonding needs to be elicited and should cover first and subsequent separations and the quality of the mother-child relationship. The reaction of both mother (or primary caretaker) and child to separation at nursery school or preschool also needs to be assessed. Children with symptoms of anxiety (particularly separation anxiety) and their parents often have extreme reactions to separation (Husain & Kashani, 1992). Clinicians need to inquire about the child's fears, phobias, nightmares, and current worries. The child should be observed closely, particularly at the time of separation from the parents. Any family history of psychiatric illness, especially anxiety or depression, will require review.

ASSESSMENT INVENTORIES FOR CHILDREN

As with the assessment of anxiety in adults, the assessment of anxiety in children is best done with a detailed clinical interview with the child and his or her parents, combined with a self-report inventory. Depression and anxiety have been found to be related (Ollendick & Yule, 1990) when children are given self-report inventories for both depression and anxiety; therefore, it is best not to rely solely on an inventory. There are two main inventories to assess anxiety in children and adolescents: the Revised Children's Manifest Anxiety Scale (RCMAS; Reynolds & Richmond, 1984), and the State-Trait Anxiety Inventory for Children (STAI-C; Spielberger, 1973). The RCMAS is used primarily in the diagnosis of anxiety while the STAI-C distinguishes more between state and trait anxiety. These inventories can help the clinician distinguish "normal" childhood anxieties from anxiety that might require treatment.

Revised Children's Manifest Anxiety Scale (RCMAS). Castaneda, McCandless, and Palermo (1956) were the first to develop an anxiety inventory for children. They used the Taylor Manifest Anxiety Scale for Adults and restructured it for use with children. The original CMAS had 42 "yes/no" items and a lie scale, with the anxiety score being the number of "yes" responses. Reynolds and Richmond (1978, 1984) revised the scale, including 28 original items and 9 new items constituting a lie scale. The 37-item RCMAS can be given to 1st- through 12th-grade children. A multitrait-multimethod validation matrix to evaluate the construct validity of the RCMAS showed large correlations with other trait measures of anxiety (Reynolds, 1982). In addition, Reynolds and Richmond (1984) have demonstrated high construct validity as the scale measures three clinical factors: (a) physiological anxiety, (b) worry/oversensitivity, and (c) social concerns/concentration. The RCMAS has good test-retest reliability as reported by Johnson and Melamed (1979). Wisniewski et al. (1987) found test-retest reliabilities of .88 at 1 week and .77 at 5-week intervals. The RCMAS yields five scores: the total anxiety score and three scores related to the clinical factors mentioned previously. Additionally, a lie subscale score is computed. For the total anxiety score, the scaled score is a standard score with a mean of 50 and a standard deviation of 10. Scoring of the subscales reflects a mean of 10 and a standard deviation of 3. Reynolds and Richmond recommend use of their norms based upon age, ethnicity, and sex (Reynolds & Richmond, 1992).

Ollendick and Yule (1990) tested 663 children in both the United States and England between the ages of 8 and 10 years. They found a high internal consistency on the test of .84 in the British sample and .87 in the American sample. Depression and anxiety (as measured by the RCMAS) were found to be highly related in this study, which may be due to some problems in the scales themselves or to the simultaneous presence of both of these emotions in children. Ollendick and Yule and others (Hodges, 1990) have found this to be true for children, reinforcing the importance of using a good clinical interview with the scales. The RCMAS is published by Western Psychological Services: 12031 Wilshire Boulevard, Los Angeles, CA 90025-1251, telephone (800) 648-8857.

State-Trait Anxiety Inventory for Children (STAI-C). The STAI-C (Spielberger, 1973) asks children to respond to how they feel in general (trait) and currently (state). However, its ability to distinguish between trait and state anxiety has been questioned by some (Johnson & Melamed, 1979). There are 20 items that measure individual differences in anxiety. In a 1990 study by Hodges, children with anxiety disorders scored significantly higher than children without anxiety disorders. The sample consisted of 70 children, ages 6 to 13, all hospitalized for psychiatric reasons. In a 1978 study by Papay and Hedl of inner-city children, the measures of internal consistency reliability were found to be much lower for measuring trait anxiety (.59 to .63) than for state anxiety (.80 to .82). In addition, a high correlation has been reported between the RCMAS and the STAI-C (Spielberger, 1973). The STAI-C is also available from Western Psychological Services (see address on preceding page).

Case Study. David, an 8-year-old boy, was brought in by his parents. They reported that he was a very bright, lively, and verbal child, who did well in his 2nd-grade class. He did not, however, do well enough to qualify for the gifted program, as his older brother had. David's parents were both university professors and reported that, despite his age, David could occasionally become clingy when his parents went out. In addition, he seemed rather constricted and shy. At bedtime, he would worry if his toy airplanes were lined up in the proper order. The parents had no serious marital problems, or behavior problems with either child. In the family, however, a high value was placed on intellectual productivity and high grades. Upon initial interview, David seemed to be a rather shy boy whose movements and behavior were tightly controlled.

The school psychologist had already administered the Stanford-Binet (Delaney & Hopkins, 1987) to David, who received an IQ score of 128 (Superior range). This and the remainder of the battery revealed no evidence of any type of mild learning disability.

When given the RCMAS, David had a T-score on Total Anxiety of 60, and a Lie scaled score of 12. These were in the 85th and 84th percentile, respectively, which are high for his age group. On the three anxiety subscales of physiological anxiety, worry/oversensitivity, and social concerns/concentration, he received scaled scores of 12, 13, and 12, respectively. These scores indicate a moderate amount of anxiety which would be enough to affect his school performance.

Essentially, David wanted to be a "good boy" (elevated Lie scale score) and not cause problems for his family. He was quiet and well behaved. He was feeling under some pressure to do very well in school, and this pressure would be enough to cause him the anxiety he was experiencing and lower his performance. The recommendation focused on family and play therapy, with the goal for David to relax some of his strict controls.

CONCLUSION

A clinical interview is necessary for the accurate diagnosis of Generalized Anxiety Disorder. However, as the two case studies demonstrate, supplementing the clinical interview with brief anxiety screening instruments can have clinical utility. Although we did not include a case study using the STAI, or its corollary for children, we would highly recommend their use in clinical practice. Brief screening instruments not only respond to managed care issues but also allow a periodic objective evaluation of where the patient's anxiety symptoms are during the course of treatment.

HAMILTON ANXIETY RATING SCALE*

Patient's Name _____ Date of First Report _____

Diagnosis _____ Date of This Report _____

Current Therapy _____

_____

Instructions: This checklist is to assist the physician in evaluating each patient with respect to degree of anxiety and pathological condition. Please fill in the appropriate rating.

0 = None
1 = Mild
2 = Moderate
3 = Severe
4 = Severe, grossly disabling

ITEM		RATING	ITEM		RATING
Anxious Mood	Worries, anticipation of the worst, fearful anticipation, irritability.		**Somatic (Sensory)**	Tinnitus, blurring of vision, hot and cold flushes, feelings of weakness, prickling sensation	
Tension	Feelings of tension, fatigability, startle response, moved to tears easily, trembling, feelings of restlessness, inability to relax.		**Cardiovascular Symptoms**	Tachycardia, palpitations, pain in chest, throbbing of vessels, fainting feelings, missing beat.	
Fear	Of dark, of strangers, of being left alone, of animals, of traffic, of crowds.		**Respiratory Symptoms**	Pressure or constriction in chest, choking feelings, sighing, dyspnea.	
Insomnia	Difficulty in falling asleep, broken sleep, unsatisfying sleep and fatigue on waking, dreams, nightmares, night terrors.		**Gastrointestinal Symptoms**	Difficulty in swallowing, wind, abdominal pain, burning sensations, abdominal fullness, nausea, vomiting, borborygmi, looseness of bowels, loss of weight, constipation.	
Intellectual (Cognitive)	Difficulty in concentration, poor memory.		**Genitourinary Symptoms**	Frequency of micturition, urgency of micturition, amenorrhea, menorrhagia, development of frigidity, premature ejaculation, loss of libido, impotence.	
Depressed Mood	Loss of interest, lack of pleasure in hobbies, depression, early waking, diurnal swing.		**Autonomic Symptoms**	Dry mouth, flushing, pallor, tendency to sweat, giddiness, tension headache, raising of hair.	
Behavior at Interview	Fidgeting, restlessness or pacing, tremor of hands, furrowed brow, strained face, sighing or rapid respiration, facial pallor, swallowing, belching, brisk tendon jerks, dilated pupils, exophthalmos.		**Somatic (Muscular)**	Pains and aches, twitchings, stiffness, myoclonic jerks, grinding of teeth, unsteady voice, increased muscular tone.	
				TOTAL SCORE	

*Note: From "The Assessment of Anxiety States by Rating" by M. Hamilton, 1959, *British Journal of Medical Psychology, 32,* pp. 50-55. Copyright © 1959 by The British Psychological Society. Reprinted by permission.

Victoria C. Demos, PhD, is currently Assistant Professor of Psychology at Marymount College in Tarrytown, New York. In addition, she works with students at the Marymount Counseling Center. She has a private practice in New York City, where she treats young adults and adults with mild depression and anxiety. Her research interests are in the areas of individual and group treatment of anxiety and depression. Particular interests are in the area of test anxiety and fear of success. Dr. Demos may be contacted at Marymount College, 100 Marymount Avenue, Box 1370, Tarrytown, NY 10591.

Maurice F. Prout, PhD, is currently an Associate Professor at Widener University's Institute for Graduate Clinical Psychology. He holds a Diplomate in Clinical Psychology from the American Board of Professional Psychology. His interests are in the diagnosis and treatment of anxiety, mood disorders, and brief models of psychotherapy. Dr. Prout can be contacted at Widener University, Institute for Graduate Clinical Psychology, Chester, PA 19013.

RESOURCES

American Psychiatric Association. (1980). *Diagnostic and Statistical Manual of Mental Disorders* (3rd ed.). Washington, DC: Author.

American Psychiatric Association. (1994). *Diagnostic and Statistical Manual of Mental Disorders* (4th ed.). Washington, DC: Author.

Barlow, D. H., Di Nardo, P. A., Vermilyea, B. B., Vermilyea, J., & Blanchard, E. B. (1986). Co-morbidity and depression among the anxiety disorders: Issues in diagnosis and classification. *Journal of Nervous and Mental Disease, 174,* 63-72.

Beck, A. T., Epstein, N., Brown, G., & Steer, R. A. (1988). An inventory for measuring clinical anxiety: Psychometric properties. *Journal of Consulting and Clinical Psychology, 56,* 893-897.

Beck, A. T., & Steer, R. A. (1991). Relationship between the Beck Anxiety Inventory and the Hamilton Anxiety Rating Scale with anxious outpatients. *Journal of Anxiety Disorders, 5,* 213-223.

Borkovec, T. D., & Inz, J. (1990). The nature of worry in generalized anxiety disorder: A predominance of thought activity. *Behavior Research and Therapy, 28,* 153-158.

Borkovec, T. D., Robinson, E., Pruzinsky, T., & DePree, J. A. (1983). Preliminary exploration of worry: Some characteristics and processes. *Behavior Research and Therapy, 21,* 9-16.

Brown, G., & Beck, A. T. (1987). *An Evaluation of the Psychometric Properties of the Zung Self-Rating Anxiety Scale.* Unpublished manuscript, University of Pennsylvania, Philadelphia, PA.

Butcher, J. N., Dahlstrom, W. G., Graham, J. R., Tellegen, A. T., & Kaemmer, B. (1989). *Minnesota Multiphasic Personality Inventory-2. Manual for Administration and Scoring.* Minneapolis: University of Minnesota Press.

Castaneda, A., McCandless, B., & Palermo, D. (1956). The children's form of the Manifest Anxiety Scale. *Child Development, 27,* 317-326.

Clayton, P. J. (1990). The comorbidity factor: Establishing the primary diagnosis in patients with mixed symptoms of anxiety and depression. *Journal of Clinical Psychiatry, 51,* 35-39.

Craske, M. G., Rapee, R. M., Jackel, L., & Barlow, D. H. (1989). Qualitative dimensions of worry in DSM-III-R generalized anxiety disorder subjects and nonanxious controls. *Behavior Research and Therapy, 27,* 397-402.

Delaney, E., & Hopkins, T. (1987). *Stanford-Binet Intelligence Scale Examiner's Handbook: An Expanded Guide for Fourth Edition Users.* Chicago: The Riverside Publishing Company.

Di Nardo, P. A., Barlow, D. H., Cerny, J., Vermilyea, B. B., Vermilyea, J. A., Himadi, W., & Waddell, M. (1985). *Anxiety Disorders Interview Schedule-Revised (ADIS-R).* Albany, NY: Phobic and Anxiety Disorders Clinic, State University of New York at Albany.

Fankhauser, M. P., & German, M. L. (1987). Understanding the use of behavior rating scales in studies evaluating the efficacy of antianxiety and antidepressant drugs. *American Journal of Hospital Pharmacy, 44*, 2087-2100.

Gotlib, I. H., & Cane, D. B. (1989). Self-report assessment of depression and anxiety. In P. C. Kendall & D. Watson (Eds.), *Anxiety and Depression: Distinctive and Overlapping Features* (pp. 131-169). New York: Academic Press.

Hamilton, M. (1959). The assessment of anxiety states by rating. *British Journal of Medical Psychology, 32*, 50-55.

Hamilton, M. (1960). A rating scale for depression. *Journal of Neurology, Neurosurgery, and Psychiatry, 23*, 56-61.

Hodges, K. (1990). Depression and anxiety in children: A comparison of self-report questionnaires to clinical interview. *Psychological Assessment: A Journal of Consulting and Clinical Psychology, 2*, 376-381.

Husain, S. A., & Kashani, J. (1992). Anxiety disorders in children and adolescents. In *Diagnosis and Assessment of Anxiety Disorders in Children and Adolescents* (pp. 29-43). Washington, DC: American Psychiatric Press.

Jegede, R. O. (1977). Psychometric attributes of the Self-Rating Anxiety Scale. *Psychological Reports, 40*, 303-306.

Johnson, S. B., & Melamed, B. G. (1979). Assessment and treatment of children's fears. In B. B. Lahey & A. E. Kazdon (Eds.), *Advances in Clinical Child Psychology* (Vol. Two, pp. 107-139). New York: Plenum.

Kramer, J. J., & Conoley, J. C. (Eds.). (1992). *The Eleventh Mental Measurements Yearbook.* Lincoln, NE: University of Nebraska Press.

Last, C. G., & Hersen, M. (Eds.). (1988). *Handbook of Anxiety Disorders.* New York: Pergamon.

Lipschitz, A. (1988). Diagnosis and classification of anxiety disorders. In C. G. Last & M. Hersen (Eds.), *Handbook of Anxiety Disorders* (pp. 41-65). New York: Pergamon.

Litz, B. T., Penk, W. E., Walsh, S., & Hyer, L. (1991). Similarities and differences between MMPI and MMPI-2 applications to the assessment of posttraumatic stress disorder. *Journal of Personality Assessment, 57*, 238-253.

Lorr, M., Strack, S., Campbell, L., & Lamnin, A. (1990). Personality and symptom dimensions of the MCMI-II: An item factor analysis. *Journal of Clinical Psychology, 46*, 749-754.

Maier, W., Buller, R., Philipp, M., & Heuser, I. (1988). The Hamilton Anxiety Scale: Reliability, validity, and sensitivity to change in anxiety and depressive disorders. *Journal of Affective Disorders, 14*, 61-68.

McGlynn, T. J., & Metcalf, H. L. (Eds.). (1989). *Diagnosis and Treatment of Anxiety Disorders: A Physician's Handbook.* Washington, DC: American Psychiatric Press.

Ollendick, T. H., & Yule, W. (1990). Depression in British and American children and its relation to anxiety and fear. *Journal of Consulting and Clinical Psychology, 58*, 126-129.

Papay, J. P., & Hedl, J. J. (1978). Psychometric characteristics and norms for disadvantaged third and fourth grade children on the State-Trait Anxicty Inventory for Children. *Journal of Abnormal Child Psychology, 6*, 115-120.

Prout, M. F., & Demos, V. C. (1993). The diagnosis and treatment of adult anxiety disorders. In L. VandeCreek, S. Knapp, & T. L. Jackson (Eds.), *Innovations in Clinical Practice: A Source Book* (Vol. 12, pp. 65-83). Sarasota, FL: Professional Resource Press.

Reynolds, C. R. (1982). Convergent and divergent validity of the Revised Children's Manifest Anxiety Scale. *Educational and Psychological Measurement, 42*, 1205-1212.

Reynolds, C. R., & Richmond, B. O. (1978). What I think and feel: A revised measure of children's manifest anxiety. *Journal of Abnormal Child Psychology, 6*, 271-280.

Reynolds, C. R., & Richmond, B. O. (1984). *Revised Children's Manifest Anxiety Scale.* Los Angeles, CA: Western Psychological Services.

Reynolds, C. R., & Richmond, B. O. (1992). *Revised Children's Manifest Anxiety Scale (RCMAS).* Los Angeles, CA: Western Psychological Services.

Riskind, J. H., Beck, A. T., Brown, G., & Steer, R. A. (1987). Taking the measure of anxiety and depression: Validity of reconstructed Hamilton scales. *Journal of Nervous and Mental Disease, 175,* 474-479.

Rorschach, H. (1942). *Psychodiagnostics: A Diagnostic Test Based on Perception* (P. Lemkau & B. Kronenburg, Trans.). Berne: Huber. (1st German ed. published 1921; U.S. distributor, Grune & Stratton)

Spielberger, C. D. (1973). *Manual for the State-Trait Anxiety Inventory for Children.* Palo Alto, CA: Consulting Psychologists Press.

Spielberger, C. D., Gorusch, R. L., & Lushene, R. (1970). *STAI Manual for the State-Trait Anxiety Inventory.* Palo Alto, CA: Consulting Psychologists Press.

Spielberger, C. D., & Krasner, S. S. (1988). The assessment of state and trait anxiety. In R. Noyes, M. Roth, & G. D. Burrows (Eds.), *Handbook of Anxiety: Vol. 2. Classification, Etiological Factors and Associated Disturbances* (pp. 31-51). New York: Elsevier Science Publishers.

Taylor, J. A. (1953). A personality scale of manifest anxiety. *Journal of Abnormal and Social Psychology, 48,* 285-290.

Wisniewski, J. J., Genshaft, J. L., Mulick, J. A., & Coury, D. L. (1987). Test-retest reliability of the Revised Children's Manifest Anxiety Scale. *Perceptual and Motor Skills, 65,* 67-70.

Zung, W. W. K. (1971). A rating instrument for anxiety disorders. *Psychosomatics, 12,* 371-379.

CLINICAL GUIDELINES FOR THE TREATMENT OF INSOMNIA

Charles M. Morin and Cheryl A. Colecchi

Sleep complaints are often brought to the attention of clinical practitioners as the chief presenting problem, as a symptom of an underlying psychological or medical disorder, or as a comorbid condition. Pharmacotherapy is by far the most frequently used treatment modality for insomnia. There are several limitations to using sleep medications, however, and insomnia sufferers are often dissatisfied with this approach. Recognition of the mediating role of psychological factors in chronic insomnia has led to the design of several behavioral, cognitive, and educational interventions for its clinical management. This contribution describes a multicomponent treatment protocol that has been used in our sleep clinic over the past several years to treat a few hundred patients seeking treatment for insomnia of varied origins. After presenting an overview of insomnia, common etiological factors are examined, and a typical assessment protocol is outlined. A treatment protocol is described next with a special emphasis on four treatment modules: behavioral, cognitive, educational, and medication withdrawal. We conclude with a brief review of therapeutic issues and clinical guidelines to improve treatment implementation and optimize therapeutic outcome.

AN OVERVIEW OF INSOMNIA

Insomnia may encompass a variety of complaints including problems falling asleep, waking up in the middle of the night with difficulty going back to sleep, or awakening too early in the morning. Clinicians often refer to these three types of insomnia as "initial," "middle," and "late" insomnia, respectively. These difficulties in initiating and maintaining sleep are not mutually exclusive, as individuals may present more than one of these problems, and the type of problems may shift over time. Additionally, sleep quality is usually described as "light," "restless," or "unrefreshing." Along with these sleep complaints, daytime sequelae of insomnia may include fatigue or lethargy, mood disturbances, social discomfort, and performance impairments.

According to the Fourth Edition of the *Diagnostic and Statistical Manual of Mental Disorders* (*DSM-IV;* American Psychiatric Association, 1994) and the *International Classification of Sleep Disorders* (ICSD; American Sleep Disorders Association, 1990), the following conditions must be present to meet the criteria for insomnia: (a) difficulties initiating or maintaining sleep for a minimum of 3 nights per week; (b) duration of insomnia is greater than 6 months; (c) subjective report of at least one daytime sequela attributed to poor sleep; and (d) the sleep disturbances (or daytime sequelae) cause significant impairment in social or occupational functioning, or marked emotional distress. Sleep researchers have further operationalized sleep-onset and sleep-maintenance insomnia respectively as sleep onset latency or time awake after sleep onset greater than 30 minutes/night, with a corresponding sleep efficiency (ratio of time asleep to time spent in bed) lower than 85% (Lacks & Morin, 1992).

Insomnia affects nearly everyone at one time or another. It is the most common of all sleep disorders and the most frequent health complaint after that of pain. A Gallup survey (Gallup Organization, 1991) consisting of 1,950 phone interviews found that 27% of Americans surveyed reported occasional insomnia while 9% claimed having a chronic problem. According to the National Survey of Psychotherapeutic Drug Use, about 35% of the adult population is afflicted with insomnia during the course of a year (Mellinger, Balter, & Uhlenhuth, 1985). Of these, half experience their sleeping problem as serious, while the remaining perceive the problem as mild and transient.

Insomnia complaints are twice as common in women as in men, and there is a strong relationship of insomnia to age: more than 25% of people aged 65 or older report sleep disruptions (Mellinger et al., 1985). Younger adults who have insomnia tend to experience sleep onset difficulties, whereas older adults complain more about sleep maintenance problems. Children are not immune to sleep difficulties, with a substantial proportion of preschoolers, pediatric patients, and adolescents suffering from sleep disruptions (Mindell, 1993).

Chronic insomnia is a genuine clinical problem that diminishes the quality of life and causes considerable emotional, occupational, health, and economic problems. There is a strong relationship between sleep and emotional disturbances, although it is often difficult to disentangle which one causes the other. However, it is clear that those who struggle nightly with insomnia often experience mood disturbances such as irritability, tension, helplessness, and a general sense of dysphoria. Worry over sleep loss and daytime sequelae often result in performance anxiety. Longitudinal data suggest that individuals whose insomnia is left untreated for over 1 year are more likely to develop major depression than either normal controls or those whose insomnia has resolved during this time period (Ford & Kamerow, 1989). Studies have also shown that chronic sleep disturbances may impair waking functions but that the deficits are subtle and inconsistent across individuals. Insomniacs often complain about physiological problems as well, such as tension headaches, gastrointestinal problems, nonspecific aches and pains, and allergies (Kales et al., 1984). This is not surprising, because insomnia itself is hypothesized to result from somatized tension and anxiety. Economic repercussions are evident in terms of reduced productivity, absenteeism from work, and other costs associated with greater utilization of health-related services among insomniacs.

COMMON CAUSES OF INSOMNIA

Multiple factors can cause insomnia. These include psychological, medical, pharmacological, circadian, and behavioral factors. Stress, anxiety, and depression are probably the most common causes of acute insomnia. Major depression and generalized anxiety disorders are the two most frequently diagnosed psychiatric disorders among chronic insomniacs. However, many insomnia sufferers who present clinical features of depression or anxiety may not meet a diagnosable psychiatric condition. It is often difficult to determine whether insomnia or mood disturbances is the primary disorder. In many instances, anxiety may be present in the early phase of insomnia whereas learned helplessness may develop as the individual perceives he or she is losing control over the regulation of the wake/sleep cycle. Sleep and mood disturbances may also be concomitant disorders that require dual interventions. Medical illness such as arthritis, congestive heart failures, hyperthyroidism, and chronic-obstructive pulmonary diseases are almost always associated with disrupted sleep patterns. Drugs prescribed for several medical or psychiatric illnesses can produce insomnia as a side effect. Among those are the bronchodilators, steroids, some beta-blockers (e.g., propranolol), and some energizing antidepressants (e.g., Prozac). Prolonged use of hypnotic medications or withdrawal from such drugs can cause significant rebound insomnia. Substances such as caffeine, nicotine, and alcohol are all associated with difficulties initiating or maintaining sleep. Several primary sleep disorders such as sleep apnea or restless legs/periodic limb movements can produce insomnia complaints, although those conditions are more often associated with a subjective complaint of excessive daytime sleepiness. Shift work and "jet lag" produce significant disruptions of circadian rhythms which interfere with sleep at the desired time. Insomnia may also be secondary to parasomnias such as nightmares, night terrors, or sleep-walking.

THE NATURAL HISTORY OF INSOMNIA

To varying degrees, everyone is predisposed to develop transient or episodic sleep disturbances. Several predisposing factors, however, may increase the vulnerability of some individuals to develop insomnia. These factors include (a) arousability, (b) an obsessive/worrisome cognitive style, (c) presence of psychopathology, (d) a family history of insomnia, (e) a deficient sleep/wake system, and (f) demographic characteristics of being female and older. Although these predisposing factors may lower the critical threshold needed for some individuals to develop insomnia, extenuating circumstances generally precipitate an episode of insomnia in most individuals. Precipitants may include such factors as psychosocial stressors, physical illness, or other life events. When these factors have been removed or adjusted to, most people will resume their normal sleep patterns. For others, however, insomnia may become independent or functionally autonomous from its origins and develop a life of its own as perpetuating variables come into play (Spielman & Glovinsky, 1991). The most salient perpetuating factors that maintain insomnia consist of maladaptive sleep habits and dysfunctional cognitions about sleep loss and its impact on a person's life. Figure 1 depicts factors associated with the development and maintenance of insomnia.

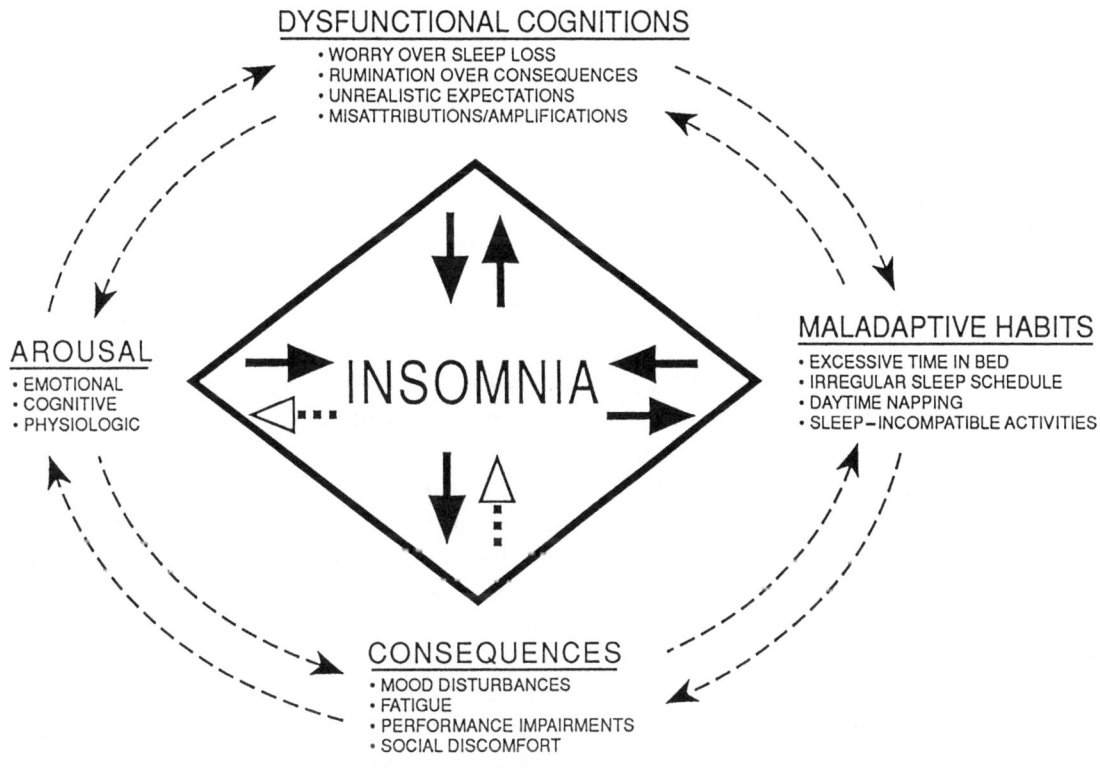

Note. From *Insomnia: Psychological Assessment and Management* by C. M. Morin, 1993, New York: Guilford Press. Reprinted with permission.

Figure 1. A Micro-Analysis of Chronic Insomnia.

Maladaptive sleep habits and dysfunctional cognitions maintain the insomnia by increasing arousal, the central mediating factor of insomnia. Maladaptive sleep habits include excessive time in bed, sleep-incompatible activities, an irregular sleep/wake schedule, and daytime napping. They result in the bed, the bedroom, and bedtime being associated with apprehension, worry, and arousal. In the long run, maladaptive sleep habits interfere with the synchronizing effect of a regular and constrained sleep/wake rhythm. Similarly, dysfunctional cognitions lead to further arousal and an almost universal tendency to try harder to go to sleep, increasing performance anxiety, muscle tension, and worry. Stressful daytime activities may also serve as activating events leading to sleeplessness at night. Daytime consequences of insomnia may include fatigue, mood disturbance, social discomfort, and performance impairments. These perceived sequelae, whether accurate or amplified, only serve to remind an individual of how miserable sleep was on the preceding night, triggering more dysfunctional cognitions about oneself and sleep and increasing maladaptive sleep behaviors. Over time, a sense of learned helplessness becomes ingrained, and insomniacs come to believe that their insomnia is uncontrollable, unpredictable, and solely attributable to external causes.

In summary, chronic insomnia generally begins with situational sleeping difficulties related to stressful life events. However, even after the stressful event has disappeared or the individual has adapted to it, the insomnia is perpetuated by maladaptive sleep behaviors and dysfunctional cognitions that increase arousal. The insomniac becomes progressively more absorbed by the sleep problem and by its presumed impact on daytime functioning. According to this conceptual framework, learned behavioral and cognitive responses play a major contributory role in maintaining insomnia. The main implication is that, to short-circuit the vicious cycle of insomnia, treatment must focus not so much on uncovering the precipitating events but rather on altering the perpetuating conditions. The primary targets for intervention are the maladaptive sleep habits and dysfunctional sleep cognitions.

THE ASSESSMENT OF INSOMNIA

THE SLEEP HISTORY

A detailed history of the sleep problem combined with a functional analysis of its current exacerbating factors are the two most important components in the assessment of insomnia (Bootzin & Engle-Friedman, 1981; Spielman, 1986). The Insomnia Interview Schedule (Morin, 1993), a semistructured interview, is helpful to gather this information in a systematic manner. It covers the nature of the presenting complaint (i.e., problems falling asleep, staying asleep, waking up too early, nonrestorative sleep, or impairment in daytime functioning), its frequency (nights per week), and its duration (acute vs. chronic).

The current sleep/wake schedule is examined next. Typical bedtime and arising times are determined, along with the time lights are turned off and the time of the last awakening in the morning. Next, frequency and duration of daytime naps, both intentional and unintentional, are determined. It is also important to assess the variability in the sleep schedule from weekdays to weekends. After evaluating the current sleep problem, a review of its history should include age of onset, its temporal course, any precipitating events, and whether the insomnia developed abruptly or gradually. Assessing the impact of disturbed sleep on daytime functioning and quality of life is important to determine the clinical significance of insomnia, as a complaint of inadequate sleep in the absence of residual effects or distress may not necessarily be pathological. The sequelae most commonly attributed to poor sleep include daytime mood disturbances, fatigue, social discomfort, and impairment of cognitive and behavioral performance (Zammit, 1988).

Conducting a comprehensive functional analysis of antecedents, consequences, and other controlling variables is essential to understanding insomnia. Careful inquiry about the patient's prebedtime routines, sleep-incompatible activities (e.g., reading or watching television in bed), secondary gains from insomnia (e.g., an excuse for avoiding unpleasant activities), and typical responses to sleeplessness is a critical component of the evaluative process. Insomnia should never be evaluated, however, strictly as a nighttime problem. Daytime cognitions, behaviors, and affect should also be examined for their impact on sleep.

A medical history is helpful in clarifying the role of factors such as pain, anemia, respiratory problems, and hyperthyroidism on sleep. It is important to take a detailed history of drugs currently used, especially sleeping medications. This should include information about both prescribed and over-the-counter sleep aids as well as their duration, frequency, and dosage. It is also important to assess use of alcohol and psychoactive drugs and past history of substance abuse and treatment for it. Other important areas are the dietary (particularly the use of caffeinated beverages), smoking, and exercise habits and factors associated with the bedroom environment including room temperature, mattress comfort, sleep partners, quietness of the room, and darkness of the room. A review of the most common symptoms of other sleep pathology is essential to differentiate between primary insomnia and insomnia secondary to other sleep disorders. The clinician should inquire about symptoms of sleep apnea (e.g., loud snoring, pauses in breathing), restless legs and periodic limb movement (e.g., repetitive leg twitches during sleep), narcolepsy, gastroesophageal reflux (e.g., heartburn), and parasomnias (e.g., nightmares, night terrors, sleep walking/talking, and bruxism).

SLEEP DIARY MONITORING

When patients initiate a request for insomnia treatment, it is usually helpful to allow a 2-week pretreatment period of self-monitoring during which baseline data on the current sleep pattern is collected via a sleep diary. A typical sleep diary requires daily recording of the following parameters: bedtime, arising time, sleep-onset latency, frequency of nocturnal awakenings, duration of each awakening, time of last awakening, arising time, naps, medication intake, and various indices of sleep quality (see Sleep Diary, p. 193). Sleep diaries are kept throughout treatment. Self-monitoring of sleep is essential in order to determine both the severity of insomnia as well as its nature and course. Self-monitoring also allows for tracking of the patient's progress over time.

SLEEP QUESTIONNAIRES

Sleep questionnaires and symptom checklists can be used to gather preliminary information about the nature and severity of insomnia and to evaluate subjective dimensions of the sleep experience. Administration of paper-and-pencil measures is helpful as an initial screening assessment to guide the focus of the clinical interview. Although there are no standardized or widely accepted screening measures, practitioners can adapt those instruments available for research to their clinical needs.

A number of ancillary measures tapping various dimensions of insomnia are also helpful for research and clinical practice. Some self-report instruments are intended for use as a global measure of quality (Buysse et al., 1989), satisfaction (Coyle & Watts, 1991), or impairment of sleep (Morin, 1993). These subjective rating scales provide valuable information about the patient's perceptions of the sleep problem. They are particularly useful as a general index of improvement from pre- to posttreatment. For example, the Sleep Impairment Index is a 5-item measure that yields a quantitative index of sleep impairment. The patient rates (on a 5-point scale) the severity, degree of interference with daily functioning, noticeability of impairments by others, level of distress caused by sleep problem, and satisfaction with current sleep patterns. Other measures are useful to evaluate mediating factors of insomnia, such as state (Nicassio et al., 1985) and trait arousal (Coren, 1988), beliefs and attitudes about sleep (Morin, 1994), sleep-incompatible activities (Kazarian, Howe, & Csapo, 1979), and knowledge/practice of sleep hygiene principles (Lacks & Rotert, 1986). These latter measures are helpful in designing individually tailored treatment plans. For instance, the Beliefs and Attitudes about Sleep Scale is designed to tap dysfunctional sleep cognitions in five domains: misattributions about the causes of insomnia; amplifications or catastrophization about the consequences of insomnia; control over and predictability of sleep; unrealistic expectations; and faulty beliefs about sleep-promoting practices. This instrument has proved extremely useful as a therapeutic tool for conducting cognitive therapy.

PSYCHOLOGICAL SCREENING

A psychological screening should be performed on all insomnia patients because sleep disturbances are often associated with concomitant features of psychological disorders, particularly depression and anxiety. Because insomnia is more socially acceptable than other psychological dysfunctions, a person may be more inclined to acknowledge sleep problems and flatly deny the presence of other difficulties. Several psychometric screening instruments can be used to evaluate the presence of concomitant psychopathology. In our clinic, all patients are administered the following instruments: the Brief Symptom Inventory (Derogatis & Melisaratos, 1983); the Beck Depression Inventory (Beck et al., 1961); and the State-Trait Anxiety Inventory (Spielberger, Gorsuch, & Lushene, 1970) or the Beck Anxiety Inventory (Beck et al., 1988). Information from these screening instruments should be supplemented, during the interview, with a history of current and past psychiatric treatment and hospitalization, and a review of symptoms of major psychopathology (e.g., depression, anxiety disorders, adjustment disorders). Although a more thorough psychological evaluation may be necessary when major psychopathology is present, we do not advocate such evaluations with all insomnia patients as administration of other more insomnia-specific measures may be more cost-effective for treatment planning.

POLYSOMNOGRAPHY

A polysomnographic (PSG) evaluation involves all-night electrographic monitoring of sleep (EEG, EOG, EMG), respiration, EKG, oxygen desaturation, and leg movements. A PSG is essential for diagnosing and documenting the severity of such sleep disorders as sleep apnea, periodic limb movements, and narcolepsy. For insomnia sufferers, there is some controversy about the role of PSG evaluation (Edinger et al., 1989; Jacobs et al., 1988). Although some contend that a laboratory evaluation is helpful in objectively assessing the severity of the sleep problem, others argue that it is relatively expensive and may have limited clinical value for treatment planning.

A MULTICOMPONENT TREATMENT PROTOCOL FOR INSOMNIA

The psychological management of insomnia relies almost exclusively on cognitive-behavioral interventions. There is little empirical evidence supporting the efficacy of insight-oriented psychotherapy for insomnia. Several papers have recently documented the efficacy, durability, and generalizability of cognitive-behavioral interventions for insomnia (Lacks & Morin, 1992; Morin, Culbert, & Schwartz, 1994; Morin, Stone, et al., 1994). In this section we describe a multiperspective approach that integrates behavioral, cognitive, educational, and medication withdrawal components, each targeting a different facet of insomnia. The focus of these treatment modalities is respectively on maladaptive habits, dysfunctional cognitions, poor sleep hygiene, and chronic use of hypnotic medications.

CHANGING MALADAPTIVE SLEEP HABITS/REGULATING THE SLEEP CYCLE

Maladaptive sleep habits include spending excessive time in bed, developing irregular sleep schedules, using the bed/bedroom for wake/time activities, and daytime napping. In general, insomniacs use these strategies in an attempt to cope with insomnia. However, these strategies are counterproductive as the bed, bedroom, or bedtime lose their discriminative properties previously associated with sleep and develop discriminative properties associated with wakefulness, anxiety, and frustration. The main therapeutic goal is to reestablish or strengthen the associations between sleep and the stimulus conditions under which it typically occurs through the use of stimulus control procedures (Bootzin, Epstein, & Wood, 1991). In stimulus control therapy, the patient is instructed to implement the following procedures:

1. Use the bed/bedroom for sleep and sex only; do not watch TV, listen to the radio, eat, or read in bed.
2. Go to bed only when you are sleepy.
3. Get out of bed if you cannot fall asleep or go back to sleep within 10 to 15 minutes; return to bed only when you feel sleepy. Repeat this step as often as necessary.
4. Maintain a regular arising time in the morning.
5. Do not nap during the day. If it cannot be avoided, limit the nap to once a day for 1 hour or less and before 3:00 p.m.

Although these procedures may seem fairly straightforward, consistent adherence to the entire regimen requires significant effort and commitment from the patient. Because patients differ widely in their compliance with these procedures, regular therapy sessions are essential to insure diligent adherence and to problem-solve for difficulties encountered in home practice. In general, most patients find one or two of the procedures more difficult to implement than the others. For example, one patient may have no problem with postponing bedtime but may find it extremely difficult to get out of bed when unable to fall asleep within 10 to 15 minutes. Another patient may have designed the bedroom as a "headquarters," reading, talking on the phone, watching TV, or doing paperwork in bed. Still another patient may not read or watch TV in bed but, instead, takes "catnaps" throughout the evening on the sofa. By careful inquiry about the patient's compliance with each of the procedures, the clinician will soon discover which ones are most problematic. The patient should be reinforced for his or her ability to carry out the majority of the instructions. The therapy can then focus on problem solving for the most difficult procedures. In the example of the patient who falls asleep on the sofa in the evening, the therapist can help the patient to generate a list of evening activities that will be incompatible with sleep or will energize the patient (i.e., physical exercise, social events, or spending time developing a new hobby).

The problem of irregular sleep schedules and fragmented sleep is treated through the use of sleep restriction. Sleep restriction therapy consists of curtailing the amount of time spent in bed to the estimated total sleep time (TST), and then gradually increasing it until an optimal sleep duration is achieved. Originally designed by Spielman (Glovinsky & Spielman, 1991; Spielman, Saskin, & Thorpy, 1987), this treatment is based on the observation that insomniacs tend to spend excessive amounts of time in bed in a misguided effort to compensate for sleep loss and to insure adequate sleep duration. Although their TST does not vary a great deal from that of good sleepers, insomniacs spend substantially more time in bed (TIB) to achieve the same sleep duration. Sleep efficiency (SE = TST/TIB X 100) is correspondingly diminished. Sleep restriction is implemented by first calculating the individual's SE from baseline sleep diaries. If the SE falls below 85%, sleep restriction is initiated. The individual's TIB is restricted to his or her baseline TST or as close to it as the patient can tolerate. However, sleep is rarely restricted to less than 4 to 5 hours per night, regardless of how minimal the TST is. The individual chooses when he or she would like to go to bed or arise and the "sleep window" is set around this time. The sleep window is reevaluated weekly according to the individual's SE for the preceding week. It is increased by 15 to 20 minutes when SE is greater than 85% for the previous week, decreased by the same amount of time when SE is below 80%, and kept constant when SE falls between 80% and 85%. Periodic adjustments are made until an optimal sleep duration is reached. Ideally, the initial sleep window and subsequent changes in allowable TIB are determined in an empirical fashion and according to sleep diary data. However, it is not always possible or desirable to follow these rules in a rigid fashion. Adjustments are often required as a function of the patient's acceptance and willingness to comply with the prescribed regimen. The sleep window establishes the maximum amount of time the individual spends in bed, but he or she should continue to adhere to the stimulus control procedures. This may result in the individual's spending even less time in bed than the sleep restriction allows.

The main effect of sleep restriction is to produce a mild state of sleep deprivation which in turn produces faster sleep onset, improved sleep continuity, and a deeper sleep (more time spent in stages 3-4 sleep). Sleep duration is not necessarily increased, though its efficiency and quality are. Sleep restriction is a somewhat paradoxical treatment for insomnia. The cognitive contrast of trying to stay awake when one is accustomed to trying to fall asleep removes performance anxiety. This shift of attentional focus, which is analogous to that achieved by paradoxical intention, appears to be an important process variable mediating a faster sleep onset.

ALTERING DYSFUNCTIONAL SLEEP COGNITIONS

Insomnia sufferers tend to endorse a variety of faulty beliefs and attitudes about sleep. The basic premise of cognitive therapy is that such dysfunctional cognitions (i.e., beliefs, thoughts, expectations, attributions) are instrumental in perpetuating insomnia by producing negative emotional responses, physiological arousal, and maladaptive sleep behaviors. The primary goal of cognitive therapy is to guide patients to reevaluate the accuracy of their thinking about sleeplessness, its causal factors, and presumed consequences. The main issue here is not to deny the presence of sleep difficulties or their impact on daytime functioning; instead, the objective is to place insomnia into a more realistic perspective and short-circuit its self-fulfilling nature. Alterations of the underlying cognitive processes should then alleviate psychological distress, curtail bad sleep habits, and ultimately improve sleep patterns.

Dysfunctional sleep cognitions tend to cluster around the following themes: (a) misconceptions about the causes of insomnia (e.g., that insomnia is basically the result of a biochemical imbalance), (b) misattributions of all daytime impairments or problems as due to poor sleep rather than to a variety of alternative factors (e.g., circadian changes, stress in other areas of life, or a poor coping style), (c) unrealistic expectations regarding sleep requirements (e.g., the belief that 8 hours of sleep is essential to maintain adequate daytime functioning), and (d) faulty appraisal of transient sleep difficulties as reflecting a loss of personal control rather than being evaluated in terms of extenuating circumstances. The same type of cognitive errors implicated in anxiety and affective disorders (Beck et al., 1979) are also involved in insomnia: magnification, dichotomous thinking, catastrophizing, overgeneralization, and selective recall.

Before working with specific sleep cognitions, the clinician should provide patients with a conceptual framework of the interrelationship between cognition, affect, and behavior. This process is facilitated by starting off with examples unrelated to insomnia and then demonstrating how these same principles operate in the context of sleep disturbances. Education about the basic principles of cognitive therapy and the rationale for targeting beliefs and attitudes is provided. A didactic approach should be used and the language adapted to the patient's educational level and psychological sophistication. The therapist's role is to help the patient (a) identify dysfunctional sleep cognitions, (b) test their validity, and (c) replace former cognitions with more adaptive substitutes.

The Beliefs and Attitudes about Sleep Scale (Morin, 1994), a 30-item questionnaire designed to tap sleep-related cognitions, is a helpful means of uncovering the patient's dysfunctional thoughts about sleep. Daily self-monitoring of dysfunctional cognitions about sleep should supplement this information. After identifying patient-specific self-statements, their validity should be explored. Hypothesis testing, experimentation, and disconfirming evidence through recent research findings are techniques used to accomplish this objective. Other cognitive restructuring procedures consist of reappraisal, reattribution, decatastrophizing, and attention shifting. A series of vignettes which illustrates the presentation of common dysfunctional cognitions, the underlying maladaptive information processing, and specific cognitive interventions are described elsewhere (Morin, 1993). Following is a sample of a cognitive restructuring intervention designed to address a patient's concern about the consequences of insomnia:

Therapist: Let's look at one common concern people have about the consequences of insomnia. On the Beliefs and Attitudes about Sleep Questionnaire, you strongly agreed with the statement, "After a poor night's sleep, I know I won't be able to function the next day." When you have this thought, what specifically do you imagine happening as a result of the poor night's sleep?

Patient: I'll be so tired, I won't be able to get out of bed to go to work.

Therapist: Have there been times when this has happened?

Patient: A few, but usually I do get up and go to work.

Therapist: And how is it when you do go to work?

Patient: Well, usually I can make it through the day but just don't function my best.

Therapist: So it sounds like the thought of not being able to function at all is not entirely accurate. When you say you don't function at your best, what specifically are you unable to do?

Patient: Well, I can still do my work but I find it more difficult to concentrate and I sometimes make silly mistakes.

Therapist: It's true that sleep deprivation can cause people to be less alert in the daytime, but I wonder if worrying about not being able to function causes you to be more distracted because you're focusing on your concerns rather than your work?

Patient: Yes, I guess that probably happens.

Therapist: Have there been times when you've had a bad night and you have still been able to function well the next day?

Patient: Sure, particularly if something is happening that I enjoy the next day.

Therapist: We can see then that the thought of being unable to function on the day following a poor night's sleep is self-defeating because it interferes with both your motivation to go to work as well as your ability to concentrate once you get there. We know from research that people can function surprisingly well even after they've suffered a poor night's sleep; however, the thought that you will not be able to function after a poor night's sleep can be very incapacitating and self-fulfilling.

As can be seen from this brief example, the patient tends to amplify the consequence of a poor night's sleep and to exclusively attribute performance deficits to sleeplessness. In addition to pointing out that poor sleep is not necessarily followed by daytime impairments, the therapist could also explore other factors (e.g., circadian variations, worries about other problems, poor time management) that might affect mood and performance.

There are several additional dysfunctional beliefs that can be addressed in cognitive therapy. For patients who believe that 8 hours of sleep is an absolute necessity, it is important to point out that there are individual differences in sleep needs. Excessive concern about achieving these "gold standards" is likely to create or exacerbate performance anxiety. Some patients have misconceptions about the causes of their insomnia. For example, they strongly believe that their insomnia is strictly the result of biological factors such as aging, pain, or a chemical imbalance. The underlying belief is that they perceive themselves to have little control over changing their fate. Cognitive therapy must convey the notion that, regardless of whether or not these biological factors are contributing to their sleep difficulties, there are always other psychological factors that they have some control over. Changing these other factors can improve their sleep patterns.

Addressing faulty appraisal of transient sleep difficulties is especially relevant in the management of acute insomnia and for relapse prevention training. Patients who enter into therapy with acute insomnia may misinterpret the origin of their difficulties as an indication that they are losing control. They may also catastrophize about the potential implications (e.g., "I am afraid of going crazy," "I am worried about having a stroke"). Such patients are often so caught up in not sleeping that they overlook situational factors (e.g., family crisis, occupational stress, shift work) that are causing their insomnia. The clinician must then provide support, decatastrophize the situation as being temporary, and directly address those situational problems that have triggered this transient episode of insomnia. With chronic insomniacs, cognitive therapy is particularly helpful in the latter phase of treatment as a means of preventing relapse. Because most insomniacs will reexperience occasional insomnia even after successfully completing treatment, it is critical to prepare them to cope with such temporary events. The main message to convey is that virtually everyone experiences occasional sleep difficulties; they should not panic about it because it is not necessarily an indication that chronic insomnia has returned. They must learn to accept the inevitable and identify/alter those factors that have caused the temporary sleep difficulties.

In summary, cognitive therapy is helpful to give insomnia patients a more adaptive perspective of their sleep difficulties. Attitudinal changes are particularly important to short-circuit the vicious cycle of insomnia, emotional distress, and further sleep disturbances.

PROMOTING GOOD SLEEP HYGIENE

Sleep hygiene education is based on the postulate that sleep is affected by a host of lifestyle and environmental factors including diet, exercise, alcohol, tobacco, and bedroom conditions such as mattress comfort, noise and light level, and temperature. These factors are usually referred to as sleep hygiene (Hauri, 1982). A comparison of good and poor sleepers on sleep hygiene knowledge and practices revealed that insomniacs are better informed but engaged in more unhealthy habits than good sleepers (Lacks & Rotert, 1986). Although poor sleep hygiene is rarely the primary cause of insomnia, it may hinder treatment progress, and the clinician should always assess its contributory role to insomnia. The following sleep hygiene guidelines are presented to the patient:

1. Discontinue caffeine 4 to 6 hours before bedtime.
2. Avoid nicotine around bedtime and at night.
3. Refrain from using alcohol as a sleep aid.
4. A light snack may be sleep inducing, but a heavy meal too close to bedtime may interfere with sleep.
5. Do not exercise vigorously within 3 to 4 hours of bedtime. Regular exercise in late afternoon may deepen sleep.
6. Minimize noise, light, and excessive temperature during the sleep period with ear plugs, white noise, window blinds, or electric blanket/air conditioner.

Both caffeine and nicotine are central-nervous-system stimulants that interfere with the initiation of sleep; these substances also make sleep lighter and more fragmented throughout the night. Although a "nightcap" may facilitate sleep onset and produce a deeper sleep in the first third of the night, sleep interruptions and early morning awakenings are common as the alcohol is metabolized later in the night. The effects of exercise on sleep depend on its timing and the individual's physical fitness. Exercising too close to bedtime interferes with sleep onset; when practiced in the morning, it may be too remote to have beneficial effects on nocturnal sleep. The best time to exercise is late afternoon or early evening. A regular exercise regimen in a physically fit person may deepen sleep, whereas strenuous exercise is unlikely to benefit sedentary individuals and may even interfere with sleep due to muscular discomfort.

This treatment component is primarily educational in nature and involves heightening the patient's awareness of sleep hygiene factors and promoting healthier lifestyles. The clinician's role is to (a) review each of these principles, (b) gauge the patient's knowledge about it, (c) present basic facts to correct misconceptions or reinforce correct knowledge, and (d) make appropriate behavior change recommendations. As part of this therapy component, it is helpful to provide basic information about sleep stages and their cyclical pattern throughout the night. Education on basic changes in sleep over the life cycle may be sufficient to reassure some older adults who are excessively concerned about normative rather than pathological changes in their sleep patterns. Although education about sleep hygiene and basic facts on sleep should be provided to all insomnia patients as a safeguard measure, the clinician should never rely exclusively on this therapy component to treat chronic insomnia because education alone has yielded limited benefits (Lacks & Morin, 1992; Morin, Culbert, et al., 1994).

DISCONTINUING HYPNOTIC MEDICATIONS IN DRUG-DEPENDENT PATIENTS

Pharmacotherapy is the most frequently used method for treating insomnia. About 7% of the adult population use a prescribed or over-the-counter sleeping aid during the course of a year (Mellinger et al., 1985). Several classes of drugs are used as hypnotics in the management of insomnia. Those include benzodiazepines, nonbenzodiazepine hypnotics, sedating antidepressants, and over-the-counter sleep aids (Morin & Kwentus, 1988). Although an occasional hypnotic may be helpful in the management of acute insomnia, with prolonged usage there is always a risk of becoming dependent on the sleep medication. In our sleep clinic, more than 80% of insomnia patients have used a sleep aid in the month preceding their initial visit, whereas 50% meet criteria for drug-dependent insomnia.

Drug-dependent insomnia is the result of both physiological and psychological factors. Patients are typically introduced to hypnotics during periods of acute stress or illness. Over time, however, the patient develops tolerance to the medication and requires an increased dosage to achieve the same sleep-inducing effect. When the patient attempts to discontinue the medication, rebound insomnia ensues and he or she returns to the medication. The psychological dependency then comes into play with the belief that medication is necessary in order to sleep. The vicious cycle of drug-dependency is perpetuated, leaving the patient with a feeling of hopelessness. In this context, the use of sleeping pills is negatively reinforced by terminating an aversive state (i.e., sleeplessness).

Before initiating a program for medication withdrawal, the patient's motivation and readiness to discontinue medication should be assessed. A structured withdrawal program that is time-limited is essential in breaking the vicious cycle of drug-dependency. In order to enhance the perception of self-control, the patient should be allowed input on when and how the withdrawal schedule is to be introduced and implemented. Furthermore, it is necessary to enlist the collaboration of a physician or pharmacist in designing a safe withdrawal schedule. Ideally, the prescribing physician should be involved and withdrawal schedules should be individualized according to the type, dosage, frequency, and duration of drug use.

A gradual withdrawal schedule is always preferable to abrupt discontinuation in order to minimize rebound effects. The dosage should be reduced by 50% until the lowest available dosage is reached. For someone taking 30 mg of temazepam (Restoril), the dosage would be reduced to 15 mg for the first week and then to 7.5 mg the next week. Once the lowest dose is reached, drug holidays are introduced. Patients are asked to decide in advance on which nights they will skip their sleeping pills. It is usually best to introduce those holidays on weekends or other days when the patient is not too concerned about daytime performance. Once the patient is down to 2 or 3 medicated nights per week, the next step is to plan in advance on which nights a sleep aid will be used. The medication should then be taken on those nights, regardless of whether the patient thought he or she needed it or not. Unlike the more typical intermittent schedule where sleeping pills are used on an "as needed" basis, this fixed schedule weakens the association between insomnia and "pill-taking behaviors."

Table 1 (p. 190) outlines a sample withdrawal schedule for a 65-year-old patient who had been taking lorazepam (Ativan) as a sleep medication for over 16 years. He had also used flurazepam (Dalmane) and over-the-counter drugs in the past. When he came for treatment at our sleep disorders clinic, he was taking lorazepam 1 mg per night, 7 nights per week. He had made numerous attempts over the years to decrease or eliminate the medication but was unsuccessful because of a worsening of his insomnia when he did not take the drug. Due to his anxiety about discontinuing medication, he was tapered very slowly. Initially, the dosage was cut in half on selected nights. Nights at the higher dose were decreased over the next few weeks. When the patient had been stabilized across the week at the lower dosage (also the smallest dose available), the next step was

TABLE 1: A SAMPLE MEDICATION WITHDRAWAL SCHEDULE

Week	Type	Dosage (mg)	Number of Nights	Total Amount	% Dosage Reduction
Week 1	Lorazepam	1.0	7	7.0 mg	0%
Week 2	Lorazepam	1.0	7	7.0 mg	0%
Week 3	Lorazepam	1.0	6		
	Lorazepam	.5	1	6.5 mg	7%
Week 4	Lorazepam	1.0	5		
		.5	2	6.0 mg	14%
Week 5	Lorazepam	1.0	4		
		.5	3	5.5 mg	21%
Week 6	Lorazepam	1.0	2		
		.5	5	4.5 mg	38%
Week 7	Lorazepam	.5	7	3.5 mg	50%
Week 8	Lorazepam	.5	6		
		.0	1	3.0 mg	57%
Week 9	Lorazepam	.5	3		
		.0	4	1.5 mg	79%
Week 10	Lorazepam	.0	7	0 mg	100%

to introduce an increasing number of drug-free nights which he chose in advance. Finally, medication was discontinued altogether. The patient was still drug-free 3 and 12 months after leaving treatment.

The management of drug-dependent insomnia can be a challenging task for the clinician. It may require more than the typical 8 to 10 weeks for nonmedicated patients. As a general rule, the tapering schedule is introduced concurrently with all the other treatment components; with highly anxious individuals, relaxation training may also be useful. Education and support should be integral elements as well. Cognitive restructuring is particularly important in helping hypnotic-dependent patients recognize the side effects of the medication which are sometimes misattributed to sleeplessness. It is also important to inform the patient that because of persistent rebound effects, it may be a few weeks before sleep improvements become noticeable. Booster sessions are important in preventing relapse.

GENERAL PRINCIPLES OF TREATMENT

Along with the specific procedures, several contextual variables and therapeutic issues mediate insomnia treatment outcome. In this section, we describe the typical format and structure of treatment implementation, and outline clinical guidelines to improve its integrity and optimize therapeutic outcome.

STRUCTURE OF TREATMENT

Duration and Format. The complete protocol involves one or two evaluation sessions and eight therapy sessions spread over a 10-week period. The first two sessions are usually devoted to clinical assessment. A minimum of eight therapy sessions, scheduled on a weekly basis, are needed thereafter to implement all procedures, to promote maximum adherence to the regimen, and to build up self-management skills for coping with periodic insomnia likely to recur after treatment completion. Therapy is implemented on an individual basis or in a group format (five to seven people). If steady progress is made toward mid-treatment, the sessions may be spaced bi-weekly. Booster sessions are occasionally scheduled for patients whose self-efficacy remains low despite sleep improvements after completion of the intervention. It may also be necessary to extend treatment duration beyond the customary 10-week period for those with a longstanding history of sleep medication use or when insomnia is associated with psychological (e.g., anxiety, depression) or medical conditions (e.g., chronic pain).

Agenda of Therapy Sessions. Each therapy session is structured according to the following agenda: (a) review sleep diary and progress from the previous week; reinforce the patient for compliance with self-monitoring; (b) review compliance with behavioral procedures and homework; identify problems encountered during home practice; (c) design strategies for optimal treatment adherence; (d) introduce new treatment component and its rationale; (e) present didactic material supporting this new component; and (f) review homework assignment for the upcoming week.

Sequence of Therapy Components. The various therapy components are generally introduced according to the sequence presented above - behavioral, cognitive, and educational. Stimulus control and sleep restriction procedures have a quicker impact on sleep and they may foster a sense of mastery early on in treatment. When the medication withdrawal component is warranted, it can be introduced at any time during the course of the intervention. Although we generally like to begin decreasing medication intake early on, the patient's readiness, anxiety level, and self-efficacy often determine the most appropriate timing for introducing this component. The sequence of therapy components may be altered as needed. For example, if an older adult is concerned only about not getting the 8 hours of uninterrupted sleep he used to get as a younger adult, and there is no clear evidence of sleep onset or maintenance insomnia, education and cognitive restructuring may be sufficient to alleviate those concerns. Likewise, if excessive caffeine intake is a salient contributing factor, it may be necessary to implement the sleep hygiene education first as sleep improvements may be impeded otherwise.

THERAPEUTIC ISSUES

Therapeutic Alliance. A strong patient-therapist alliance is necessary because much of the treatment in cognitive-behavior therapy depends upon the patient's willingness to carry out the clinician's instructions. It is critical to show genuine concern and support for patients with sleep difficulties. Some patients perceive insomnia as a sign of weakness. They may have been told repeatedly in the past that they are probably getting more sleep than they think and, in any case, they should not worry about insomnia because it has never killed anyone. A caring attitude will facilitate the development of a collaborative relationship.

The Self-Management Approach. A cornerstone of insomnia treatment is the self-management approach. An important objective of therapy is to foster a sense of control such that patients no longer feel they are victims of a sleep problem. The main goal of this approach is to help the patient take control of his or her destiny by learning skills that will enable him or her to manage insomnia. The patient must assume an active role in the treatment. The therapist's role is one of facilitator and problem solver, giving feedback and support for change. The patient is encouraged to develop a "scientific" attitude and view procedures as an experiment to be tested out. According to this self-management paradigm, treatment is time-limited, highly structured, and focused on sleep rather than on general problems or past history. The patient is informed about his or her responsibility to attend weekly sessions, keep a sleep diary throughout treatment, and do homework assignments.

Goal Setting. Before initiating treatment, it is useful to set treatment goals. As a general rule, goals must be individualized, realistic, and operational. Goal setting keeps therapy focused and helps both the patient and the therapist to evaluate outcome. After the initial baseline period, the patient sets goals he or she would like to achieve by the end of treatment. Specific values are determined for sleep parameters (e.g., sleep onset latency, frequency of nocturnal awakenings, total duration of all awakenings combined, and total hours of sleep). Patients using sleeping aids may also set a goal for medication withdrawal or reduction. At times, patients' expectations may be unrealistic and will need to be altered by the therapist. This may occur at the outset of goal setting, or as treatment progresses and the patient is more amenable to changing unrealistic expectations. Therapy goals often need to be reevaluated and readjusted as the treatment unfolds. Patients should also be given an opportunity to review goals before the end of treatment in order to evaluate their progress.

Promoting Compliance. As with most interventions that incorporate homework assignments, problems may arise with patients' noncompliance. Although the behavioral component in the present treatment is primarily didactic and does not involve in-session rehearsal or training, clinicians often make the mistake of assuming that their job is finished after handing out the behavioral prescription. Giving a behavioral prescription without regular follow-ups will almost inevitably lead to treatment failure. Much clinical work needs to be done in remaining sessions to promote compliance.

All therapy sessions should focus first on compliance with sleep diary monitoring and with homework assignments. Failure to systematically check on those issues is likely to give the patient the message that compliance with the therapist's recommendations is not as critical to treatment outcome as initially told. After introducing the procedures and their rationale, the clinician should check on the patient's understanding and acceptance of those procedures. Then, the therapist should actively elicit patients' reactions and anticipated difficulties. Although the patient should always be encouraged to try out the procedures first, it is important to address his or her objections with an emphasis on problem solving. Each problem is taken in turn and together the patient and therapist strategize about ways to overcome the problem or remove the obstacle standing in the way of successful implementation of the procedure. For example, when a patient has difficulty staying awake until his or her prescribed bedtime, the therapist may suggest alternative activities in the evening that are more physical and active (i.e., walking, visiting, talking on the phone) rather than cognitive and passive (i.e., reading or watching TV). Several additional therapeutic issues (Chambers, 1992) and strategies for promoting compliance with treatment are discussed in more detail elsewhere.

SUMMARY

Insomnia is a prevalent problem that can diminish the quality of life and have negative repercussions on psychosocial and occupational functioning. A comprehensive evaluation is necessary to determine the nature, severity, and origin of insomnia complaints. Insomnia can be a primary or secondary disorder but, when it has become a chronic problem, psychological and behavioral factors are almost always involved in exacerbating sleep difficulties. Treatment must then focus on changing maladaptive habits and dysfunctional cognitions. A multiperspective approach integrating behavioral, cognitive, educational, and medication withdrawal components was outlined. The need to tailor this intervention to the specific needs of each insomnia patient was emphasized. To optimize therapeutic outcome, it was stressed that the clinical management of insomnia be sleep focused, goal directed, and problem-solving oriented. Clinical guidelines were provided to facilitate treatment implementation and to address issues of noncompliance.

SLEEP DIARY*

NAME: _____ WEEK: _____ to _____

	Example	Mon	Tues	Wed	Thurs	Fri	Sat	Sun
1. Yesterday, I napped from ___ to ___ (note the times of all naps).	1:50 to 2:30 p.m.							
2. Yesterday, I took ___ mg of ___ (medication) and/or ___ ounces of alcohol as sleep aid.	0.125 Halcion							
3. Last night, I went to bed and turned the lights off at ___ o'clock.	11:15							
4. After turning the lights off, I fell asleep in ___ minutes.	40							
5. My sleep was interrupted ___ times (specify number of nighttime awakenings).	3							
6. My sleep was interrupted for ___ minutes (specify duration of each awakening when sleep was interrupted).	10 5 45							
7. This morning, I woke up at ___ o'clock (note time of last awakening).	6:15							
8. This morning, I got out of bed at ___ o'clock (specify the time).	6:40							
9. When I got up this morning I felt ___ (1 = Exhausted ▼——▶ 5 = Refreshed).	2							
10. Overall, my sleep last night was ___ (1 = Very Restless ▼——▶ 5 = Very Sound).	3							

*Note. From *Insomnia: Psychological Assessment and Management* by C. M. Morin, 1993, New York: Guilford Press. Reprinted with permission.

Charles M. Morin, PhD, is an Associate Professor of Psychiatry and Psychology and Director of the Sleep Disorders Center at the Medical College of Virginia/Virginia Commonwealth University. He is a Fellow of the American Psychological Association and a Diplomate of the American Board of Sleep Disorders Medicine. He is actively involved in clinical and research activities in the field of sleep disorders, and has been funded by the National Institute of Mental Health for his research on insomnia. He has published extensively and lectured internationally on the topic. Dr. Morin may be contacted at Virginia Commonwealth University, Department of Psychiatry, P.O. Box 980268, Richmond, VA 23298.

Cheryl A. Colecchi, PhD, is a licensed clinical psychologist and research associate at the Sleep Disorders Center of the Medical College of Virginia/Virginia Commonwealth University. She specializes in the treatment of insomnia and has research interests in this area as well as the management of hypnotic-dependent insomnia. She has co-authored several papers on this topic and a book chapter on psychological assessment of older adults. Dr. Colecchi can be contacted at Virginia Commonwealth University, Department of Psychiatry, P.O. Box 980268, Richmond, VA 23298.

RESOURCES

American Psychiatric Association. (1994). *Diagnostic and Statistical Manual of Mental Disorders* (4th ed.). Washington, DC: Author.

American Sleep Disorders Association. (1990). *International Classification of Sleep Disorders: Diagnostic and Coding Manual.* Rochester, MN: Author.

Beck, A. T., Epstein, N., Brown, G., & Steer, R. (1988). An inventory for measuring clinical anxiety: Psychometric properties. *Journal of Consulting and Clinical Psychology, 56*, 893-897.

Beck, A. T., Rush, A. J., Shaw, B. F., & Emery, G. (1979). *Cognitive Therapy of Depression.* New York: Guilford.

Beck, A. T., Ward, C. H., Mendelson, M., Mock, J., & Erbaugh, J. (1961). An inventory for measuring depression. *Archives of General Psychiatry, 4*, 561-571.

Bootzin, R. R., & Engle-Friedman, M. E. (1981). The assessment of insomnia. *Behavioral Assessment, 3*, 107-126.

Bootzin, R. R., Epstein, D., & Wood, J. M. (1991). Stimulus control instructions. In P. J. Hauri (Ed.), *Case Studies in Insomnia* (pp. 19-28). New York: Plenum.

Buysse, D. J., Reynolds, C. F., Monk, T. H., Berman, S. R., & Kupfer, D. J. (1989). The Pittsburgh Sleep Quality Index: A new instrument for psychiatric practice and research. *Psychiatry Research, 28*, 193-213.

Chambers, M. J. (1992). Therapeutic issues in the behavioral treatment of insomnia. *Professional Psychology: Research and Practice, 23*, 131-138.

Coren, S. (1988). Prediction of insomnia from arousability predisposition scores: Scale development and cross-validation. *Behaviour Research and Therapy, 26*, 415-420.

Coyle, K., & Watts, F. N. (1991). The factorial structure of sleep dissatisfaction. *Behaviour Research and Therapy, 29*, 513-520.

Derogatis, L. R., & Melisaratos, N. (1983). The Brief Symptom Inventory: An introductory report. *Psychological Medicine, 13*, 595-605.

Edinger, J. D., Hoelscher, T. J., Webb, M. D., Marsh, G. R., Radtke, R. A., & Erwin, C. W. (1989). Polysomnographic assessment of DIMS: Empirical evaluation of its diagnostic value. *Sleep, 12*, 315-322.

Ford, D. E., & Kamerow, D. B. (1989). Epidemiologic study of sleep disturbances and psychiatric disorders: An opportunity for prevention? *Journal of American Medical Association, 262*, 1479-1484.

Gallup Organization. (1991). *Sleep in America.* Princeton, NJ: Author.

Glovinsky, P. B., & Spielman, A. J. (1991). Sleep restriction therapy. In P. J. Hauri (Ed.), *Case Studies in Insomnia* (pp. 49-63). New York: Plenum.

Hauri, P. J. (1982). *The Sleep Disorders*. Kalamazoo, MI: Upjohn.

Jacobs, E. A., Reynolds, C. F., Kupfer, D. J., Lovin, P. A., & Ehrenpreis, A. B. (1988). The role of polysomnography in the differential diagnosis of chronic insomnia. *American Journal of Psychiatry, 145,* 346-349.

Kales, A., Bixler, E. O., Vela-Bueno, A., Cadieux, R. J., Soldatos, C. R., & Kales, J. D. (1984). Biopsychobehavioral correlates of insomnia, III: Polygraphic findings of sleep difficulty and their relationship to psychopathology. *International Journal of Neuroscience, 23,* 43-56.

Kazarian, S. S., Howe, M. G., & Csapo, K. G. (1979). Development of the sleep behavior self-rating scale. *Behavior Therapy, 10,* 412-417.

Lacks, P., & Morin, C. M. (1992). Recent advances in the assessment and treatment of insomnia. *Journal of Consulting and Clinical Psychology, 60,* 586-594.

Lacks, P., & Rotert, M. (1986). Knowledge and practice of sleep hygiene techniques in insomniacs and poor sleepers. *Behaviour Research and Therapy, 24,* 365-368.

Mellinger, G. D., Balter, M. B., & Uhlenhuth, E. H. (1985). Insomnia and its treatment: Prevalence and correlates. *Archives of General Psychiatry, 42,* 225-232.

Mindell, J. A. (1993). Sleep disorders in children. *Health Psychology, 12,* 152-163.

Morin, C. M. (1993). *Insomnia: Psychological Assessment and Management*. New York: Guilford.

Morin, C. M. (1994). Inventory of beliefs and attitudes about sleep: Preliminary scale development. *The Behavior Therapist, 17,* 163-164.

Morin, C. M., Culbert, J., & Schwartz, S. (1994). Nonpharmacological treatments of insomnia: A meta-analysis of treatment efficacy. *American Journal of Psychiatry, 151,* 1172-1180.

Morin, C. M., & Kwentus, J. A. (1988). Behavioral and pharmacological treatments for insomnia. *Annals of Behavioral Medicine, 10,* 91-100.

Morin, C. M., Stone, J., Jones, S., & McDonald, K. (1994). Psychological treatment of insomnia: A clinical replication series with 100 patients. *Behavior Therapy, 25,* 159-177.

Nicassio, P. M., Mendlowitz, D. R., Fussell, J. J., & Petras, L. (1985). The phenomenology of the pre-sleep state: The development of the pre-sleep arousal scale. *Behaviour Research and Therapy, 23,* 263-271.

Spielberger, C. D., Gorsuch, R. L., & Lushene, R. E. (1970). *Manual for the State-Trait Anxiety Inventory*. Palo Alto, CA: Consulting Psychologists Press.

Spielman, A. J. (1986). Assessment of insomnia. *Clinical Psychology Review, 6,* 11-26.

Spielman, A. J., & Glovinsky, P. (1991). The varied nature of insomnia. In P. J. Hauri (Ed.), *Case Studies in Insomnia* (pp. 1-15). New York: Plenum.

Spielman, A. J., Saskin, P., & Thorpy, M. J. (1987). Treatment of chronic insomnia by restriction of time in bed. *Sleep, 10,* 45-56.

Zammit, G. K. (1988). Subjective ratings of the characteristics and sequelae of good and poor sleep in normals. *Journal of Clinical Psychology, 44,* 123-130.

PRACTICE MANAGEMENT

INTRODUCTION TO SECTION II: PRACTICE MANAGEMENT AND PROFESSIONAL DEVELOPMENT

This section of *Innovations in Clinical Practice* includes contributions that address practice management and professional development. Successful practice management requires careful consideration of many important issues. Over recent years, we have recognized the need for careful planning and practice management. The contributions included in this section address several pertinent issues.

Many practitioners believe that managed care is a transitional vehicle in a series of ongoing changes in how we finance and deliver health care. While the current emphasis on managed care may appear to herald a shift, the shift is best viewed as just one more iteration within a constantly changing scene. Marc Frankel and John Feely provide their perspective on what features of health care financing will stay the same and what features will likely change in the next decade.

Money matters are a troublesome piece of practice for some therapists. William Herron provides a picture of the history of the struggle to balance a genuine interest in serving people with the need to earn a living. The contribution provides guidelines for effective fee practices that can be customized to fit within the range of therapists' feelings about money.

Though sexual harassment has been illegal since the adoption of the Civil Rights Act of 1964, it is only recently that meaningful remedies have been made available to victims of harassment. Sexual harassment has become one of the most common employment discrimination issues. Lilli and David Friedland bring readers up to date on this important issue.

Traditionally, mental health professionals have interacted with lawyers, courts, and legal processes with trepidation. Much of the conflict between mental health professionals and lawyers arises from either a lack of awareness of or respect for the ethical standards, professional parameters, and business practices of the two professions. In the last contribution of this section, William Foote describes a model interdisciplinary agreement between psychologists and attorneys that has been adopted in New Mexico and that has enhanced cooperation between the members of these two professions.

MANAGED CARE: WHAT'S NEXT?

Marc T. Frankel and John M. Feely

The impetus for a contribution on post-managed care practice emerges from our belief that managed care is a transitional vehicle occupying an interval in a series of ongoing changes in how we finance and deliver health care. In short, the march of change never stops. We envision no static order rising out of the current health care chaos. Even the current national health care reform initiative, only in its infancy as we write, will simply further a process that has no culmination. We expect mental health practitioners of all varieties to continue riding the "white water" of change far into the future. There are those (cf. Bergquist, 1993) who see this inherent instability as the hallmark characteristic of post-modernity in general. Although no one can predict the future of health care delivery, the recommendations we make are based on our assumptions of what will happen to the health care delivery system in the future.

Post-managed care practice will continue many of the trends mental health practitioners are already encountering: briefer therapies, incorporation of the medical model into standards of care, integrated systems of treatment delivery, and decreasing payment for units of service. By "post-managed care," we mean that traditional features of managed care such as utilization review and preauthorization procedures will largely disappear. Such icons of the late 1980s and early 1990s are irrelevant to a world where providers are responsible not for *episodes* of care but for *outcomes*. Thus, the pivotal question guiding post-managed care practice is how to achieve the maximal outcome with the least resources.

Managed care practice is concerned mostly with technological and economic factors; that is, with modalities of therapy (e.g., inpatient vs. outpatient) and with cost for units of service (e.g., per-diem rates or charge per therapy hour). Accordingly, those at the forefront of managed care practice have emphasized less intensive and costly therapies as alternatives to inpatient confinement, and have focused on negotiating significant reductions in provider rates.

By contrast, we believe that the essential issue for post-managed care practitioners is architectural: creating the organizational forms appropriate for achieving optimal outcomes. The process of creating an organizational form is vital to individual practitioners, provider groups, and institutions alike. Most, if not all, extant provider organizational forms (e.g., solo practice, group affiliation, hospital-employed, etc.) are inadequate means of optimizing outcome with expenditure of the least resources. Although the post-managed care medical marketplace clearly appears to be dominated by large groups of mental health providers incorporating virtually all points on the continuum of services, not all practitioners are appropriate members of such groups. Further, not all existing or proposed groups possess the blend of organizational, psychological, and clinical qualities necessary for thriving practices.

For those providers or groups not interested in or appropriate for group formation, some opportunity exists for finding niche markets outside mainstream health care. For example, Kovacs

(1989) suggests that psychologists position themselves outside the health care system as vendors of services (e.g., education) that consumers are willing to purchase out-of-pocket. Still others will find clinical niches built around specialties that are not offered within the national health structure (e.g., psychoanalysis). We caution readers that although these and other niches will exist and may be quite appealing, their revenue streams are small, and only a handful of providers will make a living in this manner.

It is our objective in this contribution to describe a process whereby practitioners can evaluate the opportunities open in their markets and can then test the viability of their post-managed care strategies. We intend this material to be practical; its best use is not in the reading but rather in the doing. It is through careful completion of the worksheets and consideration of the findings that providers will derive maximal benefit. We further caution that the process we describe here is meant to be replicated time and time again. Clinicians must constantly survey the emerging market. Stability of practice may be a terminal illusion, the quest for which will ultimately mean disaster.

Figure 1 is a flow chart depicting the process whereby practice reformation takes place. Individuals and groups determine first their readiness for post-managed care practice before considering decisions about practice options. Thus, the Readiness Phase of our model consists of focused questioning of the provider, scrutiny of industry trends and implications, and analysis of the local and regional market picture. Armed with these data regarding the practitioner and the market, our Decision Phase contains tools for testing the viability of competitive options and for "tinkering" with the provider's product mix and delivery system. In the Form Phase, individuals and groups explore issues of organizational architecture critical to the success of post-managed care ventures.

We expect that most readers will take the main pathway through the model defined by the bold lines and arrows in Figure 1. Others, for reasons we will discuss, will enter the Readiness Phase at alternative points, and may select a recursive pathway following "tinkering." Alternative routes

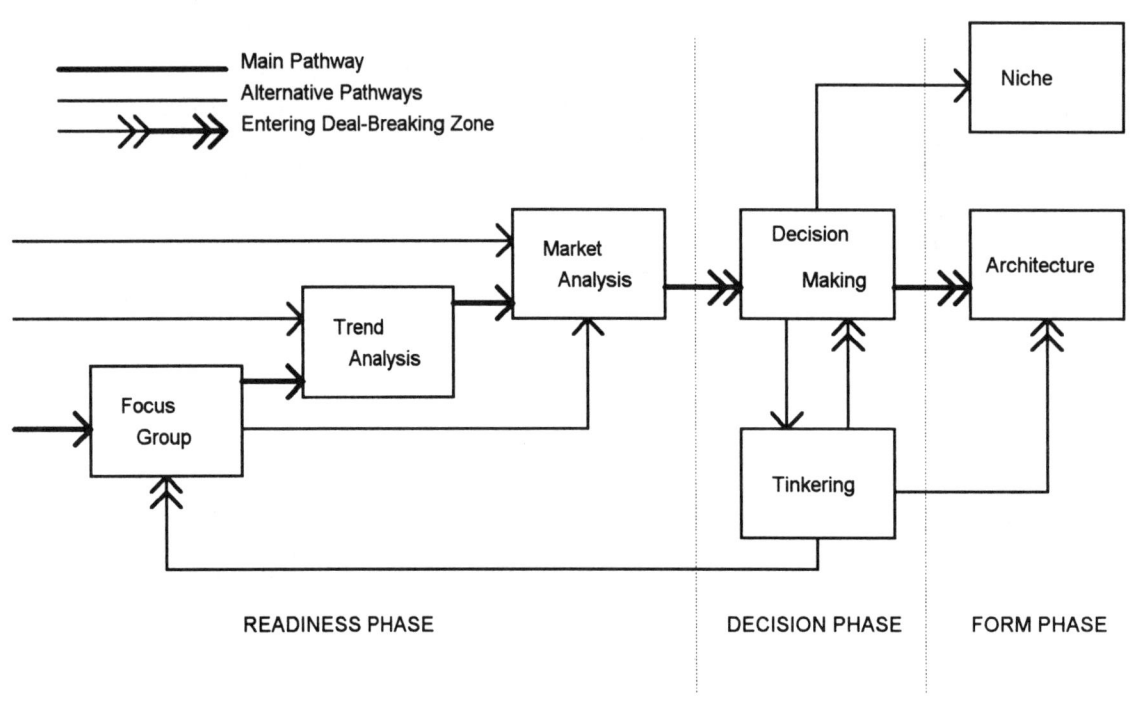

Figure 1. Process flow chart for practice reformation.

are described by thinner lines and arrows in our figure. Especially important are Deal-Breaking Zones, where critical choices and cohesion must occur. Entries to such boxes on the chart are delineated by double arrows.

Our approach is driven by a three-part strategy: (a) Gather the best data; that is, dynamic information that cuts across traditional boundaries and is timely; (b) establish a philosophical framework for making decisions; and (c) practice the integration of the pieces; that is, build models that permit analysis of various combinations of provider, market, and product attributes. This strategy is similar to that described by Fuller (1993) for use in plotting change alternatives in major corporations. The strategy is made user-friendly by way of several exercises and tools to facilitate and structure the process of creating and choosing among options.

STARTING THE PROCESS: FOCUS QUESTIONS

The point of departure for analyzing post-managed care practice options is the set of focus questions listed on pages 211 and 212. These questions may be answered by individual practitioners seeking to direct their own practices, or may alternatively be addressed by groups of providers collectively. Category 1 is a set of highly specific questions designed to focus attention on operational data and practice patterns essential to making informed decisions about business options. Category 2 contains a checklist of items comprising a continuum of care likely to be part of future integrated delivery systems in health care. Category 3 inquires about providers' beliefs and histories with collaborative and managed health care ventures.

To maximize the value of these questions, it is often useful for groups to use an external consultant as facilitator to moderate a focus group of providers or institutional constituents. This is the first of three data collection phases of the model, and it is the only one that is aimed internally; that is, collecting and analyzing information about the provider. The other two data collection steps, trend analysis and market analysis, are aimed externally, involving examination of data about factors outside the provider members. All members of the provider constituency should prepare answers to the questions.

GROUP RESPONSES

We recommend that groups of providers working their way through our model answer the focus questions separately and then meet to compare their responses. The most obvious analysis for groups to perform is to assess the degree of convergence or divergence in their responses. Neither convergence nor divergence are, alone, positives or negatives for a group considering a new venture. A group with convergent interests may offer too narrow a range of services to be marketable as an integrated delivery system. By the same token, a divergent group may work together well so long as each member's core needs are served by the venture.

It would be presumptive and risky for us to suggest "correct" responses to each item. Presumptive in that such assertions would imply that we know best what will succeed and fail in the fluid future marketplace. Risky since our likelihood of hitting the mark is low given the enormous range of providers and markets in the United States. Instead, we suggest that each clinician in the group thoroughly understand his or her unique characteristics and then participate in assessing the market for its needs and wants (see the following sections on "Industry Trends" and "Market Analysis"). We will have more to say about the match between groups, their products, and markets in the "Decision Making and Tinkering" section of this contribution.

INDIVIDUAL RESPONSES

The individual provider's responses are useful in determining the amount of internal work necessary to initiate a new business venture. In many cases these responses may tilt the decision-making process in one direction or another. For example, a provider with a strong preference for solo practice, high need for autonomy, and skills marketable outside the health care delivery system may not find group affiliation to be a desirable option. On the other hand, a provider with a strong solo practice preference, a high need for autonomy, and minimal skills apart from health care practice may be better served addressing his or her own issues, impeding group affiliation. A significant mismatch between provider beliefs and expectations and new business options, although not an absolute contraindication to the venture, raises warning flags that should be addressed prior to investment of time and money.

Further complicating the picture is the fact that an apparent close fit between clinician factors and a particular option may be without viability if there are few purchasers in the market. As noted previously, subsequent phases in the model will include collection of data about the market environment and a method of evaluating the overall goodness-of-fit between provider, market, and product factors.

INDUSTRY TRENDS

The dominant trends in behavioral health care are being driven by a changing health care system. These changes have affected providers not only in how and what they charge for services, but also in how they design and market their services. The major trends have three general implications for providers in the near future: (a) Fee-for-service payment will diminish as managed care evolves, (b) providers and managed care programs will be difficult to tell apart, and (c) delivery systems "without walls" will continue to develop.

In order to survive, providers must do more than just stay abreast of the current and changing course of behavior health care. They must anticipate and understand the personal and organizational implications of those changes. Every major shift has a multitude of predictable and unpredictable consequences on individual providers and groups. Perhaps the most stunning impact will be in the organizational architecture arena, where health care is transitioning out of its status as the last cottage industry.

To help readers focus their attention proactively on a handful of trends, we include the Megatrend Impact Worksheet, as shown on pages 213 and 214. Although we have used this instrument successfully with solo and multiple providers, we find there to be an enhanced impact when the task is completed by a group. Even if the members have no intention of affiliating or practicing together, the benefits of opening a discourse with colleagues about these trends are immeasurable.

For each identified trend on the Megatrend Impact Worksheet, readers are to think deeply about how the changes affect the *organization* of their practices and about its *personal* impact. By organization we mean things having to do with architecture of the delivery system. Staying with the metaphor, think in terms of form and function. The essential question is: *What organizational form best satisfies the function demanded by the changing industry?* What architectures make possible true integrated delivery of all points on the continuum of care? How are the providers to affiliate? What are the legal and tax implications of each alternative? In generating options, we encourage readers to consider alternatives other than traditional solo practice or a loose confederation of friends forming a like-minded group (see the section on "Organizational Architecture" later in the contribution).

With regard to personal impact, each clinician must consider the fit between his or her own preferences and style and the emerging choices. It is of no benefit in the long run to adopt a business and clinical strategy that is markedly at odds with your natural inclinations. Some of the most unhappy and tortured individuals we counsel in our clinical work are people who selected occupations antithetical to their personal interests. Clearly, solo practice does not appeal to everyone. Yet for those who find it comfortable to work alone, collaborating in a multispecialty group may require significant personal adjustment. Although there are probably few outright contraindications in the match between personal and organizational implications, we advise readers to think through the meaning of major industry trends prior to deciding on how to meet the challenge.

For illustrative purposes, we use the health care industry trends most operative as we write. Readers are advised to update the list to reflect our industry's fluid environment. It is our experience that clinicians, especially solo practitioners, are relatively unaware of these trends. Few publications targeted at providers include much review and analysis of recent developments on the business front. Perhaps the most impressive impact of the federal and state health care reform initiatives is the amount of attention paid to this industry by the media. In the past, health care has made news around great clinical advances or innovations (e.g., major organ transplantation and pharmacotherapies). Today, nearly every issue of the *Wall Street Journal* contains articles exclusively reporting health care business events (e.g., mergers and acquisitions, litigation, and health care financing). The local business periodical in our city, the *St. Louis Business Journal,* recently began a new regular section entitled "Money and Medicine."

The industry is fluid and fast-changing. Providers need to gather intelligence data continuously, covering a wide array of considerations. The data should go beyond conventional approaches that consider only reimbursement and treatment issues. In an emergent market driven by factors such as human resource utilization, knowledge, software, and biomedical technology, these topics must be constantly studied as well.

Readers are strongly advised to spend a few hours in a major medical reference library scanning the contents of publications geared toward health care managers and executives. Attendance at two or three national conferences can also yield valuable trend data. As psychologists, we have witnessed an explosion of sessions on health care practice developments at the American Psychological Association's annual meeting. The trends with the most impact on your practice may be only slightly discernible at this writing. Thus, it is critical that you apply the process we describe to the trends you detect now, and in your analysis at a later date.

MARKET ANALYSIS

Understanding characteristics of the provider members and studying industry trends will prepare participants in this process to analyze their local and regional markets. Important questions include: Who are our customers? What is our product line and what unique value does it offer to the consumer? Who are our competitors? In relation to our competitors and the market, what are our strengths, weaknesses, opportunities, and threats? What are our strategies and related action steps, target dates, and responsible parties?

Four instruments are used to systematically collect these data. We recommend their completion as follows:

SEGMENT ANALYSIS WORKSHEET (SAW)

Available information exists to obtain a general market assessment, including the demand for specific products, demographics, utilization trends, and practice patterns. More specifically, the provider will determine the needs and wants of its customers by using the Segment Analysis Worksheet (SAW), shown on page 215. Example key market segments may include the community, managed care organizations, employers, medical and surgical physicians, professional referral sources, those willing to pay out-of-pocket, and so forth. Using the SAW, the provider examines each market segment for its specific needs and wants. Brainstorming sessions, key customer group interviews, and formal customer focus groups will measurably increase the information acquired and heighten its validity. For each customer segment need or want, the SAW process asks for related customer or provider issues and the implications of those issues for the provider. For example, a large employer seeking to contract directly with a single behavioral provider might want 24-hour physician assessment for all prospective patients. A resultant human resource issue for the provider is how to staff such an intensive level of service across a broad geographical region. One implication for a group comprised entirely of nonphysicians is that they must arrange medical coverage around the clock in order to bid competitively for this contract.

We suggest the provider suspend completion of the lower portion of the SAW (strategies, action steps, time frames, and responsible parties) until after finishing the following three tools. The additional information from the other instruments will help focus strategy development on those options likely to be most viable.

PRODUCT LINE ANALYSIS (PLA)

The second step in learning market conditions is to conduct an internal assessment of the providers extant product line. Using the Product Line Analysis (PLA) shown on page 216, the provider determines what its different behavioral treatment-related services and products are and how much appeal they have to the different market segments. Within groups, individual providers know their own skills and specialties, but frequently lack comprehensive knowledge of the continuum of skills and specialties of other clinicians with whom they affiliate. After providers complete their product line listings, the cumulative list is entered on the PLA. Individually, each provider rates each service or product on a 10-point scale for each market segment, estimating its importance in satisfying customers' wants and needs ("0" means of no importance and "10" means of maximal importance). Referring back to the Segment Analysis Worksheet is helpful. Data from provider members compute into mean ratings and rank orders of value for each market segment. At a glance, the individual or group sees how appealing its services are to the current market, realizes the existing gaps on the continuum of its product line, and decides how to focus its business development resources.

COMPETITIVE ADVANTAGE ANALYSIS (CAA)

As the provider gains understanding of its customers and its own product line, it begins investigating the competition. Think carefully about your competitors market position, market share, product lines, customer groups, and marketing tactics. Local and regional hospital associations track inpatient utilization trends and are valuable sources of competitor data. Using the Competitive Advantage Analysis (CAA) tool shown on page 217, the provider develops a study of its individual competitors, networks, and institutional health care entities. The provider then acknowledges the strengths of each competitor and looks for vulnerabilities existing with or resulting from those strengths. For example, preeminence in a market as an inpatient provider may suggest a clinical, philosophical, or financial weakness in outpatient care. Continuing the analysis competitor by competitor, potential niches and exploitable advantages soon emerge along with an increased understanding of the competitive forces sharing the marketplace.

STRENGTHS, WEAKNESSES, OPPORTUNITIES, AND THREATS ANALYSIS (SWOT)

Having assessed the market, its own product line, and the competition, the provider undertakes a critical self-appraisal to know where it stands today. Using the tool shown on page 218, providers analyze their strengths, weaknesses, opportunities, and threats (SWOT). As a result of that process, they are in a position to build on their strengths, minimize weaknesses, maximize opportunities available in the dynamic market, and develop the means to constantly monitor the threats emerging from continually changing industry trends.

As it determines its position in the market and options for repositioning, the provider begins evaluating its strategic choices. It decides whether there is a fit for the current or modified organization in the marketplace, or whether it would be better to design a new architecture to pursue new business ventures. Returning at this point to the Segment Analysis Worksheet (SAW) suspended earlier, the provider develops strategies as it considers its ability to change, the barriers to overcome, the varied resources required to make the necessary changes, and the market potential of a new or restructured venture. Lastly, successful execution of the strategies demands development of objective and measurable action steps with responsibility for time frames assigned to accountable parties.

DECISION MAKING AND TINKERING

The decision-making process is really a test of the goodness of fit between the provider, the requirements of the market, and various practice options. The goal is to maximize the degree of fit, where each linkage is of equal importance. A close fit between provider skills and expectations and a particular option will be useless if there is no market for the product. Clinicians may, for instance, be highly interested in and skilled at psychoanalysis, but find little market within the health care system. Thus, staying with this scenario, the providers must either find a viable market outside health care or search for a better fitting option. In this way, decision making is one of the more critical of the deal-breaking zones.

To inform the process of decision making, we employ two tools: the Product Evaluation Scale and the Product Grid, depicted on pages 219 and 220. These instruments are to be completed for each product option generated by the market analysis, or under consideration by the provider. The Product Evaluation Scale contains items related to *external* and *internal* goodness-of-fit factors, rated according to a 5-point scale. External factors have to do with the availability of reimbursement (e.g., viability of the market in an economic sense), the ability of the provider to meet applicable regulatory requirements, the general level of demand for the product in the geographical area served by the provider, and the potential for the group to take market share away from competitors. These factors are largely outside the group, and are most closely associated with the fit between the market and the product.

Internal factors, by contrast, are attributes of the solo clinician or group, and are associated with the fit between the provider and the market. These factors have to do with the fit between a proposed product and existing products and mission, the suitability (or adaptability) of the provider's physical plant, the availability of capital required for market entry, and the potential for recruiting or retraining staff as needed for the service.

Complete the scale by rating each external and internal factor on a 1 to 5 scale, indicating degree of favorableness. Subtotals are obtained by adding the ratings for each of the four factors within internal and external dimensions. For example, a rating on External Factor 1, "Availability of Reimbursement," of "4" would correspond in scoring to 4 points. Subtotal scores will thus range between "4" and "20." Total scores, the combined subtotal scores, will range from "8" to "40." The percentage is obtained by dividing the total score by the maximum possible (40), to yield a ratio corresponding to the Scale at the left-hand bottom of the form.

As we have already mentioned, the ratings on both external and internal dimensions must be high in order for an option to truly be viable. Too low a rating means that the fit may not survive the inevitable stress of market entry and operation. For example, a relatively weak fit between provider and product may, even in the face of a high degree of market-product congruence, be insufficient to withstand the stress of capital investment, sweat equity, and collaboration.

The second tool, the Product Grid, is useful in juxtaposing external and internal factors in a graphical way. By plotting the external and internal raw scores as coordinates on the grid, providers can rate their options as highly attractive, no go, or requiring tinkering. For example, an internal raw score of "11," taken from the Product Evaluation Scale, coordinated with an external raw score of "16," would place the product slightly into the "High Attractiveness" quadrant. Obviously, the most highly attractive ventures (and there may be several) are those with the highest fits. Ideas with weak fits on both external and internal dimensions probably are not worth further effort. Those with mixed ratings (e.g., quadrants one and three) are candidates for a process we call "tinkering."

TINKERING

Some products may, with modification, be viable options for the provider. Tinkering may take the form of (a) retooling, (b) recomposition, or (c) reworking.

Retooling. Retooling refers to the acquisition of new skills or knowledge by existing members of the provider group. Such knowledge may be clinical (e.g., learning time-limited treatment methods for panic disorder) or operational (e.g., developing business systems necessary for tracking fully at-risk managed care contracts). Retooling may require considerable investment of both time and money. Thus, it is important that this step not be taken lightly; that is, those on the provider side must be highly committed to the effort in order to justify the cost.

Recomposition. An alternative or an adjunct to retooling, recomposition involves changing the members of the provider piece in order to achieve a beneficial result for the practice. Rather than, or in addition to, adding knowledge and skills through learning, the provider may elect to recruit new members already expert in the desired techniques. For example, at its simplest, a group of nonphysicians may choose to recruit one or more psychiatrists to join the collaboration, rather than retooling by sending themselves through medical school. To take a more likely case, it is infinitely easier and less costly for a group of providers to bring a hospital system into the alliance for purposes of providing inpatient care than to build, license, and operate the beds themselves. Where expertise is rare or expensive in terms of time or money, we strongly recommend recomposition as a way to rapidly bring new products to market.

Another use of recomposition is to extrude members who would make the collective unattractive to the market. For example, a psychiatrist who routinely posts high inpatient utilization numbers as a result of his or her philosophy of care may unwittingly place a group at a disadvantage in attracting large employer contracts. Recomposition may offer the remaining members of the group an opportunity to bring an integrated delivery system to market, and simultaneously allow the physician to pursue a niche in long-term hospitalization.

Reworking. Both the retooling and recomposition options rest on the assumption that the provider's plans are viable in the extant and emergent regional market. Reworking involves modification of the plans or product to increase the fit between internal and external factors. The philosophy behind a provider's idea might be sound, as in the case of offering a sole-source, direct-contract bid to a major employer in a metropolitan area. Yet, the location of the hospital member on one margin of the geographical area, and the clustering of individual providers near the institution, may be less attractive than a more diversely located competitor. Reworking, in this example, would involve opening new locations (moving existing providers) or recruiting practitioners elsewhere in town (adding the tool of recomposition).

We expect many clinicians to iterate several times between the decision making and tinkering portions of the model. The most appropriate view of tinkering is as an opportunity to enhance the goodness-of-fit between provider, market, and product. Think of tinkering as a way to "fine tune" the idea, much in the way that one adjusts a television set to improve reception and picture clarity.

ORGANIZATIONAL ARCHITECTURE

Although it is likely that the most viable practice model of the near future will be some form of group affiliation, numerous options exist for organizational architecture. Among the models now appearing are Physician-Hospital Organizations (PHOs), Medical Service Organizations (MSOs), and Physician Organizations (POs). The nomenclature of these models reflects the fact that they have evolved in medical settings with physicians and hospitals. Many of the same concepts are applicable to nonphysician providers as well. We strongly embrace the "form follows function" concept for selecting an organizational type; that is, the form ultimately selected by a group of providers must match the functions demanded of the group by the market.

Even though group practice alternatives may be highly appealing to the market, some providers may emerge from the previous "Decision Making" phase of our model not yet ready or interested in this option. For a variety of personal and professional reasons, providers may strongly desire solo practice or affiliation with a smaller, less aggressive business organization. These individuals will move into niches of opportunity, most of which will exist outside the United States' health care delivery system. These niches are small markets, focusing on services and products that consumers are willing to purchase even without health insurance benefits. Of course, there will likely always be a "Harley Street" for therapists exclusively accepting fee-for-service (cash) payment. An even smaller number of therapists will make a living delivering mental health care to those few remaining individuals with indemnity model health insurance.

In this section, we will first define issues related to group practice formation. Our intent is to focus the reader's attention on critical topics for thought when selecting an organizational form and to offer our recommendations as to the match between form and function. Next, we will address niches, with particular attention to logistical issues in starting and maintaining a niche practice.

GROUP PRACTICE MODELS

The two main issues groups face are *ownership* and *governance*. Ownership refers to who supplies and controls the capital assets of the group and thus derives most of the financial benefit (if any) from the group's work. Governance pertains to decision-making authority over multiple aspects of group operation (e.g., contracting, clinical quality, utilization management, and empanelment of providers).

Ownership. Creating and marketing any functional mental health group requires a significant investment of capital. An enormous amount of work must be done (and dollars spent) prior to acceptance of the first patient:

1. Preparation of legal documents for the group practice.
2. Negotiation and contracting with affiliated providers.
3. Creation of credentialing and recredentialing criteria.
4. Development of utilization management protocols and technique.
5. Marketing to large-scale purchasers.
6. Negotiation of contracts with payors.

The preceding partial list gives some sense of the hours of work and thus amounts of money required for creating a viable group venture. If members of the group are unwilling or unavailable to do much of this work themselves, they must contract with consultants, attorneys, and marketers to get the job done. In any event, we believe that most ventures will require more than $100,000 before securing the first contract.

Recognizing that ownership (control over capital) is different from governance (control over operations) allows us to consider the merits of three ownership models without confusing the group's financial arrangements with its clinical affairs. The first model, Group Ownership, is the case where individual members of the provider group themselves invest money up front in order to capitalize the venture. In return for this investment, the owners will receive shares in the business and are thus entitled to receive a distribution of the profits (or assume liability for the loss). The main advantage to this model is complete control for providers over all aspects of the business. Its disadvantages include demanding a payment up front from members and the risk of antitrust or inurement problems with the federal government.

A second model, the Single Entity approach, places one individual (or organization) in the position of sole owner, with providers affiliating by way of a contract. For example, a hospital may agree to provide all the start-up capital and back up the group against operational loses. Individual psychiatrists, psychologists, and so on, will then affiliate by a contract with the venture and may, in fact, choose to contract with numerous such ventures within a regional market. Provider compensation may be taken in the form of fees for services rendered, sharing in a percentage of the revenue stream, or profit sharing. Nonetheless, control over the capital, and thus the profit, rests with the single owner entity. The principle advantage of this approach is the limitation or removal of financial liability from individual practitioners. In turn, of course, the providers may participate less in reaping any financial benefits.

A third approach is the Corporation/Employee model. In this organizational form, a person or company agrees to capitalize and own the venture, with providers affiliating as employees of the owner. This approach is currently embodied by groups such as American Biodyne and United Behavioral Systems. Profits accrue to the shareholders in the owning corporation, and providers receive the usual set of benefits associated with employment (salaries, health insurance, pension plans, etc.). The principle advantages of this approach are the separation of providers still further from financial affairs (and from possible tax or legal complications) and the positioning of the venture for the rapidly emerging time when practices themselves are commodities to be bought and sold. An example of this last point is the recent acquisition of American Biodyne and Preferred Health Care by other corporations. Its disadvantages are loss of autonomy and loss of control by providers.

Tables 1 and 2 (pp. 208 and 209) itemize the issues associated with each of the ownership models. No one model is "best" in that it represents the optimal form for all ventures. Selection of a form must follow a careful group introspection about the function and the needs of individual participants in the group. We believe that all three models, including many hybrids, will prosper in the post-managed care environment.

TABLE 1: SUMMARY MATRIX OF ORGANIZATIONAL MODEL BENEFITS/ISSUES

Issues	Group Ownership	Corporation/ Employee	Single Entity
Administration/Management			
Administrative Simplicity	√	x	♦
Amount of Management Expertise Required	x	x	√
Preservation of Existing Cultures	♦/x	x	x
Marketing			
Appeal to Employers	x	√	♦
Financial/Legal			
Start-Up Costs (Capital)	√	♦	♦
Profitability	x	√	√
Risk	√	♦	♦
Economies of Scale Benefits Derived	x	√	♦
Legal Complexity	√	x	♦
Intangibles			
Creation of Synergy	√	√	♦
Trust Among Providers	High	Moderate/Low	Low
Trust Between Potential Partners	Low	Not Applicable	High

x Disadvantage
√ Minor Benefit
♦ Major Benefit

Governance. Regardless of where financial control rests, clinicians may retain significant operational and clinical control through adoption of provider-centered governance structures. Organizational bylaws can, for example, assign responsibility for provider credentialing, clinical protocol adoption, and utilization management to committees with a majority of provider members. Contracting decisions regarding new business opportunities may be similarly handled by a committee of providers and owners.

This check-and-balance approach insures a strong provider voice in operational and clinical decision making. Although few psychologists, psychiatrists, or social workers show much interest in governance at present, we strongly encourage providers to take an assertively active role in leading group affiliations. Even when ownership rests exclusively with a for-profit corporation and the providers are all employees, we believe that oversight of clinical decision making can be reserved for a committee of clinicians.

Going a step further, given the preparadigmatic nature of our field, we encourage multidisciplinary participation in governance. Just as it is important to balance the financial and clinical voices, it is also important to balance the viewpoints of psychiatrists, psychologists, and other disciplines. Because we believe that knowledge has power only when shared, there is value in allowing clinical and operation decisions to arise out of a dialogue among all interested parties.

NICHE MODELS

Despite our admonishments that niches will be small and that relatively few providers will make a living this way, we expect a high level of interest in this path. This interest reflects the similarity of this model to traditional practice, with its high level of autonomy, independence, and self-determination. For some time, Kovacs (1989) has been writing about niching (he uses the term "fee-for-service") as an alternative to health care practice. Central to this concept is that providers will sell services and products that others are willing to purchase with cash. In this way, practitioners will operate retail businesses, with product mixes determined by market forces.

TABLE 2: SUMMARY MATRIX OF ORGANIZATIONAL MODEL LEGAL ISSUES

Issues	Group Ownership	Corporation/ Employee	Single Entity
State Insurance Regulation	(Depends on Contract with Payor)		
Antitrust Exposure for Clinicians	x	♦	♦
Medicare Fraud Exposure	x	√	√
Private Inurement and Tax Exposures	♦	♦	x
Federal and State Securities Regulations	x/√	x/√	x/√
Financial and Other Liabilities	x	♦	♦

x   Disadvantage
√   Minor Benefit
♦   Major Benefit

Note:
1. Benefits and disadvantages exist to all organizational models. No disadvantage is absolute and may well be compensated for by the kind of contract created between parties, the kind of corporation/partnership employed, and the way in which all parties draw compensation from the revenue stream.
2. This matrix is offered for illustrative purposes only and does not in any way, nor is it intended to, offer legal advice.

Building on this last point, we stress that few nichers will succeed without a careful assessment of their local market. The driving energy behind any retail venture is demand, not whether the service/product is "needed" or results in a higher social good. It is in responsiveness to the market that nichers are distinguished from current mental health practitioners. Accordingly, marketing activity itself will be much more intense than most of us presently experience.

Niche Selection. As stated before, selection of niches is driven by an assessment of islands of opportunity within the local market. Think about creating products related to the mental health field but outside the usual insurance benefit structure (e.g., workplace dysfunctions, affair repair, forensic assessment, couples communication training). Rather than selling therapy time on an open-ended basis, practitioners might sell education and assessment as a package product.

Moving farther afield from clinical practice, consultation may be a viable niche for some providers. There are numerous markets for psychological services that are not exclusively clinical in nature. For example, the growing field of organizational development (OD) consulting extensively uses "therapy" techniques (e.g., group facilitation, conflict resolution, and communication training). Many mental health professionals, especially doctorally trained psychologists, are knowledgeable about data collection methodologies (e.g., focus groups, surveys, and interviews). These devices are all of value in the OD environment.

We suggest that clinicians select niches that capitalize on their extant strengths and skills. Thus, a clinical psychologist with extensive experience in testing and assessment of adults might pursue a niche practice in either forensics or outplacement counseling. Both of these specialties build on the clinician's already strong assessment background. Similarly, another psychologist, with several years experience as an operational manager of a hospital, might enter the niche of management consultation.

We caution the reader against a too-optimistic forecast of niche possibilities. Entering a niche may be relatively easy, but maintaining a thriving practice will require extensive marketing and business management activity, skills that are not widely distributed throughout the clinician population. Perhaps the most important criterion for a successful niche venture is the entrepreneurial inclination of the principle.

CONCLUSION

We have described a process designed to assist providers in making the transition to a post-managed care marketplace. Because simply being on the list of providers will no longer be sufficient for viability in practice, and because many of the features of managed care are likely to disintegrate in the face of new collaborative ventures such as integrated delivery systems, we believe no clinician of any type is protected from change. Rather than propose a practice model that we think will be successful, our approach is to be consultative rather than advisory. We think the most exciting practice options are to be found in the imaginations of practicing psychologists, social workers, counselors, and others. Our best effort, therefore, is to help readers unleash and develop their own ideas.

Two points are so important as to bear repeating here. First, practice assessment and reformation are best thought of as continuous and must be replicated periodically to insure currency amid fluidity. Second, the ultimate test of any product idea is in the market; that is, are there sufficient purchasers nearby to buy the product or service? We encourage readers to think broadly, both inside and outside traditional health care systems, about potential purchasers and products.

We want to hear from you. If you apply our process to your individual practice or group, please write and share with us your comments and suggestions. We try to continuously rethink and redesign our consultations in light of our clients' experiences. Your thoughts are welcome. Because of the fluidity of our industry, any resources we might list today may well be obsolete by the time you read this contribution. Feel free to write us for a current bibliography and listing of key resource materials.

FOCUS QUESTIONS

CATEGORY 1: PRACTICE PATTERNS

1. What is your average inpatient length of stay for psychiatry and chemical dependency cases (for physicians); or, what is your average number of outpatient sessions for a given therapy episode (for all providers)?

2. What contracts do you presently have with Health Maintenance Organizations (HMOs), Preferred Provider Organizations (PPOs), or Physician-Hospital Organizations (PHOs)?

3. What is your weekly average number of billable hours?

4. What is your current excess capacity (e.g., ability to absorb new cases)?

5. What is your net (after expenses) income expectation from your practice?

6. How do you expect your net income to change in the first and second year of a new venture?

7. What are your top five referral sources?

CATEGORY 2: CONTINUUM OF CARE

Check the applicable box reflecting your status with each modality of therapy.

Therapy Modality	Direct Experience	Access Available	Unavailable
Day Office Hours			
Evening Office Hours			
Weekend Office Hours			
Day Hospitalization			
Evening Hospital			

Therapy Modality	Direct Experience	Access Available	Unavailable
Emergency Triage			
Home Care			
Family Therapy			
Adult Inpatient			
Child Inpatient			
Adolescent Inpatient			
Chemical Dependency			
Consultation/Liaison			

CATEGORY 3: PRACTICE ORIENTATION

1. Describe your experience with "at-risk" contracting.

2. How tolerant are you of the trappings of managed care (e.g., utilization review, preauthorization procedures, benefit limitations, etc.)?

3. How tolerant are you (or do you think you might be) of others continuously monitoring and measuring your clinical behavior?

4. What is your ideal practice scenario? Write a story that describes such a practice with particular attention to issues of autonomy, collegial relationships, money, practice location, number of hours at work each week, number of weeks of vacation annually, number of days for conferences and continuing education, number of days for consulting and teaching, and paperwork.

MEGATREND IMPACT WORKSHEET

BEHAVIORAL HEALTH CARE MEGATRENDS	PERSONAL AND ORGANIZATIONAL CHANGES AND IMPLICATIONS
Managed Care Dominance Currently 48% of Americans with health care are enrolled in managed behavioral health programs. Of this number, 18% are in EAPs, 38% are in utilization review/case management programs, 36% are in network-based programs, and 8% are in integrated (EAP/managed care) programs.	
Integration of EAPs and Managed Health Care Over the past 6 years, the functions provided by "employee assistance" and "managed behavioral health" programs have grown increasingly similar. EAPs have added utilization review capabilities, provider network arrangements, and claims payment capabilities. Managed care programs are now providing "employee help lines," referrals to community resources, and management consultation.	
Growth in Capacity of Managed Behavioral Health Programs It is accepted that there is more capacity (inpatient and outpatient providers) than there is funding to pay for treatment. However, there has also been a rapid growth in the number of managed behavioral health care vendors (fewer than 20 in 1985 to over 400 in 1992). This situation has led to price-based competition among vendors, aggressive expansion of vendors into new markets, and financial instability of many programs.	
Period of Mergers and Acquisitions As a result of an expanding market for managed behavioral health services at a time of great price competition, a period of mergers and acquisitions has started (e.g., Mecco Containment purchased Personal Performance Consultants, Inc. as well as American Biodyne in 1992, making it the third largest managed behavioral health entity in the country). More industry consolidation is likely until price competition abates and market expansion wanes.	

MEGATREND IMPACT WORKSHEET (Continued)

BEHAVIORAL HEALTH CARE MEGATRENDS	PERSONAL AND ORGANIZATIONAL CHANGES AND IMPLICATIONS		
Growth of "Carve-Out" Concept Payers of all types are adopting the "carve-out" concept - creating separate plans for behavioral health benefits.			
Increasing Performance-Based Contracting Increasingly, payment for behavioral health services is being based on some measure of performance. Over the past 3 years a host of performance measures have started to be used, such as recidivism/relapse, patient satisfaction, patient access, and administrative efficiency. The growing link between performance and payment will focus providers on outcome measurement.			
Integration of Behavioral Health Benefits With "Human Risk Management Programs" An integration of the management of medical benefits with workers compensation and disability benefits is starting to occur in large corporations. As the focus of managed behavioral health becomes more long term, "wellness" and health promotion will also become an integral part of most programs. The EAP component of managed behavioral health programs should be able to coordinate corporate health promotion activities.			
Public Sector Payers Adopt Managed Behavioral Health Concepts Recent trends suggest that many of the public sector funding sources for behavioral health services may soon adopt managed care models. Already, many proprietary managed behavioral health programs are looking to state programs for an area of market expansions.			

SEGMENT ANALYSIS WORKSHEET

MARKET SEGMENT:

Needs/Wants	Issues	Implications

Strategies	Action Steps	Time Frame/Responsible Party

PRODUCT LINE ANALYSIS

Products*	Community	Managed Care	Medical Physicians	Employers	Total	Comments
Psychiatric Inpatient Units						
Psychiatric Day Outpatient Treatment						
Psychiatric Evening Outpatient Treatment						
Psychiatrist Office Services						
Psychologist Office Services						

*These are examples of the kinds of products providers may include on this form.

COMPETITIVE ADVANTAGE ANALYSIS

COMPETITOR:

Competitor Strengths	Competitor Vulnerabilities
Exploitable Advantages	

STRENGTHS, WEAKNESSES, OPPORTUNITIES, AND THREATS ANALYSIS

Weaknesses	Threats
Strengths	Opportunities

PRODUCT EVALUATION SCALE

External Factors		1 (Unfavorable)	2	3	4	5 (Favorable)
1	Availability of Reimbursement					
2	Ability to Meet Regulatory and Licensure Requirements					
3	Product Demand					
4	Potential to Take Market Share from Competitors					

Subtotal _____

Internal Factors		1 (Unfavorable)	2	3	4	5 (Favorable)
1	Fit with Mission and Product Lines					
2	Physical Plant Suitability					
3	Capital Requirements					
4	Staff Recruitment or Retraining Potential					

Subtotal _____

Total _____

Percentage _____

Scale

80% to 100% = High Success
60% to 80% = Good Success
50% to 60% = Revisit/Reformulate
< 50% = No Go

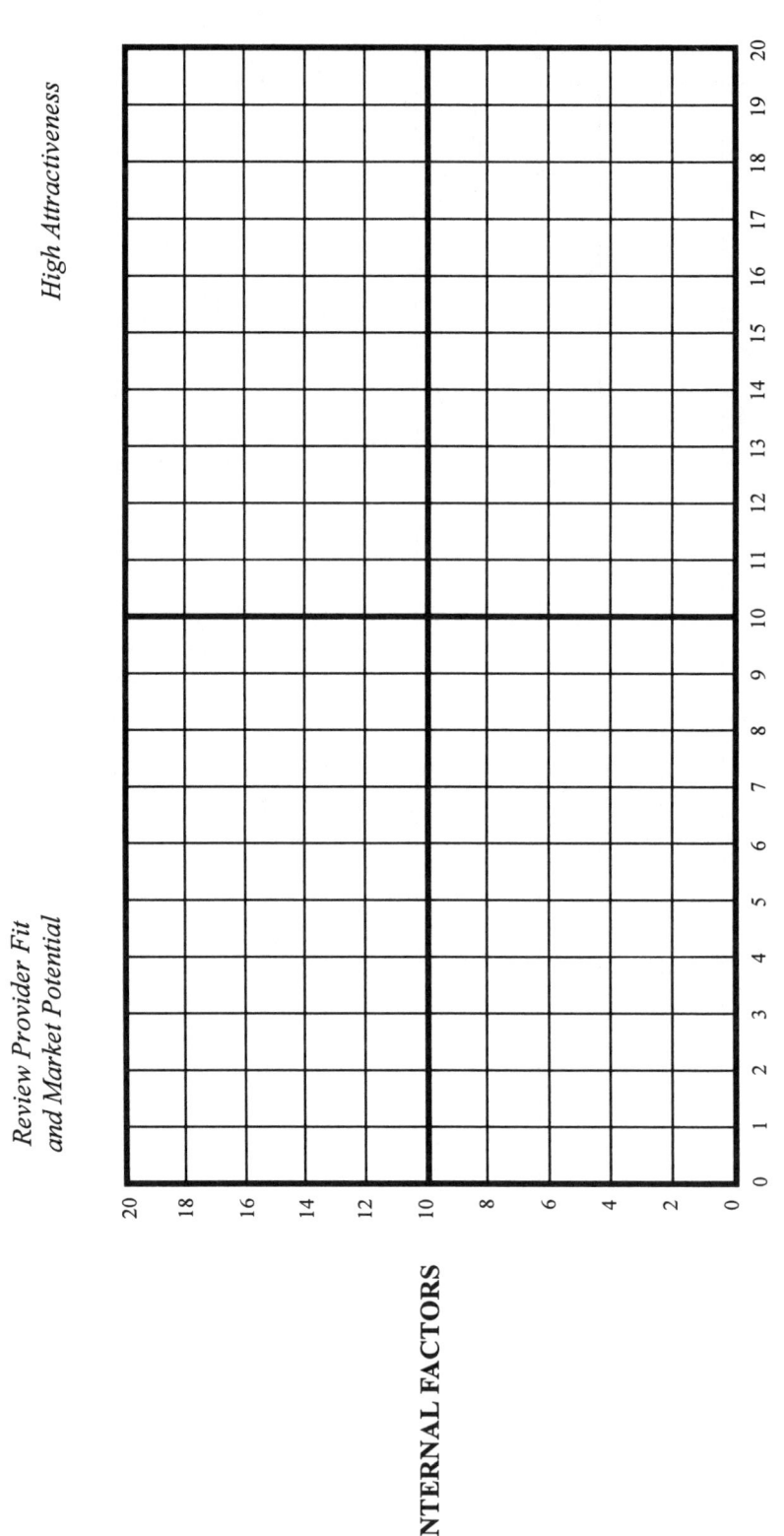

Marc T. Frankel, PhD, is a practicing clinical psychologist and senior partner in Leadership Innovation Associates. Dr. Frankel's doctoral degree is from Emory University, and he has worked in management and administration at several St. Louis area hospitals. He is president-elect of the Society for Psychologists in Management. In addition to organization development consultation, Dr. Frankel's clinical specialties are individual and couples psychotherapy. Dr. Frankel may be contacted at Leadership Innovation Associates, 131 West Monroe, Suite 4, St. Louis, MO 63122.

John M. Feely, PhD, is a practicing clinical psychologist and senior partner in Leadership Innovation Associates. Dr. Feely received his doctorate from St. Louis University, and has broad experience developing and directing clinical programs. Dr. Feely has consulted on numerous human resource-related organizational development projects. His clinical specialties include individual and couples psychotherapy, and chemical dependency treatment. Dr. Feely may be contacted at Leadership Innovation Associates, 131 West Monroe, Suite 4, St. Louis, MO 63122.

RESOURCES

Bergquist, W. (1993). *The Post-Modern Organization: Mastering the Art of Irreversible Change.* San Francisco, CA: Jossey-Bass.

Fuller, M. B. (1993). Business as war. *Fast Company, 1,* 42-51.

Kovacs, A. (1989). Here comes the iceberg. *The Psychotherapy Bulletin, 24,* 11-14.

DEALING WITH FEES IN PSYCHOTHERAPY

William G. Herron

Money has always been a problem for psychotherapists. Contributors to this start with balancing a genuine interest in serving people regardless of monetary returns with the need to make a living. This difficulty is increased by an idealized role image of selfless service. Another factor is the questioning of psychotherapeutic services as really belonging in the "for pay" category considering their prominent humane characteristics. Also, there are allegations that therapists charge too much, exemplified in the growth of managed mental health care. Then, most people have feelings about money that are reflected in their personal uses of money - acquiring it and/or spending it. Therapists are no exception.

The major issue is the development of comfortable, appropriate ways of handling fees for providing psychotherapeutic services. The focus is on private practice, because, although all psychotherapists, regardless of settings, may have feelings about money matters, private practitioners are most directly affected by the fee structures that exist for their patients. Paradoxically, the managed care emphasis on the cost of services has forced therapists to be more open about their monetary interests. It is now even more apparent that fees can be a significant source of discomfort. Unfortunately, whenever that is the case there is a potential for therapists' dilution of the quality of the therapeutic process.

This contribution is designed to remedy these problems by providing guidelines for effective fee practices that can be customized to fit within the range of psychotherapists' feelings about money. Therapists' roles in regard to fees are discussed first, followed by patients' roles, and concluding with the different fee policies that can be used to enhance the value of psychotherapy for patients and therapists.

THERAPISTS

ROLE DEFINITION

Psychotherapists are paid service providers. This means that psychotherapy is considered a viable profession and that, wherever possible, which will be in most cases, therapists expect and attempt to collect a reasonable fee for their services. This is a necessary conceptual beginning for anybody attempting to make their living as a therapist. The degree to which this premise is accepted will largely determine the degree of economic success of the practitioner.

The provision of some low-cost or free service is included in the role definition, but with the understanding that it will be limited by the realities of each psychotherapist's economic needs. Because psychotherapists live and work with a market economy, they have a personal need to get paid for their work. How much pay is reflective of the particular lifestyle desired by each therapist. Based on the fee survey by *Psychotherapy Finances* (1992), indicating an $80 median fee for individual psychotherapy and a $62,000 net income for full-time private practice, psychotherapists are mainly middle-class professionals.

At the same time that psychotherapists seek and receive money for their services, some still have a need to downplay their desire for money in favor of the image of selfless helper to whom acquiring money is always relatively incidental. The reality of economic interest is avoided in accord with a long and continuing history of fee guilt which has been documented in major reviews of fee issues (Herron & Welt, 1992; Klebanow & Lowenkopf, 1991; Krueger, 1986). Therapists want to get paid, yet question the implications for their image if this desire is quite visible, with some even questioning the validity of getting paid "just to listen to someone else's problems."

The latter attitude reflects confusion about what psychotherapists actually do. It is essential to recognize that they render a specialized professional service that is different from any other helping behavior, even when it appears to overlap help given freely by a friend, relative, or any kind of concerned person. Psychotherapists have learned distinctive theories and techniques that are in turn applied to solving people's mental health problems. They are paid then for their competence as problem-solving experts.

Of course it is true that certain personal qualities of therapists are displayed in service delivery, and that these qualities, such as warmth, respect, and understanding, are not generally conceptualized in the society as actions for which one ought to get paid. However, these personality characteristics are not what psychotherapists are paid for, nor are they what other professionals who have reasons to show these traits in their work, such as physicians and attorneys, get paid to provide.

Nonetheless, relationship behaviors that may be freely given in social situations are at times mistakenly identified as the work of psychotherapists. Then the appearance of the therapeutic process is thought of as the actuality and essence of psychotherapy with the result that therapists feel guilty about being paid for what they begin to believe should be given away. Related guilt-inducing possibilities include the relative uncertainty of therapeutic work, the relative intangibility of results, and the possibility of failure.

Although the role of the psychotherapist in regard to fees has been defined here, confusion and accompanying guilt are quite understandable. When psychotherapy was formally recognized as remunerative work, which appears to have occurred with the advent of psychoanalysis, the fee was depicted as a necessary symbol of patients' motivation (Freud, 1913). The message was that the fee had to be there primarily because it helped the patient, and only secondarily was of benefit to the therapist. The fee was a "necessary sacrifice" (thereby also providing a scale to determine the size of fees), without which patients would lack the resolve to really work in their therapy. As a result, psychotherapy without some fee that indicated sacrifice, even in low-cost services, was long thought to be ineffective if attempted. In addition, the motive for fee collection by therapists was to help patients, not themselves. This approach clearly supported a particularly altruistic image of psychotherapists.

However, the increasing use of third-party payments for psychotherapy altered the sacrificial tone of fee transactions in that patients often did not make significant fee payments, and at times paid nothing directly. Furthermore, a review of the literature regarding the effect of fees on psychotherapy indicated that patients can benefit from psychotherapy without paying fees (Herron & Sitkowski, 1986). Of course, it remains probable that fees can have motivational value for patients, but the major motivational impetus is really for therapists. This tended to be obscured at first by insurance coverage which deflected much of the need for therapist-patient discussion about payment that could have illustrated the therapist's needs. Now, managed care puts a spotlight on costs and on the monetary interests of therapists that indeed were there, and will remain there. Thus, the effect of fees on psychotherapy appears to be primarily a function of therapists' satisfaction with what they are being paid.

Achieving career satisfaction for therapists is a complex issue when discomfort is experienced in getting what is desired in payment from patients. Based on therapists' income, it would not seem that they have much, if anything, to feel guilty about. Not only are therapists primarily middle class, but private practice is so time and labor intensive that income has a fairly modest ceiling. In addition, current approaches to funding mental health service put downward pressure on fees. It is just not a viable way to get rich. It is a way to make a comfortable living, but the heavily competitive flavor of today's marketplace for mental health services puts a damper on the degree. Still, the primary reason for psychotherapy remains doing intriguing, special, helpful work that also provides an acceptable standard of living. It is true that some individuals have been able to use the field of psychotherapy in various creative or innovative ways to make notable incomes, but they are relative exceptions, and it was usually not accomplished by seeing patients hour after hour. Practicing psychotherapy is simply not a place that the greedy would be prone to find a home.

Given all this, why the problems with fees? It could be because some therapists are guilty most of the time, and all therapists are guilty some of the time, about getting paid *at all* for what they do. Although it should not, it clashes with a helping image of which they are justifiably proud. The ethical obligation to serve the needy has been well respected. This is exemplified in the frequency of sliding-scale fee policies based on patients' abilities to pay and in the large number of therapists who provide some low-cost or free service (Welt & Herron, 1990).

However, the key qualifier is "some," because extreme maintenance, or even extreme provision, of low-cost or free service would put most therapists in a financial bind. In turn, they are likely to be resentful of their patients and do ineffective psychotherapy. Translating the helping image into the reality of predominantly low-fee practice is not viable for most therapists, and therefore not for most patients either. It is not how most therapists practice, but seeking equilibrium in the area still haunts the development of effective practice.

At this point some readers may be quite in agreement, while others may feel fee issues are not so much a problem. Although some therapists are better with fees than others, the existing literature supports the idea that there is indeed a significant, extensive problem which too often goes unrecognized or, if recognized, is given restricted attention (Bishop & Eppolito, 1992). Clinical evidence is also readily available. As a therapist, simply ask yourself how you would feel (or did feel) if a patient asked you, "If I cannot pay, will you see me?"

The solution lies in accurately defining the role of psychotherapist as a paid helper and integrating that role in the therapist's personality. Payment is not a negative reflection on the help provided or on the personality of the helper. Instead it increases the probability of a better helping experience, particularly in private practice where payment motivates therapists. Also, the type of help provided by psychotherapy is different from help provided without a fee by any well-meaning person. The distinctive services involved justify charging for therapy and define the profession for all disciplines included as psychotherapists.

MONETARY TRANSACTIONS

The starting points for any therapist are beliefs in the distinctive validity of the services and the appropriate necessity of payment for the services. Without these, an effective therapeutic role is in jeopardy. Assuming then that these concepts are basically in place, the psychotherapist is ready to deal with the particulars of the monetary transactions in therapy.

Money is generally an uncomfortable topic for the society. There are unwritten rules which indicate that people should be discreet about showing interest in money. It is considered improper to ask others how much they earn, or what their possessions cost, as well as talking about how much one makes or how much one's car or home cost. Appearing greedy or stingy is frowned upon, as is the flamboyant display of wealth. Moderation is the favored course, in line with the moralistic equation of money with evil. At the same time, this is a capitalist country with a market economy where most people have a deep and abiding interest in money. Signs and symbols of money are everywhere, as is the need for money.

Therapists have to wade into this confusing, distorting, and threatening thicket of ambivalence and make money as much a part of the therapeutic discourse as any other significant topic. It is an ongoing struggle to create this type of open therapeutic environment because money has a "taboo" status for so many people (Krueger, 1986). Although therapists can learn what their role ought to be, they still have the task of working with their mixed feelings about implementing the role. Continued evaluation is needed of how financial transactions involving therapy are being carried out. Even therapists who are relatively comfortable with money matters can be made uncomfortable by a particular patient's financial concerns or a shift in their own economic situations.

Therapists' attitudes may be balanced or extreme, the latter being most problematic for the progress of therapy. One extreme is an obsession with getting the fee, which can give the appearance of "being in it for the money," even when that is not the case. This approach tends to result in poor timing, insensitivity to patients, and dissension.

For example, a patient is in tears at the end of a session. She usually pays the therapist at this point, but, being distraught, she starts to leave without paying. The therapist stops her and asks for the payment. Another situation is disagreement as to whether or not the patient paid a particular bill. The patient believes that he did, but the therapist's records indicate otherwise. Instead of politely asking the patient to reevaluate his records, or considering the possibility that she, the therapist, did not record the payment, she insists she is owed the money. A third situation is having a go-between, such as a secretary, collect the fees and make sure that patients pay, including chiding them if they do not. This keeps the money issue as far removed from the therapist, and the therapy, as possible, giving illusory relief to a money-anxious therapist who is making it harder for patients to discuss money issues in therapy.

Some therapists in this category may be avaricious, but most are not. They are just worried about their ability to consistently collect fees because they know they can be manipulated in this regard. Rather than deal with this problem in a specific and therapeutic way, they impose rather rigid procedures on all their patients. Such an approach has the unfortunate effect of costing these therapists money, because, although some masochistic patients may endure, most patients will react negatively and go elsewhere.

The other extreme is that the therapist is manipulated into a personally undesired fee arrangement where the therapist gets less than he or she wants. This usually comes about because the helping role is being distorted by the therapist's need to demonstrate apparent selflessness. The most complete form of this extreme would be that the therapist accepts whatever fee arrangements each patient wants. Milder forms would be compromises between patient and therapist desires that are actually unappealing to the therapist and, as a result, likely to cause resentment for the therapist.

These situations tend to occur when the fee is being based on the patient's ability to pay. The patient then has the opportunity to negotiate the fee and can utilize whatever vulnerability the therapist has to get bargain rates. However, if the therapist is going to dislike the result, it is unlikely that the service will turn out to be a bargain because the quality of it may suffer. A key ingredient is how the therapist feels about doing the work. Fee arrangements that really do not satisfy a therapist pose the threat of sabotaging therapy.

Therapists are responsible for establishing and maintaining reasonable fee policies. Such policies take into account the feelings of providers and consumers as well as the reality of the marketplace. What patients themselves, and increasingly their insurance plans, are willing to pay dictates to a major extent the fees that can be charged. The market provides a framework for realistic expectations about income. Knowing this, therapists can price themselves within a range that is designed to bring them a desired income and market their services accordingly. After setting this goal, therapists have to actively pursue the payment of fees. There needs to be sufficient flexibility so that therapists can cope with variations in patients' payment patterns, including failures to pay as well as needs for reductions and delays. Factored in is the willingness to accept a certain number of low-fee patients, but that number should not be so high as to unduly limit income. In essence, staying with the realities of one's markets and their congruence with one's needs provides for balanced, reasonable fee policies.

One shifting reality that bears special consideration is the increasing presence of managed mental health care. This approach restricts the flexibility of therapist-patient fee negotiations. Generally, if the therapist is a designated provider for the plan, he or she has agreed to accept a set fee, most of which comes from a third party. Therapists still have to collect something from the patient, but it is usually a small amount that is not likely to present much of a collection problem. Collecting the rest, however, often requires assertiveness and persistence, and is usually the responsibility of the therapist. Managed care companies may have restrictive guidelines on what services will be reimbursed, so it can be a struggle to get full payment. However, therapists' monetary interests are exposed to relatively anonymous employees of third-party payers rather than patients, so the helping image may not appear as tarnished in the money-seeking process. If therapists are in accord with the managed care philosophy, and follow the rules, stability of payment and patient supply are good possibilities. However, the total fee is usually lower than what the therapist customarily charges, and it is a set fee. Thus, unless volume is high, income will be lower. Managed care appeals to monetary security, but even that is possible only if therapists practice as expected, and for many therapists this becomes too restrictive, thus making security questionable over time.

The alternative is to be an outside-the-network provider, which means the patients get less coverage and are paying a fee negotiated with their therapists. This approach allows therapists to retain their fee structures, but it can require them to explain to patients why they are not part of the network that would make therapy less expensive for patients. This highlights therapists' desires for money, which could make some therapists quite uncomfortable. Managed care is creating a situation in which therapists have to choose between being approximately equivalent to a salaried employee with a set income and limited room for monetary growth, and being an independent practitioner with freedom to set fees, but with a limited patient supply. The first alternative makes money less of a visible issue between therapist and patient, while the second increases its visibility, so they have different appeals according to therapists' personal feelings about money matters.

PATIENTS

ROLE DEFINITION

Patients generally come to psychotherapy with an understanding that they are the people in need of help, and that therapists will provide that help for a fee. What it means to be a patient will vary based on the personality styles of each. Essentially this will be symbolized in the degree to which any patient cooperates with the therapy program. Patients will expect their therapists to explain, in as much detail as possible, what the patients' problems are and what they are to do, in and out of therapy, to solve these problems. Explanations of the treatment method should include payment procedures, because these are part of the treatment process. Also, because patients will understandably be focused on what is bothering them, it is likely that fee policies will need to be explained more than once.

At times patients will accept the role of payer with greater ease than therapists accept their role of asking for and receiving payment. Patients are accustomed to paying for health services and do not tend to differentiate psychotherapy to the same extent as therapists. However, acceptance of the role does not mean that they like it, or that they will not complain. The likelihood of patients "resisting" payment in some fashion is high. They bring their attitudes, concerns, and conflicts about money to psychotherapy and display them in reaction to each therapist's suggested monetary arrangements.

If a therapist tends to be vague or hesitant about fee policies, patients are provided with an opportunity to do the same in their payment patterns. A small number of patients see the pursuit of payment as primarily their concern, but most do not. The role of patient is to wait for the therapist to both describe and, when necessary, to pursue compliance with fee policies. In addition, the role of the patient includes discretion as to what is revealed in therapy, with expectations that the therapist will facilitate discussions about important but discomforting topics. Money is of course one of these, and that means therapists cannot wait for patients to make it easy to discuss financial matters. In addition, because most forms of therapy involve repeated visits, even if the course of treatment is relatively brief, negative feelings about payment have a chance to accumulate. This suggests that almost any patient over time will be likely to alter payment procedures and expect that this will be understood and, in turn, accepted by the therapist. Typical examples are "forgetting" the check and "needing a bit more time" this month.

In the current market environment, patients have become more serious about being informed consumers. The advantages for therapists in this trend are that patients are identifying themselves in advance as prepared to pay for services, as well as having a more detailed view of the probable activities that constitute therapeutic process and outcome. This facilitates therapists' presentations regarding fees as part of the therapeutic process. The disadvantages are that patients' information comes from diverse sources, and some of these involve distortions about psychotherapy. Thus more patients now arrive with false ideas than before when they may have had less knowledge. The current situation can be vexing because therapists' attempts to correct the incorrect may be categorized by patients as defensive incompetence. In the fee area, for example, a patient may believe that payment is always negotiable and that only the foolish pay what therapists ask.

Another area of patient confusion is an unawareness of both the specific details required by third-party payers and the consequences of not revealing such information, namely discontinuance of reimbursement. Actually insurance carriers, and more often their agents, managed care entities, have in many ways assumed the characteristics of patients. They have expectations that affect payment, including a limit on what they will pay, how long they will pay, and standards to be met, such as medical necessity, in order to get payment. The extent to which patients are involved with managed care then becomes a major factor in defining the role because limits are set for the patient prior to seeing any therapist. Some patients are aware of them, whereas others tend to learn the details of their health plans only after they have initiated contact with a therapist.

Patients also now have a more apparent interest in accountability on the therapist's part than they did. This means that therapists need to be open to discussing the value to be received by patients for the money spent. Although the focus on competence in cost terms does make some psychotherapists uncomfortable, patients do expect therapists to respond to such evaluations. This clarifies the "business" aspect of psychotherapy, and in so doing illustrates that the nature of the relationship is a professional one in which both parties have clearly defined roles.

Although people may act as if they accept all the aspects of their role as seekers of help, including paying a fee, it is quite likely that they may want types of relationships that deviate from the therapeutic, such as social relationships. The presence of the fee serves to define the boundaries of the relationship. Patients are protected from therapists distorting the relationship in an exploitative way, and therapists are clearly identified for patients as being paid helpers. The fee makes it clear to patients that therapists have a responsibility to perform in a professional, therapeutic manner, to do their job in contrast to any other type of relating that might be in the fantasy of either patient or therapist.

MONETARY TRANSACTIONS

Although patients understand that they are going to pay for therapy services, the particulars of payment are not so well known. In contrast to the way most health services are now paid for, namely to a member of an office staff rather than to the service provider, payment will usually be made directly to the therapist, particularly in individual practices. The monetary exchange will be a direct one in most instances; even in situations where that is not the case, such as a clinic, there is usually a direct discussion with the therapist regarding payment. Many patients are not prepared for this, particularly if the discussion involves details of their income which may be necessary for the provider to establish the appropriate fee. The situation requires tact and consideration on the therapist's part as well the ability to get the necessary information and establish the fee arrangements.

This initial dialogue constitutes a payment contract between the provider and the consumer. The contract may be a written one, but the usual procedure is verbal. This means that the manner in which the contract is explained and then put into practice will set the tone for monetary transactions for the course of the therapy. Although each patient will approach the contracting process somewhat differently, what is depicted here tends to be the usual patient style, namely a relatively high level of anxiety and self-preoccupation that often results in not completely understanding the monetary arrangements. If there are uncertainties, vague areas, or omissions on the therapist's part when presenting these matters, then the possibilities of distortions are increased. These distortions most often take the form of delaying or reducing payment, which in turn causes the therapist to have to reintroduce the topic. Consequently, it is of great value to establish a clear contract from the start. Some repetition may still be necessary as a result of patients being understandably distracted, but when therapists know they have been explicit, then they are more comfortable about subsequent discussions. Also, a frank style about money matters from the therapist provides a model for the open discussion of all money matters by the patient.

It is likely that patients will have an idea of the "going rate" for psychotherapy in their area, including a differential between providers by discipline, namely, that psychiatrists will charge the highest fees. Some patients shop therapists, interviewing a number with preestablished criteria for their fit with a therapist, one of those criteria being the fee. Some patients want to negotiate and feel that they have accomplished something positive for themselves if they get a therapist to reduce his or her fee. However, the shoppers and the bargainers seem unaware that getting the cheapest therapy may work to their disadvantage. Sometimes therapists charge less because they are lacking competence in some fashion, or intend to cut corners. Then, in striking a bargain patients run the risk that a therapist will not be satisfied with the situation and that this dissatisfaction will affect the therapy. None of this means that the higher the fee the greater the competence, but it does mean that fees are performance incentives. Patients are better off if they recognize this and, in choosing a therapist or continuing with one, put their emphasis on competence rather than cost, assuming that the requested fee is indeed one they can afford.

In addition, therapists can be sensitized to whether or not the fee is a problem for a patient, because there can be a "barrier effect" (Herron & Welt, 1992) where fees serve as ostensible reasons for patients who are in need to avoid either beginning or continuing psychotherapy. People may say they cannot afford to begin therapy or continue in therapy because it is too expensive, when they are actually looking for an "acceptable" reason to avoid or discontinue psychotherapy. Therapists then should be willing to provide a rationale for their fee policies as well as being willing to suggest other resources for patients if satisfactory arrangements cannot be worked out with them.

It is also likely that patients will have some confusion about their insurance coverage. Therapists who do not actively investigate this and clarify payment procedures involving insurance will be creating potential difficulties for themselves and their patients. It is not practical to view insurance payments to therapists as solely the patient's responsibility. Insurance companies ask for information from providers and in certain situations are making direct payment to providers. The most likely situation is that there will be a sharing of activities between patients and therapists in making sure that payments are made in a timely and appropriate fashion. However, although therapists can assist patients in dealing with insurance companies, the payment relationship essentially remains between patient and therapist.

Even where the contract is definitely in place and being adhered to consistently, patients attempt to deviate from it from time to time. There are a multitude of reasons for doing this, ranging from just not liking to pay, to having had an unpleasant session, to displaying feelings toward the therapist that are displaced from significant others. Patients do not enter therapy with this in mind, but as the process unfolds, the fee becomes a convenient way to express something to the therapist. Sometimes this is a positive statement that is relatively easy for a therapist to explore, such as overpayment or payment in advance. More often it appears as an indicator of hostility. At times this may just be verbal descriptions of the patient's limited financial resources, or doubts about how long the patient can continue in therapy due to the cost, or envy of what the patient believes is a lifestyle that the therapist is achieving at the patient's expense. These are designed to make the therapist feel sorry for the patient and alleviate the financial burden, but they are not direct requests. Their indirect nature makes it easier for the therapist to focus on the feelings involved. In these instances, patients often want empathic understanding rather than direct action.

More discomforting are instances where patients do not acknowledge what they are doing with the fee and the therapist has to appear confrontative. Another possibility is a direct request for a change in the fee or in the payment arrangements where the therapist has to sort out the legitimacy of the patient's expressed need. In essence, is it a manipulation that is designed to satisfy a psychic need or is it a necessary financial exigency? If the former, it can be worked out without the fee having to be changed, but the therapist may appear to the patient as distrustful and only interested in payment somewhere in the process. Therapists should not be deterred by the possible patient projections, but they can be, and are manipulated. Still more difficult is when the patient's need is legitimate, therapy is in process, and the therapist feels an obligation to respond to the need but does not like the reduction in income. This type of situation makes the point that all therapists will need to be flexible about their fee policies at least some of the time. Also indicated is the need for accepting attempted and actual changes in fee policies over time. Therapists generally recognize this when it comes to raising fees, and they expect patients to understand that need and pay higher fees. At the same time, patients can expect that therapists will in turn be as responsive as possible to patients' changing financial circumstances. All in all, patients can be quite good about meeting therapists' financial needs, as long as therapists are willing to view the fee as part of the therapeutic process and treat it accordingly.

FEE POLICIES

There are three general categories of fee policies: sliding-scale, fixed, and the hybrid of managed care. There are also various procedures, such as the handling of vacations, cancellations, and missed sessions; the raising and lowering of fees; payment schedules; compensation for extra session services such as phone calls and completing insurance forms; and debt collection, that will also be considered in this section.

SLIDING SCALES

This has been the most common policy in which the fee is based on the ability of the patient to pay (Herron & Welt, 1992). Used frequently in public service and training facilities, it is limited only by the extent of the agency's funding. In private practice it is more limited because each therapist can afford only a certain number of low-fee patients, and a sufficient range of fees is required to provide a balance that will insure a reasonable income.

The advantages of such a policy are that it is in the mainstream, appears fair, and gives patients and therapists opportunities to negotiate. The disadvantages are that it requires a detailed exploration of patient finances by therapists in order to set an accurate fee, and both groups may find this distasteful so that it is often carried out carelessly, in turn distorting the fee; it penalizes the wealthy; and it leaves therapists vulnerable to having their feelings, and performance, dependent on what patients are paying, so that higher paying patients are more valuable to therapists than low-fee patients. Therapists may want to hold on to high-fee patients longer than necessary and turn over low-fee patients quickly, or they may, out of guilt, take an excessive number of low-paying patients and continually resent it. Satisfactory sliding-scale operations will be conducted by therapists who are comfortable with obtaining accurate financial information from patients and are able to maintain an appropriate range of fees that satisfies their economic needs. These therapists have to be willing to provide the same quality of service to all and to be selective about their patient load based on fees paid.

Sliding scales really only slide to a point, particularly when they are moving downward. Some therapists adopt modified versions of this, in that they say they have flexibility, but they narrow the range to middle- and high-fee patients. Other therapists give a fee, usually quite high, which they tell patients is their usual fee, but they will take less, and usually do. These "sort of" adaptations to need reflect considerable ambivalence by therapists which needs reevaluation if their fee policies are truly going to be effective.

Fee variability includes the issue of raising or lowering fees in accord with the needs of therapists as well as patients. In a sliding scale, therapists would need to monitor their patients financial situations, with fees adjusted accordingly, and they would need to keep patients aware that their fees could increase as well as decrease. There is the possibility of patients hiding, or overlooking, financial improvement while highlighting any financial problems. Therapists can deal with this by having periodic financial reviews with their patients. However, some patients may resent this, and so some therapists may avoid it, but they then miss opportunities to justifiably increase their income from existing patients.

Although sliding-scale fees are popular, they are the most difficult to carry out with precision. Also, even though they appear to be patient focused, they require periodic inquiries about money from therapists, and that may cause patients to view therapists as overly concerned with money. Then, because a fee range is needed, therapists have to be selective on economic grounds or suffer, so this approach really requires giving money a lot of attention. Because this bothers a significant number of therapists, they tend to be lax in their use of the method, generally to their economic detriment.

FIXED FEES

The advantages of this approach are that it guarantees a set return based on the number of patients seen, and, because all patients pay the same fee, there is no economic reason to favor one patient over another. It is easier to provide quality service to all. Also, monetary negotiations are simplified and need to be reopened by the therapist only if he or she needs more money. At the same time, the therapist is frank about a personal need for a certain amount of money, thus indicating that an interest in money is acceptable for patients as well.

The disadvantages are that some patients may perceive the therapist as more interested in their money than in them. In addition, there is no room in this approach for low-fee patients, which could make many therapists uncomfortable. More of a problem is that patients who incur financial problems have no room to negotiate fee relief. The result is that most therapists who use this approach actually modify it, so there can be ambivalence here as well. They make some room for needy patients, but do not regularly accept them and prefer to refer them. They do provide flexibility for patients already being seen who run into financial difficulties. A common arrangement is fee suspension, either in part or completely, with the understanding that the rest is owed to the therapist to be paid when the patient can do so. Of course it is possible that will never happen, but therapists who have experimented with this arrangement report that they usually do get the full payment (Hofling & Rosenbaum, 1986). Another possibility is reducing the frequency of the patient's visits.

Fixed-fee arrangements work best for therapists who are comfortable with their need for money and are willing to be definitive with their patents. A certain amount of flexibility is also necessary, namely exceptions to the rule that make therapeutic sense to the therapist so that any decrease in income is compensated for by the reward of service. It does not work well with therapists who are guilty about their fees, or vulnerable to economic manipulation, but are trying the approach because of its potential consistency and the lesser need to continually evaluate patient finances. Their difficulties will appear if they want to raise fees, because the logic clearly involves therapist need, or if patients attempt to negotiate fees. The negotiating that does take place is really within the patient who has to decide whether or not this therapist is worth the fee charged. The therapist rests on stated personal competence without offering fee options and lets the patient decide. Of course, for this to work, it is necessary to keep fees in line with market conditions, so a moderate to relatively high fee will provide the greatest consistency.

MANAGED CARE

The types of fee policies just described may be mere remembrances for therapists by the year 2000 if health care trends follow the course they now seem to be on. A brief look at the history of payment for psychotherapy is useful to illustrate what is happening. In the early stages of the independent practice of psychotherapy, direct payments from patients to therapists was the norm. Existing insurance coverage was limited in terms of both amount (generally less than payment for other health services) and providers (usually only psychiatrists). This picture changed dramatically on both counts so that there was a large increase in the number of people who had insurance for psychotherapy provided by a number of disciplines. This had the effect of categorizing therapy as a definite health service that met the criteria of "medically necessary," and it created a dependency on payment sources other than patients themselves. Although the continuing rise in overall health costs was due to inpatient services, including mental health (Herron, 1992), psychotherapy was targeted for cost reduction. The reduction agent has become one or more forms of managed care.

Managed care takes the view that past practices were inefficient by being both longer than necessary and too costly per session. Thus insurance payments for mental health are managed to reduce these alleged inefficiencies. All managed care companies claim that they do not sacrifice quality for cost savings, but therapists have sharply disagreed (Shulman, 1988). Thus far the dissent has not had that much influence on policy because there is sufficient disagreement among therapists so that significant support has been provided to meet the cost-cutting desires of employers who actually fund insurance. The need for accountability is agreed upon by all, but the arbitrary solutions are not. However, at the moment the burden of proof appears to be on those who disagree with managed care, which, in turn is increasing its reach. The president's proposal for national health care that is now available reinforces that trend.

Some managed care plans are less restrictive than others, but the main thrust is to provide an incentive for patients to go to the least costly provider. This is usually accomplished by getting a certain number of providers to agree to see patients for a set fee, customarily lower than the providers' before-the-plan fees, to provide progress reports as designated by management, which is usually quite often, and to terminate patients according to management's impression that treatment is no longer needed, meaning that most psychotherapies are to be brief. Therapists in the plan have little discretion as to fees and treatment methods. Patients have a limited co-payment, which therapists collect directly, while the rest of the fee, namely most of it, has to be authorized by and collected from the managed care companies. This is a fixed-fee approach, but the fee is fixed to meet the companies' needs, not the therapists'.

The lure to patients is their minimal out-of-pocket expense, but disillusionment can set in if they want to continue in therapy beyond the "cure point" established by the company. They cannot unless they pay for it all themselves, and even then they will have to switch therapists, because the therapists in the plan may be contractually prohibited from continuing with them for a fee, regardless of who pays for it. This feature is designed to discourage therapists from turning short-term patients who have insurance coverage into long-term patients who directly pay the therapist. Also, patients do not have a real choice of therapists, an issue that seems particularly problematic given the significant relationship component of psychotherapy.

The lure to psychotherapists is that they will get a steady supply of patients at set fees, thus stabilizing their income. However, due to the lower fee schedule they will actually have to work more hours to maintain the same income they would have if the patients were seen in the traditional fee models. Also, in-plan providers have experienced disappointment with the number of patients they get, and the plans have discretion as to the providers they use. Providers who contest managed care's treatment coverage decisions, or those who continually use the maximum number of sessions available to patients, may find themselves discontinued as plan providers. Also, therapists who feel obligated to continue with patients whose benefits have been terminated may have to do this for no fee if they want to remain within the plan.

It is also possible to be an outside-the-plan provider for a patient in a managed care plan. The patient will then have a significantly larger co-payment, namely the difference between whatever the plan pays - usually a fixed fee for a maximum number of sessions, such as $30 each for 30 sessions per year - and the fee charged by the therapist. The therapist still has to do the paperwork, primarily to get approval for the coverage that is available, but all fees are collected from the patient who in turn collects whatever the insurance pays. Patients have freedom to choose any licensed psychotherapist, but it costs them more to do this; they can continue with that therapist after they have used all their benefits for the year, but again at a cost. Although therapists remaining outside the plans can indeed set fees and procedures, such as duration of therapy, the extensive presence of managed care puts economic pressure on all therapists, particularly in regard to the duration of therapy.

Even with procedural flaws removed, the philosophy of managed care supports a limited view of mental health that also appears to appeal to most funding policy makers. It is a "good-enough" approach operating at the level of necessity in contrast to other levels of mental health that can also be attained through psychotherapy, namely the levels of improvement (more than what is just necessary to function) and potentiality (striving for one's personal ideal). The basic position is that those who want more than the fundamental level will have to pay for it themselves. Therapists who view this policy as problematic to ultimately disastrous for the health of the society are going to have to work very hard to educate all involved to a broader view of mental health.

In the meantime, it appears as though a two-tier system is in process. In the first tier will be all the people in some type of managed plan, probably the majority of the population, and therapists who are part of these plans and receive fixed fees set by the plans. In the other tier will be patients, probably a minority, who, even if they use the plans to some degree, will seek providers of their choice and pay the difference. However, a significant number of these patients will be more cost-conscious than ever and expect therapists to respond accordingly. For example, if national health insurance were to provide psychotherapy coverage at a set fee for a stipulated number of sessions, which is likely if outpatient psychotherapy is included, it is possible that many people may see this as the standard rather than a minimum designed to do at least something for mental health. They will then expect psychotherapists to follow this standard, and, if they do not, therapists will have to explain their stance, knowing that only some of the potential patients will accept it.

It seems clear that the fee policy landscape will change, and is already doing so, taking more of the fee-setting control away from therapists and patients and putting it in the hands of care managers. Therapists are going to have to adapt, even if they are trying to alter the management approach. Some will adapt by conforming to managed care, and others will stay away from it as much as possible while still being competitive. Their pitch will be that better care requires a higher price, but they will be facing the probability of becoming price-competitive or they will have too limited a patient supply.

FEE POLICY AND PROCEDURES

A key feature in having an ongoing effective fee policy is its initial establishment. Thus whatever policy the therapist has decided upon, including participation in managed care, it is crucial to explain all the details to each patient and to make sure that they are understood. In managed care situations this may have to occur in the first session and, in any case, within the first few sessions with the strong possibility of the need for repetition.

The fee per session will be considered first, then the timing of payments. Cash flow is helped by getting paid at each session, but patients need a variety of possibilities based on their own manner of receiving funds. Thus most practices have a mixture of payment patterns: some once a week, some every other week, some monthly, and some floating but tied to agreed-upon times, as when insurance checks are received by the patients. Flexibility is necessary, but balanced with a payment plan for each patient that serves as a reference point for therapists and patients (Herron & Welt, 1992).

Sessions that are missed without any prior notice from the patient are usually charged for, and so are cancellations, although some therapists do not charge if notice is given sufficiently in advance, or they offer make-up sessions. Patients are usually urged to take their vacations when therapists do, but if that is not going to be the case, then arrangements can be made to make up the missed sessions. The basic idea is to have patients come to whatever number of sessions would be available to them during a specific course of therapy, even if the specific dates are not always the same day in a week, or consistently once a week. Most insurers will not pay for missed sessions, so whenever that is the case patients would need to be informed that they have total cost responsibility. Therapists in managed care plans usually will not get paid for missed sessions as they cannot charge patients directly for the total fee.

The important concept in these matters is to have a logical, consistent policy that all patients understand. The specifics will vary in each therapist's practice, because patients need to be charged according to the therapeutic and market realities of the practice. Ancillary services, such as phone calls and paperwork, are generally part of the package that comes with per-session charges. A case can be made for trying to charge for phone time if it tends to be essentially another session, although the issue certainly needs clarification with the patient. Charging patients or third-party payers for paperwork would probably be futile, because insurance carriers expect it and are moving toward electronic filing, which means increased overhead for providers in terms of equipment. In addition, some phone contact with reviewers from managed care companies is becoming routine. Thus overhead costs in terms of both service time and equipment are increasing with the potential for offsetting fee increases.

In all the money matters involved in practicing psychotherapy there are going to be indications of therapists' personal feelings and attitudes about money. These are a mixture of monetary realities and fiscal fantasies. Therapists who are struggling economically will be particularly sensitive to the loss or lack of income, and their fee policies are likely to reflect a certain desperation. In contrast, the more affluent therapists may show a certain annoyance and insensitivity in their approaches to monetary arrangements. A balanced, reasonable approach is advocated, but this will be possible only if therapists keep the personal factor in mind and periodically examine their fee policies to validate their appropriateness. The ideal is to effectively mesh clinical, fiscal, and ethical concerns in treating each patient. That ideal is translated from an abstract conception to specific therapist-patient transactions in which the therapist bears the responsibility for how money matters are handled.

CONCLUSIONS

The subject of money has been a sensitive and problematic area for therapists and continues to be, although there is an increasing openness about exploring it, in and out of psychotherapy. The contribution of therapists and patients to making money an avoided topic have been noted, along with various solutions. The fee is the monetary transaction in therapy that is a prime pathway for consideration of all money matters. Fee policies have been discussed in detail, with special consideration given to the changes that are effected by the growth of managed care. It is clear that the field is in a transition phase in regard to the economic return that can be expected from the practice of psychotherapy as well as the type of therapy that is going to represent mainstream practice. The most likely possibility is greater control of funding by agents other than patients and therapists, with brief therapy the favored mode of treatment. Blueprints for the future, besides that just mentioned, have been described elsewhere (Herron, Eisenstadt, et al., 1994; Herron, Javier, et al., 1994). At the moment, economic return is less of an incentive for independent practice than it was, and that trend is likely to continue with some form of fee capitation a strong possibility in any national health plan. Because quality of care can also be seriously affected, it is of utmost importance that all psychotherapists get involved in the development of funding policies. The inescapable fact is, money matters.

William G. Herron, PhD, is Professor, Psychology Department, St. John's University, Jamaica, New York, and in private practice in Woodcliff Lake, New Jersey. He is Senior Supervisor and Training Analyst, Contemporary Center for Advanced Psychoanalytic Studies, Livingston, New Jersey, Fellow of the American Psychological Association, and Diplomate in Clinical Psychology of the American Board of Professional Psychology. An Editorial Consultant for the journal, *Psychotherapy,* he is coauthor of *Issues in Psychotherapy, Narcissism and the Psychotherapist,* and *Money Matters: The Fee in Psychotherapy and Psychoanalysis.* Dr. Herron may be contacted at 5 Pascack Road, Woodcliff Lake, NJ 07675.

RESOURCES

Austad, G. S., & Berman, W. (Eds.). (1991). *Psychotherapy in Managed Health Care: The Optimal Use of Time and Resources.* Washington, DC: American Psychological Association Press.

Bak, J. S., Weiner, R. H., & Jackson, L. J. (1992). Managed mental health care: Should independent practitioners capitulate or mobilize? *The Independent Practitioner, 12*(1), (2), (4), 31-35, 75-80, 159-164.

Bishop, D. R., & Eppolito, J. M. (1992). The clinical management of client dynamics and fees for psychotherapy: Implications for research and practice. *Psychotherapy, 29,* 545-553.

Freud, S. (1913). On beginning the treatment. In J. Strachey (Ed.), *The Standard Edition of the Complete Psychological Works of Sigmund Freud* (Vol. 12, pp. 123-144). London: Hogarth.

Herron, W. G. (1992). Managed mental health care redux. *Professional Psychology: Research and Practice, 23,* 163-164.

Herron, W. G., Eisenstadt, E. N., Javier, R. A., Primavera, L. H., & Schultz, C. L. (1994). Session effects, comparability, and managed care in the psychotherapies. *Psychotherapy, 31,* 279-285.

Herron, W. G., Javier, R. A., Primavera, L. H., & Schultz, C. L. (1994). The cost of psychotherapy. *Professional Psychology: Research and Practice, 25,* 106-110.

Herron, W. G., & Sitkowski, S. (1986). Effect of fees on psychotherapy: What is the evidence. *Professional Psychology: Research and Practice, 17,* 347-351.

Herron, W. G., & Welt, S. R. (1992). *Money Matters: The Fee in Psychotherapy and Psychoanalysis.* New York: Guilford.

Hofling, C. K., & Rosenbaum, M. (1986). The extension of credit to patients in psychoanalysis and psychotherapy. In D. W. Krueger (Ed.), *The Last Taboo: Money as Symbol and Reality in Psychotherapy and Psychoanalysis* (pp. 202-217). New York: Brunner/Mazel.

Klebanow, S., & Lowenkopf, E. L. (Eds.). (1991). *Money and Mind.* New York: Plenum.

Krueger, D. W. (Ed.). (1986). *The Last Taboo: Money as Symbol and Reality in Psychotherapy and Psychoanalysis.* New York: Brunner/Mazel.

Lasky, E. (1984). Psychoanalysts' and psychotherapists' conflicts about setting fees. *Psychoanalytic Psychology, 1,* 289-300.

Margenau, E. (Ed.). (1990). *The Encyclopedic Handbook of Private Practice.* New York: Gardiner.

Psychotherapy Finances. (1992). Survey report. *Psychotherapy Finances, 17*(12), 1-8.

Shulman, M. E. (1988). Cost containment in clinical psychology: Critique of Biodyne and the HMOs. *Professional Psychology: Research and Practice, 19,* 289-307.

Welt, S. R., & Herron, W. G. (1990). *Narcissism and the Psychotherapist.* New York: Guilford.

WORKPLACE HARASSMENT: WHAT MENTAL HEALTH PRACTITIONERS NEED TO KNOW

Lilli Friedland and David Friedland

Sexual harassment has received a lot of attention over the past few years. This is not because there is anything new about the presence of sexual harassment in the workplace. In fact, this harassment has been occurring for many years, as have other forms of unfair discrimination. Though sexual harassment has been illegal since adoption of the Civil Rights Act of 1964, it is only recently that meaningful remedies have been made available to victims of harassment. Availability of remedies and the visibility provided by highly publicized charges of sexual harassment have stimulated a major surge in litigation. Sexual harassment has become a popular topic in both print and electronic media. Employers are developing policies concerning workplace harassment and investing in training programs in attempts to provide a harassment-free work environment, as required by law.

The Equal Employment Opportunity Commission (EEOC) published guidelines in 1980 (Equal Employment Opportunity Commission, 1980) defining sexual harassment. However, though sexual harassment was recognized as a violation of the Civil Rights Act, the sanctions available under the Civil Rights Act did not encourage victims of harassment to file complaints. There was no provision for assessment of compensatory or punitive damages, and the available remedies carried no assurance that the victim's situation would be improved as a result of lodging a complaint. As a result, relatively few complaints were filed.

With the passage of the Civil Rights Act of 1991, substantial compensatory and punitive damages became available for sexual harassment victims, putting teeth in the law and providing incentive for attorneys to represent alleged victims of harassment. This fact, coupled with the publicity resulting from the sexual harassment allegations accompanying the Clarence Thomas confirmation hearings, encouraged many individuals to seek relief from sexual harassment. Sexual harassment has become one of the most common employment discrimination issues.

A BROADER VIEW OF WORKPLACE HARASSMENT

Since the passage of the Civil Rights Act of 1964, there has been a focus on reducing illegal discrimination in the workplace. The Civil Rights Act made it illegal to discriminate on the basis of race, gender, national origin, or religion in compensation, terms, conditions, or privileges of employment. Since passage of the Americans With Disabilities Act, people with disabilities have been added to the protected groups covered by the Civil Rights Act.

Harassment on the basis of any of these protected categories is illegal if it creates a hostile work environment that hampers the ability of individuals to carry out their work or if it results in different work standards for people on the basis of the protected category. Though harassment on the basis of race, national origin, religion, and disability are also illegal, harassment on the basis of gender has resulted in far more complaints and lawsuits than have the other categories. In addition, because of its nature, sexual harassment is sufficiently different from other types of discriminatory harassment to deserve its own definition.

To clarify the law on workplace harassment, the EEOC published *Proposed Guidelines on Harassment Based on Race, Color, Religion, Gender, National Origin, Age, and Disability* (EEOC, 1993). These proposed guidelines make it clear that any form of harassment on the basis of these categories that is severe enough to alter an individual's working conditions or terms of employment is a form of employment discrimination.

DEFINITIONS

SEXUAL HARASSMENT

Section 703(a)(1) of the Civil Rights Act states, in part, that it is unlawful for an employer to discriminate against any individual with respect to compensation, terms, conditions, or privileges of employment, because of that individual's race, color, religion, sex, or national origin. In its Sex Discrimination Guidelines, EEOC interpreted Title VII to mean that unlawful sexual harassment exists when unwelcome sexual advances, requests for sexual favors, and other verbal or physical conduct of a sexual nature alter the terms or conditions of employment. There is considerable reason to believe that sexual harassment is related to power motives (Cleveland & Kerst, 1993). Cleveland and Kerst examine how power is related to sexual harassment and explore the concept of power as contributor to sexual harassment. They suggest ways in which research can clarify the extent to which power can explain sexual harassment.

Two main types of sexual harassment are recognized: quid pro quo harassment, and hostile work environment harassment.

Quid Pro Quo. This type of harassment involves coercion, or making submission to demands or acquiescence to sexual advances a term or condition of employment. Quid pro quo harassment exists when submission to demands or acquiescence to sexual advances is used as a basis for an employment decision, thus making acquiescence to these demands a term or condition of employment.

In some cases, a claim of sexual harassment may be made if individuals other than the complaining party receive benefits from granting or acquiescing to sexual advances or demands. In some instances, this practice creates a reasonable presumption that such acquiescence is required for advancement, or other benefits of employment, even if the person who is complaining was not asked to grant sexual favors.

Hostile Work Environment. This type of sexual harassment is often more subtle, and probably more common, than quid pro quo harassment. It involves the creation of a work environment that is offensive, intimidating, or hostile to individuals on the basis of gender. The concept here is that the environment created interferes with the ability of the complaining party to work effectively, therefore altering the conditions of employment on the basis of gender. This type of harassment has been alleged in many work environments which have been traditionally male, and in which the work environment has acquired characteristics that are offensive to many women. One example is the posting of calendars with pictures of nude women, or prevalence of jokes or language that is offensive to most women, which tends to create a work environment that most women would consider to be hostile. This type of work environment may create an additional burden of stress and anxiety for women, as opposed to men.

It very often occurs in some jobs that have been traditionally male that the men resent the introduction of women into the work force. This may result in hostility that becomes expressed as harassment. Fire departments, police departments, mining companies, construction companies, and other work environments where the work force has traditionally been predominantly male have provided many examples of this type of harassment.

CHARACTERISTICS OF SEXUAL HARASSMENT

Severe or Pervasive. In addition to being unwelcome, the harassment must be severe or pervasive. This position was reinforced by the U.S. Supreme Court in the cases of *Meritor Savings Bank v. Vinson* (1986) and *Harris v. Forklift Systems* (1993). The court ruled that sexual harassment violates Title VII of the Civil Rights Act because it alters the terms, conditions, or privileges of employment based on an employee's sex. It is not necessary to prove that the victim suffered economic harm.

Under the Supreme Court standards, the harassment must be sufficiently severe or pervasive to alter the conditions of the victim's employment and create an abusive work environment. Since the *Meritor* decision, lower courts have been busy refining the concept of sexual harassment.

The concept of sexual harassment is gender neutral. This concept of gender neutrality can lead to some odd results, however. The Michigan Court of Appeals recently dismissed a case in which a cartoon depicting a female employee engaged in a sexual act with a male employee was posted in an office. The court reasoned that, because the cartoon was equally offensive to the woman and the man involved, it was gender neutral and therefore was not sexual harassment.

Some Confusion Remains. Many had hoped that the U.S. Supreme Court would clarify the definition of sexual harassment in its decision in *Harris v. Forklift Systems* (1993). As is often the case, some clarity was achieved, but with a considerable amount of vagueness. It is still difficult to define precisely what constitutes legally prohibited sexual harassment. The court has said that for workplace conduct to create an "abusive work environment" it need not result in psychological harm, but it needs to be so severe or pervasive that a reasonable person would perceive the work environment as hostile or abusive. It is also necessary for the victim to perceive the environment as hostile or abusive. Note the use of the word "or" rather than "and." Conduct that is severe, but not pervasive, may constitute harassment if it is severe enough, and conduct that may not be as severe may still constitute harassment if it is pervasive enough. The *Harris* decision specifically rejects the idea that the conduct must be severe enough to seriously affect the victim's psychological well-being. The key determining factor is whether the conduct is sufficient to alter the terms or conditions of employment on the basis of some prohibited factor. If the victim perceives the environment as being hostile or abusive, and other reasonable people would also perceive it as hostile, then the conduct causing this condition is harassment, even if there is no psychological injury. This may change the role of the practitioner as expert in harassment cases. Previously, the question of psychological harm was central to proving that harassment occurred. Since *Harris*, proof of psychological harm is not necessary, but it still may be important in determining the amount of damages to be assessed against the employer or the perpetrator.

HARASSMENT THAT IS NOT SEXUAL IN NATURE

It is clear that the Civil Rights Act prohibits harassment in the workplace on the basis of other factors in addition to gender. In fact, there is an increase in lawsuits involving harassment on the basis of race, religion, and other categories. In a recent case (*Rogers v. Western-Southern Life Insurance Company*, 1993), an African-American insurance agent was awarded $100,000 in back pay because he resigned his job after enduring a racially hostile work environment in the insurance company where he worked.

The *Proposed Guidelines on Harassment Based on Race, Color, Religion, Gender, National Origin, Age, and Disability* (EEOC, 1993) define harassment as follows:

> Harassment is verbal or physical conduct that denigrates or shows hostility or aversion toward an individual because of his/her race, color, religion, national origin, age, or disability, or that of his/her relatives, friends, or associates, and that:
>
> (i) Has the purpose or effect of creating an intimidating, hostile, or offensive working environment;
> (ii) Has the purpose or effect of unreasonably interfering with an individual's work performance; or
> (iii) Otherwise adversely affects an individual's employment opportunities.

According to the proposed guidelines, harassing conduct includes epithets, slurs, negative stereotyping, or threatening, intimidating, or hostile acts that relate to race, color, religion, gender, national origin, age, or disability. Harassing conduct also includes posting of written or graphic material that denigrates or shows hostility or aversion toward an individual or group on the basis of any of these categories. Age is included, even though age is not a category covered by the Civil Rights Act, because EEOC is charged with enforcement under the Age Discrimination in Employment Act.

As of this writing, the *Guidelines on Harassment* had not yet been adopted in final form. There is controversy over the wording of the guidelines to insure that they do not step beyond the law as defined by the U.S. Supreme Court in the *Harris* case. There is also concern that by regulating behavior on the job, the EEOC may violate basic free speech rights.

Ultimately, the *Guidelines* will be published. It is clear, however, that harassment in the workplace on any basis covered by the Civil Rights Act will be prohibited. It is clear from the *Harris* decision that that is what the U.S. Supreme Court intends when it states, "When the workplace is permeated with 'discriminatory intimidation, ridicule, and insult,' . . . 'that is sufficiently severe or pervasive to alter the conditions of the victim's employment and create an abusive working environment,'. . . Title VII (of the Civil Rights Act of 1964) is violated."

SOME LEGAL ISSUES OF IMPORTANCE TO PRACTITIONERS

RETROACTIVITY OF THE 1991 AMENDMENTS TO THE CIVIL RIGHTS ACT

Until recently there was considerable difference of opinion among the federal courts concerning whether the Civil Rights Act of 1991 should apply retroactively in pending legal cases where the events complained about occurred prior to enactment of the Act in November of 1991. The U.S. Supreme Court recently resolved this issue in its decision in the case of *Landgraf v. USI Film Products* (1994). The court ruled that the Act should not apply retroactively, but should apply only to events that took place subsequent to November of 1991, the date the Act was signed into law.

PSYCHOLOGICAL HARM

Of major importance to practitioners is the issue of whether the victim must be able to show that he or she suffered psychological harm as a result of the harassment. Although, as indicated, the court made it clear that it is not necessary to prove that the victim suffered psychological harm, such a showing is likely to be important in determining the amount of the damages to be paid to the victim.

Practitioners are likely to play a major role in assessing whether psychological harm resulted from the harassment. Practitioners will be asked to perform psychological assessments of alleged victims of harassment and will be called upon to serve as experts in litigation.

DAMAGES

One of the most important changes to result from passage of the Civil Rights Act of 1991 is the introduction of compensatory and punitive damages to be paid to victims of workplace harassment. Even though there is a cap on the maximum amount payable in damages, the maximum amount payable per plaintiff is substantial. The maximum amount available under the amendment is $300,000 per plaintiff for the largest employers. Although this amount is substantial, it is especially large in the case of class action lawsuits, in which there may be many plaintiffs.

CLASS ACTIONS INVOLVING WORKPLACE HARASSMENT

In class action cases, damage awards under federal law can be much higher than in individual cases. In May of this year the first decision in a class action lawsuit alleging sexual harassment was issued against a mining company in Minnesota (*Jenson v. Eveleth Taconite Company*, 1994). Although damages in this case have not yet been assessed, they could be as high as $30 million, because there are 100 named plaintiffs.

PERVASIVENESS OF THE PROBLEM

Surveys have shown sexual harassment to be a widespread problem. Sixty percent of the 900 female attorneys participating in a recent federal government study said they had experienced sexual harassment during the previous 5 years. Most of the harassment was attributed to other attorneys and clients. In a study of sexual harassment in medical training, Komaromy et al. (1993) found that 24 of 33 female and 11 of 49 male medical residents reported that they had been sexually harassed at least once during their training. The women were more likely than the men to have been physically harassed, and their harassers were of higher professional status. Nineteen of the women and five of the men said that the experience created a hostile environment or interfered with their work performance, but only two of the women, and none of the men, reported the experiences to an authority.

Although most victims of sexual harassment are female, there are also male victims. A survey conducted by Northwestern University found that nearly one-fifth of men surveyed in the Chicago area said they had been sexually harassed in the workplace at some time during their careers.

ISSUES IN DEFINING HARASSMENT

The prevalence of sexual harassment, coupled with the differences in perception of sexual harassment between men and women (Saal, Johnson, & Weber, 1989; Stockdale, 1993; C. Struckman-Johnson & D. Struckman-Johnson, 1993), signals an urgent and widespread need for training. Complaints of harassment are sharply increasing. Evidence suggests that many men have little understanding of the point of view of women concerning this problem. The EEOC announced last year that they were conducting a study to identify industries where sexual harassment is most prevalent in order to target those industries for compliance activity. The EEOC also plans to develop technical assistance for employers to aid them in resolving the problem.

One difficulty with the concept of sexual harassment is that it is subjective. The courts are struggling with the task of defining conditions under which victims may be compensated and perpetrators punished. In the process of defining sexual harassment, a number of key issues are yet to be resolved.

REASONABLE WOMAN VERSUS REASONABLE PERSON

Many have argued that sexual harassment involving female victims requires that the conduct at issue be viewed from the perspective of the "reasonable woman" (*Ellison v. Brady*, 1991). There is an inherent assumption in the reasonable woman standard that what is acceptable for most reasonable men may be unacceptable to the reasonable woman. Events that would not offend or damage a reasonable man may offend or damage a reasonable woman. There was a major split in the federal courts of appeal on this issue that was finally resolved by the U.S. Supreme Court in the *Harris* case. In its decision in this case, the court adopted the concept of a reasonable person.

The *Harris* decision appears to have cleared up the vagueness of the concept of the "reasonable woman." However, the EEOC, in its proposed guidelines on workplace harassment, takes the position that the term "reasonable person" incorporates the perspective of the victim, which some see as an attempt to return to a "reasonable woman" or "reasonable victim" standard in sexual harassment cases.

Because of the differences in perceptions between alleged perpetrators and alleged victims, the problem of harassment becomes complicated. Under the "reasonable victim" standard, illegal harassment need not be obvious to the alleged perpetrator for the victim to successfully claim harassment has occurred. This makes training especially important for employers. Training to sensitize employees to the perceptions of others should reduce the incidence of workplace harassment. In addition, by providing such training, the employer gains some protection from being held liable for actions of the employee.

As the courts gain experience with the concept of the reasonable person, employers and courts will gradually come to understand their obligations in the area of harassment. For example, in *Burns v. McGregor Electronic Industries, Inc.* (1992), a federal trial judge stuck by his original decision in a case in which the Eighth Circuit Court of Appeal had ordered him to reconsider his opinion. He concluded that the sexual harassment and unwelcome sexual advances were not so unpleasant as to force the alleged victim to resign. The judge based his opinion on the plaintiff's personal history, her appearance on the stand, her manner of dress, her "pierced, bejeweled nipples," her tattoo, and the fact that she had posed nude for two motorcycle magazines. The Circuit Court rejected the judge's reasoning in this case and reversed his decision, indicating that the sexual advances of her boss were unwelcome because they came from him, and that was sufficient to constitute sexual harassment. The victim's personal history did not preclude her from finding her boss's behavior offensive.

In another case (*Trotta v. Mobil Oil Corp.*, 1992), the court found that the behaviors complained of were not serious enough to be considered sexual harassment by a reasonable woman.

In *Fisher v. Tischler*, a case brought under California state law, the court concluded a woman who claimed sexual harassment by a physician was not a reasonable woman, and that she saw sexual innuendo in innocent affection among other staff. Her claim of sexual harassment was weakened by the fact that no other female staff took her side and, in fact, other women testified in defense of the doctor who was charged with harassment.

PSYCHOLOGICAL ISSUES

A large volume of research has examined the differences between men and women in their perceptions of many phenomena. The volume of psychological research regarding sexual harassment is increasing rapidly. It has been well established that women and men differ substantially in their perceptions of whether particular observed behaviors constitute sexual harassment. There are also differences in the degree to which men and women perceive the behavior of women, or their manner of dress, to be contributing factors in determining whether male behavior constitutes sexual harassment in particular situations. There are also differences between women in their tendency to perceive particular situations as sexual harassment as a result of their own experience.

MISPERCEPTION OF FRIENDLY CUES

Men tend to misperceive friendly cues from women in ways that influence their labeling of behavior as harassing. For example, in observing videotaped scenes of women interacting with men, male observers tend to perceive the woman's behavior as sexier than do female observers (Stockdale, 1993). This tendency suggests that men will often fail to perceive situations as sexually harassing when women observing the same situation will tend to perceive sexual harassment to have occurred.

Workman and Johnson (1991) found that when a model wore heavy or moderate cosmetics, males tended to rate her as more likely to be sexually harassed than if she did not wear cosmetics. Women rated the likelihood of sexual harassment lower than did males regardless of the cosmetics worn by the model.

Some recent research suggests that, although men may perceive women's friendly behavior as more sexy than do women, this tendency may be unrelated to their perceptions of whether behaviors are sexually harassing. In other words, sexual harassment, like rape, may be motivated by factors other than sex or sexual attraction. Although some instances of sexual harassment may be simply the result of innocent misreading of friendly cues, this research suggests that even though a man may initially misread friendly cues as indicating sexual interest, a reasonable man should be able to discern when his response to this perceived interest is not welcomed by the woman and cease making advances. Similarly, when a man perceives cues that indicate that off-color jokes or other types of sexually related office behavior are offensive to women, a reasonable man may cease the behavior. In such an instance, even though the friendly cues from the woman are initially misread, no sexual harassment will take place. Sexual harassment is most likely to occur when the man fails to perceive, or ignores, cues that his sexually related behavior is unwelcome or offensive.

Clearly, some instances of sexual harassment reflect hostile intent. This has been most clear in incidents that have occurred in nontraditional jobs, where hazing or other activities have occurred with the intent to create a hostile environment due to resentment on the part of some men toward the presence of women in particular types of jobs. In other instances, the harassment is clearly related to sexual interest. Some instances of harassment that appear on the surface to be motivated by sexual interest may turn out on closer examination to be influenced by power motives. The motives for sexual harassment are of key importance for the development of harassment policies and in developing training programs regarding sexual harassment. These motives will certainly be of interest in litigation and are likely to influence the award of damages.

USE OF STUDENTS VERSUS EMPLOYEES IN RESEARCH ON HARASSMENT

In evaluating research on sexual harassment, it is appropriate to exercise some caution. Many of the studies have been conducted in an academic context, using students and faculty as subjects. A number of studies that have compared the reactions of students to those of actual employees have found that male and female employees differ less in their perceptions of harassment than do male and female college students (Baker, Terpstra, & Cutler, 1990). It may be that the students in these studies are dealing with the question of sexual harassment in the workplace from a hypothetical standpoint. Studies using actual employees are more likely to reflect actual workplace conditions than are studies using college students.

SCALE DEVELOPMENT

There have been a number of efforts to develop scales to assess tendencies for individuals to sexually harass others (Bartling & Eisenman, 1993; Pryor, 1987). These efforts are still young, but there is building evidence that questionnaires and inventories will be developed that will be useful in measuring propensity to engage in sexual harassment.

ROLES FOR THE PRACTITIONER

TESTING AND ASSESSMENT

The *Harris* decision has removed the requirement to prove psychological harm in order to prove sexual harassment. It is clear, however, in the legal language of the decision, that understanding the implications of the "reasonable victim" or "reasonable person," "idiosyncratic" reaction, or "hostile environment" requires an understanding of the psychological environment of the work situation as well as the individual's unique psychological reaction, both preexisting and current, to the sexually harassing incidents. In order to assess these individual and environmental dimensions, the psychological expert is essential. Typically, punitive damages are substantially higher with demonstrated psychological consequences. According to Hadsell (1992), the most important factor in maximizing the damages the plaintiff can collect would be the evidence that demonstrates the anquish and anger that they suffered as a result of the harassment.

Emotional effects on the individual can best be ascertained from both the clinical interview and psychological testing by the practitioner. The information garnered from clinical interviews and testing is necessary to formulate an accurate assessment. It is important to remember that licensed clinicians are the only mental health professionals trained in development and research of tests. The "scope of practice" in many states recognizes only the testimony of licensed practitioners in the areas of giving and interpreting psychological tests. Other mental health professionals may receive the necessary and appropriate courses in the statistics and psychological test construction and interpretation that may permit them to ethically administer and interpret the tests. It is recommended that the psychological testing and interviewing be conducted on at least two occasions so that the practitioner can evaluate the preliminary information from the first interview and tests and use the results to follow up with additional testing and interview questions.

THERAPY AND COUNSELING CONSIDERATIONS

Victims of harassment progress through stages of feelings as a result of the stress caused by the harassment. According to Salisbury et al. (1986), these stages include confusion/self-blame, fear/anxiety, depression/anger, and disillusionment. History of prior victimization may affect the vulnerability and perception of stress the victim experiences. As a consequence of this past history as well as the individual's experienced stress, it is recommended that the therapist conduct the clinical interview with open-ended questions that cannot be construed as leading the client or patient in any way. Leading questions suggest a particular answer, and it is desirable to obtain unbiased, reliable, and relatively undistorted information from the client. Many times, clients, when talking about workplace harassment, feel overwhelmed in describing their feelings and in understanding the significance of their experiences.

It is important to elicit the client's responses, associations, and understandings of the situation to achieve an understanding of the client's reality. This may be done with gentle probing designed to detect the client's reactions without challenging the client's interpretations. It is helpful to use "why" questions or "what do you think. . . ?" questions to elicit the client's perception. It is also helpful to use the client's vocabulary to give a sense of empathy. Caution should be exercised in this regard because clients frequently misconstrue this understanding to be agreement with their perception. This particularly complicates the role of the clinician if the case goes to trial and the client hears the responses to questions asked by counsel which may be construed as "not being on my side." Care needs to be exercised also in summarizing what the client states because it is sometimes perceived as "putting words into my mouth." It is also wise to steer away from legal phrases such as "sexual harassment," "retaliation," "hostile environment," and so forth. It is recommended that the clinician ask clients to state in their own words their perceptions, feelings, behaviors, and beliefs regarding all the incidents. It is easier to develop understanding of clients' reality if they are more specific in the details they give. It is not uncommon for a client to come in and say "I am a victim of sexual harassment," which is a legal definition and does not give the therapist any insight into the feelings or experiences of that individual.

Therapeutic intervention for victims of sexual abuse includes individual, group, and family therapies. Salisbury et al. (1986) suggest that a group therapy setting is more effective than individual treatment for coping with the specific effects of sexual harassment because clients can use the group to help in understanding their experience, sort through legal and employment decisions, and learn new coping skills. The authors differentiate sexual harassment victims from victims of crimes in that harassment primarily affects economic and career well-being. There are also secondary effects on private relationships and physical well-being. Clinicians note that conjugal complications frequently arise. Many victims are hesitant to bring up these factors in therapy because of a sense of privacy or shame, or because their lawyers recommended that they not discuss these issues. The clinician may find that receiving input from the marital partner or "significant other" about the effects on the emotional and sexual aspects of the relationship may be helpful. The role of the therapist may appear to be compromised or complicated by involvement in other aspects of the case. It is advisable for the clinician to consider the therapeutic complications that may arise from the therapist's involvement in court proceedings. Many clinicians have commented about their difficulties shifting from the role of the treating therapist to that of the forensic professional testifying regarding the clinical issues in court. This is awkward for some therapists and needs to be considered prior to accepting this kind of case.

Gosselin (1984) and Crull (1982) also point out that sexual harassment is a form of stress inflicted on a person while at work. The way in which an individual responds to the stress is affected by personality traits, ability to resist the stressor, and conditions present in the work environment. The victim often experiences feelings of vulnerability and has a need to reconstruct aspects of self-concept. Clinicians often note that the feelings of victimization, helplessness, fear, and rage over time can erode even positive self-images and self-respect. The appropriate role of the clinician is to facilitate the growth of support networks and internal coping strategies, and to review work-related problems to facilitate the development of alternative beliefs and behavioral skills. Frequently the victim of sexual harassment cases feels very alone or misunderstood. Keeping this in mind, the clinician needs to gently develop the therapeutic relationship with a focus on trust issues and disclosure of feelings. It is important for the therapist to encourage discussion of feelings and promote the victim's ability to request assistance from whatever support group the individual has. If there is none, group therapy, in addition to individual, might be advisable even sooner than usual. It is important to remind the victims of sexual harassment that even good friends and caring family members may not have the patience to hear the feelings and details of these incidents and stresses repeated many times. It is common for friends and family to feel or respond, "You've already said that, now you have to get on with your life" well before the victim is ready. It is for this reason as well as the feeling of relief that others have shared similar experiences that group therapy is recommended often.

Woody and Perry (1993) discuss the family therapy implications of sexual harassment. The stress of harassment has negative impact on job productivity and motivation, but the emotional impact also spills over into the family. There are emotional and physical reactions to the stress of the harassment that result in effects on self-perception, interpersonal relatedness, and sexuality. The fallout of one family member affected by sexual harassment can disrupt or alter the entire family system. The therapist may become involved in working with other family members. Even if the therapist can meet with the family only a time or two, discussing the long-term recovery that is typical plus the normalcy of the victim's response can promote more acceptance and support within the family system. The clinician can point out frequently to family members that victims need to repeat their feelings and talk about their stresses many times for many months. It is helpful to the family when the therapist can explain that this is part of the process to work through the feelings of victimization. They can point out that the only and best thing the family can do is to respond to the victim's needs with unconditional listening and support during these times. The therapist reduces the stress and promotes greater understanding in the family when he or she discusses some of the common symptoms of the victim - such as lowered sex drive, more anxiousness, mood swings, sleep disturbances, fear and paranoid-type responses, feeling disoriented, and so on.

It is important to remember that many individuals are experiencing stress and anxieties due to numerous economic and psychological realities that are byproducts of the sexual harassment. These symptoms need to be differentiated from the direct effects of the sexual harassment. Some of the typical symptoms victims experience are stress reactions to the trial, the pressures of multiple doctor appointments, financial difficulties if victims are not working or are on stress leave, or not being able to understand the lack of understanding or support from family or colleagues. These normal stress responses must be differentiated from reactions to alleged sexual harassment. The practitioner typically evaluates victims' comments and assesses their responses. The psychological interview attempts to obtain a reliable history, observe the appropriateness of the behavior, and ascertain the client's social and professional functioning. Psychological tests are typically used to ascertain characteristic style with confronting stress, susceptibility to stress as a trait versus a state, tendency toward malingering, and underlying deeper psychological characteristics.

Psychological tests assist in the confidence of the diagnosis and evaluation. A basic battery usually includes a personality assessment using the MMPI (Minnesota Multiphasic Personality Inventory), the Beck Depression Scale (designed to be used on two separate occasions to ascertain change in time), a sentence completion test such as the Rotter, a symptom checklist such as the SCL-90, and the Millon. If necessary, a projective test, such as the TAT (Thematic Apperception Test), may be used to ascertain deep-seated personality characteristics, or the Rorschach inkblot test used to test clients' ability to perceive reality. Examples of typical tests given when particular diagnoses are suspected follow:

Depression	**Stress**	**Anxiety**
MMPI	MMPI	MMPI
Millon	Millon	Millon
Beck (administered twice)	Beck Depression	Beck Depression
Sentence completion	Sentence completion	Sentence completion
Symptom checklist	Symptom checklist	Symptom checklist
Wechsler Intelligence Test	Wechsler Intelligence Test	Projective tests such as the TAT
Projective tests such as the TAT	Projective tests such as the TAT	Taylor Manifest Anxiety Scale

When psychological damage was required to substantiate sexual harassment cases, it had been common to employ the diagnosis of Post-Traumatic Stress Disorder (PTSD) in the past, when the *DSM-III-R* (American Psychiatric Association, 1987) was used. With the publication of the *Diagnostic and Statistical Manual of Mental Disorders - 4th edition* (DSM-IV; American Psychiatric Association, 1994), the diagnosis of PTSD changed to require that the client or patient experience, witness, or be confused by an event or events that involves actual or threatened death or serious injury or a threat to the physical integrity of the self or others, and so forth. This essential requirement does not apply in most workplace or sexual harassment cases. Therefore it is likely that the following diagnosis will be used in the future to justify psychological damage: Generalized Anxiety Disorder, 300.02. This diagnosis is characterized by excessive anxiety and worry occurring for the majority of 6 months about the work performance, the person finds it difficult to control the worry, and the anxiety and worry are associated with three or more of the following six symptoms: restlessness, easily fatigued, difficulty concentrating or mind going blank, irritability, muscle tension, and sleep disturbance. Social Phobia, 300.23, is a possible diagnosis for workplace harassment. Social Phobia is characterized by marked and persistent fear of social or performance situations in which embarrassment may occur. This response may take the form of situationally bound or situationally predisposed panic attacks. Adults may recognize that their fear is excessive or unreasonable. Usually the situation is avoided, although sometimes endured with dread. This diagnosis is appropriate only if the avoidance, fear, or anxious anticipation of encountering the social or performance situation interferes significantly with the person's daily routine or occupational functioning, or if the individual is markedly distressed about having the phobia. Symptoms must persist at least 6 months. Panic Disorder Without Agoraphobia, 300.01, and Panic Disorder With Agoraphobia, 300.21, are other possible diagnoses. Both of these diagnoses are characterized by recurrent, unexpected panic attacks, and at least one of the attacks has been followed by one or more of the following for at least 1 month: persistent concern about having additional attacks, worry about the implications of the attack or its consequences, and a significant change in behavior related to the attacks. Obsessive-Compulsive Disorder (OCD), 300.3, requires there to be recurrent intrusive thoughts, but these are experienced as inappropriate and not related to the experienced traumatic event. The obsessive thoughts of the OCD are not merely excessive worries about everyday real-life problems, but often take the form of urges, impulses, and images as well as thoughts. Obsessive-Compulsive Disorder needs to be differentiated from Generalized Anxiety Disorder, anxiety reactions, or trauma stress reaction. The trauma stress reaction may exhibit similar symptoms which may or may not reach the level of threshold for PTSD. Some of the characteristics of this reaction, as described in *Post-Traumatic Therapy and Victims of Violence* (Ochberg, 1988), are as follows:

1. Shame: deep embarrassment often characterized by deep humiliation.
2. Self-blame: exaggerated feelings of responsibility for the trauma despite obvious evidence of innocence.
3. Subjugation: feeling belittled, dehumanized, lowered in dominance, powerless as a result of the trauma.
4. Morbid hatred: obsessions of vengeance and preoccupation with hurting or humiliating the perpetrator.
5. Paradoxical gratitude: positive feelings toward the perpetrator ranging from compassion to romantic love.
6. Defilement: feeling dirty, disgusted, tainted, and in extreme cases as rotten and evil.
7. Sexual inhibition: loss of libido, reduced capacity for intimacy.
8. Resignation: a state of broken will or despair, often associated with repetitive victimization or prolonged exploitation.
9. Second injury or second wound: re-victimization through participation in the criminal justice, health, and other systems.
10. Socioeconomic status downward drift: reduction of opportunity or lifestyle and increased risk of victimization due to psychological, social or vocational impairment.

When a client claims psychological damage, it is necessary to go into the mental health history of the individual. The possibilities of both malingering and vulnerabilities due to previous mental health problems such as childhood sexual abuse need to be explored by the therapist. Assessment of preexisting conditions or premorbid personality is important to determine other factors which may explain the client's perceptions. Some clinicians have noted that earlier sexual abuse, especially that which has not been "processed" by discussing and releasing the feelings with a clinician, family, or friend, may make the client more overly sensitive in his or her response to perceived workplace harassment. Part of the mandate is to assess how the client may be responding idiosyncratically, or differently than the reasonable person or woman would have responded under these circumstances. It is conceivable that the earlier childhood experiences when the client felt helpless and impotent to effect change may be unconsciously reexperienced and the individual may not assert himself or herself. Nonetheless, the focus is how the normal or reasonable person would have responded to the precipitating events.

The clinician has a broad array of treatment alternatives available once the diagnosis has been made. The alternative treatment modalities assume preexisting coping skills and a modicum of psychological health. Ochberg (1988) suggests several paradigms to be used to account for symptoms, apparent post-traumatic maladjustment, and related problems. Some of these that are appropriate for the issue of workplace harassment are victimization, autonomic arousal, and negative intimacy.

Victimization is the experience of feeling deliberately, unjustly harmed or coerced by another human being. The victim characteristically feels like a loser, humiliated and diminished. The therapist can explain and forewarn the patient of the expected feelings, anticipated course of healing, and the working through of the shame and ostracism experienced as a result of the experience.

The great majority of trauma victims experience autonomic nervous system activation. The pattern and type of anxiety need to be defined in terms of PTSD, generalized anxiety, panic, or phobia because of the specific psychotherapeutic medication and desensitization therapies that may be used.

Negative intimacy refers to the sensation experienced by many patients of one's personal space or person being invaded. Feelings of self-loathing or disgust are often expressed by the patient. The therapist and the patient need to address, examine, and discuss the disgust and degradation felt by the patient. The diagnosis of the victim's disorder is based on clinical evidence and determines the treatment paradigm. The therapist may choose from a variety of treatment modalities, including medication, education, individual and/or group psychotherapy, and family intervention. Usually a combination of these modalities is advised. Studies indicate the involvement of the family frequently promotes healing and support. Therapy groups for patients facilitate the acceptance of feelings and reactions of victims and the building of trust.

EXPERT WITNESS AND LITIGATION CONSULTING

In the event of sexual harassment litigation, attorneys need mental health practitioners to serve as consultants. Even though the *Harris* decision states clearly that psychological harm need not be shown to make a case of sexual harassment, monetary awards may be much greater if such harm is shown. Both the attorney for the plaintiff and the one representing the employer will need to hire practitioners to conduct assessments to determine the degree of psychological harm, if any, that may have resulted from the alleged harassment. As a consultant in litigation, the practitioner's role is to educate the attorneys and the court and to evaluate the work situation and the alleged victim and communicate findings in an understandable way to attorneys and the court. Because of potential for conflict of interest, it is not appropriate for the practitioner to serve as psychotherapist and litigation consultant for the same client.

The expert witness should be brought in at the earliest stages of the legal case to facilitate assessing the strengths and weakness in both sides of the case. The expert serves an early role in helping the attorneys gain a clearer view of their options in handling the case by making them aware of psychological and technical issues that need to be considered in the case. This early assistance may be critical to the attorney in establishing his or her strategy for the case, and in some cases may be instrumental in decisions to settle the case. The expert assists the attorney in reviewing the facts of the case and identifying areas for further inquiry. The expert's special knowledge can be used to frame precisely worded questions during the discovery process that will yield information desired by the attorney.

The expert serves a crucial role in assisting the attorney in the examination of opposing experts. In this role, the expert provides critical assistance in formulating questions and suggesting areas for future inquiry. During testimony of opposing experts, the practitioner suggests follow-up questions and possible fruitful avenues of questioning for the attorney. The expert is also essential in interpreting the answers provided by opposing experts. Because of their professional knowledge, experts serve an important role in educating attorneys, judges, and juries in the issues relevant to the case. In this role, the expert must be able to discuss the issues of the case in lay terms, so that the decision makers in the case can make informed judgments.

The expert must be aware of the hazards of the expert role. The attorneys in the case each present one-sided arguments, while the judge or jury must weigh the arguments on both sides so that they can reach their decision. The expert is caught in the middle and may be tugged off center by the attorneys as they try to persuade the judge or jury. The expert must maintain his or her objectivity throughout this process. The adversarial nature of the litigation process, and the fact that the expert may have limited access to information, can present serious problems.

Typical and appropriate questions to be asked of the therapist are:

1. What is the diagnosis of the client? Axis, I, Axis II, Axis III, Axis IV, and Axis V. What is the basis for this diagnosis? What psychological tests did you have a psychologist administer and interpret to make the diagnosis? If the test administrator was not a licensed clinical psychologist, what training has he or she had in the development, construction, interpretation, and administration of psychological tests? Other mental health professionals would be practicing out of their range of competence if they gave and interpreted the tests without specific training and education.
2. What are the clinician's credentials or knowledge in the area of sexual harassment? What qualifies this professional as an expert in the field? Has the professional taken or given courses in this field? Has the professional published any books or chapters on this subject? Has the professional previously given expert testimony in this area?
3. What is the relationship of the diagnosis to the workplace/sexual harassment that is claimed?
4. How would the clinician distinguish preexisting conditions (e.g., psychological and physical symptoms from previous normal workplace, family, and personal life stresses) from those claimed? How would the clinician distinguish the nonjob-related conditions that the individual may have undergone from the claimed stresses?
5. What are the essential elements of therapy for an individual who feels he or she is a victim of sexual/workplace harassment? In what ways is the clinician's treatment consistent with the above-mentioned elements?
6. Is the client's diagnosis permanent and stationary? If not, what conditions would be necessary to be fulfilled for the diagnosis to be permanent and stationary? Is more psychological treatment necessary? If so, how much more therapy is anticipated in order to achieve the permanent and stationary condition (this is affected by the premorbid conditions)?
7. Where in the therapeutic progress notes are the specific incidents that prompted the diagnostic conclusions reached? Where in the therapeutic treatment notes are specific clinical interventions mentioned that focus on the processing of the emotions and developing insights to help the client achieve the goals listed above?
8. How would you as a clinician interpret specific incidents claimed by the client? Could there be other interpretations? How would you explain the client's lack of assertiveness or the fact that the client apparently did not use established grievance procedures? Is this consistent with his or her lifetime behavior patterns, or with the client's behavior in other areas of life? If not, why not?

An expert who allows himself or herself to be lured into making statements that are not supported by the known facts of the case risks losing credibility and possibly suffering damage to his or her reputation. Both plaintiff and defendant attorneys may, either intentionally or inadvertently, put pressure on the expert to provide opinions that fit the attorney's litigation strategy. It is the responsibility of the expert to maintain objectivity, though there may be some pressure to overstate the data or even to make statements that rely on unproved assumptions. The expert must maintain objectivity and balance throughout this process and avoid becoming emotionally invested in the issues. Overstating the data may not only be hazardous to the expert's reputation but may also be damaging to the case.

WHAT SHOULD EMPLOYERS BE DOING?

Simply put, employers are obligated to insure a harassment-free workplace. Employers must provide employees with means to safely register complaints. Complaints must be investigated, and progressive disciplinary steps must be established for perpetrators of harassment. The disciplinary system must include discharge as a final resort, and the employer must be prepared to carry out discipline uniformly and fairly.

ORGANIZATIONAL ASSESSMENT OF SEXUAL HARASSMENT RISK

Organizations and industries differ in risk factors for sexual harassment. Sexual harassment may be motivated by a variety of organizational factors. To reduce the risk of sexual harassment incidents that can give rise to complaints and lawsuits, training programs and policy development should be preceded by an assessment of the organizational risks that could result in sexual harassment complaints. Sexual harassment policies must address the unique needs and conditions of the organization for which they are intended. The assessment should include an examination of attitudes toward sexual harassment.

INFORMAL LINES OF COMMUNICATION

One important factor in organizational success is access to informal lines of communication. Workplace harassment can be an important factor in determining whether members of protected groups have access to these lines of communication.

A survey by Stroock and Stroock and Lavan, a law firm specializing in labor and employment issues (BNA Labor Daily, 1994), found that the most important factors in deciding who gets promoted are the informal factors that are not normally included on official evaluations, according to 54% of the respondents. The important factors include such things as office politics, contact and familiarity with the candidate, integrity, loyalty, personality, and ability to develop new business. If women or members of other covered groups are not afforded an equal opportunity to develop the relationships needed for advancement, they will not be successful in achieving promotions.

The report recommends five steps to help increase access to informal workplace activities:

1. Adopt and communicate clear policies prohibiting discrimination.
2. Educate all employees about equal employment opportunity laws.
3. Insure that women and other protected group members get equal opportunities to be included in lunches, client meetings, and other networking opportunities vital to advancement.
4. Adopt in-house grievance procedures of dispute-resolution mechanisms and "open door" policies to facilitate airing of problems.
5. Use "Mentor" or "Big Sibling" programs to aid in developing junior-level employees.

DEVELOPMENT OF SEXUAL HARASSMENT POLICY

Policies must address the unique aspects of the organization. For example:

- When women work in nontraditional jobs, ingrained practices, such as pin-up calendars and off-color jokes, may create a hostile environment.
- Resentment from males toward females in nontraditional jobs may come out in the form of sexual harassment. This has been a problem for many police and fire departments and other traditionally male environments. Assessment of attitudes is especially critical for the development of policies for these types of organizations.
- Jobs in which business travel is common may present risks when male and female employees travel together on work assignments.
- Jobs in which female employees must deal with clients in social situations or other environments where the likelihood of sexual advances is increased should include training for the employees involved.

Although some provisions of sexual harassment policies are generic, and may be obtained from published sources or labor attorneys, it is essential to remember that the policy is useless if it does not affect the behavior of employees. Special emphasis should be given to the risk factors that are particular to the organization involved and to the special issues identified in the assessment of sexual harassment risk.

Recommended Components of Policy. The *Guidelines on Harassment* currently proposed by the EEOC include a statement suggesting that prevention is the best tool for the elimination of harassment. Employers should take all steps necessary to prevent harassment from occurring, including having an explicit policy against harassment and clearly and regularly communicating this policy to employees. The communication should explain sanctions for harassment. Steps should be taken to sensitize supervisory and nonsupervisory employees to issues of harassment and inform employees of their right to raise the issue under Title VII of the Civil Rights Act, the Americans with Disabilities Act, the Age Discrimination in Employment Act, and the Rehabilitation Act. Effective complaint procedures should be implemented for employees to make their complaints known to management without fear of repercussion or retaliation.

Prompt and Appropriate Response. One of the most important factors in determining the success of steps taken by the organization in response to charges of harassment is the promptness and appropriateness of steps taken to resolve the problem. If the organization takes all harassment allegations seriously by promptly investigating them and taking steps to resolve the problem, chances of avoiding legal action or prevailing in the event of litigation are greatly increased. A successful policy of prompt and appropriate response will also reduce the incidence of harassment problems, because it results in communicating the fact that harassment will not be tolerated.

In a recent case (*Carmon v. Lubrizol Corp.,* 1994), the company showed the court that it had promptly handled harassment charges by conducting prompt investigations and taking steps to insure that appropriate discipline was carried out and that steps were taken to prevent recurrence of the problem. When the plaintiff appealed the decision and failed to present a plausible reason for the appeal, the court ordered the plaintiff and her attorney to pay the company's legal fees and court costs for the appeal.

TRAINING PROGRAMS FOR MANAGERS, SUPERVISORS, AND EMPLOYEES

If the reasonable man thinks differently from the reasonable woman, many men may not recognize when their behavior crosses the line into the area of sexual harassment. Men must be educated to understand the reasonable woman's point of view, and women must be educated concerning the man's point of view.

Sexual harassment perpetrators are found at all levels of the organization. Even clients can be sexual harassment perpetrators. Training and information dissemination is needed at all levels of the organization. In the case of clients, the employer is still at risk if the employee involved brings the problem to the attention of management. There are steps that management can take to deal with this problem through policy development and training.

BE PROACTIVE!

Every organization that has more than a few employees must accept the fact that some instances of sexual harassment will probably occur. Fortunately, there are steps that prudent organizations can take to drastically reduce the risk of being assessed monetary damages. Programs to address sexual harassment through development of clear policies and education of the work force will not only reduce the legal risk of the employer but, if properly implemented, will have a positive impact on morale, particularly for female employees.

CONCLUSIONS

There is little doubt that sexual harassment is a major problem for employers. The behavior of individual employees who are not sensitive to the problem, or who have not been educated concerning proper conduct, can place organizations in a position of major financial risk. Unlike some other human resources problems, sexual harassment can be perpetrated by any employee in the organization and, in some cases, by clients or customers.

Fortunately, there are actions that employers may take that can drastically reduce their exposure to sexual harassment claims and that will improve the organizational climate in which their employees work.

Lilli Friedland, PhD, ABPP, is a clinical psychologist and a consultant to business and organizations. She has consulted to legal counsel in numerous sexual harassment lawsuits. Dr. Friedland is President-Elect of Division 46 (Media Psychology) of the American Psychological Association (APA), and Co-Editor of the *Amplifier*, the Division 46 newsletter, for the past 3 years. She is a member of the Public Information Committee of the APA, a member of the Board of Psychology for the State of California, and is a past president of the Los Angeles County Psychological Association. Dr. Friedland may be reached at 2080 Century Park East, Suite 1403, Los Angeles, CA 90067.

David Friedland, PhD, is Director of Consulting Services for Friedland Psychological Associates. He has over 20 years of experience in the human resources field, working with both public and private sector employers. Dr. Friedland earned his BA and MA degrees in psychology, and earned his PhD in measurement and evaluation from the University of Southern California. He is active in numerous professional organizations and often speaks before professional groups concerning issues in personnel assessment and human resources management. He has published articles in his field and is listed in Who's Who in California and Who's Who in the West. Dr. Friedland can be contacted at 2080 Century Park East, Suite 1403, Los Angeles, CA 90067.

RESOURCES

American Psychiatric Association. (1987). *Diagnostic and Statistical Manual of Mental Disorders* (3rd ed. rev.). Washington, DC: Author.

American Psychiatric Association. (1994). *Diagnostic and Statistical Manual of Mental Disorders* (4th ed.). Washington, DC: Author.

Baker, D., Terpstra, D. E., & Cutler, B. (1990). Perceptions of sexual harassment: A reexamination of gender differences. *Journal of Psychology, 124,* 409-416.

Bartling, C. A., & Eisenman, R. (1993). Sexual harassment proclivities in men and women. *Bulletin of the Psychonomic Society, 31,* 189-192.

BNA Labor Daily. (1994, March 3). *Women Who Lack Access to Communication Lines Miss Out on Senior Management Positions.* Washington, DC: Bureau of National Affairs.

Burns v. McGregor Electronic Industries, Inc. (January 30, 1992). CA 8, 90-2504, 955 F.2d 559.

Carmon v. Lubrizol Corp. (March 31, 1994). CA 5, 92-2964.

Cleveland, J. N., & Kerst, M. E. (1993). Sexual harassment and perceptions of power: An underarticulated relationship [Special issue: Sexual harassment in the workplace]. *Vocational Behavior, 42,* 49-67.

Crull, P. (1982). Stress effects of sexual harassment on the job: Implications for counseling. *American Journal of Orthopsychiatry, 5293,* 529-544.

Ellison v. Brady. (January 23, 1991). 9th Circuit Court of Appeal (924 F.2d 872, CA 9, 89-15248).

Equal Employment Opportunity Commission. (1980). *Sex Discrimination Guidelines* (29 CFR 1604). Washington, DC: U.S. Government Printing Office.

Equal Employment Opportunity Commission. (1993, October 1). *Proposed Guidelines on Harassment Based on Race, Color, Religion, Gender, National Origin, Age, and Disability* (Federal Register 58 FR 51266). Washington, DC: U.S. Government Printing Office.

Gosselin, H. L. (1984). Sexual harassment on the job: Psychological, social and economic repercussions. *Canada's Mental Health, 32,* 21-24.

Hadsell, B. (1992). *Maximizing Damages in a Sexual Harassment Case from the Plaintiff's Perspective.* ALI-ABA Course of Study: Employment Discrimination and Civil Rights, Co-sponsored by the California Continuing Education of the Bar, Los Angeles, CA.

Harris v. Forklift Systems. (November 9, 1993). U.S. S. Ct., 92-1168.

Komaromy, M., Bindman, A., Haber, R., & Sande, M. (1993). Sexual harassment in medical training. *New England Journal of Medicine, 328,* 322-326.

Jenson v. Eveleth Taconite Company. (December 16, 1991). D.C. Minn., 5-88-163, 139 FRD 657.

Landgraf v. USI Film Products; Rivers v. Roadway Express. (1994). U.S. S. Ct., 64 FEP Cases 820 and 842.

Meritor Savings Bank V. Vinson. (1986). U.S. S. Ct. *aff., rem.* 40 FEP Cases 1822.

Ochberg, F. M. (1988). *Post-Traumatic Therapy and Victims of Violence.* New York: Brunner/Mazel.

Pryor, J. B. (1987). Sexual harassment proclivities in men. *Sex Roles, 17,* 5-6.

Rogers v. Western-Southern Life Insurance Company. (December 17, 1993). CA 7, 93-1125.

Saal, F., Johnson, C., & Weber, N. (1989). Friendly or sexy? It may depend on whom you ask. *Psychology of Women Quarterly, 13,* 263-276.

Salisbury, J., Ginorio, A., Remick, H., & Stringer, D. (1986). Counseling victims of sexual harassment [Special issue: Gender issues in psychotherapy]. *Psychotherapy, 23,* 316-324.

Stockdale, M. S. (1993). The role of sexual misperceptions of women's friendliness in an emerging theory of sexual harassment [Special issue: Sexual harassment in the workplace]. *Journal of Vocational Behavior, 42,* 84-101.

Stockdale, M. S., & Saal, F. (1991). Persistence of men's misperceptions of friendly cues across a variety of interpersonal encounters. *Psychology of Women Quarterly, 15,* 463-475.

Struckman-Johnson, C., & Struckman-Johnson, D. (1993). College men's and women's reactions to hypothetical sexual touch varied by initiator gender and coercion. *Sex Roles, 29,* 371-385.

Trotta v. Mobil Oil Corp. (April 8, 1992). D.C. Southern New York, 90 Civ. 5663, 788 F. Supp. 1336.

Woody, R. H., & Perry, N. W. (1993). Sexual harassment victims: Psycho-legal and family therapy considerations. *American Journal of Family Therapy, 21,* 136-144.

Workman, J. E., & Johnson, K. K. (1991). The role of cosmetics in attributions about sexual harassment. *Sex Roles, 24,* 759-769.

AN INTERDISCIPLINARY AGREEMENT BETWEEN PSYCHOLOGISTS AND ATTORNEYS: A MODEL FOR PSYCHOLOGY-LAW INTERACTION

William E. Foote

Traditionally, psychologists have interacted with lawyers, courts, and legal processes with some trepidation (Barton & Sanborn, 1978). Their concerns arise in part from differences between psychological and legal paradigms (Melton et al., 1987). These differences may be unresolvable, as the goals, methods, and theoretical bases of the two fields have been quite disparate. However, much of the conflict between psychologists and lawyers arises from a lack of either awareness of or respect for the ethical standards, professional parameters, and business practices of the respective professions.

To address these issues, members of the New Mexico Psychological Association (NMPA) and the New Mexico Bar Association (NMBA) worked together to develop an interdisciplinary agreement. This document was designed to function as an educational tool for both disciplines rather than a legal standard for legal or psychological practice. Since the associations adopted the resulting accord, psychologists and lawyers in New Mexico have enjoyed more amicable relationships and smoother professional interactions.

In this contribution, I will first discuss the issues that seem to cause the most concern to psychologists and lawyers. Then I will discuss the agreement that NMPA and NMBA devised and adopted.

SOURCES OF PSYCHOLOGY-LAW CONFLICTS

From the perspective of psychologists, some aspects of the psychological-legal interface are especially troublesome. Many psychologists have been concerned about the confidentiality of patient information in legal settings. Informed consent has also been an issue, as have the business and professional aspects of lawyer-psychologist relationships.

CONFIDENTIALITY

In the usual contexts of professional practice, psychologists are aware of their duty to maintain the confidentiality of communications from patients (DeKraai & Sales, 1984; Miller & Thelen, 1987). This long has been a tenet of ethics in psychology (American Psychological Association [APA], 1992) and is recognized by practitioners of many disciplines as an essential element of successful consultation and intervention (Appelbaum et al., 1984; Austin, Moline, & Williams, 1990).

A related concern focuses upon the use of psychological test instruments. Not only do the test data and responses fall under the constraints of confidentiality noted previously, but psychologists are also protective of test stimuli, protocols, and manuals (American Educational Research Association, 1985; APA, 1992). Maintaining the confidentiality of raw test data is essential in preventing people who are not trained to interpret the information from misusing it. Protecting the test instruments is also critical in preventing these materials from passing into the public domain. Such general knowledge would allow potential examinees to be tutored on responses for the tests or at least would compromise the usual assumption that patients are naïve to the test materials (Tranel, 1994).

These concerns of psychologists about patient and test confidentiality encounter a legal process dedicated to bringing such information under judicial scrutiny. As a matter of legal tradition and state and federal law, and as a function of the rules of evidence, the adversarial process demands that all possible relevant information be brought to the finder of fact (Federal Rules of Evidence, Rule 501). Only with complete information may the judge, jury, or other legal tribunal adequately weigh the issue before the court.

Against these demands, psychologists have few means of preserving confidentiality. Although some patient-therapist communications may be privileged, in most practical situations any privilege has been waived by the patient's use of the mental condition as a basis for a claim or defense (DeKraai & Sales, 1982; Shah, 1969). This waiver calms the concerns of most psychologists about confidentiality as an ethical issue, because patients usually sign appropriate releases of information. Nevertheless, some fears persist about maintaining the integrity of ongoing psychotherapy, because the psychologist's public discussion of previously private information may well result in harm to the therapeutic alliance (Corcoran, 1988; Dubey, 1974).

Maintaining the confidentiality of test materials in legal settings is a concern largely unresolved (Tranel, 1994). Psychologists who receive a subpoena that includes a request for "raw test data" are forced into a choice of violating ethical standards or facing sanctions of the court for contempt. Although a witness who responds to a valid court order generally is protected from other legal sanctions (e.g., proceedings from a state professional licensing body), ethical consequences may still ensue.

INFORMED CONSENT

Ethical standards require psychologists to obtain informed consent from a patient before they initiate a clinical procedure. The most recent APA *Ethical Principles* (1992) states in Section 4.02: "Psychologists obtain informed consent to therapy or related procedures, using language that is reasonably understandable to participants" (p. 1605). Such informed consent procedures are relatively routine in the usual contexts of psychotherapy or evaluations.

In forensic referrals, the context may not be so evident to the client. Some evaluations are "friendly" and may be requested by the lawyer working on the client's side of the case (in civil cases, the plaintiff's counsel; in criminal, the defense attorney). Other evaluations are conducted in a more adversarial context, as the examining psychologist may be hired by the prosecutor or the defense counsel. Whatever the origin of the referral, the client should be fully informed about the evaluative procedures that will be used and the probable use of the evaluation results.

As noted earlier, clients should be advised that in almost any forensic context, the usual protection of confidentiality does not apply. Psychologists complain that the referring counsel may not properly advise the client before the evaluation. In some cases, the examining psychologist may assume the advice has already been given. The overall outcome is that the client may be confused, frightened, or angry, resulting in an aborted, or at least distorted, evaluation.

PROFESSIONAL ISSUES

A third area of concern in the psychology-law interface is the professional and business relationships of the lawyer and psychologist. These relationships are most likely to be problematical when the psychologist is asked to serve as an expert witness. Some psychologists complain of delayed payment or no payment for their services. Others have been asked to enter into unethical "contingency fee" arrangements (Shapiro, 1991). Psychologists find that their schedules become chaotic when lawyers inaccurately predict the time or date when the psychologist is expected to testify. And they complain about "hardball tactics" that lawyers use, such as relying on subpoena powers to intimidate psychologists (Brodsky, 1991).

On the other hand, lawyers have been concerned about the excessive fees that some psychologists charge for deposition or trial testimony. At times, lawyers argue, psychologists have been so unwilling to testify that lawyers have had to resort to the use of subpoenas to bring an ostensibly favorable witness into court. And when psychologists do testify, lawyers are often befuddled by psychological jargon and the apparent inability of some psychologists to translate their findings into comprehensible language.

Professionals from both fields are irked by the trespass of the other into their domain. Psychologists are appalled by lawyers exercising their role as "counselors at law" by doing psychotherapy or counseling. Lawyers find psychologists who give legal advice likewise troublesome, as that advice is prone to error and may interfere with the ongoing lawyer-client relationship.

THE STATEMENT OF PRINCIPLES

HISTORY

The psychology/law conflicts outlined previously were evident to New Mexico psychologists and lawyers by the mid-1980s. As a result, Frank Spring, a member of NMPA who is also a lawyer and a member of NMBA, proposed the development of an interdisciplinary agreement to allow for more effective interprofessional interaction. NMPA contacted NMBA and a joint committee comprised of equal numbers of psychologists and lawyers was formed to discuss the elements necessary for such an agreement. After a year of work, the committee produced the finished document which was accepted by the NMPA Executive Board in early 1986 and the Board of Bar Commissioners in August 1986 (see pp. 259-261).

CONTENT

The interdisciplinary agreement contains six sections. Section I recognizes that both lawyers and psychologists hold the welfare of the client as the most important goal of the principles. Section II limits the intrusion of psychologists into the territory usually claimed by lawyers. Section III limits the intrusion of lawyers into territory usually claimed by psychologists.

Section IV is a more comprehensive section dealing with the responsibilities of attorneys. This section recognizes the concerns of psychologists about the scheduling of deposition and court testimony. Lawyers are reminded to discuss fees and to properly compensate psychologists for their time in forensic cases. Lawyers are advised to become familiar with the psychological literature related to their cases and to be familiar with the rules and laws concerning confidentiality. Finally, lawyers are asked to prepare their clients for interaction with psychologists.

Section V outlines the responsibilities of psychologists, beginning with a discussion concerning the necessity of maintaining confidentiality. Later sections remind psychologists that they are to turn over records in a timely manner when they receive appropriate informed consent, and that they are to provide reports of their evaluations within similar time constraints.

A critical part of this section dealing with psychological testing materials states: "Secured instruments, such as Rorschach or TAT cards, testing manuals or other copyrighted materials, should only be forwarded to certified psychologists retained by the requesting attorney." This deals well with the concern described previously about the release of raw test data to unqualified people.

The next part of this section deals with the need for the psychologist to obtain informed consent from the client before initiating a psychological evaluation. Psychologists are then asked to confer with the lawyers retaining them as a means of educating counsel about a particular client or, more generally, about a body of psychological knowledge. Preparation for testimony and the psycho-legal context of that testimony is the focus of the next part of Section V. Psychologists are reminded to provide only testimony and to leave the representation of the client up to the lawyer.

The final part of Section V focuses on psychological fees. This section skirts antitrust issues as it attempts to place limitations upon the fees that psychologists may charge for evaluation and testimony. This section was provided as a guideline for both psychologists and lawyers to determine what constitutes "customary and ordinary" fees.

Section VI provides for a grievance procedure. However, in the 7 years since the adoption of the agreement, the convening of a grievance committee has not proved necessary.

USE OF THE STATEMENT OF PRINCIPLES

This document may serve as a model for other state psychological associations to negotiate with their bar associations to produce a similar agreement. Similarly, it may provide a basis for the American Psychological Association and American Bar Association to discuss a national agreement to facilitate psychologist-attorney interactions.

At a less grandiose level, the statement provides a group of expectations for members of both professions. It clarifies the demands of the respective professions and serves as a basis for the resolution of disputes. And it suggests that the interface between psychology and the law need not be a barrier that reduces the effectiveness of either psychological or legal services. Rather, it may be a channel through which information flows for the benefit of the client.

STATEMENT OF PRINCIPLES RELATING TO THE RESPONSIBILITIES OF ATTORNEYS AND PSYCHOLOGISTS AND THEIR INTERPROFESSIONAL RELATIONSHIPS

Adopted August 30, 1986, by the Board of Bar Commissioners of the State Bar of New Mexico

These principles should govern the interprofessional relations of psychologists and attorneys.

I. THE PATIENT-CLIENT

The welfare of the patient-client is the paramount and joint goal of these principles.

II. PSYCHOLOGISTS AND THE LAW

1. Psychologists shall refrain from giving legal advice.
2. Psychologists shall refrain from interfering with established lawyer-client relationships.

III. ATTORNEYS AND PSYCHOLOGICAL CARE

1. Attorneys shall refrain from giving psychodiagnostic opinions.
2. Attorneys shall refrain from interfering with established psychologist-patient relationships.

IV. AN ATTORNEY'S RESPONSIBILITIES

An attorney's responsibility is always first to his* client. However, in his relationship with psychologists, an attorney has the following responsibilities:

1. *Testimony:* An attorney should keep the psychologist informed as to the status of the litigation and in particular inform him sufficiently in advance of:

    a) deposition and trial settings;
    b) vacated deposition and trial settings; and
    c) pre-trial settlements.

2. *Fees:* The services of a psychologist in a legal matter involve the consumption of the psychologist's time and the utilization of his facilities and his expertise. As a result, the attorney shall make proper arrangements with all involved psychologists beforehand for payment for the psychologist's services either directly by his client or by the attorney himself through the advancement of costs.

    An attorney is not expected to advance costs for psychologist services involving treatment.

    An attorney who requests information from a psychologist solely to advance his knowledge of psychology is responsible personally for prompt payment of those services.

---

*Use of the male pronoun throughout this document follows the conventional style of the New Mexico statutory construction. It is understood to refer to both males and females.

3. *Background:* An attorney should attempt to familiarize himself with the psychological literature in order that he may have some initial understanding of the problem and so that he might be able to specify the information requested from the psychologist and understand the psychologist's explanation and report.

4. *Confidentiality:* An attorney must know the applicable law relating to confidentiality in the psychologist-patient relationship, such as the psychotherapist-patient privilege, Rule 504, New Mexico Rules of Evidence and the disclosure of information provision of the New Mexico Mental Health and Developmental Disabilities Code, N.M.Stat.Ann. Section 43-1-19 (1978). The attorney shall refrain from asking a psychologist to disclose confidential information other than as provided by law.

5. *Client Preparation:* An attorney should inform his client as to the nature and purposes of any psychological evaluation and should identify the potential uses of information to be gathered during the evaluation.

V. A PSYCHOLOGIST'S RESPONSIBILITIES

A psychologist's primary responsibility is always the well-being of his patient. The psychologist must maintain the confidentiality of patient communications as provided by New Mexico law. The psychologist acting as psychotherapist must claim the psychotherapist-patient privilege on behalf of his patient, recognizing that this privilege may be waived or excepted under New Mexico law. In any event, the psychologist must obtain a valid authorization from his patient or the patient's guardian before confidential information may be disclosed. A psychologist involved in the legal process has the following responsibilities:

1. *Records:* Given a valid authorization, the psychologist should promptly transfer information from his records to the requesting attorney. Psychologists have no proprietary interest in test or interview responses, whether written, taped, or otherwise recorded.

2. *Reports:* Given a valid authorization, reports covering a summation of psychological facts and opinions, and their significance shall be furnished upon request by the treating psychologist or the psychologist specifically engaged to do such work. The attorney should specify the items he wishes covered in that report.

3. *Psychological Testing Materials:* Secured instruments, such as Rorschach or TAT cards, testing manuals, or other copyrighted materials, should be forwarded only to certified psychologists retained by the requesting attorney.

4. *Psychological Evaluations:* Before evaluating a person, the psychologist must inform the person of the nature and purposes of the psychological evaluation and must identify the potential uses of the information to be gathered during the evaluation.

5. *Conferences:* Given a valid authorization, attorneys may confer with psychologists either to:

    a) gain psychological information on a topic of the attorney's interest, or
    b) discuss psychological aspects of the case of a particular client with the treating psychologist or with one engaged to render such opinions. This may include a discussion of testimony that may be elicited at trial.

6. *Testimony:* Psychologists may be requested to testify either in court or by deposition. Cooperation between both attorneys and psychologists should allow for setting of court or deposition testimony for mutual convenience; while a subpoena may be necessary, it is not a substitute for direct communication between the attorney and psychologist for purpose of setting a time for testimony.

A psychologist should familiarize himself with the basic requirements of court procedure.

A psychologist should limit his testimony to his opinion and its basis. He should leave the representation of his patient and advancement of the patient's interest to the patient's attorney.

7. *Fees:* Psychologists may use the expenditure of their time, office facilities, and funds as a basis for arriving at a reasonable fee for services rendered pursuant to these principles. If an attorney fails to give timely notification of a change in the scheduled time for the psychologist's services, which makes the psychologist unavailable for other remunerative work, the psychologist may charge for the time set aside. A reasonable fee for the psychologist's time spent in preparation for testimony by deposition or in the courtroom is the same rate charged for usual psychological services. A reasonable fee for deposition or courtroom testimony is no more than double the usual rate for psychological services.

VI. GRIEVANCE PROCEDURE

Any grievance regarding the Principles set forth above shall be referred to a grievance panel for hearing. The State Bar of New Mexico and the New Mexico Psychological Association will each provide six committee members and one co-chairman to serve on grievance panels which will be composed of two lawyers, two psychologists, and one co-chairman. The co-chairman will alternate in chairing grievance panels. The chairman for a grievance panel will choose two panel members from each profession. Grievance panels are intended to resolve disputes arising out of the Principles set forth above; they are not intended as a substitute for the bodies governing the ethical conduct of the respective professions. Breaches of the ethical code of either profession or violations of law are to be referred to the appropriate body for consideration.

William E. Foote, PhD, is a psychologist in private practice in Albuquerque, New Mexico. His is primarily a forensic practice in which he consults in both criminal and civil cases. A diplomate in forensic psychology since 1984, Dr. Foote has taught psychology-law classes in both the Psychology Department and Law School of the University of New Mexico. Both mental health and legal groups have requested his participation in workshops. He has been active in the New Mexico Psychological Association, serving as ethics chair, president, legislative chair, and currently, APA council representative. Recently, he began a 3-year term on the APA Ad Hoc Committee on Legal Issues. Dr. Foote may be contacted at 1400 Central Avenue, S.E., Suite 3200, Albuquerque, NM 87106-4811.

RESOURCES

American Educational Research Association, American Psychological Association & National Council on Measurement in Education. (1985). *Standards for Educational and Psychological Testing.* Washington, DC: American Psychological Association.

American Psychological Association. (1992). Ethical principles of psychologists and code of conduct. *American Psychologist, 47,* 1597-1611.

Appelbaum, P. S., Kapen, G., Walters, B., Lidz, C., & Roth, L. H. (1984). Confidentiality: An empirical test of the utilitarian perspective. *Bulletin of the American Academy of Psychiatry and Law, 12,* 109-116.

Austin, K. M., Moline, M. E., & Williams, G. T. (1990). *Confronting Malpractice.* London: Sage.

Barton, W. B., & Sanborn, C. J. (Eds.). (1978). *Law and the Mental Health Professions: Friction at the Interface.* New York: International Universities Press.

Brodsky, S. L. (1991). *Testifying in Court.* Washington, DC: American Psychological Association.

Corcoran, K. J. (1988). The relationship of interpersonal trust to self disclosure when confidentiality is assured. *The Journal of Psychology, 122,* 193-195.

DeKraai, M. B., & Sales, B. D. (1982). Privileged communications of psychologists. *Professional Psychology, 13,* 372-388.

DeKraai, M. B., & Sales B. D. (1984). Confidential communications of psychotherapists. *Psychotherapy, 21,* 293-317.

Dubey, P. (1974). Confidentiality as a requirement of the therapist: Technical necessities for absolute privilege in psychotherapy. *American Journal of Psychiatry, 131,* 1093-1096.

Melton, G. B., Petrila, J., Poythress, N. G., & Slobogin, C. (1987). *Psychological Evaluations for the Courts.* New York: Guilford.

Miller, D. J., & Thelen, M. H. (1987). Confidentiality in psychotherapy: History, issues, and research. *Psychotherapy, 24,* 704-711.

Shah, S. (1969). Privileged communications, confidentiality and privacy: Privileged communications. *Professional Psychology, 1,* 56-59.

Shapiro, D. L. (1991). *Forensic Psychological Assessment.* Boston: Allyn and Bacon.

Tranel, D. (1994). The release of psychological data to nonexperts: Ethical and legal considerations. *Professional Psychology: Research and Practice, 25,* 33-38.

INTRODUCTION TO SECTION III: ASSESSMENT INSTRUMENTS AND OFFICE FORMS

This section of *Innovations* includes various instruments, checklists, and forms for practitioners to use in collecting and organizing information. It reflects the goal of our series to share useful assessment materials. Although some of the items included here have been formally developed and normed, others were designed for informal application and should not be used as formal instruments. We have included them here because we feel they can be used effectively by practitioners to collect information from their clients. We also wish to alert readers to the fact that a number of practical instruments and forms are available in other contributions in this volume. Specifically, the contributions in Section I by Chris Coleman, Alice Friedman, and Donna Gates (pp. 55-72); Ruby Takushi Chinen and Linda Berg-Cross (pp. 151-166); and Victoria Demos and Maurice Prout (pp. 167-178) provide useful forms. In Section II, the contribution by Marc Frankel and John Feely (pp. 199-221) includes a form for clinicians to use. In Section IV, the contribution by Thomas and Mary Grant (pp. 339-356) includes forms for both clinicians and clients.

The value of forms and instruments depends upon their appropriate application by the clinicians who use them. It is important to emphasize that they are not necessarily designed to generate the types of inferences often associated with more formalized tests that have a long history of use. Readers should recognize the potential as well as the stated limitations to these materials and use them in accordance with accepted ethical principles. It is assumed that anyone who uses these instruments will have a general clinical knowledge of the area being evaluated.

Given the limitations noted previously, we have attempted to insure that the materials that follow include sufficient information to allow readers to evaluate their appropriate application. Certain basic information and instructions have been included with each contribution and, when necessary, the Resource sections contain references to more detailed studies. Readers who wish to use such material are advised to obtain the additional resources. If there is a desire to use the material for research purposes, most authors would appreciate being contacted so that data may be shared.

The first contribution in this section, by Patricia Petretic-Jackson, Genell Sandberg, and Thomas Jackson, presents an empirically derived scale that assesses the manner in which individuals attribute blame for domestic violence in our society. The Domestic Violence Blame Scale (DVBS) has several potential applications, including serving as a pre-/post-treatment assessment measure for both victims and perpetrators of spousal violence and for assessing the biases that law enforcement and health professionals may have regarding the causes of domestic violence.

The next contribution, also authored by Thomas Jackson and several colleagues, presents a scale that assesses the manner in which individuals attribute blame for violence in our society. The results of this scale include five blame factor scores and demonstrate differences between groups of individuals who have or have not been exposed to violence. In contrast to the first contribution in this section on the DVBS which addresses domestic violence, the Violence Attitudes Scale (VAS) can be used to assess violence attitudes in general.

Some managed care companies have indicated that they will hire only those clinicians who can provide client profiles and data on client satisfaction with services. Chris Stout presents a client satisfaction survey that collects information on clinical and nonclinical issues, and includes the client's own perceptions regarding therapeutic outcomes.

The last contribution in this section, by John Rudisill, is a checklist that clinicians can use to monitor clinical and administrative activities with patients. The checklist will help to insure that therapists have attended to the various details that accompany quality care.

THE DOMESTIC VIOLENCE BLAME SCALE (DVBS)

Patricia Petretic-Jackson, Genell Sandberg, and Thomas L. Jackson

INTRODUCTION

Prior to 1970, wife abuse/domestic violence was perceived as a private, family problem that affected only a small, unique group of women (Davis, 1987). However, research conducted by investigators within the social and legal sciences in the last 25 years has indicated that wife abuse is a serious social and clinical problem of epidemic proportions affecting women in intimate relationships (American Psychological Association Task Force, 1984; Walker, 1984).

It has been estimated that each year over 3 million married couples in the United States experience one or more severe physical assaults, and that the percentage of battering nonmarried couples (cohabiting and dating) may be even higher than that for married couples (Stets & Straus, 1989). Over 1 million battered women seek medical attention each year for injuries inflicted by their partners, and increasing numbers are served at community women's shelters. The problem is one faced by women in all segments of society.

Despite the scope of the problem, wife abuse has suffered from "selective inattention" (Gelles, 1980) compared to other forms of family violence which involve parent-to-child abuse. Wife abuse is often informally sanctioned as a legitimate form of violence within our society (Hofeller, 1982). Although, in part, such abuse reflects a general acceptance of using physical punishment as a means of controlling the behavior of individuals within a family (Gelles & Strauss, 1988), Martin (1985) argues that wife abuse has unique aspects which differentiate it from other forms of family and societal violence. Because many batterers believe it is their right to control their partners by any means, including physical battering, they believe that no societal limits on such violent behaviors directed toward a partner exist. Misconceptions concerning the nature of domestic violence held by many nonabusive individuals also permit wife abuse to go undetected and untreated. Stereotypes of batterers and battered women lead to minimization of the problem; thus, abusive behavior may not be labeled as such.

Our definition of the family as nonviolent and nurturant results in a "perceptual blackout" of violence that occurs in "normal" families (Gelles, 1974). Minimization is more likely if characteristics of the abusive situation, abusive partner, or abused woman do not adhere to common stereotypes. The man who has battered his partner may not appear to be a "mentally disturbed abuser." The battered woman may not act like a defenseless, innocent victim. The family may not be of lower socioeconomic status or its members uneducated. Such misperceptions regarding family violence permit individuals to construct fictions in which wife abuse is defined as a problem that occurs in "other people's families."

Findings of several surveys of public attitudes toward wife abuse confirm that widespread misperceptions of wife abuse exist. Community surveys suggest that many individuals hold erroneous, stereotyped beliefs about battered women (Ewing & Aubrey, 1987). Many people are quick to blame the woman for a violence episode in an intimate relationship (Hillier & Foddy, 1993). In ongoing battering relationships the questions "Why doesn't she leave?" and "What did she do to provoke him?" are more frequently asked than "Why does he continue to batter and abuse her?" and "Why didn't he choose to deal with his anger in another way?" Several surveys of health and mental health professionals have found that some service/care providers similarly demonstrate nonsympathetic and victim-blaming attitudes toward victims of domestic violence (P. W. Easteal & S. Easteal, 1992; Hall-Apicella, 1983).

In contrast to a victim-precipitation model of battering, individuals may explain the male's abusive behavior as due to mental illness. This perception is consistent with a psychopathology model of battering found in the clinical literature (Hamberger & Hastings, 1988). Clinicians treating batterers often find that the majority of men referred for treatment meet criteria for *DSM-IV* Axis II personality disorders. Based on Millon Clinical Multiaxial Inventory (MCMI) scores (Millon, 1983), Hamberger and Hastings (1986) found that schizoidal/borderline, narcissistic/antisocial, or passive dependent/compulsive diagnoses were common in their sample of male batterers, although no single abuser personality was found. Current thinking among professionals working with batterers is that, as with other forms of violence involving intimates, wife abuse involves a multiplicity of interacting causal factors (Hamberger & Lohr, 1989; Thorne-Finch, 1992). Treatment of the male batterer in which there is a deliberate focus on the battering is a relatively new field (Sonkin, Martin, & Walker, 1985). Although a diversity of treatment programs for batterers now exist (Caesar & Hamberger, 1989), a growing consensus is that battering behavior, along with its associated features, is best conceptualized as behavioral in nature (e.g., skill deficits in anger management and communication skills), such that cognitive-behavioral interventions are most effective.

Several measures currently exist that directly assess male responses to the demands of an intimate relationship and, more specifically, the nature of their anger (e.g., Conflict Tactics Scale [Straus, 1979]; Anger Scale [Novaco, 1975]). Such measures are often used in combination with more global measures (MCMI; Millon, 1983).

Clinicians working with male batterers often find that such men fail to view themselves as having problems. In fact, many believe that their abusive treatment of their partners was justified. Such clinical anecdotal evidence is supported by group studies of abusive males. For example, Cantos, Neidig, and O'Leary (1993) found that violent men attributed their violence to external causes, most often blaming their wives for the violent episodes. Abusive men were less likely to justify their abusive behavior for the latest than for the first episode of violence. Thus, it appears that batterers consider several variables when evaluating their abusive behavior. Consequently, one limitation of existing measures used to assess abusive males is the failure to assess in a standardized fashion batterers's attitudes regarding the relative importance of partner, self, situational, and societal factors in motivating abuse. Additionally, existing measures were not designed for use by nonviolent couples or adults not currently in a relationship. This is unfortunate because such groups are logical targets of relationship violence prevention and educational programming.

Those working with battered women know that the psychological impact of wife abuse on its victims can be enormous and often complicates the physical trauma. Walker (1984) labeled the cluster of symptoms she observed in her battered clients the Battered Woman Syndrome (BWS) and categorized BWS as a subcategory of Post-Traumatic Stress Disorder (PTSD). It is likely that between 40% and 80% of women seeking treatment for battering will meet clinical criteria for PTSD (Houskamp & Foy, 1991; Kemp, Rawlings, & Green, 1991).

Symptomatic criteria for PTSD listed in the *Diagnostic and Statistical Manual of Mental Disorders* (American Psychiatric Association, 1994), as well as other problems of comorbidity, reflect behavioral, emotional, and physical symptoms commonly observed in response to psychological distress (Dutton, 1992). In addition, battered women frequently exhibit cognitive distortions that involve a sense of invulnerability, self-blame, an increased tolerance for abusive behavior ("normalizing" the violence), and an inability to identify the cognitive inconsistency of abuse within an intimate relationship.

Several measures have been used to assess the response of battered women to their battering experience (see Dutton, 1992; Petretic-Jackson & Jackson, in press, for a review). Assessment is supplemented with more global measures (MMPI-2; Butcher et al., 1989). Clinicians working with battered women note that many cognitive distortions relate to self-blame. Many battered women believe that their abusive treatment by their partners is justified by their own behavior or the circumstances of the assault. Such clinical anecdotal evidence is supported by group studies of battered women. In these studies battered women ascribed blame to both themselves and their partners, as well as to some aspect of their interaction within the relationship (Andrews & Brewin, 1990; Holtzworth-Munroe, 1988). They blamed their partners more and themselves less when the violence was of greater severity (Cascardi & O'Leary, 1992). It appears that self-blame is more likely when the woman is still in the relationship, and tends to involve behavioral rather than characterological attributions. Existing assessments used with battered women are limited by the general absence of standardized measures that adequately assess cognitive sequelae. Because behavioral self-blame is a common reaction, assessing attitudes regarding the relative importance of partner, self, situational, and societal factors in motivating abuse would be valuable in evaluating such self-blame.

The assessment of blame in wife abuse using a multidimensional scale has potential value, particularly given what is known about justifications offered for abuse by both batterers and battered women living in these relationships. A number of questions remain unanswered. To what extent are wives seen to be the instigators of their own abuse? Is the relationship between the batterer and his partner perceived to be responsible for abuse? Do abusive and nonabusive males, as well as abused and nonabused females, differ in their perceptions of the contributory roles assigned to different causal factors? To what extent is alcohol seen as a contributory versus a causal factor? Could different patterns of blame for abuse among batterers or battering victims predict differential amenability to treatment? Do attributions of blame affect attitudes about the appropriate target populations for prevention and treatment services?

THEORETICAL PERSPECTIVE

Since the 1970s a number of models have been developed in an attempt to explain family violence. Although parent-to-child violence has been the major focus in the theoretical literature, several conceptualizations of wife abuse have been offered in the last 20 years. They can be subsumed under one of the following broad categories: psychological (including emphasis on personality, social learning, and/or psychodynamic aspects of the batterer), family systems, feminist/sociological, and integrative approaches (Caesar & Hamberger, 1989). Common to each of the models is an attempt to understand the development of the abusive male in terms of both past and present influences. Each of the models varies in the emphasis it places on offender, situational, offender-victim relationship, and societal-cultural variables in explaining the causes of wife abuse.

The model of wife abuse developed by Walker (1979, 1984) focuses on a three-phase cycle theory of battering. In Phase 1, the tension-building stage, minor battering incidents occur. Minimization is common among women at this stage. In Phase 2, the acute battering incident occurs. Both the batterer and the battered woman accept the fact that anger is "out of control." The trigger for this incident is rarely the woman's behavior. It is more likely an external event coupled with the internal state of the man. The last phase involves contrite, loving behavior by the batterer. The batterer may appear sorry and guilty. He believes he can control his behavior, and also that he has "taught her such a lesson" that she will change her behavior and so he "will not be tempted to beat her" again (Walker, 1979, p. 66). According to Walker, the phases vary in time and intensity both within and between couples. Situation events often influence timing.

It also appears that the transition model of child abuse developed by Wolfe (1985) has much in common with Walker's model and accurately describes the course of battering. As with physical child abuse, a multiplicity of causal factors are hypothesized to contribute to the development and maintenance of battering. In the initial phase, the batterer's contributory role is emphasized. Batterer vulnerability, or diminished coping skills, creates a diathesis for wife abuse. Such vulnerability is thought to be influenced by family-of-origin and other social learning experiences. A man at risk for physically abusing his partner brings a reduced tolerance for stress and the disinhibition of aggression to the relationship. The coping skills of these men are taxed by current life stresses. The demands of an intimate relationship provide just one of many stressors in the batterer's environment. Often a perceived sense of loss of control creates the setting for coercive control of one's partner. In chronic cases of abuse, batterers show a pattern of more habitual arousal and aggression. Coercive and violent behaviors are reinforced because they tend to reduce unwanted partner behaviors, and the batterer temporarily regains a sense of control.

The multiple causal factors of domestic violence perpetrated against women by their partners (Sonkin et al., 1985) bears some correspondence to the causal factors of other forms of interpersonal violence. Clinical researchers have sampled various lay and professional groups for their attributions of blame for rape, incest, and child physical abuse. The theoretical model that guided the development of causal models in other areas of interpersonal violence was initially developed by Brodsky (1976). Blame is conceptualized as multidimensional in nature and is distributed among victim, perpetrator, situational/contextual, and societal factors. Scales assessing the distribution of blame for rape (Ward, 1980), incest (Jackson & Ferguson, 1983), and child physical abuse (Petretic-Jackson, 1992) have validated Brodsky's multidimensional model. These scales have been used with different groups in educational, preventive, and treatment contexts.

DEVELOPMENT OF THE DOMESTIC VIOLENCE BLAME SCALE (DVBS)

The Domestic Violence Blame Scale (DVBS) was designed to assess blame attribution for domestic violence/wife abuse in an effort to assess whether the levels of blame assigned to the battering victim (e.g., wife) and the batterer, as well as situational variables and societal attitudes supporting wife abuse, would follow the pattern established with rape and incest blame. The DVBS has existed as a clinical research scale for approximately 7 years. It has also been used in clinical settings and applications, with the requisite psychometric precautions, during that time.

The DVBS is a 23-item self-report questionnaire (see pp. 272-275). An item pool of 32 items was generated using the rational-empirical method following a survey of the wife abuse literature. A number of items in the preliminary 32-item scale corresponded to items on existing standardized rape and incest blame scales. These items represented victim, perpetrator, societal, and situational variables common to the different forms of abuse. The remaining items addressed unique aspects of wife abuse with regard to these four variables.

Item format followed the model used in existing interpersonal violence blame attribution scales. Items were scored using a 6-point scale with "1" representing strong disagreement and "6" representing strong agreement with the statement in question. The definition of domestic violence provided with the DVBS was restricted to physical assault or violence between marital partners and identified the husband as the assailant and the wife as the victim.

The DVBS was administered to 424 young adults (mean age = 21.5 years). Respondents were predominantly single, Caucasian, and from Midwestern backgrounds. Following administration of the scale to the entire group, half of the sample had their 32-item preliminary DVBS scores subjected to factor analytic procedures. Based on these analyses, 23 items were retained. This procedure yielded four blame factors. Using the 23-item version of the DVBS, the remaining questionnaires were subjected to factor analytic procedures for cross-validation purposes. Because the results of this analysis supported the initial factor analytic procedure, all questionnaires were then combined and the 23-item DVBS was subjected to another factor analysis. Four meaningful, independent attributional blame factors were extracted as had been predicted, accounting for 48% of the data variable variance.

This sample provided normative data for the DVBS. The multidimensional nature of blame distribution obtained with domestic violence confirmed that previously obtained with rape and incest blame. The final DVBS factor structure, based on the responses of the combined standardization and cross-validation samples, is composed of four blame factors: Situational Blame, Perpetrator Blame, Societal Blame, and Victim Blame.

The first or Situational Blame factor is defined by five items that assign blame for wife abuse to situational or contextual variables. Individuals scoring high on this factor consider various family conditions and the abuser's use of alcohol/drugs as important contributors to spousal violence.

The second factor (Perpetrator Blame) is defined by five items that pertain to husband blame. Individuals obtaining high scores on this factor believe that battering husbands are mentally ill/psychologically disturbed, unable to control their violent behavior, learned violent behavior from aggressive fathers, and should be locked up for abusing their wives.

Six items associated with the third DVBS factor (Societal Blame) assign blame to societal values. Individuals scoring high on this factor consider the amount of sex and violence in the media, wives being regarded as property, a male-dominated society, and wife beating as acceptable masculine behavior in marriage as contributing to the occurrence of spouse abuse.

Seven items associated with the fourth factor are consistent with the construct of Victim Blame. Individuals scoring high on this factor believe that wives encourage or provoke domestic violence, deserve physical assaults, and exaggerate the effects of domestic violence. They also believe that the rise of the "women's movement" has contributed to increased wife abuse.

Mean factor scores for the combined samples as well as for health care professionals are presented in a subsequent section of this contribution. These scores indicate the absolute magnitude of blame ascribed to the four blame factors and provide a relative rank ordering of blame for victim, perpetrator, and contextual factors. A comparison of relative factor score means obtained by men and women indicates different patterns of overall order, or ranking, of blame assignment as well as differences in the individual factor score magnitudes. In terms of relative blame factor rankings, females blamed the husband most for wife abuse, followed by situational variables. Males, however, placed the greatest blame for wife abuse on situational variables, and the husband was assigned a secondary degree of blame. Society was ranked third by both males and females. Finally, wives were blamed the least by both sexes. When blame factor means for the total sample were calculated, situational variables were blamed most, followed by the husband, society, and the wife. This pattern of ascribing more blame to situational as opposed to husband factors represents the only form of interpersonal violence wherein offenders for crimes committed against women are not assigned the most blame. Clearly, domestic violence is viewed as a unique form of interpersonal violence by the lay public, with the perceived dynamics differing from rape and incest. Unlike rape and incest blame, in domestic violence, the defined perpetrator of the crime is not held the most responsible for its occurrence. Comparing scores of males and females for each factor indicated that males rated situational variables as significantly more important than did females. Females blamed both the batterer and societal variables to a greater extent for wife abuse than did males. Finally, despite the fact that both males and females had ascribed the least amount of relative blame to the victim, males blamed the victim to a significantly greater extent than did females.

SCORING

A scoring template is presented following the actual DVBS in this contribution (p. 275). We have found it helpful to present the factor scores as means, corresponding to the 6-point format. In this way, the higher the score, the more weight or blame is assigned to the factor in question.

For clinical use, individual item analysis may prove to be useful. However, given the face validity of items, the absence of a "lie" scale, and limited clinical norms for an abusive sample, the validity of using factor scores for predicting clients at risk of abuse or of determining the severity of risk for clients in treatment for wife abuse is questionable.

For the purposes of comparison, the total normative sample obtained the following factor mean scores: Situational Blame = 4.2; Perpetrator Blame = 4.1; Societal Blame = 3.4; and Victim Blame = 2.2. Factor scores for various professional groups are provided in the section below.

APPLICATIONS

The DVBS is designed for use in both research and clinical settings. However, at this point in its development, the efficacy of its use as a standardized clinical tool has not yet been fully established. Both adult nonabusive professional and lay public norms are available as standards of comparison.

The DVBS has been used in several studies of adults sampled from professional populations. Psychologists, physicians, and mental health professionals have been administered the scale. In a surprising lack of contrast to the normative sample, both regional and national samples of mental health professionals ($N = 153$; $N = 437$) (Petretic-Jackson, Sandberg, & Jackson, 1994; White & Petretic-Jackson, 1992) and physicians ($N = 145$) (Tarver & Jackson, 1992) obtained factor mean scores and rankings similar to the standardization sample. Factor means for mental health professionals were: Situational Blame = 4.3; Perpetrator Blame = 3.7; Situational Blame = 3.7; and Victim Blame = 1.9. For physicians, the factor score means were: Situational Blame = 4.5; Perpetrator Blame = 4.0; Societal Blame = 3.3; and Victim Blame = 2.1.

Male physicians and mental health workers obtained higher victim blame scores. Male physicians also made fewer mental health referrals. Correspondingly, mental health workers with higher victim blame scores made fewer referrals for ancillary services (shelters, legal assistance) and were less likely to develop a protection plan for victims. Greater victim blame was associated with a greater likelihood to utilize systems as opposed to individual therapy, while greater societal blame was associated with utilization of individual treatment. Thus attitudes regarding victim blame are associated with different case disposition and choice of interventions in treatment.

College students, mental health professionals, and physicians obtained quite similar factor mean scores and virtually identical blame factor rankings, suggesting similar attributions across the three groups. Again, unlike blame distribution for rape and incest, where the perpetrator is ascribed the most blame, respondents assign the most blame for the occurrence of domestic violence to situational variables, followed by the perpetrator, society, and the victim.

The emergence of four separate, psychologically meaningful factor constructs from the DVBS provides empirical support for the hypothesis that distribution of blame in domestic violence is multidimensional. As in other crimes of violence against females, such as rape and incest, domestic violence blame is distributed among offender, victim, societal, and situational factors. However, for male respondents in the standardization and cross-validation groups, as well as health and mental health care professionals in subsequent surveys, the order in which the four factors were assigned degree of blame differed significantly from that found in blame distribution studies involving rape and incest. In the present study, contextual/situational variables (e.g., unstable homes, social isolation, alcohol and drug abuse) were assigned the most blame, whereas in crimes of sexual abuse against females, the offender was held the most responsible (Jackson & Ferguson, 1983; Resick & Jackson, 1981). However, this pattern shows a closer correspondence with findings on blame attributions for child physical abuse (Petretic-Jackson, 1992). Although child victims of family physical violence are assigned less absolute blame than adult victims of such violence, the relative pattern of assigning blame is similar. In both wife physical abuse and child physical abuse, situational variables are assigned the most blame.

The results of our surveys of health and mental health professionals have important clinical implications. Individuals who provide services to victims of spouse violence and their abusing partners may hold beliefs that could influence the type, quality, and appropriateness of services they offer. The gender of the service provider as well as adherence to victim-blaming attitudes has a direct impact on their choice of interventions and use of ancillary services, and thus warrants further consideration. Knowledge of distribution of blame in marital violence by medical, legal, and mental health service providers of both sexes has concrete and practical applications for improving service delivery.

The DVBS can also serve as a valuable pre-post assessment instrument in the treatment of battered wives and violent husbands, although the DVBS should not be used as the sole means of assessing changes in the attribution of blame for wife abuse. The clinician may use the DVBS as only one tool in a comprehensive assessment battery which also includes a variety of standardized behavioral and personality measures.

Therapist-client discussion of the responses on a DVBS administered prior to treatment may serve a therapeutic function. For example, items on the Victim Blame factor might be used with battering males to initiate discussion concerning common misperceptions of a partner's behaviors. Victim blame item responses can be used to assess victim self-blame. Similarly, discussion of situational triggers could initiate discussion of stressors and specifically to identify client misperceptions regarding alcohol use as a causal factor. Perceptions of the abusive male regarding control are useful initiating discussion of the cognitive-affective link in abuse.

The DVBS can be used as a clinical tool to assess attitude changes which occur both during and following treatment. For victims, changes in self-blame over the course of treatment can be determined by comparing scores on the victim factor as well as relative shifts in other factors over the course of treatment. Similarly, the tendency of batterers to minimize responsibility and inappropriately focus blame on the victim and/or external circumstances (i.e., alcohol) could be assessed in a standardized fashion by examining both individual item as well as scores for victim, offender, and situation factors. Changes in batterers' scores over time could also serve as evidence that the treatment goal of accepting responsibility for violence is being met.

Given that the Domestic Violence Blame Scale is an attitude survey, one could argue that there are no "right" or "wrong" scores. It does seem reasonable to believe, however, that attitudes affect behavior, and DVBS scores were related to treatment and referral practices in two professional groups. This would argue that professionals could use the DVBS to serve the best interests of their clients. In light of current treatment approaches to battering, therapists could use the scale to assess client progress toward the treatment goal of increased responsibility taking on the part of batterers and the goal of decreased self-blame on the part of victims.

DOMESTIC VIOLENCE BLAME SCALE (DVBS)

In this survey, domestic violence is defined as physical assaults or violence between marital partners. For the purposes of this survey, the husband will always be the *assailant,* and the wife will be the *victim*. Listed below are several statements sometimes used to account for domestic violence. Please indicate your agreement/disagreement with or perception of the frequency of these statements on the six-point scale accompanying each item. While some of these items might be offensive to you, please remember that they do not represent facts per se, but are attitudes often used to account for the occurrence of domestic violence. If you agree with a statement, please place an X over the blank that corresponds to the degree of your agreement. If you disagree with a statement, place an X over the blank that corresponds with the amount you disagree.

For example:

A. Most tooth decay is caused by a lack of careful brushing.

| Strongly Disagree | 1 | 2 | 3 | 4 | X 5 | 6 | Strongly Agree |

An X above the 5 would indicate a strong amount of agreement. Please answer the following questions based on your opinion only. There are no right or wrong answers.

1. The amount of sex and violence in the media today strongly influences the husband to physically assault his wife.

| Strongly Disagree | 1 | 2 | 3 | 4 | 5 | 6 | Strongly Agree |

2. Domestic violence is a result of wives being regarded as property by our society.

| Strongly Disagree | 1 | 2 | 3 | 4 | 5 | 6 | Strongly Agree |

3. A husband who physically assaults his wife should be locked up for the act.

| Almost Never | 1 | 2 | 3 | 4 | 5 | 6 | Almost Always |

4. A husband who physically assaults his wife is "mentally ill" or psychologically disturbed.

| Strongly Disagree | 1 | 2 | 3 | 4 | 5 | 6 | Strongly Agree |

5. Domestic violence can be mainly attributed to peculiarities in the husband's personality.

| Strongly Disagree | 1 | 2 | 3 | 4 | 5 | 6 | Strongly Agree |

6. It is the wife who provokes the husband to physically assault her.

| Almost Never | 1 | 2 | 3 | 4 | 5 | 6 | Almost Always |

7. Domestic violence is the product of a male-dominated society.

| Strongly Disagree | 1 | 2 | 3 | 4 | 5 | 6 | Strongly Agree |

8. Wives encourage domestic violence by using bad judgment, provoking the husband's anger, and so on.

| Almost Never | 1 | 2 | 3 | 4 | 5 | 6 | Almost Always |

9. Wives are physically assaulted by their husbands because they deserve it.

| Almost Never | 1 | 2 | 3 | 4 | 5 | 6 | Almost Always |

10. Domestic violence can be avoided by the wife trying harder to please her husband.

| Almost Never | 1 | 2 | 3 | 4 | 5 | 6 | Almost Always |

11. Domestic violence is more likely to occur in unstable homes.

| Strongly Disagree | 1 | 2 | 3 | 4 | 5 | 6 | Strongly Agree |

12. Domestic violence is more likely to occur in families with poor interpersonal relationships.

| Strongly Disagree | 1 | 2 | 3 | 4 | 5 | 6 | Strongly Agree |

13. The husband's abuse of alcohol and drugs causes domestic violence.

| Almost Never | 1 | 2 | 3 | 4 | 5 | 6 | Almost Always |

14. Domestic violence occurs because society accepts it in marriage.

| Strongly Disagree | 1 | 2 | 3 | 4 | 5 | 6 | Strongly Agree |

15. Domestic violence is more likely to occur in slum or "bad" areas.

| Strongly Disagree | 1 | 2 | 3 | 4 | 5 | 6 | Strongly Agree |

16. As stress on the marriage increases, so does the probability of domestic violence.

| Strongly Disagree | 1 | 2 | 3 | 4 | 5 | 6 | Strongly Agree |

17. Domestic violence is more likely to occur in families that are socially isolated from the community.

| Strongly Disagree | 1 | 2 | 3 | 4 | 5 | 6 | Strongly Agree |

18. Husbands who physically assault their wives cannot control their violent behavior.

    Strongly ____ ____ ____ ____ ____ ____ Strongly
    Disagree   1   2   3   4   5   6   Agree

19. Husbands who physically assault their wives had dominant, aggressive fathers who also engaged in domestic violence.

    Strongly ____ ____ ____ ____ ____ ____ Strongly
    Disagree   1   2   3   4   5   6   Agree

20. The rise of the "women's movement" and feminism has increased the occurrence of domestic violence.

    Strongly ____ ____ ____ ____ ____ ____ Strongly
    Disagree   1   2   3   4   5   6   Agree

21. Wives exaggerate the physical and psychological effects of domestic violence.

    Strongly ____ ____ ____ ____ ____ ____ Strongly
    Disagree   1   2   3   4   5   6   Agree

22. In our society, it is a husband's prerogative to strike his wife in his own home.

    Strongly ____ ____ ____ ____ ____ ____ Strongly
    Disagree   1   2   3   4   5   6   Agree

23. Husbands physically strike their wives because in our society this is defined as acceptable masculine behavior.

    Strongly ____ ____ ____ ____ ____ ____ Strongly
    Disagree   1   2   3   4   5   6   Agree

SCORING TEMPLATE FOR THE DVBS

Note: Sum item scores within each factor to obtain the factor total score. Divide by the number of items on factor to yield factor mean score.

FACTOR	ITEM NUMBER	SCORE	TOTAL	MEAN
Situational Blame	11	_____		
	12	_____		
	13	_____		
	15	_____		
	17	_____		
	Total for Situational Blame Factor		_____ ÷ 5 =	☐
Perpetrator Blame	3	_____		
	4	_____		
	5	_____		
	18	_____		
	19	_____		
	Total for Perpetrator Blame Factor		_____ ÷ 5 =	☐
Societal Blame	1	_____		
	2	_____		
	7	_____		
	14	_____		
	16	_____		
	23	_____		
	Total for Societal Blame Factor		_____ ÷ 6 =	☐
Victim Blame	6	_____		
	8	_____		
	9	_____		
	10	_____		
	20	_____		
	21	_____		
	22	_____		
	Total for Victim Blame Factor		_____ ÷ 7 =	☐

Patricia Petretic-Jackson, PhD, is currently an Associate Professor in Clinical Psychology at the University of Arkansas. She completed her doctoral work in developmental psychology at Bowling Green State University and post-doctoral lateral retraining in clinical psychology at the University of South Dakota. Prior to her present position, she was on the faculty at the University of South Dakota. She has specialized in clinical treatment of victims of family violence for the last 10 years. Dr. Petretic-Jackson may be contacted at Psychology Department, University of Arkansas, Fayetteville, AR 72701.

Genell Sandberg, PhD, is currently in private practice at Parkview Psychological Services in Sioux City, Iowa. She received her doctoral training in clinical psychology at the University of South Dakota, and completed a post-doctoral fellowship at the University of Washington. Dr. Sandberg can be contacted through the first author.

Thomas L. Jackson, PhD, is Professor and Director of Clinical Training in the Department of Psychology at the University of Arkansas. Dr. Jackson may be contacted at Department of Psychology, 216 Memorial Hall, University of Arkansas, Fayetteville, AR 72701.

RESOURCES

American Psychiatric Association. (1994). *Diagnostic and Statistical Manual of Mental Disorders* (4th ed.). Washington, DC: Author.

American Psychological Association Task Force. (1984, November). In A. S. Kahn (Ed.), *Victims of Crime and Violence: Final Report of the APA Task Force.* Washington, DC: Author.

Andrews, B., & Brewin, A. (1990). Attributions of blame for marital violence: A study of antecedents and consequences. *Journal of Marriage and the Family, 52,* 757-767.

Brodsky, S. (1976). Sexual assault: Perspectives on prevention and assailants. In M. Walker & S. Brodsky (Eds.), *Sexual Assault: The Victim and the Rapist* (pp. 1-8). Lexington, MA: Lexington Press.

Butcher, J. N., Dahlstrom, W. G., Graham, J. R., Tellegen, A. M., & Kaemmer, B. (1989). *MMPI-2: Manual for Administration and Scoring.* Minneapolis, MN: University of Minnesota Press.

Caesar, P. L., & Hamberger, L. K. (1989). *Treating Men Who Batter: Theory, Practice, and Programs.* New York: Springer.

Cantos, A. L., Neidig, P., & O'Leary, K. D. (1993). Men's and women's attributions of blame for domestic violence. *Journal of Family Violence, 8,* 289-302.

Cascardi, M., & O'Leary, K. D. (1992). Depressive symptomatology, self-esteem and self-blame in battered women. *Journal of Family Violence, 7,* 249-259.

Davis, L. V. (1987). Battered women: The transformation of a social problem. *Social Work, 32,* 306-311.

Dutton, M. (1992). *Empowering and Healing the Battered Woman.* New York: Springer.

Easteal, P. W., & Easteal, S. (1992). Attitudes and practices of doctors toward spouse assault victims: An Australian study. *Violence and Victims, 7,* 217-228.

Ewing, C. P., & Aubrey, M. (1987). Battered women and public opinion: Some realities about the myths. *Journal of Family Violence, 2,* 257-264.

Follingstad, D., Neckerman, A., & Vrombrock, J. (1988). Reactions to victimization and coping strategies of battered women: The ties that bind. *Clinical Psychology Review, 8,* 373-390.

Foy, D. W. (1992). Introduction and description of the disorder. In D. W. Foy (Ed.), *Treating PTSD: Cognitive-Behavioral Strategies* (pp. 1-12). New York: Guilford.

Gelles, R. (1974). *The Violent Home: A Study of Physical Aggression Between Husbands and Wives.* Beverly Hills, CA: Sage.

Gelles, R. (1980). Violence in the family: A review of research in the seventies. *Journal of Marriage and the Family, 42,* 873-885.

Gelles, R., & Strauss, M. (1988). *Intimate Violence: The Causes and Consequences of Abuse in the American Family.* New York: Simon & Schuster.

Hall-Apicella, V. (1983, August). *Exploring Attitudes of Mental Health Professionals Toward Battered Women.* Paper presented at the annual convention of the American Psychological Association, Anaheim, CA.

Hamberger, L. K., & Hastings, J. E. (1986). Personality correlates of men who abuse their partners: A cross-validation study. *Journal of Family Violence, 1,* 323-341.

Hamberger, L. K., & Hastings, J. E. (1988). Characteristics of male spouse abusers consistent with personality disorders. *Hospital and Community Psychiatry, 39,* 763-770.

Hamberger, L. K., & Lohr, J. M. (1989). Proximal causes of spouse abuse: A theoretical analysis for cognitive-behavioral interventions. In P. L. Caesar & L. K. Hamberger (Eds.), *Treating Men Who Batter: Theory, Practice, and Programs* (pp. 53-76). New York: Springer.

Hart, B. (1993). Battered women and the justice system. *American Behavioral Scientist, 36,* 624-638.

Hillier, L., & Foddy, M. (1993). The role of observer attitudes in judgments of blame in cases of wife assault. *Sex Roles, 29,* 629-644.

Hofeller, K. H. (1982). *Social, Psychological and Situational Factors in Wife Abuse.* Palo Alto, CA: R. & E. Research Associates.

Holtzworth-Munroe, A. (1988). Causal attributions in marital violence: Theoretical and methodological issues. *Clinical Psychology Review, 8,* 331-344.

Houskamp, B. M., & Foy, D. W. (1991). The assessment of posttraumatic stress disorder in battered women. *Journal of Interpersonal Violence, 6,* 367-375.

Jackson, T. L., & Ferguson, W. P. (1983). Attribution of blame in incest. *American Journal of Community Psychology, 11,* 313-322.

Kemp, A., Rawlings, E., & Green, B. (1991). Post-traumatic stress disorder (PTSD) in battered women: A shelter sample. *Journal of Traumatic Stress, 4,* 137-148.

Martin, D. (1985). Domestic violence: A sociological perspective. In D. J. Sonkin, D. Martin, & L. E. A. Walker (Eds.), *The Male Batterer: A Treatment Approach* (pp. 1-32). New York: Springer.

McCann, I. L., Sakheim, D., & Abrahamson, D. (1988). Trauma and victimization: A model of psychological adaptation. *The Counseling Psychologist, 16,* 531-594.

Millon, T. (1983). *Millon Clinical Multiaxial Inventory Manual.* Minneapolis, MN: Interpretive Scoring Systems.

Novaco, R. W. (1975). *Anger Control: The Development and Evaluation of an Experimental Treatment.* Lexington, MA: Lexington Books.

Petretic-Jackson, P. A. (1992). The Child Abuse Blame Scale-Physical Abuse (CABS-PA): Assessing blame for child physical abuse. In L. VandeCreek, S. Knapp, & T. L. Jackson (Eds.), *Innovations in Clinical Practice: A Source Book* (Vol. 11, pp. 315-324). Sarasota, FL: Professional Resource Press.

Petretic-Jackson, P., & Jackson, T. L. (in press). Mental health interventions with battered women: Professional attitudes, assessment techniques, treatment strategies, and case illustrations. In A. Roberts (Ed.), *Helping Battered Women: New Remedies.* New York: Oxford Press.

Petretic-Jackson, P., Sandberg, G., & Jackson, T. L. (1994). *Mental Health Professionals' Spouse Abuse Blame Distribution: Correlates to Duty to Warn.* Manuscript submitted for publication.

Resick, P. A., & Jackson, T. L. (1981). Attitudes toward rape among mental health professionals. *American Journal of Community Psychology, 9,* 481-490.

Sonkin, D. J., Martin, D., & Walker, L. E. A. (1985). *The Male Batterer: A Treatment Approach.* New York: Springer.

Stark, E., & Flitcraft, A. (1988). Personal power and institutional victimization: Treating the dual trauma of woman battering. In F. M. Ochberg (Ed.), *Post-Traumatic Therapy and Victims of Violence* (pp. 115-151). New York: Brunner/Mazel.

Stets, J., & Straus, M. (1989). The marriage license as a hitting license: A comparison of assaults in dating, cohabiting, and married couples. In M. Pirog-Good & J. Stets (Eds.), *Violence in Dating Relationships: Emerging Social Issues* (pp. 33-52). New York: Praeger.

Straus, M. A. (1979). Measuring intrafamily conflict and violence: The conflict tactics (CT) scales. *Journal of Marriage and the Family, 41,* 75-88.

Tarver, D., & Jackson, T. L. (1992, August). *Physician Blame Attribution in Domestic Violence Cases.* Paper presented at the annual convention of the American Psychological Association, Washington, DC.

Thorne-Finch, R. (1992). *Ending the Silence: The Origins and Treatment of Male Violence Against Women.* Toronto: University of Toronto Press.

Walker, L. E. A. (1979). *The Battered Woman.* New York: Harper & Row.

Walker, L. E. A. (1984). *The Battered Woman Syndrome.* New York: Springer.

Ward, M. (1980). *Attribution of Rape Blame Scale.* Unpublished manuscript, University of South Dakota, Vermillion, SD.

White, P., & Petretic-Jackson, P. (1992, August). *Psychologists' Patterns of Blame Attribution for Wife Abuse.* Paper presented at the annual meeting of the American Psychological Association, Washington, DC.

Wolfe, D. (1985). *Child Abuse: Implications for Child Development and Psychopathology.* Newbury Park, CA: Sage.

THE VIOLENCE ATTITUDES SCALE (VAS)

*Thomas L. Jackson, Richard D. Dienst, Terry L. Efird,
Brenda D. Mobley, David A. Schroeder, April D. Hout,
Julleah C. Montecillo, and Andrea L. LaBine*

The incidence of violent crime in the United States continues to attract increasing professional and public attention. Statistics from the Uniform Crime Reporting Program (U.S. Department of Justice, 1994) indicate that violent crimes such as murder and nonnegligent manslaughter, robbery, forcible rape, and aggravated assault have, for the most part, steadily increased in the last decade. The incidence of violent offenses in 1993 was over 15% higher than 5 years ago, and 40% greater than a decade ago. Data compiled in 1993 indicated that the nation's cities were the most dangerous areas, although suburban and rural living environments were also significantly affected by violence (U.S. Department of Justice, 1994).

Of additional importance is the public's perception of the occurrence of violent crime. Recent public media survey polls find between 55% and 65% of the respondents feel afraid for their safety because of perceived increases in violent crime. Clearly, the American public has become sensitive to the problem of violence in our society.

The psychological consequences of being a victim of crime can be enormous (Ellis, Black, & Resick, 1992). Post-Traumatic Stress Disorder (PTSD) is reportedly exhibited by up to two-thirds of crime victims, with even higher PTSD symptomatology among victims of rape and incest. The PTSD symptoms most frequently and consistently reported by crime victims include fear, anxiety, depression, and vegetative complaints (Ellis et al., 1992). Victims of violent crime are not the only ones affected by violence. Those individuals who are related to or in close contact with actual victims of an assault can also suffer significant symptomatology (Jackson, in press).

The increases in violent crime, the public's heightened awareness of and sensitivity to violence, and the significant negative impact of violence on victims provided the impetus for the development and cross-validation of the Violence Attitudes Scale (VAS; see pp. 285-289). The VAS can be used to delineate violence blame attitudes, to delineate the presence of PTSD and other related symptoms, and to provide clinicians with clear evidence of therapeutic progress in victims and perpetrators of violence. The VAS can also be used in forensic processes and assessment of professional and institutional attitudes and biases involving violent crime.

ATTITUDES TOWARD VIOLENCE

In recent years the American public has come to believe that assaultive behaviors are multidetermined. Essentially, the public often perceives the perpetrator as being driven to commit violent acts due to economic pressures, an impoverished upbringing, violent subcultures, and so on. The public also appears to assign some degree of responsibility for crimes to society, to situations, and, to a lesser extent, the victim for dangerous behaviors or bad judgment. This multidimensional approach to responsibility was first hypothesized with regard to the crime of rape (Brodsky, 1976). Rape blame was posited to be distributed across not only perpetrator factors, but also societal, situational, and victim blame dimensions. Several studies have provided validation for the multidimensional nature of blame distribution for rape, incest, and domestic violence (e.g., the Jackson Incest Blame Scale [JIBS; Jackson & Ferguson, 1983], the Attribution of Rape Blame Scale [ARBS; Resick & Jackson, 1981], and the Domestic Violence Blame Scale [DVBS; Petretic-Jackson, Sandberg, & Jackson, 1994]). These scales allow for comparisons of relative levels of blame for the specific crimes of rape, incest, and domestic violence distributed to victims, perpetrators, and situational and societal factors. For example, for the crimes of rape and incest, both lay public and professional samples have been found to distribute blame across (in order from most to least blamed) offender, situational, societal, and victim factors. For the crime of domestic violence, results derived from lay public and professional samples indicated that situational variables were blamed most for the occurrence of relationship violence, followed closely by the offender, society, and the victim. Additionally, significant gender differences have been found for rape, incest, and domestic violence blame, with males evidencing significantly less offender blame and significantly greater victim blame than female respondents. This finding generalizes across samples of college students, attorneys and judges, mental health professionals, and physicians (Jackson & Sandberg, 1985; Morris & Jackson, 1989; Resick & Jackson, 1981; Tarver & Jackson, 1992). These scales have been utilized to aid in jury selection, expert witness testimony, forensic evaluations of perpetrators' attitudes, and the assessment of the severity of negative effects on victims.

The ability to assess perceived blame for violent crime in general using a multidimensional scale may have significant potential descriptive value, because previous research in sexual assault has found that blame distribution patterns are affected by gender and assault history. The consequences of the assaults, attorney and judge sentencing preferences, and health care professional treatment practices may also be influenced by different levels and rank orders of blame factors (Jackson & Sandberg, 1985; Morris & Jackson, 1989; Resick & Jackson, 1981; Tarver & Jackson, 1992). For example, as sexual assault victim blame increases, preferred prison sentences for perpetrators decreases (Jackson & Sandberg, 1985; Morris & Jackson, 1989). Finally, educational programs can significantly modify blame distribution, increasing perpetrator blame and decreasing victim blame for the occurrence of sexual assaults (Jackson et al., 1989). Taken together, the preceding findings suggest that an empirically derived violence blame scale might prove helpful in such arenas as the development of victim treatment protocols and offender education, and relapse-prevention programs. Such a scale could also offer forensic experts additional information regarding the complexity of perceptions of culpability for violence, enhancing their effectiveness with regard to forensic evaluations and expert witness testimony.

DEVELOPMENT OF THE VIOLENCE ATTITUDES SCALE (VAS)

The development of the VAS was accomplished in two parts. The first, or standardization study, used 308 subjects and utilized an 80-item scale. Following initial factor analysis, the scale was revised to its current 38-item format and cross-validation was accomplished using 301 subjects. The resulting 5-factor VAS is felt to be psychometrically sound and yields substantive information regarding a respondent's blame distribution pattern for violence. Violence blame distribution was also found to be significantly associated with previous exposure to violence, gender, and relevant criminal behavior and adjudication histories.

THEORETICAL UNDERPINNINGS OF THE ORIGINAL ITEM POOL

Previously mentioned blame distribution scales (ARBS, JIBS, & DVBS) have relied on Brodsky's (1976) model for the multidimensionality of rape blame. However, the crimes of rape, incest, and domestic violence share a common characteristic not necessarily found in violent crime in general - prior relationship between the victim and the perpetrator. Perpetrators and victims in the crimes of incest and domestic violence, by definition, have a preexisting relationship, either by blood, marriage, or dating history. Violent crimes, however, do not necessarily possess the characteristic of a perpetrator-victim familiarity. For this reason, the original item pool construction for the VAS was not constrained by Brodsky's four blame factors. Rather, the authors developed an 80-item pool using a rational test construction method, based on existing literature dealing with factors that contribute to the occurrence of violent crime. Items were scored on a 6-point, forced choice continuum, with a rating of 1 representing strong disagreement and a rating of 6 representing strong agreement with the specific blame item.

STANDARDIZATION AND CROSS-VALIDATION OF THE VAS

The initial 80-item Violence Attitudes Scale (VAS) was administered to 308 undergraduate university students. Demographically, 54% of the sample were female, 46% were male, and the mean age of the sample was 20.8 years. The majority (84%) of the sample were Caucasian. Factor analysis of the initial scale revealed five factors, utilizing 38 of the original 80 items, accounting for approximately 50% of the variance. These results, which demonstrated multidimensional blame distribution for violence as well as the impact of gender and prior victimization on violence blame, led to the following cross-validation attempt of the 38-item VAS.

Three hundred and one additional university subjects participated in the cross-validation of the revised VAS questionnaire. Forty-seven percent of these subjects were male, 53% female, and 88% Caucasian. Their mean age was 20.3 years. Thirty-two percent of the subjects reported having been personally exposed to violent crime, 58% reported that a friend had been exposed, and 34% reported that a family member had been exposed. A total of 76% of the subjects reported having had some direct or indirect exposure to violent crime. These figures were consistent with the standardization sample.

Factor analytic procedures were performed on the 38 questionnaire items to reassess the basic dimensionality of the scale, resulting in the extraction of five factors, accounting for 44% of the variance.

The final five VAS factors corresponded to the blame dimensions (in rank order, from most strongly endorsed):

1. Preferred criminal sanctions and perpetrator consequences
2. Societal and family values
3. Perpetrator internal characteristics
4. Gang-related issues and ethnicity
5. Victim blame

These derived factors comprise the VAS in its final form.

VAS BLAME FACTORS

Factor one, the Perpetrator Consequences factor, consists of nine items sampling attitudes toward the consequences of violent crime and ascribing the occurrence of violent crime to insufficient punishment for perpetrators. Individuals scoring high on this factor advocate stricter laws and harsher punishment to decrease violent crime, believe in capital punishment, and generally subscribe to a strong retributive model of incarceration. Low scorers believe that lengthy incarceration and decreased privileges for violent perpetrators do not significantly decrease the incidence and prevalence of violent crime.

Factor two, the Social Morality factor, includes eight items wherein the blame for violent crime is placed on social values and norms. High scorers on this factor associate the occurrence of violent crime with increased divorce rates, substance abuse, unhealthy societal morals, a decreased emphasis on family values, and the stressful nature of our society.

Factor three, the Perpetrator factor, incorporates seven items that assign the blame for violent crime to offender characteristics. High scorers tend to believe that such internal characteristics as low tolerance for frustration, poor anger control, alcohol and substance abuse, and loss of control lead to an increase in violent crime.

Factor four, the Ethnicity factor, is defined by seven items that assign blame for violent crime to ethnic minority involvement. Individuals scoring high on this factor believe that ethnic minorities are involved in a large portion of the violent crimes that are committed in our society.

The final factor, Victim Blame, is comprised of seven items that place the blame for violent crime on the object of the violence. Individuals who score high on this factor tend to believe that victims bring violent crimes upon themselves, can avoid these situations, and deserve to be victimized because they use bad judgment and place themselves in danger.

SCORING THE VAS

A template for scoring the VAS can be found following the presentation of the VAS (p. 289). Because items do not overlap across the factors, the means of the five independent factors are obtained. Items are scored using the 6-point, forced-choice rating, with higher scores representing greater overall blame. The sum of the ratings for the items on each factor is divided by the number of items in that factor. The higher the mean score for the factor, the greater the responsibility or blame the individual places on that construct for the occurrence of violent crime.

For comparisons, the cross-validation derived factor means were: Perpetrator Consequences = 4.6; Social Morality = 4.2; Perpetrator = 4.1; Ethnicity = 3.6; and Victim = 2.7. The extent to which a client's or subject's scores differ from these means depends largely on the presenting complaint and/or progress in treatment. Typically, the goals of treatment would involve decreasing inappropriate Victim blame, increasing Perpetrator blame, and further exploring the other factors regarding violence in our society. Clinically, it is important to consider blame factor mean rankings as potentially indicative of biases, inappropriate self-blame, or externalization of blame. Individual item analysis may also prove to be useful in a clinical setting.

The use of the VAS in *voir dire* proceedings is probably self-explanatory and would differ only according to whether it was being used by prosecution or defense experts.

ADDITIONAL VIOLENCE BLAME FINDINGS

In addition to the five factor scores derived from the VAS, several other significant findings from this research should be considered. Foremost among these findings, alluded to in the scoring section, are blame factor rankings. The present, combined samples assigned the most blame to the Perpetrator Consequences factor, followed by the Social Morality, Perpetrator, and Ethnicity factors. They placed the least blame on the Victim factor, but, as in previous blame distribution research, they did not hold the victim completely blameless. Conversely, recently collected data from an incarcerated felon sample (Efird & Jackson, 1994) found both violent and nonviolent felons placing greater blame for violence on perpetrator characteristics and social morality, and reported significant disagreement that harsher perpetrator consequences would decrease violent crime.

The relationship between gender, prior victimization, and VAS factor structure must also be considered when using the VAS. For the present samples, analyses of variance were performed on the five obtained VAS blame factors and factor means were compared across the gender and prior exposure to violence variables.

The Analysis of Variance (ANOVA) performed on the Perpetrator Consequences factor demonstrated a significant difference for prior victimization level, $F(3,284) = 4.62, p < .01$. Although all groups agreed that harsher consequences should be imposed on perpetrators, individuals who had been personally exposed to violence believed this to a lesser degree than did the group with no prior violent crime exposure. Essentially, victims of violence preferred lighter perpetrator sentences than nonvictims. Although this finding may seem counterintuitive, we believe it stems from the aforementioned inappropriate self-blame that victims of assaults often exhibit. This self-blame symptom is seen most often in victims of sexual assault, but now seems at least indirectly supported in the area of violent crime in general. Victims of violence apparently prefer less punishment for perpetrators because they blame themselves for their own victimization. Again, these issues are believed to be important to the therapy process and support our contention that the VAS may serve a useful role in treatment.

A significant gender difference was also found on the Ethnicity factor, $F(1,284) = 11.61$, $p < .001$, with men blaming ethnic minorities for violent crimes significantly more than did female respondents.

The significant Social Morality gender difference, $F(1,284) = 4.96, p < .027$, indicated that, although both males and females tended to agree that a decrease in societal values has led to an increase in violent crime, males endorse this belief to a lesser degree than females.

Finally, the Victim blame dimension yielded a significant gender difference, $F(1,284) = 24.11$, $p <. 001$. Although both males and females disagreed with statements indicating that the victim was to blame for the violence, males placed significantly more blame on the victim for the occurrence of violent crime than did females.

DISCUSSION AND APPLICATIONS

It is clear that distribution of blame for violent crime is multidimensional. Among subjects in these two samples, the perpetrator is not viewed as the sole cause of violence. Blame for violence was distributed among Perpetrator Consequences, Social Morality, Perpetrator, Ethnicity, and Victim factors.

Further, the manner in which an individual perceives violence and distributes blame for violence varies depending on gender and previous exposure to violence. In a study of incarcerated violent and nonviolent felons, the VAS was able to differentiate between these groups on several dimensions.

Importantly, men and women also differ on the degree of violence blame involving Ethnicity, Social Morality, and Victim factors. Differences on the Social Morality factor indicated that although both men and women tended to agree that a decrease in societal values led to increased violent crime rates, men believed this to a lesser degree than women.

The significant gender difference regarding Ethnicity involved men placing significantly greater blame for violence on ethnic minorities than did women. Great care should be taken in the generalization of this result in that the vast majority of the 600 respondents (85%) in these studies were Caucasian. Clearly, more research related to this factor is required before strong conclusions can be drawn. If, however, "perception is everything," then this finding lends credence to concerns regarding ethnic divisions and racial stereotypes, and should be interpreted accordingly with Caucasian clients.

Finally, with regard to Victim blame, men blamed the victim of violent crime more than women. This finding is consistent with the sexual assault blame distribution literature (Acock & Ireland, 1983; Jackson & Plane, 1987; Resick & Jackson, 1981). Given that the majority of health and mental health care professionals, and judicial and law enforcement personnel, are male, it may be important to increase educational and empathy-training experiences for these professionals in order to decrease possible biases, and aid them in providing sensitive and fair treatment for victims of violent crime.

As for violence history, previous personal exposure to violence was associated with significantly lowered preferred perpetrator consequences. Again, we believe this is a result of inappropriate self-blame. This finding has clear implications for jury selection or *voir dire* examinations, and for the treatment and education of both victims and perpetrators of violence.

Finally, a larger proportion of the present samples had been directly or indirectly exposed to violent crime (roughly 75%) than might have been expected based on reported crime statistics alone. This is of particular significance in light of research indicating that large percentages of violence victims exhibit PTSD and related symptoms. Careful interviewing of clients at first presentation may elicit previously unrevealed violence exposure information, which could then have relevance to the interpretation of VAS scores and to subsequent treatment goals. When previous exposure to violence is detected it is recommended that the VAS be administered to determine the violence blame distribution pattern of the client or client's significant others. Based on the resulting VAS scores, treatment goals might include cognitive behavioral techniques designed to modify inappropriate self-blame or externalization of blame.

Implications for forensic evaluations are twofold. First, psychologists might consider including the VAS in their evaluations of alleged perpetrators or victims. Externalization of blame by perpetrators or inappropriate self-blame by victims have diagnostic and testimony implications. Secondly, persons involved in jury selection or *voir dire* procedures may wish to consider the multidimensional nature of blame for violent crime and how the effects of gender and previous exposure to violence might influence perpetrator and societal blame attitudes.

In summary, the VAS is an empirically derived instrument with acceptable psychometric properties that delineates the distribution of blame for the occurrence of violent crime in our society. It is suggested that use of the VAS be considered with general clinical populations as well as during forensic processes.

VIOLENCE ATTITUDES SCALE (VAS)

In this survey violence is defined as physical assault between two or more people. For the purposes of this survey, the assailant or initiator of the violence will always be the *perpetrator,* and the person being assaulted will be the *victim.* Listed below are several statements sometimes used to account for the occurrence of violence. Please indicate your agreement or disagreement with these statements on the six-point scale accompanying each item. While some of these items might be offensive to you, please remember that they do not represent facts, but are attitudes often used to account for the occurrence of violence. If you agree with a statement, please place an X over the blank that corresponds to the degree of your agreement. If you disagree with a statement, place an X over the blank that corresponds with the amount you disagree.

For example:

A. Most tooth decay is caused by a lack of careful brushing.

Strongly Disagree   1   2   3   4   __X__ 5   6   Strongly Agree

An X above the 5 would indicate a strong amount of agreement. Please answer the following questions based on your opinion only. There are no right or wrong answers.

1. People are victims of crime because they deserve it.

Strongly Disagree   1   2   3   4   5   6   Strongly Agree

2. Violent offenders need to be dealt with more harshly.

Strongly Disagree   1   2   3   4   5   6   Strongly Agree

3. Victims of violence should be held responsible for actions which place them in jeopardy.

Strongly Disagree   1   2   3   4   5   6   Strongly Agree

4. As alcohol or drug abuse increases so does violent crime.

Strongly Disagree   1   2   3   4   5   6   Strongly Agree

5. Violent perpetrators suffer from a low frustration tolerance.

Strongly Disagree   1   2   3   4   5   6   Strongly Agree

6. Ethnic minorities are responsible for most of the violent crime in the country today.

Strongly Disagree   1   2   3   4   5   6   Strongly Agree

7. Violence is a product of a morally unhealthy society.

Strongly Disagree   1   2   3   4   5   6   Strongly Agree

8. Violent perpetrators lose their temper easily.

| Strongly Disagree | 1 | 2 | 3 | 4 | 5 | 6 | Strongly Agree |

9. As poverty increases so does violence.

| Strongly Disagree | 1 | 2 | 3 | 4 | 5 | 6 | Strongly Agree |

10. People can avoid violence by staying out of dangerous situations.

| Strongly Disagree | 1 | 2 | 3 | 4 | 5 | 6 | Strongly Agree |

11. Ethnic minorities commit more violent crimes than Caucasians.

| Strongly Disagree | 1 | 2 | 3 | 4 | 5 | 6 | Strongly Agree |

12. As divorce rates increase so does violence.

| Strongly Disagree | 1 | 2 | 3 | 4 | 5 | 6 | Strongly Agree |

13. Whenever a person is frustrated, that person will act violently.

| Strongly Disagree | 1 | 2 | 3 | 4 | 5 | 6 | Strongly Agree |

14. Violent crimes in which minorities are victims are almost always perpetrated by minorities as well.

| Strongly Disagree | 1 | 2 | 3 | 4 | 5 | 6 | Strongly Agree |

15. Stricter laws will decrease violent acts.

| Strongly Disagree | 1 | 2 | 3 | 4 | 5 | 6 | Strongly Agree |

16. Victims provoke violence by using bad judgment.

| Strongly Disagree | 1 | 2 | 3 | 4 | 5 | 6 | Strongly Agree |

17. Due to an overly tolerant philosophy in our society, violent crime rates have increased.

| Strongly Disagree | 1 | 2 | 3 | 4 | 5 | 6 | Strongly Agree |

18. Feelings of loss of control lead to violent crime.

| Strongly Disagree | 1 | 2 | 3 | 4 | 5 | 6 | Strongly Agree |

19. Violent crime is common in areas in which there is a high percentage of ethnic minorities.

   Strongly Disagree   1   2   3   4   5   6   Strongly Agree

20. Murderers should be executed.

   Strongly Disagree   1   2   3   4   5   6   Strongly Agree

21. There is a strong relationship between alcohol/drug usage and violent acts.

   Strongly Disagree   1   2   3   4   5   6   Strongly Agree

22. An angry person will be a violent person.

   Strongly Disagree   1   2   3   4   5   6   Strongly Agree

23. Due to the decreased emphasis on family values, there is a high rate of violent crime.

   Strongly Disagree   1   2   3   4   5   6   Strongly Agree

24. People who commit violent crimes should not be allowed to be released on parole.

   Strongly Disagree   1   2   3   4   5   6   Strongly Agree

25. Violent crime is more likely to occur in slum or "bad" areas.

   Strongly Disagree   1   2   3   4   5   6   Strongly Agree

26. There are certain types of people who become victims of violence.

   Strongly Disagree   1   2   3   4   5   6   Strongly Agree

27. Due to the stressful nature of our society, there are high crime rates.

   Strongly Disagree   1   2   3   4   5   6   Strongly Agree

28. Violent offenders should be allowed less privileges in prison.

   Strongly Disagree   1   2   3   4   5   6   Strongly Agree

29. Whenever a person behaves violently, it is because the person was frustrated.

   Strongly Disagree   1   2   3   4   5   6   Strongly Agree

30. There is a relationship between present morality and the incidence of violent crime.

    Strongly Disagree   1   2   3   4   5   6   Strongly Agree

31. People set themselves up to be victimized.

    Strongly Disagree   1   2   3   4   5   6   Strongly Agree

32. Punishing perpetrators is the only way to reduce violent acts.

    Strongly Disagree   1   2   3   4   5   6   Strongly Agree

33. Minority group members are usually at fault when involved in violent crimes.

    Strongly Disagree   1   2   3   4   5   6   Strongly Agree

34. The rate of violent crime is directly related to our societal values.

    Strongly Disagree   1   2   3   4   5   6   Strongly Agree

35. People who commit violent crimes should be imprisoned for their offenses.

    Strongly Disagree   1   2   3   4   5   6   Strongly Agree

36. As the number of unstable and/or chaotic homes increases, so does the amount of violent crime.

    Strongly Disagree   1   2   3   4   5   6   Strongly Agree

37. The death penalty should be enforced in every state.

    Strongly Disagree   1   2   3   4   5   6   Strongly Agree

38. A high percentage of perpetrators are members of an ethnic minority.

    Strongly Disagree   1   2   3   4   5   6   Strongly Agree

SCORING TEMPLATE FOR VAS

Note: Sum item scores within each factor to obtain the factor total score. Divide by the number of items on factor to yield factor mean score.

FACTOR	ITEM NUMBER	SCORE	TOTAL	MEAN
Consequences of Violence	2	____		
	15	____		
	17	____		
	20	____		
	24	____		
	28	____		
	32	____		
	35	____		
	37	____		
	Total for Consequences of Violence Factor		____ ÷ 9 =	☐
Social Morality Blame	7	____		
	12	____		
	21	____		
	23	____		
	27	____		
	30	____		
	34	____		
	36	____		
	Total for Social Morality Blame Factor		____ ÷ 8 =	☐
Perpetrator Blame	4	____		
	5	____		
	8	____		
	9	____		
	13	____		
	18	____		
	29	____		
	Total for Perpetrator Blame Factor		____ ÷ 7 =	☐
Ethnic Minority Blame	6	____		
	11	____		
	14	____		
	19	____		
	25	____		
	33	____		
	38	____		
	Total for Ethnic Minority Blame Factor		____ ÷ 7 =	☐
Victim Blame	1	____		
	3	____		
	10	____		
	16	____		
	22	____		
	26	____		
	31	____		
	Total for Victim Blame Factor		____ ÷ 7 =	☐

Thomas L. Jackson, PhD, is Director of Clinical Training in the Department of Psychology at the University of Arkansas. Dr. Jackson may be contacted at the Department of Psychology, 216 Memorial Hall, University of Arkansas, Fayetteville, AR 72701.

Richard D. Dienst, MA, is a Psychology Intern at the U.S. Medical Center for Federal Prisoners in Springfield, MO. Mr. Dienst can be contacted through the first author.

Terry L. Efird, PhD, is a psychologist at the Ozark Guidance Center at Springdale, AR. Dr. Efird may be contacted through the first author.

Brenda D. Mobley, PhD, is the Director of the Psychological Clinic within the Department of Psychology at the University of Arkansas. Dr. Mobley can be contacted through the first author.

David A. Schroeder, PhD, is the Chair of the Department of Psychology at the University of Arkansas. Dr. Schroeder may be contacted through the first author.

April D. Hout, MA, is a doctoral student in the Department of Psychology at the University of Arkansas. Ms. Hout can be contacted through the first author.

Julleah C. Montecillo, BA, is a doctoral student in the Department of Psychology at the University of Arkansas. Ms. Montecillo may be contacted through the first author.

Andrea L. LaBine, BS, is a doctoral student in the Department of Psychology at the University of Arkansas. Ms. LaBine can be contacted through the first author.

RESOURCES

Acock, A. C., & Ireland, N. K. (1983). Attribution of blame in rape cases: The impact of norm violation, gender, and sex-role attitude. *Sex Roles, 9,* 179-193.

Brodsky, S. L. (1976). Sexual assault: Perspectives on prevention and assailants. In M. Walker & S. Brodsky (Eds.), *Sexual Assault: The Victim and Rapist* (pp. 1-8). Lexington, MA: Lexington Press.

Efird, T. L., & Jackson, T. L. (1994). *Incarcerated Felons' Blame Distribution for Violence.* Manuscript submitted for publication.

Ellis, L. F., Black, L. D., & Resick, P. A. (1992). Cognitive-behavioral treatment approaches for victims of crime. In L. VandeCreek, S. Knapp, & T. L. Jackson (Eds.), *Innovations in Clinical Practice: A Source Book* (Vol. 11, pp. 23-38). Sarasota, FL: Professional Resource Press.

Jackson, T. L. (Ed.). (in press). *Acquaintance Rape: Assessment, Treatment, and Prevention.* Sarasota, FL: Professional Resource Press.

Jackson, T. L., & Ferguson, W. P. (1983). Attribution of blame in incest. *American Journal of Community Psychology, 11,* 313-322.

Jackson, T. L., Petretic-Jackson, P. A., Ostrowski, M., & Keller, J. (1989, August). *Acquaintance Rape Attitude and Information Change Through Education and Empathy.* Paper presented at the annual convention of the American Psychological Association, New Orleans, LA.

Jackson, T. L., & Plane, T. (1987, May). *Attribution of Rape Blame Among Native Americans.* Paper presented at the annual convention of the Midwestern Psychological Association, Chicago, IL.

Jackson, T. L., & Sandberg, G. (1985). Attribution of incest blame among rural attorneys and judges. *Women and Therapy, 4,* 13-22.

Morris, Y., & Jackson, T. L. (1989, August). *Midwestern Attorneys' Blame Attribution and Sentencing Preferences in Rape.* Paper presented at the annual convention of the American Psychological Association, New Orleans, LA.

Petretic-Jackson, P. A., Sandberg, G., & Jackson, T. L. (1994). The Domestic Violence Blame Scale (DVBS). In L. VandeCreek, S. Knapp, & T. L. Jackson (Eds.), *Innovations in Clinical Practice: A Source Book* (Vol. 13, pp. 265-278). Sarasota, FL: Professional Resource Press.

Resick, P. A., & Jackson, T. L. (1981). Attitudes toward rape among mental health professionals. *American Journal of Community Psychology, 9,* 481-490.

Tarver, D., & Jackson, T. L. (1992, August). *Physicians' Blame Attribution in Domestic Violence Cases.* Paper presented at the annual convention of the American Psychological Association, Washington, DC.

U.S. Department of Justice. (1994). *Uniform Crime Reports for the United States: 1993 Preliminary Annual Release.* Washington, DC: U.S. Government Printing Office.

A CLIENT SATISFACTION SURVEY

Chris E. Stout

Managed care has had a dramatic impact on outpatient mental health care (Stout, 1992c). Among other things, clinicians now must demonstrate efficiency in terms of number of sessions of treatment and in demonstrable outcomes (Stout, 1992b, 1992d). Some managed care entities have indicated that they will hire only those clinicians who can provide client profiles and data on client satisfaction with services (Kantera, 1993). The author has developed the following form to facilitate collection of client satisfaction data.

The Client Satisfaction Survey (pp. 294-295) collects information on clinical and nonclinical (e.g., appointment scheduling, courteousness of office staff) issues, and includes the client's perceptions of improvement. Such data, in contrast to diagnosis or the number of sessions, may aid in determining standards of care or value-to-treatment ratios. This survey should also be supplemented with a self-administered symptom screening device such as the Symptom Checklist-90-Revised (Derogatis, 1983), to further examine the presence or severity of symptoms. Such screening devices should be conducted pre- and post-treatment for comparison purposes (Stout, 1993a).

The benefits of establishing such a system of data collection are manifold. As noted earlier, such data permit clinicians to assess the effectiveness of interventions. The data can be aggregated for trends and patterns (Hinton & Stout, 1993). Comments from clients may be useful in clarifying and interpreting the numeric ratings. Costs in terms of time and money are minimal, and office staff can easily be trained to incorporate these forms into patient contracts and databases which can then be used to market the practice to managed care companies (Stout, 1992a, 1992d, 1993a).

Before using this form, clinicians must obtain informed consent from clients. Clients' approval for satisfaction surveys must be obtained as part of an overall informed consent form regarding treatment, record keeping, finances, and so on, or it may be obtained with a separate form such as the one presented on page 296.

Clinicians are encouraged to edit and adapt these forms for their practices.

Innovations in Clinical Practice: A Source Book (Vol. 13)

CLIENT SATISFACTION SURVEY

Dear Client,

At this point you have completed your use of services from this provider. We value your honest input concerning what your experiences have been with your therapist. Please take a few minutes to complete this survey form and return it in the attached self-addressed stamped envelope. Your opinion is important for helping us to insure the highest quality of services possible. Thank you for your time.

Your Therapist's Name: _____

Approximate Number of Sessions: _____

How would you rate the following? (Please circle your answer and comment specifically on items rated 3 or 4. Comments on items rated 1 and 2 would be appreciated.)

	Strongly Agree	Mildly Agree	Mildly Disagree	Strongly Disagree
1. I had no difficulty obtaining a convenient appointment time.	1	2	3	4
Comments: _____				
2. My therapist discussed and clearly explained my treatment plan.	1	2	3	4
Comments: _____				
3. I was treated courteously by office staff.	1	2	3	4
Comments: _____				
4. I have benefited from the services provided to me.	1	2	3	4
Comments: _____				
5. My presenting problem has been resolved.	1	2	3	4
Comments: _____				
6. My work/school performance has been improved.	1	2	3	4
Comments: _____				
7. My billings and fee payments were managed to my satisfaction.	1	2	3	4
Comments: _____				

	Strongly Agree	Mildly Agree	Mildly Disagree	Strongly Disagree
8. The care provided by my therapist was beneficial.	1	2	3	4

Comments:_____

	Strongly Agree	Mildly Agree	Mildly Disagree	Strongly Disagree
9. If a friend or family member needed counseling, I would recommend my therapist.	1	2	3	4

Comments:_____

10. What was the most beneficial part of your treatment?

_____

11. What did you dislike about your treatment?

_____

12. What would you recommend to improve our services?

_____

13. Please provide any further comments:_____
_____
_____
_____

Thank you for your input.

Your Name (Optional):_____

INFORMED CONSENT FORM

Name (Print):_____

Age:_____ Client ID #:_____

- I hereby consent to being involved in the Client Satisfaction Survey.

- I understand that I will not be identified by name or in any report or summary of this survey.

- I understand that I may withdraw consent and discontinue participation in this survey at any time and that this will have no bearing on my status in my treatment.

- I understand that I may decline participation in this survey and that doing such will not be cause to deny or alter any indicated services to me.

- This survey meets the regulatory standards set forth by the U.S. Department of Health and Human Service Regulations concerning the protection of participants.

- I understand that this questionnaire will cause me no discomfort or risk. There are no medical or physical procedures or tests. All I will be asked to do is complete one very brief questionnaire which deals with my opinions and has no right or wrong answers. I understand that there are no tests of any sort.

- I understand that I and the practitioner can expect the following benefits:

  (a) Improved treatment at _____ clinic.
  (b) Addition to general knowledge of mental health care.

- If I have any questions about this survey, I can contact Dr. _____ (123-456-7890).

_____   _____
(Client's Signature*)   (Date)

_____   _____
(Parent's or Guardian's Signature*)   (Date)

_____   _____
(Witness' Signature* and Printed Name)   (Date)

*Signatures required: Adult client (18 or over) and witness; parent (or guardian) and child plus witness, if child is 12 through 17; parent (or guardian) and witness, if child is under 12 or patient judged incompetent.

Route:

Original - Client Chart   Copy - Client

Chris E. Stout, PhD, is Chief of Psychology and Associate Administrator of Forest Hospital in Des Plaines, Illinois, and Executive Clinical Director of the Forest Academies throughout Illinois. He has written over 250 articles and published seven books. He is past consultant to the White House on national education matters and has appeared on numerous television, radio, and cable programs. Dr. Stout can be contacted at Forest Hospital, 555 Wilson Lane, Des Plaines, IL 60016-4794.

RESOURCES

Derogatis, L. (1983). *Symptom Checklist-90-Revised.* Towson, MD: Clinical Psychometric Research.

Hinton, J., & Stout, C. E. (1993). Patient satisfaction. In M. B. Squire, C. E. Stout, & D. M. Ruben (Eds.), *Current Advances in Inpatient Psychiatric Care: A Handbook* (pp. 41-52). Westport, CT: Greenwood.

Kantera, A. (1993). Interview, preferred healthcare. *Psychotherapy Finances, July,* 5.

Ruben, D. M., & Stout, C. E. (1993). *Transitions: Handbook of Managed Care for Inpatient to Outpatient Treatment.* New York: Praeger.

Stout, C. E. (1992a). Automated collection, storage, retrieval seen as benchmark. *The National Psychologist, 1,* 17.

Stout, C. E. (1992b). How to give managed care the data it wants. *Addiction and Recovery, May/June,* 22-23.

Stout, C. E. (1992c). Managed care and the human touch: Are they compatible? *Chicago Medicine, 95,* 24-26.

Stout, C. E. (1992d). You can give managed care the data it wants without hiring a statistician. *The Psychotherapy Letter, 4,* 1, 6.

Stout, C. E. (1993a). *Advances in Outcomes Management.* Des Plaines, IL: Forest Health Systems.

Stout, C. E. (1993b). Managed care needs system for measuring treatment efficacy. *The Psychotherapy Letter, 5,* 8.

CLINICAL AND ADMINISTRATIVE MANAGEMENT CHECKLIST

John R. Rudisill

This checklist is designed to help practitioners be sure that they have attended to the various details that insure quality care for their clients and prevent problems with insurance companies, managed care organizations, and regulatory agencies (see pp. 300-304). Consistent and careful use of this type of checklist will give practitioners instant feedback on the extent to which they have completed various clinical and administrative tasks in a timely fashion. In addition, adherence to a checklist will help practitioners attend to often forgotten details such as thanking referral sources.

This checklist presents a model for this type of form; individual practitioners and group practices will undoubtedly need to modify, add, and delete items to "fit" the checklist to their particular offices. Solo practitioners without secretaries or office managers may elect to keep a copy of the checklist in each client's file and review the checklist before and after each session and whenever any event occurs that requires an action. Group practices, and practices where there are administrative support services, may decide to keep a copy of each client's checklist in a central file or three-ring binder where some designated staff person can review them regularly, complete tasks that are their responsibility, and alert the clinician or other staff members when they have failed to complete one of their required tasks.

Various items on the checklist require completing various forms, instruments, and letters (e.g., telephone contact forms, intake forms). If you do not already use such materials in your practice, you should seriously consider developing them. Samples of a wide variety of forms, letters, and instruments appear throughout the 13 volumes of this series, *Innovations in Clinical Practice: A Source Book*. Additional forms are available from other publishers, Employee Assistance Programs (EAPs), and managed care organizations. You may also want to consult with colleagues about the forms they use in their practices. To help you understand the general content of each form and letter, the author has included a brief note after some items that require completion of this type of document.

Innovations in Clinical Practice: A Source Book (Vol. 13)

CLINICAL AND ADMINISTRATIVE MANAGEMENT CHECKLIST

Client Name:_____ File #:_____

INSTRUCTIONS:

1. The staff person completing each item on this checklist must initial and date the item on the line to the left of the item!
2. When a task is required but not yet completed (e.g., a future date for sending a managed care or insurance report, a referral to be made at a future date), the date for completing that task should be noted to the right of the item and the item should be circled. When the task is completed, the person completing the task should date and initial on the line to the left of the item.

WHEN CLIENT FIRST CONTACTS/CALLS THE OFFICE:

_____ Complete referral form (*Note:* Referral forms typically include the name of client(s), date of birth, name of spouse/parents, addresses, telephone numbers, referral source, brief description of the problem, and information regarding any third-party payers.)

_____ Briefly explain office policies, payment arrangements, and what client can expect in first session.

_____ Set up client file and any related computer management files (e.g., initial entry in a billing, insurance, or case management program).

_____ Mail client any materials typically mailed before first session (e.g., intake form, consent forms, problem checklists, insurance authorization forms, office policies, directions to office).

_____ Contact insurance company, Employee Assistance Program (EAP), or managed care company to determine extent of coverage, determine co-payment required, obtain preauthorization (if needed), and determine any managed care requirements or limits.

_____ Document all insurance and billing information in insurance records on this client and note dates/sessions for reports, reauthorization, and similar tasks on this checklist.

_____ Send thank-you letter to referral source.

_____ With client's written consent, contact referral source regarding reason for referral.

_____ Other unique issues, needs, or requirements for this client (describe and initial/date when completed):

WHEN CLIENT FIRST VISITS THE OFFICE:

_____ Have client complete:

    _____ Intake form
    _____ Social and medical history form
    _____ Insurance authorization forms
    _____ Details of prior treatment form
    _____ Consent for treatment and/or testing
    _____ Consent to obtain information form
    _____ Consent to release information form (if needed)
    _____ Consent to audio/video record sessions (if needed)
    _____ Form listing charges and services likely not to be covered by insurance with agreement of client responsibility
    _____ Acknowledgment of receipt of office policies

_____ Photocopy insurance cards and other information needed to obtain reimbursement.

_____ Give client office policies brochure.

_____ Inform client of information received from his or her insurance company, EAP, or managed care company regarding extent of coverage, limitations, requirements, and exclusions.

_____ Other unique issues, needs, or requirements for this client (describe and initial/date when completed):

IN FIRST SESSION:

_____ Develop documentation of initial treatment plan and review with client.

_____ Discuss any appropriate referrals to other caregivers with client and receive appropriate consents and authorizations to contact those caregivers (e.g., referral to psychiatrist, primary care physician, treatment program, diagnostic testing).

_____ Obtain information to allow you to write a detailed chart note including social/medical history, presenting problems, and diagnosis (at the very least, a tentative diagnosis for first insurance claim filing).

_____ Other unique issues, needs, or requirements for this client (e.g., testing ordered, prescriptive instructions to client). Describe and initial/date when completed. Circle if assigned but not completed:

AFTER FIRST SESSION:

_____ Write a detailed chart note including social/medical history, presenting problems, and diagnosis (at the very least, a tentative diagnosis for first insurance claim filing).

_____ Update file with information obtained prior to and during first session.

_____ Update insurance, managed care, and billing systems with information obtained prior to and during first session (*Note:* There are numerous manual and computer software systems for tracking this information):

      _____ Name of guarantor of account
      _____ Name of insurance company (including address, phone number, and contact person
      _____ Policy and group numbers
      _____ Deductible
      _____ Co-payment required
      _____ Allowable fees and services
      _____ Authorization and preauthorization requirements
      _____ Other unique billing/insurance requirements for this client (list below with descriptions, date/session required, circle, and initial/date when completed):

_____ File first insurance claim.

_____ Enter billing information on first session.

_____ Give feedback to referral source (if client signed consent for this release of information).

_____ Make all referrals and order all procedures as indicated from first session.

_____ Other unique issues, needs, or requirements for this client (e.g., testing ordered, prescriptive instructions to client). Describe and initial/date when completed. Circle if assigned but not completed:

DIAGNOSTIC/TREATMENT SESSIONS
(Photocopy as many sheets as needed - each session should be documented):

SESSION # _____ DATE: _____

_____ Review treatment plan and revise as necessary.

_____ Discuss any appropriate referrals to other caregivers with client and receive appropriate consents and authorizations to contact those caregivers (e.g., referral to psychiatrist, primary care physician, treatment program, diagnostic testing).

_____ Write a detailed chart note including problem identification, progress toward treatment goals, and changes in diagnosis (note below for change on insurance records):

      _____ Change in diagnosis: _____

_____ Check client's progress toward completing any prescriptive instructions given in last session.

_____ Other unique issues, needs, or requirements for this client (e.g., testing ordered, prescriptive instructions to client). Describe and initial/date when completed. Circle if assigned but not completed:

      *   *   *   *   *

SESSION # _____ DATE: _____

_____ Review treatment plan and revise as necessary.

_____ Discuss any appropriate referrals to other caregivers with client and receive appropriate consents and authorizations to contact those caregivers (e.g., referral to psychiatrist, primary care physician, treatment program, diagnostic testing).

_____ Write a detailed chart note including problem identification, progress toward treatment goals, changes in diagnosis (note below for change on insurance records):

      _____ Change in diagnosis: _____

_____ Check client's progress toward completing any prescriptive instructions given in last session.

_____ Other unique issues, needs, or requirements for this client (e.g., testing ordered, prescriptive instructions to client). Describe and initial/date when completed. Circle if assigned but not completed:

DURING LAST SESSION:

_____ Discuss progress in reaching treatment goals established in treatment plan (initial revisions).

_____ Process termination issues:

        _____ Unresolved issues
        _____ Relationship issues
        _____ Reasons/clues client may want to seek further treatment or referral
        _____ Other issues (list):

_____ Give client copy of therapy evaluation/client satisfaction survey.

AFTER LAST SESSION:

_____ Write detailed progress note and closing summary.

_____ Send progress note to referral source (with client's written consent).

1 MONTH POST-TERMINATION:

_____ Call client to review current status and follow up on any pending referrals.

_____ Document conversation with client in chart/file.

6 MONTHS AFTER TERMINATION:

_____ Send client post-treatment evaluation survey.

John R. Rudisill, PhD, ABAP, is currently Professor and Director, Division of Applied Psychology, Department of Family Medicine, School of Medicine, Wright State University in Dayton, Ohio. Prior to this, he was Behavioral Science Director, Departments of Family Medicine and Psychiatry. His training is in clinical psychology with special interests of individual/family psychotherapy, and organizational consultation. He has published numerous articles ranging from psychotherapy supervision to psychological consultation for outplacement firms. In 1992, he received the School of Medicine Teaching Excellence Award for his work in behavioral science. Dr. Rudisill may be contacted at 601 Edwin C. Moses Boulevard, Dayton, OH 45408.

ADDITIONAL RESOURCES

American Association for Marriage and Family Therapy. *AAMFT Forms Book*. Washington, DC: Author.

Innovations in Clinical Practice: A Source Book. (See "Cumulative Index" for all volumes or the "Subject Index" for each volume; look under "Forms and Instruments"). Sarasota, FL: Professional Resource Press.

Small, R. F. (1993). *Maximizing Third-Party Reimbursement in Your Mental Health Practice* (2nd ed.). Sarasota, FL: Professional Resource Press.

Zuckerman, E. L., & Guyett, I. P. R. (1992). *The Paper Office 1* (rev. 1992 ed.). Pittsburgh, PA: The Clinician's ToolBox.

COMMUNITY INTERVENTIONS

INTRODUCTION TO SECTION IV: COMMUNITY INTERVENTIONS

Although the primary focus of the *Innovations in Clinical Practice* series is on clinical interventions, we have always included this section because of our belief that practitioners are at risk for selecting unnecessarily narrow roles that may limit their potential influence on the community. Mental health professionals are, in fact, in excellent positions to address a diversity of problems that are sometimes overlooked by traditional clinicians. We have included three contributions in this realm that take the practitioner out of the typical role in the office.

The first one, by P. Gregg Blanton, provides a manual for time-limited group treatment with separated couples. The program is designed for use with individuals in the predivorce stage (between the time of considering divorce and actually completing the divorce decree).

For many psychologists, going to court has meant testifying in support of one side or the other in either a civil or criminal suit. There are less stressful opportunities in litigation that do not involve getting on the witness stand, such as working as a litigation consultant. The focus of this contribution, by Robert Ellis, involves consulting with attorneys on how to cross-examine neuropsychologists.

The final contribution in this section addresses the evaluation and treatment of motorists convicted of driving while intoxicated (DWI). Thomas and Mary Grant describe a program they have directed in New York for several years. The contribution focuses on the diagnostic issues involved in assessing DWI offenders and on providing group psychotherapy programs.

INTRODUCTION TO SECTION IV
COMMUNITY PHYSIOLOGY

A MANUAL FOR TIME-LIMITED GROUP TREATMENT WITH SEPARATED COUPLES

P. Gregg Blanton

This manual (see pp. 310-321) is designed for use in the group treatment of individuals in the predivorce stage, that is, the period in the divorce process which begins with the initial consideration of divorce as an option and ends with the divorce decree. The training manual was designed to (a) address the specific needs of individuals in the predivorce stage of the divorce process; (b) focus on what may be the most prominent divorce adjustment task, that of resolving ambivalent feelings; and (c) incorporate a family systems perspective of divorce.

In a study designed to examine the usefulness of this group treatment model for predivorced individuals, 56 participants were randomly assigned to either the experimental or the control group. Group treatment consisted of six sessions, which revolved around the training manual. The Fisher Divorce Adjustment Scale (FDAS; Fisher, 1978a) was used to measure the dependent variables of anger (i.e., a strong feeling of antagonism), attachment (i.e., the emotional involvement and affectional bonds with the spouse), and ambivalence (i.e., simultaneous feelings of attachment to and anger toward the spouse). The FDAS was administered as a pretest and as a posttest. Results of the study indicated that the experimental group, relative to the control group, significantly increased their levels of adjustment in the areas of anger, attachment, and ambivalence. That is, participants in the experimental group felt less anger toward and less emotional connection to the spouse by the end of treatment.

There are a few guidelines for selecting group members. Criteria for admission to the group are that (a) the individual must be separated or considering separation, and (b) the court date for a legal divorce decree cannot precede completion of the program. The group member decides whether or not to participate in the group with his or her spouse.

The following manual (pp. 310-321) takes group participants through a structured process. The group meets once a week for 6 consecutive weeks. A session lasts for 1 hour and 30 minutes. Each session revolves around that week's chapter from the training manual. Discussion is facilitated by the group leader who is skilled and experienced in leading groups.

A program designed specifically for predivorced individuals is desirable for several reasons. An early intervention in the divorce process may prevent crisis-related difficulties. Healthy adjustments to the predivorce tasks may prevent many divorce-related difficulties. Predivorce treatment also addresses the needs of many individuals who will eventually decide not to divorce.

The program seems to be particularly beneficial for individuals who (a) are in the early stages of the divorce process, (b) are vacillating between the decision to divorce and the decision to improve the marriage, (c) are interested in brief therapy, and (d) have not traditionally participated in divorce adjustment groups (e.g., males, separated couples, nonseparated couples).

A PROGRAM FOR SEPARATED COUPLES

PREFACE

THE PURPOSE OF THIS PROGRAM

This manual is written for couples who are separated or are considering separation. You have not as yet divorced, but one or both of you are considering divorce as an alternative to a dissatisfying marriage. Separations are usually temporary and significant. In a relatively short period of time, you will make decisions that will significantly change your life. The important question is: Will your life be better or worse after this separation? The main purpose of this program is to assist you in making the changes that are necessary preconditions for a successful divorce or reconciliation.

Ultimately, the decision to divorce or to reconcile is yours as a couple. However, regardless of your decision, a healthy outcome will depend upon how you complete the following separation tasks: (a) understanding and resolving the emotions related to separation, (b) understanding and sharing responsibility for the marital decline, (c) completing the grief process, (d) resolving mixed feelings of anger and attachment, and (e) completing the decision-making process. This program will help you address these issues.

Achieving a successful outcome to the separation transition requires a motivation for things to get better and also a great deal of work. This program will introduce you to the tools necessary for completing your tasks. In addition, you will be working together with others going through the same difficult time. You will learn from and support each other as you go through this crisis period together.

A DESCRIPTION OF THE PROGRAM

Participants in Program. This program is designed for a maximum of 16 individuals who are separated or are considering separation. The court date for these individuals should not occur before the completion of the program.

Length of Program. The group will meet once a week for 6 consecutive weeks. A session will last for 1 hour and 30 minutes.

Typical Meeting Sequence

- *Preparation.* Group members will prepare for each session by reading the appropriate chapter from the training manual.
- *Reviewing the Chapter.* For the first 15 minutes, the group leader will review the concepts in the chapter assigned for that session.
- *Group Discussion.* The group will discuss questions that follow the chapter assigned for that session. Group discussion will last 1 hour and 15 minutes.

HOW THE GROUPS WILL FUNCTION

Role of the Group Leader. The group leader is skilled and experienced in leading groups. The leader is present to structure the sessions, facilitate constructive discussion, and provide encouragement.

Rules for Group Discussion

- Give everyone a chance to talk
- Maintain confidentiality
- Join in the discussion as desired
- Take responsibility for yourself
- Protect members from physical threats, intimidation, and undue peer pressure

CHAPTER 1: SEPARATION CREATES A CRISIS

SEPARATION DISTRESS

Whether you are separated or considering separation, you are more than likely in a state of crisis. A crisis is accompanied by feelings of distress, which vary in intensity, duration, and quality from person to person. Some of the symptoms of separation distress that you may be experiencing are:

- Difficulty concentrating
- Tension
- Sadness
- Yearning to be with your spouse
- Anger
- Apprehensiveness
- Worry
- Difficulty sleeping
- Change in eating patterns
- Despair

Several factors affect the level of distress that you are feeling. Separation that occurs after a reasonably satisfactory marriage is usually more painful than one that occurs after a dissatisfying marriage. The separation is more disruptive for individuals who have integrated marriage into their emotional and social lives. This generally takes around 2 years, so separations in the first or second year of marriage may be less distressing. Some people believe that the spouse responsible for the separation experiences less emotional discomfort than the noninitiator, but separation distress appears in both individuals. The difference is in the kind of pain felt by each. The one who initiated the separation tends to feel guilty, whereas the noninitiator tends to feel more rejection. It seems that those with the least separation distress are those who have a new love. By shifting their attachment feelings to a new figure, they may escape separation distress.

FACTORS IN A CRISIS

What led up to this crisis? Separation, in and of itself, does not necessarily create a crisis. The event of separation produces a crisis when combined with other contributing factors:

1. *Hardships.* The hardships that accompany separation increase and intensify your difficulties. For example, what economic, housing, legal, and parental hardships are you already experiencing or likely to experience? You are likely to experience greater distress if you have more actual or potential hardships.
2. *Resources.* Personal, family, and community resources provide some protection against the harmful effects of separation. Finances, education, physical health, psychological health, family support, and the help of friends are all valuable resources. With them, you will feel more capable of facing the demands and threats of separation. Without them, you will feel more overwhelmed by separation-related difficulties.
3. *Perceptions.* How do you view your marital situation? If you believe the separation has a purpose or value, then you will be able to cope better with your difficulties. However, you will be more likely to fall apart if you perceive the separation as a horrible, a terrible, and an unbearable experience.
4. *Prior Strains.* Is your separation being added on to existing stressors? Have you recently lost your job or had a child? If so, you are likely to experience your situation as more demanding and difficult. Difficulties have a way of piling up. Fewer prior strains will make it more possible for you to cope with the demands of separation.

CRISIS: A TURNING POINT

A crisis by its very definition only lasts for a short while. Sooner or later, you will reorganize and your crisis will end. The question is: When your separation crisis is over, will your life be better or worse? Neither divorce nor marriage is inherently better or worse. Your life could be worse off if you continue in an unsatisfactory marriage. Deciding to divorce, but failing to successfully end your marital relationship and resolve feelings of anger, guilt, and grief, will also produce negative outcomes. However, you can decide to make the necessary changes that can produce positive outcomes for everyone involved, whether the decision is divorce or reconciliation. In a crisis, both positive and negative outcomes are possible. The choice is up to you.

DISCUSSION QUESTIONS

1. Which hardships have occurred and could occur because of this separation?
2. Identify the resources (e.g., family support, friends, groups, etc.) that you can rely upon during this time of distress.
3. Do you have other stresses going on in your life at the present time?
4. Do you believe that your life will be better or worse after this crisis? What could you do to make it better? Worse?

CHAPTER 2: UNDERSTANDING YOUR EMOTIONS

THE STAGES OF DIVORCE

Separation, or thinking about separation, is accompanied by a multitude of painful feelings. It is important that you understand these emotions. To understand them, however, you must know something about the divorce process.

Divorce is not an event, but a process that takes place in three stages over a period of approximately 3 years:

1. *Stage 1.* The first stage begins when one or both spouses begin to consider divorce as an alternative to relationship difficulties. Because the couple have not as yet chosen divorce as the solution to their marital dissatisfaction, this period is also referred to as the decision stage. This stage may begin years before the couple separate. During this stage, the marriage partners are becoming more aware of their differences, and they begin to dwell more upon the negative aspects of the relationship. The erosion of the marriage will begin to manifest itself in a variety of ways (e.g., criticalness, avoiding one another, disrespect, uninvolvement, extramarital affair). This stage ends when one partner moves out or files for divorce.
2. *Stage 2.* This stage begins with the decision to separate and ends when the legal divorce decree is granted. This period is referred to as the restructuring stage, because the couple now begin to make the necessary legal, emotional, financial, social, and parental arrangements that are essential for making the transition from marriage to singlehood.
3. *Stage 3.* Following the legal decree, each individual continues with the difficult task of defining a new identity. Each person continues the process of reorganizing his or her life. Gradually, a new self emerges, one different from the one he or she was. The divorce process ends when the individual attains a fairly stable and autonomous identity and lifestyle.

THE EMOTIONAL PROCESS OF DIVORCE

Everyone going through the divorce process feels pain. However, the intensity, duration, and timing of these feelings are different for each individual. Each spouse is on his or her own emotional track. The two spouses are not moving side by side. Instead, they are at different points on the track, moving at their own pace.

The emotional track that you are on is greatly influenced by whether or not you initiated the separation (or talks of separation). It is sometimes difficult to define which spouse is more responsible for the separation, because the husband and wife may alternate concerning who is going to initiate the separation. However, in the majority of divorces, one partner wants out more than the other. This person is determined to separate, whereas the other opposes it or reluctantly acquiesces. The first person is called the initiator, while the other person is called the noninitiator. It is not necessarily the initiator who files for the divorce. In the following discussion, we will examine the typical emotional processes of the initiator and noninitiator. I will organize this discussion around the first two divorce stages.

THE INITIATOR'S EMOTIONAL PROCESS

1. *Stage 1 of the Divorce Process.* Early in Stage 1, the initiator begins to consider the possibility of separation. This person is angry at the spouse for unfulfilled needs and unmet expectations. The spouse is blamed for creating a dissatisfying relationship. As the initiator imagines the multitude of losses that could result from separation and divorce, he or she experiences feelings of grief. This individual feels intense guilt over the impact that the separation decision will have upon the family. Even though the relationship is no longer rewarding, feelings of attachment may be present to a significant degree. Attachment refers to a sense of being bonded to the other, a sense that home is where the other is.
2. *Stage 2 of the Divorce Process.* Sometimes, the initiator feels relief, euphoria, and freedom soon after the separation. The euphoria may gradually change to a feeling of normalcy, but it tends to be replaced by lingering feelings of guilt, anger, and attachment. However, by Stage 2, these ambivalent feelings are beginning to subside. The initiator begins to recognize his or her own contributions to the marital breakdown. Working through feelings of grief, anger, and attachment, the initiator experiences a sense of acceptance of the divorce. This person is in a good emotional state to proceed to the final stage of divorce.

THE NONINITIATOR'S EMOTIONAL PROCESS

The emotional process of the noninitiator is somewhat different:

1. *Stage 1 of the Divorce Process.* During this stage, the noninitiator denies the possibility of separation. This person clearly is not experiencing the same feelings as the initiator in Stage 1 of the divorce process. The noninitiator's spouse is far ahead in the emotional process.
2. *Stage 2 of the Divorce Process.* Once the separation occurs, the noninitiator feels intense hurt. The rejection strikes a severe blow to self-esteem. The noninitiator experiences ambivalent feelings of anger and attachment. Because of the attachment, the noninitiator may want to win the spouse back. Initially, if feelings of anger are repressed, the noninitiator may feel depressed. Once the noninitiator gives up on winning back the spouse, intense feelings of anger begin to surface. The noninitiator attacks and blames the spouse for the marital problems. Realizing the present and potential losses, the noninitiator begins to feel grief. Gradually, this person begins to acknowledge his or her own contributions to the marital breakdown. As the noninitiator's feelings of anger and attachment begin to subside, this spouse begins to be in a good place emotionally. This person is now emotionally prepared for the last stage of divorce.

THE IMPORTANCE OF THE EMOTIONAL PROCESS

The previous discussion described a couple who successfully completed the emotional process. Each partner worked through ambivalent feelings, resolved feelings of grief, and recognized contributions to the marital breakdown. Both the initiator and the noninitiator accepted the decision to divorce. They were emotionally prepared for the legal divorce. They will use the divorce as an opportunity to grow as individuals and as a postdivorce family. Many couples do not make the emotional adjustments necessary for a successful legal divorce. One or both partners may feel reluctant about the decision to divorce. This reluctance is usually connected to continuing feelings of anger and attachment. Ambivalent feelings in only one spouse may make it difficult for the individuals to reach legal agreements concerning property and custody. If this couple divorce, intense conflict may follow them beyond the legal decree. Feelings of anger and resentment may interfere with the well-being of these individuals and their children. They may be worse off after the divorce.

DISCUSSION QUESTIONS

1. In which stage of the divorce process are you as a couple?
2. Are you the initiator or noninitiator? How would your spouse answer this question?

3. How long did you and your spouse deliberate over the decision to separate?
4. Where are you in the emotional adjustment process? Your spouse?

CHAPTER 3: WHY MARRIAGES GO BAD

ESTABLISHING RESPONSIBILITY

How many times have you asked yourself the question: "What happened to my marriage?" You wonder how the love that was once present could now be so totally lost. It may be difficult for you to identify the events leading up to the separation and the causes of your marital problems. However, whether you divorce or reconcile, it is psychologically important for you to organize a story of how your marriage deteriorated. By organizing and writing your history, you can move from confusion to understanding and growth.

One issue you probably want to settle is who was responsible for what. Early in the emotional divorce process, each spouse allocates blame to the other spouse: "You caused our marriage to fall apart." This is a natural and normal approach to take. However, maintaining this view eventually interferes with the emotional divorce process. A unilateral approach, one that holds the other spouse entirely responsible for the deterioration of the marriage, prevents personal and marital growth. In order to emerge from this separation transition a better person, it is essential that you examine your role in the deterioration of the marriage. Assuming responsibility for your portion of the problem enables you to move forward without repeating the same mistakes in a future relationship, whether with your present spouse or someone else.

MARITAL LIFE CYCLE

Examining the deterioration of your marriage requires some understanding of the marital life cycle. The marital life cycle has three predictable stages:

1. *Stage 1.* The first stage is also called the preparental stage. It begins with preparations for marriage and ends with pregnancy.
2. *Stage 2.* Beginning with pregnancy and ending when the last child leaves home, this is the parental stage. This phase has the highest divorce rate.
3. *Stage 3.* The final stage is referred to as the postparental stage. Marital satisfaction tends to increase during this phase, after the couple adjust to the absence of children. The marital life cycle ends with the death of a spouse.

MARITAL TASKS

Each stage of the marital life cycle requires the completion of certain tasks if the marriage is to be lasting and satisfactory. Some of these are basic tasks, whereas others are special. (I will discuss the differences between these two types of tasks later.) The completion of these tasks is essential. As a couple successfully complete the tasks of one stage, they become better prepared to meet and resolve the tasks of the next stage. However, difficulties accomplishing the tasks of one stage negatively affect the couple's ability to meet changing needs at the next stage.

BASIC MARITAL TASKS

Some basic tasks must be addressed throughout the marital life cycle. Instead of being accomplished once and for all time, these tasks must be addressed at each stage of the marital life cycle if the marriage is to remain vital and satisfactory.

1. *Commitment.* Commitment refers to how much the partners value the relationship and intend to maintain and continue the relationship. In Stage 1 (preparental), the couple form an initial commitment. The challenge of Stage 2 (parental) is to maintain this bond while coping with the difficulties of raising children. Commitment during Stage 3 (postparental) enables each partner to support the other in his or her attempts to find meaning, satisfaction, and productivity in later life.

2. *Caring.* Caring refers to the emotional attachment between the two spouses. Once again, in Stage 1, the couple forms an initial attachment. Throughout Stage 2, the couple must work to maintain this emotional closeness. This emotional attachment continues in Stage 3 despite declining physiological functioning.
3. *Communication.* Communication refers to the ability to share both verbally and nonverbally. Workable patterns of communication are being established in Stage 1. Throughout Stage 2, communications are being reexamined and deepened. The challenge of this stage is for the couple to continue intellectual and emotional sharing. In the final stage, deepening communication allows for the examination of critical issues such as loss, loneliness, and death.
4. *Conflict.* Conflict refers to the ability to recognize and deal with interpersonal disagreements. In Stage 1, the couple are learning how to resolve conflicts by compromising. A common conflict of Stage 2 emerges when the wife begins to establish her individual identity after being identified for so long as the husband's wife and the children's mother. Another common conflict occurs over how to dispose of child-care responsibilities and household chores, if both spouses work full-time. The continuing struggle is to reconcile their separate desires and needs. In Stage 3, the couple must find ways to face the inevitable losses (e.g., loss of job, death of friends, declining health, etc.) of later life.

SPECIFIC TASKS

Even though the basic tasks are addressed throughout the marital life cycle, special tasks must be completed at specific stages. Failure to successfully complete these tasks contributes to marital decline. I will organize this discussion around the three marital stages.

The special tasks of Stage 1 are:

1. *Building a Satisfactory Sexual Relationship.* Inherent in this task is the ability to express affection separate from as well as part of sexual activity.
2. *Establishing the Primacy of the Spousal Relationship.* This task requires an alteration of relationships with friends and extended family. These relationships must be redefined so that they do not compete with the spousal relationship. This issue also pertains to work or career. Are you married primarily to the job or to your spouse?
3. *Forming Appropriate Ties to Families of Origin.* As the couple work to define themselves as separate from their respective families of origin, the marriage partners want to resolve old and prevent new extended family problems. Problems such as being distant, overinvolved, or conflictual with the extended families puts too much emotional pressure on the couple. Unresolved extended family problems - not the specific marital conflicts on which the spouses may focus - are behind most marital problems. It is the couple's task to be independent from, yet maintain caring ties to, their respective families.
4. *Adapting to the "Real" Spouse.* Romantic love, by definition, causes the lover to perceive the loved one as more than he or she actually is. There is an inevitable disillusionment as one's perceptions of the spouse change. The challenge is to adapt to the fact that the spouse is different from what you originally expected. Hopefully, you learn to accept and appreciate the way your spouse really is.

The special tasks of Stage 2 are:

1. *Fulfilling Parental Roles as a Couple.* Now the couple must work together to make room for a child. Attention, nurturance, and caring must now be shared with a third person. Parental roles and responsibilities must be defined, negotiated, and accepted. It is important that the couple avoid the problem of one parent becoming too close to the child, creating emotional distance between the spouses.
2. *Developing Together.* Even though each spouse continues to develop individually, it is important that the couple keep enough in common. If interests diverge too greatly, the partners may develop in two completely different directions. The result is that they may wind up with too little left in common.
3. *Dealing With Midlife Crisis.* One or both spouses may experience a midlife crisis during this stage. This crisis involves a reevaluation of major issues, such as career and marriage. The couple must be able to renegotiate the marriage relationship.

The special tasks of Stage 3 are:

1. *Refocusing on the Marriage.* For many years, the couple directed much of their attention toward the children. The couple must restructure their marital relationship now that their parental responsibilities have ceased.
2. *Adapting to Retirement.* For so long, the home was the wife's domain. Now that the husband is retired, he must be incorporated into the household. The challenge is to avoid confusing their roles and responsibilities. Separate chores and activities need to be established.

MUTUAL RESPONSIBILITY

As you have examined the stages and tasks of the marital life cycle, you have probably identified difficulties that you and your spouse had in adapting to and adjusting to new developmental changes. Hopefully, you do not hold your spouse or yourself totally responsible for the marital failure. In most cases, the deterioration of marriages is close to a 50-50 responsibility. By accepting your own responsibility, you are using the separation crisis as an opportunity for positive growth.

DISCUSSION QUESTIONS

1. Where are you in the marital life cycle?
2. Which basic tasks were not successfully completed in your marriage? Successfully completed?
3. Which special tasks were not successfully completed? Successfully completed?
4. In terms of the emotional divorce process, are you blaming one person (e.g., your spouse or yourself) or both people for the marital problems?
5. What do you need to do to make a future relationship (e.g, reconciliation or remarriage) a successful one?

CHAPTER 4: DEALING WITH YOUR LOSSES

LOSS OF LOVE

Whether you divorce or reconcile, you have experienced a significant loss: the loss of love. When you got married, you were in love with your spouse, but now, almost every component of your initial love has faded. What are these components of love?

1. *Idealization.* This is a sense that the other person is good and capable. You perceive the loved object as possessing as many positive qualities as possible.
2. *Trust.* This refers to a belief in the other's commitment.
3. *Identification.* This is the sense of being associated with the other. Whatever affects this person in some way also affects you.
4. *Complementarity.* The loved object is perceived as possessing capacities that you lack. Associating with the other person gives you a sense of completeness.
5. *Attachment.* This refers to a bonding to the other that produces feelings of security and ease when the other is present. The result is a feeling of no longer being lonely.

As your marriage deteriorated, almost every component of love came under attack. Rather than dwelling on the positive qualities of the other, one or both spouses started to think negatively of the other. Disappointments and betrayals converted trust into distrust and disrespect. Instead of feeling identified with and supported by the other, the other became viewed as critic and competitor. Feelings of being completed by the other gave way to feelings of being diminished by the relationship. Feelings of attachment were the most resistant to attack. Attachment may have continued despite feelings of anger and resentment toward the other.

ADDITIONAL LOSSES

If you divorce, in addition to the loss of love, you will experience many other significant losses. You may lose your home and other prized possessions. Long-cherished friends may fall by the wayside as you enter the world of singles. The dreams of a shared future with your spouse must be relinquished. If you have children, your relationship with them will undergo changes. You will probably experience temporary or permanent financial difficulties as you adjust to a new lifestyle. These and other losses and changes occur as one makes divorce adjustments.

GRIEF

Whenever you suffer the loss of something significant, you must grieve that loss. Many people are surprised to find out that grief is a necessary part of the divorce process. Many people are reluctant to do the grieving because it is emotionally painful, and they do not want to let go of the old relationship. However, in order to emerge from the separation transition a better person, you must mourn your actual and potential losses.

STAGES OF GRIEF

Grief is part of the emotional divorce process, which we discussed in Chapter 2. Grief itself is a process that progresses through five stages. You need to understand these stages in order to effectively work through your grief:

1. *Denial.* The first reaction to separation or the thought of separation is denial. It is a sense of, "This is not happening to me." You may feel emotionally numb, because you are repressing your feelings. Or you feel depressed, because you are repressing your anger. You may act as if nothing is happening, and you may avoid telling your friends and family about what is happening.
2. *Anger.* Feelings of anger are now turned outward. As you work through your anger, a few reminders may be helpful. First, realize that feelings of anger are normal and natural and learn positive ways of expressing this anger. Second, understand that feelings of loss are often underneath the anger. Verbalizing these feelings of loss may help diffuse the anger. Finally, reach the point of forgiveness. Forgiveness is letting go of the anger - toward yourself and your spouse. Forgive yourself and the other for contributing to the marital breakdown.
3. *Bargaining.* Before you work through your anger to forgiveness, you will go through a stage of bargaining. Bargaining is an effort to hold onto the marital relationship for the wrong reasons. The individual in this stage wants to avoid the difficulties, unhappiness, and loneliness of single life. Therefore, this person may try to get the other person to come back. The spouse may say something like, "I will do anything if you will just come back." This person is willing to settle for second best, instead of choosing to have a successful divorce or marriage.
4. *Depression.* This depression is accompanied by feelings of sadness and crying as the person lets go of the old relationship. It is accompanied by questions like, "What is my purpose in life?" and "Is this all there is to life?" This is a final letting go, the dark before the dawn. It is comforting to know that this stage does not usually last a long time.
5. *Acceptance.* You have completed the grief work when you feel free from the emotional pain of grief. You no longer feel emotionally tied to the past relationship. You have let go of that experience.

THE IMPORTANCE OF COMPLETING THE GRIEF PROCESS

As you have read this chapter, you have probably identified where you are in the grief process. Hopefully, you have resolved to experience the feelings associated with grief work and complete the grief process. As you are working through the grief process, you may sometimes find yourself moving forward and sometimes find yourself in an earlier stage. Regressing to a prior stage for a short period of time is not uncommon. However, it is important to avoid getting stuck at one stage so that you do not move forward in the process. The consequences of getting stuck are too great. You will remain emotionally tied to your past marital relationship, with all of its negative emotions. In order to grow into the future, in order to enter into a new relationship, you must complete the grief process.

DISCUSSION QUESTIONS

1. What have been or will be your greatest losses associated with separating?
2. What stage of the grief process are you in?

3. The initiator is typically further along in the grief process than the noninitiator. Compare where you are in comparison to your spouse.
4. Does this present loss of love bring up any other losses from your past?
5. How do you express the anger you have toward your spouse? Are you expressing your anger appropriately?
6. How will you keep from getting stuck in the grief process?

CHAPTER 5: MAKING A DECISION

DECISION-MAKING STEPS

The separation period can be a time of great ambivalence. One or both partners may feel torn between whether to get out of or to stay in the marital relationship. Even the initiator often has mixed feelings about the decision to divorce. The relationship is unsatisfactory, but you may still feel attached to your spouse. These feelings may make it difficult for you to make a decision.

For the outcomes of the separation to be positive, however, it is essential that you make a stable decision. Ultimately, the decision is yours, but I do want to introduce you to a decision-making process that may be helpful. The steps to making a balanced decision are as follows:

1. *Decide to Decide.* The risks of not changing are too great. Remaining in an unsatisfactory marriage is detrimental to both spouses and the children. Decide to either constructively divorce or rebuild a solid marriage. Decide to get out of a state of ambivalence.
2. *Gather Information.* The only way you can deal with your fear of the unknown is with knowledge. Do not make the mistake of walking blindly into the future. Become aware of the consequences of divorce. Give yourself enough time to search thoroughly for pertinent information.
3. *Weigh the Alternatives.* This simply refers to examining the pros and cons of each alternative. You may want to create a balance sheet and fill in positive and negative anticipated consequences of each alternative. This step will help you stabilize your decision.
4. *Make a Decision.* After you have made your decision, you may face a lot of negative feedback. Others may dislike and resist your decision. If their reactions cause you doubts about your decision, do not view this as a defeat. It merely means that you may need to temporarily regress to an earlier step. Remember, the most important step is the first one.

MUTUAL DECISION

In addition to making a stable decision, it is also to your advantage to reach a mutual decision. Often, one spouse will passively allow a unilateral decision. However, regardless of who initiated the separation (or talks of separation), both partners need to take control of and responsibility for the final decision. A one-sided decision usually results in unhealthy divorce outcomes.

You may be in a marital situation where only one spouse is ambivalent. The other spouse has no reluctance about the decision to divorce. In that case, a divorce will more than likely occur. The challenge, therefore, is for both spouses to make the decision to divorce. If you are the noninitiator, think about the consequences if you fail to take control of the situation. Think about the implications of staying emotionally tied to a person who no longer loves you. It will be terribly difficult and painful for you to let go of this relationship, but the outcome of your doing so will be best for everyone. Take that first step toward a decision. Decide to decide.

Often, both spouses are ambivalent about the decision to divorce. Do we divorce or do we work on our marriage? You may lean more toward divorce if (a) you are able to resolve your attachment to the other, (b) one spouse is unwilling or unable to work on rebuilding the marital relationship, and (c) the advantages of divorce outweigh the benefits of marriage. Or you may be pulled toward reconciliation because (a) enough love and attachment still exist, (b) both spouses are willing and able to address identified problems, (c) negative feelings can be resolved, and (d) the advantages of marriage outweigh the benefits of divorce.

After you and your spouse have each gone through the decision-making steps, you may both reach the same decision If so, you can both cooperate for a constructive future. However, if only one spouse decides for a divorce, the other spouse must painfully accept the reality of an inevitable divorce. Hopefully, this person can decide to let go of the relationship in order to achieve a divorce with healthy outcomes for everyone involved.

DISCUSSION QUESTIONS

1. Are you ambivalent about the decision to divorce? Is your spouse?
2. Have you started the decision-making process? If so, where are you in the process?
3. If you are not making a decision, identify your reasons for not doing so.
4. What actions on your part would assist you in making a mutual decision with your spouse?

CHAPTER 6: A SUCCESSFUL POSTSEPARATION RELATIONSHIP

Eventually you will move through the separation transition into a postseparation relationship. Regardless of your eventual status, married or divorced, it is beneficial to have a successful relationship with your present spouse. However, many partners act in such a way as to produce dysfunctional outcomes. In this chapter, we will examine ways to achieve positive outcomes, as opposed to negative ones. The components of a functional postseparation relationship are as follows:

1. Accept your contributions to the marital disintegration.
2. Let go of the past.
3. Redefine your attachment.
4. Resolve the anger and conflict.
5. Restructure your relationship.
6. Make the best interests of the children a top priority.

ACCEPT YOUR CONTRIBUTIONS

Blaming one person, yourself or your spouse, for the marital deterioration is normal early in the emotional divorce process. However, just as it takes two people to make a marriage work, it typically takes two to cause it to fail. As you acknowledge your part in the marital problems, you will build a bridge for a better postseparation relationship. In addition, you will be able to learn from your past mistakes. You can resolve to learn new patterns of relating that will make a future relationship more successful.

LET GO OF THE PAST

Resolve to complete the grieving process so that you can disentangle yourself from the past relationship. By working through your losses, anger, and depression, you can reach a point of forgiveness and acceptance. You can forgive yourself and your spouse for past mistakes. Once you do that, nothing can keep you hooked into your past. You will be free to enter into a future relationship, whether with another person or with your spouse, with no damaging emotional ties to the old relationship.

REDEFINE YOUR ATTACHMENT

If you decide to reconcile, you will probably want to reexamine your attachment to your spouse. In the past, did you rely too much on the other for security? Did your at-homeness with that person restrict you from developing interests and activities of your own? Did your sense of ease with your spouse lull you into taking him or her for granted? Did you become overly dependent on the other? If so, you will want to redefine and work at establishing a healthier attachment.

If you decide to divorce, you will want to resolve your feelings of attachment to your present spouse. Ongoing attachment will interfere with your divorce adjustment process. However, as you let go of your feelings of attachment to your spouse, remember that some aspects of attachment to a former spouse can have positive consequences. You do not have to hate your spouse to get a divorce. It is possible to develop an amicable friendship. However, this friendship must develop over time, as you drop spousal ties and learn to work together as parents.

RESOLVE THE ANGER AND CONFLICT

Without a doubt, you have been hurt and disappointed by your spouse, and feelings of anger are normal. However, in order to have a functional postseparation relationship, you must work through your feelings of anger and reach a point of forgiveness. It is too risky to reunite without resolving the anger and conflict. Ongoing conflict will destroy your marriage and psychologically harm your children.

If you decide to divorce, you must also work through your feelings of anger toward your ex-spouse. If either partner does not resolve his or her anger, family members will suffer. The children are hurt because they get caught in their parents' struggle. Children also suffer from decreasing contact with the nonresidential parent, who wants to avoid conflict with the other parent. The spouses also suffer because the anger keeps them emotionally attached to each other. As a result, they find it difficult to move forward and establish new, constructive relationships.

Because of its adversarial nature, the legal system many times perpetuates feelings of anger. Instead of resolving the anger toward the spouse, court battles promote intense hatred and resentment. The legal divorce can turn into a win-lose battlefield that prolongs and intensifies the conflict. You may want to consider divorce mediation as an alternative to this adversarial system.

RESTRUCTURE THE RELATIONSHIP

If you decide to reconcile, you cannot afford the risk of returning to old relationship patterns. You will need to redefine your roles, expectations, and relationship. You will need to learn new patterns of behavior. As you examined the marital life cycle, you probably identified areas of your relationship that need restructuring. You may need to work on one or several of the following areas: (a) commitment, (b) caring, (c) communication, and (d) conflict. Reconciliation is a difficult process, and you may want the assistance of a marriage counselor.

If you are terminating the marital relationship, you will continue having a parent-parent relationship with your spouse. Restructuring the postmarital relationship means that you terminate marital roles while redefining the parental roles. Postdivorce adjustment is more constructive if you can mutually decide on these parental roles. You will need to define when and how each parent continues to relate to the children. Making joint decisions about the children seems to foster constructive postdivorce adjustment. If you find it difficult to imagine this type of postmarital relationship, think of it as a brand new relationship, in which you and the children's other parent are just starting to do business together. This business relationship between divorced parents usually works.

THE BEST INTERESTS OF THE CHILD

Whether you reconcile or divorce, you will continue to be your children's parents. Hopefully, for their sakes, you will maintain your parental responsibilities. Regardless of your marital status, divorced or married, the same parenting principles apply. First, keep children out of the middle. Children suffer from having to take sides with one parent against the other. Second, children need ongoing contact with each parent. Do not interfere with your child's relationship with the other parent. It is their relationship, and they deserve a chance to make it work. Finally, protect children from ongoing parental conflict. Children should not have to listen to intense conflict or hear one parent denigrate the other. Whatever you decide, keep your child's best interests foremost in your minds. They deserve either a healthy nuclear family or a healthy postdivorce family.

CONCLUSION

You also deserve a functional family. Neither marriage nor divorce, in and of itself, will bring you a better future. Either one can make your life better or worse. It depends on what type of marriage or divorce you decide to create. Whatever you decide or have decided to do, I hope this manual has assisted you in the direction of personal and family growth.

DISCUSSION QUESTIONS

1. Do you still feel emotionally tied to the old relationship? If so, what keeps you attached? Is anger keeping you attached?

2. What changes do you want to make in the way you and your spouse parent?
3. How do you want your postseparation relationship to be different from your preseparation one?
4. Of the concepts addressed in this manual, which one has meant the most to you?
5. How have you changed as a result of this group experience?
6. What have you learned about yourself as a result of this experience?
7. Which aspects of this program have been helpful? Not helpful?

P. Gregg Blanton, EdD, received his Doctorate in Counseling and Guidance from East Texas State University. He has over 10 years experience as a counselor. Dr. Blanton currently works as a full-time counselor at the University of South Carolina at Spartanburg. He has conducted a limited private practice in marriage and family therapy since 1991. He is happily married and lives with his wife and two daughters. Dr. Blanton may be contacted at 189 Converse Circle, Spartanburg, SC 29302.

RESOURCES

SUGGESTED READINGS FOR GROUP PARTICIPANTS

Fisher, B. (1978b). *When Your Relationship Ends.* Denver: Eastwood Printing.
Gardner, R. (1971). *The Boys and Girls Book About Divorce.* New York: Bantam Books.
Krantzer, M. (1974). *Creative Divorce.* New York: Signet.
Ricci, I. (1980). *Mom's House: Dad's House.* New York: Collier Books.
Rofes, E. (Ed.). (1982). *The Kids' Book About Divorce: By, For & About Kids.* New York: Vintage Books.
Smoke, J. (1976). *Growing Through Divorce.* Irving, CA: Harvest House.
Trafford, A. (1982). *Crazy Times: Surviving Divorce.* New York: Bantam Books.
Wallerstein, J., & Blakeslee, S. (1989). *Second Chances.* New York: Ticknor & Fields.
Weiss, R. (1975). *Marital Separation.* New York: Basic Books.

ADDITIONAL REFERENCES*

Ahrons, C., & Rodger, R. (1987). *Divorced Families.* New York: W. W. Norton.
Brown, E. (1976). A model of the divorce process. *Conciliation Courts Review, 14*(2), 1-11.
Fisher, B. (1978a). *Fisher Divorce Adjustment Scale.* Boulder, CO: Family Relations Learning Center.
Fisher, B. (1978b). *When Your Relationship Ends.* Denver: Eastwood Printing.
Kaslow, F. (1984). Divorce: An evolutionary process of change in the family system. *Journal of Divorce, 7,* 21-39.
McCubbin, H., & Patterson, J. (1983). Family transitions: Adaption to stress. In H. McCubbin & C. Figley (Eds.), *Stress and the Family* (pp. 5-25). New York: Brunner/Mazel.
McGoldrick, M. (1988). The joining of families through marriage: The new couple. In B. Carter & M. McGoldrick (Eds.), *The Changing Family Life Cycle* (2nd ed., pp. 209-234). New York: Gardner.
Nichols, W. (1988). *Marital Therapy.* New York: Guilford.
Peck, J., & Manocherian, J. (1988). Divorce in the changing family life cycle. In B. Carter & M. McGoldrick (Eds.), *The Changing Family Life Cycle* (2nd ed., pp. 335-369). New York: Gardner.
Ricci, I. (1980). *Mom's House: Dad's House.* New York: Collier Books.
Storm, C., & Sprenkle, D. (1982). Individual treatment in divorce therapy: A critique of an assumption. *Journal of Divorce, 5,* 87-97.
Turner, N. (1985). Divorce: Dynamics of decision therapy. In D. Sprenkle (Ed.), *Divorce Therapy* (pp. 27-38). New York: Haworth.
Weiss, R. (1975). *Marital Separation.* New York: Basic Books.

---

*Many of the concepts in this manual grew out of ideas from the listed references.

LITIGATION CONSULTING: PREPARING ATTORNEYS TO CROSS-EXAMINE NEUROPSYCHOLOGISTS

Robert H. Ellis

For many psychologists, "going to court" has meant taking the witness stand to provide expert testimony in support of one side or the other in either a civil suit or a criminal action. An increasing number of psychologists are discovering, however, that there are less stressful opportunities in the courtroom that do not involve getting on the witness stand. These opportunities involve working with one side or the other as a litigation consultant. As an example, attorneys are turning to psychologists for consultation in helping them construct profiles for questioning and selecting jurors. Another developing area, and the focus of this contribution, involves consulting with attorneys faced with the prospect of cross-examining well-trained and experienced neuropsychologists. Neuropsychologists are highlighted because, as a specialty, they spend more time in court as experts than any other group of psychologists and, as a consequence, are usually the best prepared and the most difficult to cross-examine.

The cross-examination of an expert witness, if well prepared, can be the most effective tool in the presentation of a case. When an attorney presents an expert witness, it is expected that the testimony will support the attorney's position. But when an attorney can demonstrate that the basis (the facts or the logic) of the opposing attorney's expert is faulty, the impact is quite dramatic and can have a powerful effect on the jury. However, challenging an expert is risky business: If the expert is able to counter each of the cross-examination thrusts with authority, the expert's position will be enhanced and the cross-examiner's diminished. To mount an effective cross-examination of a neuropsychologist, then, an attorney must be conversant in neuropsychology. It is the rare attorney, however, who has the expertise in testing, evaluation, and neuropathology necessary to mount an effective cross-examination of an experienced neuropsychologist without help.

In one sense, it is more straightforward to take part as an expert: One evaluates the individual, prepares with the attorney, presents one's findings during the direct examination, and then defends oneself during the cross-examination. As a litigation consultant, however, it is not so straightforward: One must anticipate what the neuropsychological evidence will look like; one must understand both the evaluation instruments and their underlying logic at least as well as the expert; one must be familiar with the critical literature (i.e., knowing the weaknesses of the various instruments and evaluation strategies); one must examine the data and preliminary testimony looking for any errors of logic, omission, assumptions, and so forth; one must communicate all of this information to the attorney in such a way that he or she can use it to cross-examine the expert in a clear and understandable manner; and then one must be prepared for any surprises.

Before continuing, it should be noted that although the emphasis in this brief overview is on cross-examining the neuropsychologist as if he or she has been incompetent in the evaluation of the plaintiff or is exaggerating the extent of the plaintiff's injuries, I do not imply that neuropsychologists do so on a regular basis. The relationships between the brain and behavior are very complex, and it requires a great deal of training and experience to untangle the various factors, internal and external, that go into maintaining those relationships. As a consequence, it is easy even for the best trained person to overlook a factor that may be contributing to an individual's problems.

More importantly, however, the demand for well-qualified neuropsychologists is a lot greater than the supply and there are, therefore, many psychologists posing as qualified neuropsychologists who have no business taking the witness stand. The only assurance that a professionally competent evaluation has been conducted is provided by a thorough cross-examination of the evaluator and the evaluation. In short, effective cross-examination, and the expectation of a comprehensive cross-examination, will improve the quality of both the expert's work and the litigation itself.

If the potential litigation consultant is coming from a clinical background, he or she must be prepared for a shock in making the transition to an adversarial environment. Years of training designed to minimize critical evaluation will have to be abandoned when entering the world of litigation. Effective litigation consulting requires an ability to see potential weaknesses in all aspects of another's work. On the other hand, those potential litigation consultants with a more experimental background will experience less transitional trauma because of the adversarial structure inherent in the scientific method. But they, too, should be prepared for culture shock and the need to give up accepted practices of collegiality.

The practice of providing consultation to attorneys preparing to cross-examine psychologists (and psychiatrists) was first popularized with the publication in 1970 of *Coping With Psychiatric and Psychological Testimony* by Jay Ziskin. Since then, three successive editions of the book have appeared (Ziskin, 1975, 1981; Ziskin & Faust, 1988). The most recent edition is now in three volumes with David Faust (a psychologist) as co-author. Faust and Ziskin teamed with James Hiers (a lawyer) in 1991 to write a book specifically directed toward cross-examining neuropsychologists: *Brain Damage Claims: Coping With Neuropsychological Evidence*. At a minimum, anyone contemplating litigation consulting should have ready access to the latest editions of these two books. There are other resources (a few of which are listed at the end in the "Resources" section), but these two are primary.

To help the potential litigation consultant better understand how to help an attorney develop the foundation for an effective cross-examination, this contribution is organized as follows: "The Logic of Litigation" describes the playing field and includes a description of the major players; "Preparing the Strategy" provides a review of the fundamentals in developing a plan of attack; and, "The Cross-Examination: 20 Questions" outlines a list of specific questions that should be addressed during either the discovery or the cross-examination along with a discussion indicating how each can be used as part of an overall strategy.

THE LOGIC OF LITIGATION

In preparing to become a litigation consultant, one must, of course, have a strong background in both evaluation and the specific content area. At present, there are no specific or proposed guidelines for those functioning as litigation consultants in the area of neuropsychological testimony. It is a newly evolving field with little defined structure from either the psychological or the forensic professions. For those considering consulting in this area, the minimum background should include a grounding in neuropsychology from either the clinical or the experimental perspective and a thorough understanding of test construction, statistical evaluation, and experimental design. Of probably equal importance, however, the potential litigation consultant must be willing to establish a presence in the marketplace so that when an attorney is in need of a consultant, he or she will know how and where to contact the consultant.

Given that preparation, the next most important skill is understanding the litigation process. Litigation is not as simple as it is usually portrayed in the media. It is helpful to think of it as a form of structured warfare, much like a chess game. Thus, there is a prescribed environment in which moves are made, there is a set of specific rules determining which moves can and cannot be made, there is a strict sequence of alternating moves, and then there is the war itself which starts before the first piece is moved and continues until the last piece is taken from the board. As in real life, the game is often won or lost before it even begins: It is estimated that 97% of all litigation is settled prior to the trial rather than continuing to a jury decision. If the litigation consultant prepares the attorney well, the foundation for a favorable settlement can be established well in advance of the trial, thereby saving time, emotional wear and tear, and expense for all parties involved.

Typically, litigation begins when an individual (the plaintiff) receives a brain trauma because of someone else's purported negligence. The focus of the suit against the negligent person is that the negligence has resulted in permanent brain damage that will compromise the quality of the rest of the victim's life. In some situations, the medical evidence is clear enough to establish that the individual has received a permanent head injury and the neuropsychologist is brought in as an expert to establish the extent to which that injury has affected the individual's behavior. In other situations, the medical evidence is unclear and the neuropsychologist is brought in to establish that there has been brain damage as well as permanent effects on the plaintiff's behavior. It should be noted that as soon as the plaintiff's attorney decides to use an expert neuropsychologist, the defendant's attorney must, by law, be notified. At that point, the defendant's attorney should contact a neuropsychologist to act as a litigation consultant because the game has begun.

In order to make the argument of negligence to the jury, the plaintiff's attorney develops a "theory" of what has happened to the plaintiff such that an award for negligence is justified. The attorney will attempt to "prove" this theory by presenting "facts" to the jury that support the claim of negligence. Facts play the key role in the trial. Facts can only be established by witnesses, lay and expert, who present them under oath from the witness stand. No other facts can be considered in a trial so it is important that witnesses be available to present all the facts that go to build each attorney's theory. It is the jury's duty, as "trier of fact," to determine which facts represent the truth. The judge's purpose is to interpret the law for the jury and to insure that the two attorneys follow the rules of protocol and evidence. In a trial without a jury, the judge takes on the roles of both judge and trier of fact.

Each attorney's facts are established during the direct testimony. The plaintiff's attorney is allowed to call each of his or her witnesses first to establish the case for negligence. It is at this point that most neuropsychologists give their testimony as an expert witness. After the plaintiff's attorney has presented his or her witnesses, the defending attorney will try to refute the plaintiff's theory by presenting an alternative theory supported by a different set of "facts." The defending attorney will also use witnesses (but may choose not to, especially if he or she feels that the other attorney's case can be destroyed in cross-examination). On occasion, the defending attorney will use an expert neuropsychologist to establish that either the plaintiff was not permanently damaged or that the plaintiff's neuropsychologist was wrong in his or her interpretation of the several tests given to the plaintiff.

Because the facts presented by the two attorneys will be different and incompatible, it will be up to the jury to determine which set of facts is a better reflection of the truth. To better help the jury determine which set is more accurate, both attorneys are given the opportunity to question witnesses right after their direct testimony to the jury. This is the cross-examination. Within the structure of a trial, facts are challenged in two different ways. The most effective way is to attack them as they are being presented, during the cross-examination, because the source is then being attacked as well as the veracity of the fact. The second way to challenge a fact is for the opposing attorney to call a witness who presents testimony that contradicts or refutes the first witness's facts. This second type of attack is not as compelling because it comes later (sometimes by several days) and often results in a question of "She said, he said" or "Expert A was more sure of himself/herself than expert B." The cross-examination, then, can be a critical tool for the defendant.

A key but generally unfamiliar part of the examination of the expert witness is the discovery process. Discovery occurs prior to the actual start of the trial. Because each attorney has the right to know in advance what evidence (facts) will be brought up by the opposing attorney, that attorney is allowed to "discover" that evidence by a variety of means. Thus, if one side decides to use an expert, the other side must be immediately notified of that decision and all materials developed by that expert then made available for scrutiny by the other side. At the simplest level of discovery, the attorney can simply ask for any written material, such as reports, testing results, and so forth, that the expert has developed. More typically, the attorney will require that the opposing expert show up at a specific time and place (at the requesting attorney's expense) to be "deposed," that is, for formal questioning under oath and with an official record being kept. The value of this "examination before trial" is that the attorney can ask for the facts that the expert will be presenting during the trial. (The expert does not have to volunteer any information beyond any report that has already been made available, but questions must be answered.) The attorney can also attempt to pin the expert down to limiting statements of fact during the examination that can then be used during the trial. Another value of the discovery examination is that the attorney can ask the numerous detailed questions required of a thorough cross-examination without boring and possibly alienating the jury. Also, by examining the expert before the actual testimony, blind alleys and land mines can be identified and avoided before they embarrass the attorney in front of the jury. Further, because the examination is taken under oath, it can be brought up during the trial if the expert's memory needs a bit of "prompting." Finally, a thorough examination before trial can signal the plaintiff's attorney that the litigation is being taken seriously, that the opposing attorney is well prepared, and that there will be a thorough cross-examination when the case goes to trial. As such, a thorough pretrial examination often leads to a reasonable settlement.

This sketch of the logic of a trial is presented to make several points: First, that it is strategically more effective to attack the expert directly rather than relying on a counterexpert. Secondly, the cross-examiner actually has two opportunities to examine the expert, and the key to an effective cross-examination is laid during the discovery examination.

PREPARING THE STRATEGY

In chess, the purpose of the match is to checkmate the king. Similarly, the purpose of the cross-examination is to find a pattern of weaknesses in the testimony of the expert and thereby impugn the credibility of that expert. As in chess, success is rare without a systematic plan that helps one find, develop, and exploit specific weaknesses. Gone are the days when an attorney could count on impugning the naïve witness through confusion, intimidation, and logical traps. A strategy is necessary, too, for a not-so-obvious reason: Given the respect accorded the "expert" in our culture, small errors in the expert's testimony will tend to be overlooked by the jury. To convince the trier of fact that the expert's testimony should be questioned, it will be necessary for the cross-examining attorney to demonstrate a *pattern* of error.

The necessity of establishing a pattern of error with the cross-examination follows from the basic reason why an expert is allowed to give testimony in the first place. It is expected that, as a highly educated professional, the expert will bring a level of training and expertise to the courtroom that goes beyond the understanding of the layperson. Accordingly, the expert is expected to help the trier of fact to better understand the facts of the case (in addition to providing facts), and that can only be accomplished if the expert gives competent and independent testimony. If the cross-examiner is able to demonstrate a pattern of incompetence or bias by the expert, the argument can then be made to the jury that a basic trust has been violated and that the expert's testimony should be disregarded.

The development of a strategy is aided by the fact that the cross-examining attorney has two opportunities to question the expert, once during the discovery and then again during the cross-examination. Questioning during the discovery is designed to uncover as much information as possible without disclosing the fact that possible errors have been identified. If a pattern of incompetence or bias is revealed, the wise cross-examiner waits until the cross-examination itself to confront the expert with the findings in front of the jury. Of course, the attorney may suggest in meetings with his or her counterpart that there are "problems" to help speed up a negotiated settlement.

The structure of the expert's cross-examination is guided by the key points that the plaintiff's attorney will be attempting to establish through the testimony of the neuropsychologist. From the standpoint of the plaintiff, the goal of the suit will be to prove that (a) there is brain damage, (b) the brain damage did not exist before the purported negligent act, (c) the brain damage had a negative effect on the plaintiff's ability to function independently, and (d) the damage and its effects are permanent. Accordingly, the cross-examiner and litigation consultant will attempt to establish that (a) there is no brain damage, it is minimal, or the plaintiff is exaggerating; (b) there are events in the plaintiff's past (e.g., seizures, alcohol use, exposure to toxins) that could account for the present problem as well as, or in addition to, the purported negligence; (c) the reason it appears the plaintiff has problems is that the expert reported only the data that suggested a problem and ignored those tests and test results that would indicate no problems; and (d) there is no evidence suggesting that the purported problems are permanent in nature and require the level of support indicated by the expert. The cross-examiner may not be able to establish all four of these points, but if at least one is established then the chances of the defendant being forced to make a large settlement are reduced considerably.

When a neuropsychologist is asked to evaluate a plaintiff, the first step should be to collect a thorough history of the individual. The purpose of the history is two-fold. First, the expert will attempt to establish that there is behavioral evidence (and, hopefully, earlier testing scores) indicating a change in the person's behavior and personality from before the accident to the present. Second, the neuropsychologist will argue that there are no other factors in the victim's background (such as a prior head injury or a history of substance abuse) that could account for the person's present status. A discussion of the requirements for a thorough history and how it should be approached in the cross-examination is presented in more detail under Questions #2 and 17 in the next section.

In the next step of the evaluation, the neuropsychologist will give an extensive series of tests to the plaintiff to establish an empirical basis for the problems claimed in the suit. The quality of that testing must be examined in detail and, in fact, may make up the bulk of the questions during the discovery and cross-examination.

The litigation consultant helps the attorney examine the quality of the testing from three different angles: (a) questioning the selection of the tests used to assess the post-accident status of the plaintiff, including both the reputation of those tests within the profession and the extent to which they meet professional standards for reliability, validity, and norms; (b) questioning the extent to which the expert followed strict procedural protocol in administering the tests and collecting data from the plaintiff; and, (c) questioning the rationale used by the expert to develop conclusions regarding the extent of the damage, the cause of the damage, and the permanence of the damage. The structure of the questions used to examine this category of questions is presented in Questions #3 to 11 in the next section.

After the history and the testing have been examined in detail, the cross-examiner's next task will be to question the care with which the expert protected the evaluation against sources of distortion. The most obvious source of such error is the distortion contributed by a plaintiff who has the potential of realizing a great deal of money with a successful settlement or decision. This problem is recognized in the profession (Rogers, 1988) and, although it has never been successfully resolved, there are ways of minimizing its impact. A discussion of the different ways the expert can be questioned to determine if an effort was made to control for this problem is reviewed under Question #18.

A second general source of distortion is introduced when the expert makes generalizations from specific test evidence about the existence of a problem. The correspondence between test results and the existence of a problem is rarely 100%. As a consequence, there is always the chance of error when making a prediction. There are two types of prediction error: false positive (predicting that something exists when it does not) and false negative (predicting that something does not exist when it does). The probability of these two types of errors occurring is important to establish because they qualify the certainty of any prediction made by the expert. Another common error is for the expert to confuse the difference in predicting from the cause to the effect with predicting from the effect to the cause. For example, Dawes (1988) notes that 10% of chronic smokers will develop lung cancer (predicting from the cause to the effect) while 99% of lung cancer victims have a history of chronic smoking (predicting from the effect to the cause). It will be the litigation consultant's responsibility to examine the expert's predictions closely to insure that these several subtle errors have not contaminated the expert's conclusions.

As can be seen, these questions can become quite technical and, as a consequence, many evaluators pay them little attention despite the amount of time spent learning about them during their training years. Accordingly, they offer a potentially fertile source of questions for demonstrating a pattern of incompetence or bias. These sources of error are described in more detail under Questions #11, 12, and 14 in the next section.

A third source of error originates in an expert's failure to appreciate that his or her own hard-won clinical experience can be a source of distortion and error. Ziskin and Faust (1988) and Faust, Ziskin, and Hiers (1991) review a great deal of literature showing that it is a common error for experts to believe that their "clinical" experience provides them with a clinical acumen that allows them to predict results better than actuarial tables. Paul Meehl argued in 1954, with a book entitled *Clinical Versus Statistical Prediction*, that it is extremely rare for a clinician to make better predications than statistical formulae. Despite almost 40 years of effort to demonstrate otherwise, that observation is still accurate (Dawes, Faust, & Meehl, 1989). If the expert is not aware of the literature on the fallibility of "clinical experience" in making predictions about human behavior, and unwisely attempts to offer an opinion not supported by the actuarial literature, that expert can be shown, with few exceptions, to be incompetent.

This, of course, does not exhaust the ways in which an expert (or not-so-expert) neuropsychologist can introduce error unwittingly into the evaluation of a plaintiff. In the next section, a series of more detailed questions is presented and discussed. Each of these questions needs to be addressed as the foundation for a basic cross-examination. Given the brief nature of this contribution, the discussions are not complete and the reader is referred to the material listed in the "Resources" section. They do, however, offer a taste of the contribution that a well-prepared litigation consultant can provide.

THE CROSS-EXAMINATION: 20 QUESTIONS

As has been noted previously, the purpose of the cross-examination is to insure that the testimony of the expert is thorough, that the testimony meets both legal and professional standards, and that the conclusions reached by the expert follow directly from the facts that have been presented in a manner that would be acceptable to the profession. To structure the questioning of the expert, a series of 20 questions has been developed which focus on the key areas in which facts/data can be biased, corrupted, and/or misinterpreted. These questions are presented with a brief explanation describing some of the detail that should be covered in the questioning.

QUESTION #1

What Are Your Qualifications for Giving Expert Testimony in This Case? Not all people are qualified to give expert testimony, not all psychologists are qualified to give expert psychological testimony, and not all neuropsychologists are qualified to give expert neuropsychological testimony. With this first question, the purpose is to determine if the expert does, in fact, have the training and the experience to give testimony that reflects the standards accepted by the profession, that is, diplomate status. Questions that should be asked are:

- Where did you get your training?
- What kind of training was it (i.e., What was your major)?

- Was it an American Psychological Association-approved program?
- Where did you complete your internship?
- Was it an American Psychological Association-approved internship?
- Where are you presently employed?
- What are your responsibilities?
- What professional organizations do you belong to?
- Are you board certified in neuropsychology?
- Have you published any articles in the area?
- Have you conducted any research in this area as a project director?
- Are you licensed to practice psychology?
- Which states?
- Have you ever been censured or had your license suspended in any state or by any professional organization?
- Have you given testimony as a neuropsychologist before?
- What kind of experience or background do you have working with head injury cases where the injury was the same as is purported to have occurred in this case?
- What proportion of your practice is made up of forensic testimony?

The question of fees for testimony can be raised to make sure that the expert is not being paid contingent on the outcome of the litigation and to determine if the fee is outrageous (i.e., Is the expert being paid while he or she sleeps?).

QUESTION #2

What Historical Information Did You Collect from the Plaintiff? The purpose of this question is to determine if a thorough and comprehensive history was developed. Quite often, there is material in the plaintiff's past that may provide a partial explanation for the plaintiff's present problems. For example, is there a history of alcohol or substance abuse? Is there an earlier history of traumatic head injury, coma, oxygen deprivation (e.g., a near-drowning experience), concussion, or infection of the brain? The expert should be asked if he or she checked for a history of special education placement while the individual was in school (which would suggest that the plaintiff has a history of brain dysfunction). In attempting to determine if the expert made a thorough search, the following kinds of records should have been reviewed: School records, any records indicating functioning level (SAT scores, aptitude tests, or intelligence testing), any records indicating involvement with the law (and the Department of Motor Vehicles for DWI arrests), any involvement with the mental health profession (psychiatric or inpatient substance abuse treatment), any medical records, military records (discharge status can sometimes reveal a history of instability), any indications of car or motorcycle accidents, and other potential sources of head injury.

Another important historical line of questioning is to develop as detailed a picture as possible of the events leading up to, during, and immediately following the plaintiff's injury. It is not unusual that a pattern of behaviors will be found that is inconsistent with the type or seriousness of injury that is being reported by the expert.

This early point in the questioning is a good place to begin searching for patterns of bias. As the expert is answering questions about the types of historical information gathered, ask if a standardized, structured interview was used to guide the choice of questions. The point of asking this question is to determine if the expert was looking for historical information to confirm a hypothesis (conscious or otherwise) regarding the presence of brain damage. Even experts sometimes forget that it is easier and more rewarding to find confirming evidence for just about anything than it is to find disconfirming data. If it can be demonstrated that the expert looked just for confirming data, then the argument can be made that the plaintiff's test profile is incomplete and possibly biased. Without following a structured format, it is almost impossible to insure that all sources of information, supportive and nonsupportive, are examined.

QUESTION #3

What Tests Did You Administer? A specific set of questions will be asked for each test administered to the plaintiff, and so it is important to get a complete list. It is important, too, to make sure that all tests that were administered to the plaintiff are listed, not just the ones that showed positive results.

The cross-examiner will want to ask if the expert personally administered each and every test. Many neuropsychologists use master's-level psychometricians to administer the actual test, leaving the neuropsychologist to interpret the data. Although it is an accepted practice in the profession, the expert loses a degree of control over the quality of the testing and the opportunity to observe the plaintiff taking the tests. When a psychometrician is used, or when the expert is relying on data collected by another psychologist, the expert needs to be asked the following question: How can you be sure that the tests were administered appropriately? Regardless of who administered the tests, these questions should be asked to insure that the test was administered appropriately and that no information was left out: Were all questions and tasks presented? If some were not presented, which ones and why not? Were the instructions and questions read verbatim to the plaintiff or might the expert have relied on (fallible) memory to give the instructions? Were timing constraints observed and were all materials used appropriately?

In addition to determining if there were any changes in the way the testing was presented, questions about the testing environment itself need to be asked: Where was each test administered? How long did each one take? Were there breaks between tests? Was each test taken at one sitting or were there breaks during the test? What time of day was the test administered? How did the plaintiff appear before, during, and after each test? Was there any indication of fatigue, confusion, or distractibility? Did anyone help the plaintiff answer the questions, such as a friend, an interpreter, or a facilitator?

The purpose of making test-taking procedures standardized is so that individual data can be compared to groups who took the test under essentially identical conditions. When standardization procedures are not followed, the comparability of the individual to the group (the norming group) is no longer maintained and, as a consequence, the individual data is rendered meaningless. When an expert makes any changes in procedure, follow-up questions must be asked to determine if the expert took into consideration the impact of those changes on the interpretation and meaningfulness of the data.

One potential solution to this problem is to have the expert videotape the complete evaluation. The question of videotaping is being hotly debated within the profession; some fear that the presence of a camera would, itself, violate standardization conditions, while others are concerned that the testee would behave in unpredictable ways with the knowledge that a camera was recording everything. Regardless, the videotape provides a record that can be examined by all and it will become a standard practice in the near future.

QUESTION #4

For each test identified in Question #3, ask: **Why Did You Administer That Test?** The purpose of this question is straightforward: to establish whether or not the expert chose each test using systematic and consistent criteria. As in Question #2, the potential for biasing the outcome of the evaluation is quite high in the types and sequencing of tests administered to the plaintiff. The expert should be asked if a standard, fixed battery of tests such as the Halstead-Reitan Battery or the Luria Nebraska Battery was administered. This question is important because there are estimates that approximately 80% of neuropsychologists use what is called a flexible approach. That is, depending on the results of the first several tests administered (which usually include the Wechsler Adult Intelligence Scale), the selection and sequencing of the rest of the battery is left up to the discretion of the neuropsychologist. From a diagnostic and rehabilitation perspective, this approach makes sense for it is more efficient and less expensive. In addition, slight errors are not so costly and the consequences of bias not so important. In the litigation environment, however, bias and error take on much greater importance, and it is critical that all efforts to control for bias, both conscious and unconscious, be observed. Experts should understand this and use a fixed battery despite their possible preference for the flexible approach.

Question #4 must be asked in the discovery phase, and, as it is being asked, close attention should be paid to the answer for each test; even if a standard battery was used, attention should be paid to the sequence in which the tests in the battery were administered. In addition to asking why a test was given, the cross-examiner should also ask why a particular test was given at a particular point in the evaluation. If large changes in the sequencing of a standard battery's tests are noted, or if the expert used a flexible approach, the consultant should become suspicious and begin looking for a pattern that would suggest that the expert is attempting to present a biased picture or is poorly trained.

QUESTION #5

For each test identified in Question #3, ask: **What Were the Findings?** There are often errors in the translation of raw test data into standardized and norm-based conclusions. On occasion, a test will be administered and, when the results do not look interesting to the evaluator, the testing will be discarded and not reported as part of the plaintiff's evaluation. Therefore, it is important during the discovery to have the expert report on all the testing and all the data that was collected and, if possible, get access to the actual test protocols to check for scoring errors.

QUESTION #6

For each test identified in Question #3, ask: **Is This Test the Best Test for This Problem?** The selection of tests in the expert's neuropsychological battery is almost always changing as research comes up with better and more precise tests. This is one of the problems with the fixed batteries. As the batteries have grown older and developed extensive norms, clinicians have also been forced to continue using the older, original tests in the battery so that the norms would remain valid. As an example, Ralph Reitan insists (with good reason) that the older form of the Wechsler Adult Intelligence Scale continue to be used in the Halstead-Reitan Battery despite the fact that the adult form of the Wechsler was revised in 1981. This creates quite a dilemma for the expert: Should the older form with the more extensive and reliable norms be used, or should the newer and better model with the smaller norm base be used? In asking this question, then, listen carefully for the reasons why one test or sequencing of tests was chosen over another. There are often valid reasons, and these should be accepted, but on other occasions, the expert may have taken a shortcut or may not have realized that there were newer, better accepted tests available for a specific psychological process. Those latter situations provide an excellent opportunity to raise the question of incompetence.

QUESTION #7

For each test identified in Question #3, ask: **What Set of Norms Was Used to Determine How the Plaintiff Performed Relative to Brain-Damaged and Nonbrain-Damaged People?** The purpose of norms is to provide a baseline against which the behavior of the plaintiff can be compared to see if it is "normal" or out of the ordinary when compared to the general population. It is critical, therefore, that in choosing a norming group for comparison purposes, one be chosen that is as close to the characteristics of the plaintiff as possible. For example, if the plaintiff is a middle-aged, Asian female, the expert should not have used norms for white, adolescent males. One can find this error quite regularly when an evaluator uses the generic norms in the Wechsler manual and does not correct for the testee's age. Norming tables are being updated rather regularly, and one of the responsibilities of the consultant will be to stay up-to-date with the evaluation literature and be familiar with the norm profile for each of the most commonly used tests in neuropsychology.

QUESTION #8

For each test identified in Question #3, ask: **How Was This Test Validated?** Validity is the measure of how well a test is measuring what it is supposed to be measuring. In the development of any test, it is the critical question that must be answered to the potential user's satisfaction. There are a variety of ways that validity is demonstrated, and some are more acceptable than others. The litigation consultant will be required to demonstrate his or her best teaching skills in communicating these concepts to the attorney so that the attorney will be able to ask questions without having them backfire because the attorney did not understand the concept. At a minimum, the attorney should understand and be able to differentiate between predictive and construct validity.

This question will need to be emphasized if the expert has used tests that are fairly new and not yet well accepted in the profession or if the test is obscure. Most of the more popular tests have acceptable levels of validity; an extensive cross-examination on the validity of those tests will probably not prove productive. However, this question should never be completely ignored because there are differences in the levels of validity between the various tests; it will prove instructive to the jury to understand that all tests are not as good as others. On occasion, the cross-examiner may be able to demonstrate that the evidence in support of damage relies on tests that have weaker validity and that the tests with stronger validity indicated no damage.

QUESTION #9

For each test identified in Question #3, ask: **Has This Test Been Cross-Validated?** If you find that an expert has used a test that is unfamiliar or is quite new, then the question of cross-validity should be raised. In asking if a test has been cross-validated, one is asking if the research by which the test was originally validated has been duplicated by an independent researcher with a different group of individuals. It is a common phenomenon in science that new findings, despite acceptable controls used during the initial demonstration, cannot be replicated. In fact, it is the requirement for independent replication that sets science apart from the pseudosciences like astrology. Therefore, when an expert presents data from a test that is unfamiliar, it is imperative that the expert be questioned in some detail regarding how, when, and by whom the test was independently cross-validated. If that cross-validation cannot be demonstrated, the cross-examiner should bring up several examples of scientific experiments that may be familiar to the jury that looked good on first blush and then became major disappointments when the effort was made to cross-validate them.

QUESTION #10

For each test identified in Question #3, ask: **What Is the Reliability of This Test?** Reliability is a measure of the extent to which a test is consistent in measuring some trait or characteristic. To the extent that a test is not reliable, that is, it gives a different score each time that it is given, then to that extent it cannot be trusted to be measuring what it is supposed to be measuring. There are two reasons why a test is not reliable: It is either a poorly constructed test or it is trying to measure something that does not exist. Low reliability is a very strong indication that the test is not measuring what it is supposed to be measuring, that is, the test is not valid.

Reliability is one of the foundations of testing. The consultant will, of course, have a thorough understanding of the reliability literature for each of the tests that are commonly used in neuropsychological evaluations. As in the preparation for asking questions about a test's validity noted previously, the attorney may require a good deal of education to reach the point where he or she is able to ask questions that will develop good information from potentially nonresponsive or hostile expert witnesses.

QUESTION #11

For each test identified in Question #3, ask: **Would You Tell Us What the Probability of Error Was?** Although experts will give their conclusions with statements of "professional certainty" and "clinical judgment," each test result that went into those decisions will have an error rate that can be determined from the test scores. These error rates will be based on the selectivity and sensitivity of the tests. When tests are developed, they are examined to see how well they categorize each individual in a group that is made up of individuals, some of whom have the target problem and some of whom do not. The percentage of those with the target problem who are selected is a measure of the test's *sensitivity*. The percentage of those without the problem who are identified as not having the problem is a measure of the test's *selectivity*. When a test indicates that a person has the target problem and, in fact, does not, that type of error is called a *false positive* error. By the same token, when the test indicates that an individual does not have a target problem when, in fact, the individual does have the problem, that error is called a *false negative* error.

No test is perfect, and although the expert will focus on the test's accuracy, the cross-examiner should direct the jury's attention to the rate of error. One approach the attorney can use is to refer the expert back to the validation data for the particular test being reviewed and ask what those data say about the probability of making erroneous predictions. If the expert is not able to give a clear answer, the attorney can follow up with questions directed toward the expert's ability to reach a conclusion when he or she is unfamiliar with the test's error rate. If the expert is able to provide a specific measure of the test's rate of error (and the litigation consultant should have calculated this number ahead of time), the attorney may want to challenge it if it is discrepant, or he or she may use it as the basis for additional questions if it is reasonably accurate. For example, if the validity score is .82, the attorney can ask "Does this mean that 18% of the people taking the test (almost one out of five) will be misidentified by this test?" It is important to move the expert away from using technical terms like correlation, which most people do not understand, and to a basis that they do understand. When the numbers and relative proportions of mis-selected people are made concrete, the jury can begin to see that even the best of tests is not very accurate. Furthermore, by having an actual number, the attorney will have something concrete to refer back to when he or she begins asking about the effects of changed instructions and nonstandard testing procedures later in the examination.

QUESTION #12

What Are the Base Rates You Used in Arriving at Your Conclusions? "Base rate" refers to the rate at which a particular disorder or a particular symptom actually exists in the population. Without knowing both of those rates, it is impossible to make a prediction about the existence of a particular problem in a particular individual based on the presence or absence of a particular symptom (or test result). It is important to bring up this point because many experts do not pay particular attention to base rates and assume that when a test result indicates a problem, the problem exists. However, as was indicated in the description of the different types of prediction errors, the actual rate of the disorder in the population, as well as the "hit rate" of the symptom or test, has a major impact on the accuracy of predicting that problem based on the symptom or test result.

Consider the following: Assume that the rate of frontal lobe injury is 10 per 1,000 in people involved in car accidents. Assume that your test for frontal lobe injury has a hit rate of .9. If you gave the test to all one thousand accident victims you would identify 9 out of the 10 people with frontal lobe injury and miss just one. But consider the other side of the equation. Assume, for the sake of argument, that your test is also able to identify 99% of those without frontal lobe injury and misdiagnose only 1%. That 1% translates into approximately 10 people wrongly diagnosed as frontal lobe injured out of the population of 990 without the injury. Thus with a very good test, we get 19 people diagnosed as having a frontal lobe injury, only 9 of which (less than 50%) actually have the injury. It is not difficult to see how the error rate increases radically as the hit rates decrease, and there are not many psychological tests with the hit rates used in this example. It is important, therefore, that the jury understand the importance of base rate in making decisions about the presence or absence of a head injury. To put this in a somewhat facetious perspective, how many of us would be wrongly diagnosed as having an amnestic disorder because we occasionally misplace our car keys?

Many poorly trained neuropsychologists are not familiar with the problems introduced by an ignorance of base rates and so it is a good practice to ask the expert during the discovery if he or she is familiar with the concept of base rate. If the expert indicates familiarity with it, have the attorney follow up with a question asking for an explanation of its importance. In addition, an effort should be made to have the expert report the actual base rates used in reaching the various conclusions. Those data can be used to check the accuracy of the conclusions. However, if the expert indicates unfamiliarity with the concept of base rate, it will be up to the attorney as to whether further questions should be forestalled until the actual cross-examination in front of a jury.

QUESTION #13

What Are Your Conclusions? This question needs to be asked during the discovery phase of the litigation. Its importance is that it forces the expert to make a specific statement of his or her findings. Having such a statement provides the consultant with a criterion against which to evaluate the expert's logic. By knowing what the expert is trying to establish, the consultant can then examine all the data to determine if that conclusion does, in fact, follow from the data and, if so, if it is the simplest and most reasonable of the possible alternatives. In addition, having a statement by the expert on record makes it difficult for the expert to change his or her conclusions as a consequence of information developed during the examination before trial.

QUESTION #14

On What Basis Did You Reach Your Conclusion? The purpose of this question during the discovery is to identify the means whereby the expert made the leap from the pattern of test scores, historical information, and behavioral observations to his or her conclusions. The first thing that the cross-examiner should be looking for is whether the expert used actuarial tables based on reported base rates or, rather, relied on "clinical experience" as the basis for interpreting the data. As noted previously, if the expert used "clinical" or "qualitative" observations as the rationale, a line of questioning must be opened during the cross-examination showing the general unreliability and high potential for bias that are inherent within an expert's use of "clinical experience" as a basis for arriving at a conclusion. The reader is referred to both Ziskin works (Faust, Ziskin, & Hiers, 1991; Ziskin & Faust, 1988) for an extended discussion of the problems introduced when decisions are based on "clinical experience."

QUESTION #15

How Did You Control for Bias in the Evaluation? There are many ways that bias can enter into the expert's development of an opinion regarding the plaintiff's brain injury. A number of these have been noted throughout the preceding questions. They include the major sources such as the selection of tests, the degree of emphasis placed on the various test scores, the tendency to emphasize those that agree with the tester's conclusions, and the tendency to deemphasize or ignore those scores that are not consistent with the final conclusion. They also have included the more subtle forms of bias including the types of precautions taken to insure that one's personal expectations do not influence the evaluation process. It will be up to the attorney to decide whether a general question is asked directly of the expert. However, it is sometimes fruitful to ask the expert to describe how the problem of bias was addressed to see if the expert even considered it as a potential problem. If it appears that the expert was not aware of bias as a contaminating influence or arrogantly assumed that his or her "competence" eliminated the possibility of bias, then the attorney should consider systematically addressing sources of bias during the cross-examination, pointing out to the jury in each instance how bias may have affected the outcome because it was not given much consideration as a problem by the expert.

QUESTION #16

How Did You Establish That There Was a Change in Functioning? An essential demonstration in the expert's testimony is that there has been a change in the plaintiff's behavior. A theory of negligence cannot be maintained if there has been no change in the plaintiff's ability to function independently. Because the expert's evaluation is conducted only after the accident, those results cannot be used to demonstrate a change in the person's behavior. Without comparable premorbid (i.e., before the accident) testing, making the argument that there is a demonstrable cause-and-effect connection between the accident and the plaintiff's present status becomes very difficult to maintain. As noted earlier, historical information becomes very important for establishing premorbid functioning.

There are techniques suggested in the neuropsychological literature for estimating premorbid functioning in lieu of collecting a thorough history, but these techniques have never been demonstrated to be valid enough to justify their use in the legal arena. For example, there is an argument that certain scales in the intelligence scales are more resistant ("hold their value") to head injury, and if one sees a profile with the "hold" scales significantly higher than the "don't hold" scales, that is *prima facie* evidence of brain damage. Another effort to estimate premorbid intellectual functioning has been to combine those demographic variables that have been shown to correlate with intelligence (such as education and Social Economic Status) into a prediction formula. This approach has also proven to generate predictions little better than chance. These efforts using the IQ tests have proven unsuccessful despite the fact that IQ is the most researched psychological variable. Efforts to estimate premorbid functioning of other neuropsychological processes have received less attention with no better outcome.

Given the unreliability of interview-generated data, the establishment of premorbid levels without actual testing data will be one of the most difficult aspects of the expert's testimony. These sources of error and doubt should be emphasized in all cross-examinations. The arguments will be especially effective if any evidence (see next question) from before the accident can be produced indicating that there are other possible explanations for why the plaintiff appears to be brain damaged.

QUESTION #17

Have You Taken into Consideration All Conditions in the Plaintiff's Background That Could Account for the Results That You Are Reporting? There are several reasons why this question needs to be asked. First, many, if not a majority, of evaluators do not take the time to conduct a thorough background check with both the plaintiff and the plaintiff's family (nuclear and extended) to determine if there is anything in the person's background that could even partially account for his or her present status. Most evaluators, as trusting professionals trained in a caring profession, automatically assume that the accident is the cause of the problem and look no further than test data in support of that hypothesis. Second, until recently, Ralph Reitan (developer of the Halstead-Reitan Battery [HRB]) argued that all evaluations should be done "blind," that is, with no contaminating knowledge of the plaintiff's history. Apparently many experts using the HRB took his instructions literally and collected no history even after completing the assessment. Although they could say with some certainty whether the plaintiff was brain damaged or not, they were rarely able to speak to the core issue of the litigation: What was the cause?

If the expert indicates or suggests in any way that the history taking was limited, then it is imperative that the attorney collect as much background history as possible (using the legal means available to him or her). It is surprising the ease and frequency with which prior car accidents, drunk driving convictions, concussions, near-drowning experiences, poisonings, seizures, and other phenomena associated with potential brain injury show up when looked for. In addition, if the history by the expert is sketchy and nothing untoward turns up, the attorney is still able to lay the groundwork for a pattern of incompetence by going through and asking if this was checked or if that was checked and so on until it is clear that a thorough and competent effort was not made.

QUESTION #18

How Did You Control for the Possibility That the Plaintiff Was Deliberately Attempting to Distort the Test Results? After the quality of the testing has been examined, it should be clear if the expert made an effort to determine if the plaintiff was malingering or deliberately distorting the results. Any time there is a large sum of money involved, the question of distortion must be taken into consideration. The question of malingering has taken on increased importance in the last two decades since the courts began allowing head injury litigation to continue without hard medical evidence. Although that opened the door for both mild head injury cases (which can have a devastating impact on an individual's life) and neuropsychologists, it also opened the door for malingerers.

For the most part, malingerers are clumsy and end up contradicting themselves. However, given the sums involved in head injury suits, and the hope that the defendant's insurance company will settle before the going gets too intense, the possibility of malingering has to be given serious attention in every cross-examination. Malingering does not have to consist of a complete distortion of the purported injury; quite often the distortion involves only an exaggeration of symptoms. Regardless, triers of fact are very sensitive to distortion, and if the specter of distortion can be raised by showing inconsistencies in either the testing profile or the historical profile, or that the expert made no effort to control for distortion in his or her testing, then a broad charge of negligence, incompetence, and bias can be made.

There are several ways that the expert should proceed to minimize the possibility of distortion. During the first phase of the evaluation, when the plaintiff's history is being developed, a detailed search should be made for any other possible injury that could account for the present symptoms. The expert should be asked for the results of that search including a list of all the materials that were checked. The expert should also have made an effort to determine if the plaintiff has been involved in other litigation, neuropsychological and otherwise. Toward that end, the cross-examiner should expend the time, resources, and energy to develop an independent review of the plaintiff's history (as noted previously in Question #2). A second approach to detecting malingering is to see if there is any tendency on the part of the plaintiff to project an image of himself or herself that differs from how the majority of people present themselves. One of the tests routinely administered during a neuropsychological battery is the Minnesota Multiphasic Personality Inventory (MMPI), a personality test. It is rarely of much diagnostic use for detecting brain damage, but it does have the best developed series of scales for detecting the extent to which an individual tends to distort the impression, both positive and negative, that they give others. This is not a foolproof technique - a certain small percentage of honest people see themselves in idealistic ways. Good discussions are available in the many texts about the MMPI that explore the restrictions and interpretations of the several distortion scales in the MMPI (see, e.g., Pope, Butcher, & Seelen, 1993).

Another way to detect intentional distortion is to give a simple test that moderately brain injured people have been shown to pass with ease and presenting it with instructions suggesting that it is difficult. This approach is rather new and the supporting data is only now being developed; it does not yet have the acceptance in the professional community that would be required to justify its use in a litigation. The book written by Richard Rogers (1988) in the "Resources" section provides an excellent review of the various strategies.

QUESTION #19

How Did You Control for Examiner Error in the Administration of These Tests? Error can be introduced into a standardized test in a variety of ways: By changing the instructions, by changing the standard conditions under which the test is to be administered (e.g., tests like the MMPI are not to be taken home to be completed where a friend or a psychology text can be used to help answer the questions), by changing or modifying the scoring criteria, and, more often than one would expect, by simple errors in scoring. As noted earlier in the discussion regarding sources of bias, it is worth the time and effort during the discovery phase to have the expert review what was done to find simple mistakes that may have been overlooked. If the expert did not have the results checked by an independent reviewer, that oversight can be exploited in the cross-examination. If the expert used a psychometrician to give and score the testing, a simple inquiry as to whether the expert checked the data can occasionally lay the foundation for a pattern of incompetence, bias or both.

If there is suspicion that great care was not taken in the scoring of the data, the expert should be asked if he or she is familiar with the extensive research literature showing how expectations affect how people see things, allowing them to see things that do not exist and overlook things that do exist. The goal of this line of questioning is to establish that the expert is familiar with the literature on the effects of expectations (bias), yet did not invest an effort into protecting himself or herself from that possibility. If the expert is familiar with the literature and did not take a special effort to have the scoring checked independently, or if he or she is not familiar with the literature, the question of incompetence can be raised.

The expert should also be asked if any recordings of the administration of the tests, audio or video, were collected. If not, the cross-examiner should ask the expert to describe the actual testing process in as much detail as possible. Besides attempting to determine if any changes in the standard procedures were introduced, the attorney should also be attempting to determine whether the instructions were read directly from the instruction manual or if the tester relied on memory to instruct the testee. A possible source of error occurs when "examiner drift" is introduced. Examiner drift occurs when examiners begin to rely on their memories to give the instructions after repeated administrations of a test and, as a consequence, begin to introduce subtle changes in the instructions which have unknown effects on test behavior. If the expert did not read the instructions, he or she should be asked about the concept of examiner drift and to describe it for the jury (this, during the cross-examination rather than the discovery). A follow-up question should then be directed to the expert asking why more of an effort to control for changes in the instructions was not made since it is well known that small changes can have a large impact on the results and it was clear that the plaintiff was involved in litigation. Again, if the expert fails to show concern for these small details, a pattern of incompetence can be raised to the jury.

QUESTION #20

At What Point in Your Evaluation Did You Arrive at the Conclusion That the Plaintiff Was Brain Damaged? While this question is presented as the last general question, the possibility that the expert has arrived at a conclusion early in the testing regarding brain damage should be considered throughout the discovery and cross-examination. The only acceptable answer to this question is that the decision was made after all the testing was completed, all the test data were analyzed and reviewed, and all of the background information was taken into consideration. If there is any exception to this answer, then the possibility must be raised to the jury that the expert made up his or her mind early and continued with the evaluation just to collect data to support that conclusion. If so, then the evaluation was not objective and should be dismissed.

CONCLUDING COMMENT

I would like to leave the reader with two observations. First, contemplating the possibility of leaping into a new endeavor where the need and structure of one's services is defined by another profession can be daunting. By providing an overview of the cross-examination process within the structure of a brain injury litigation, it is hoped that a few of the unknowns have been eliminated.

Second, as the potential for the independent practice of clinical psychology dries up with the establishment of more and larger Health Maintenance Organizations, Preferred Provider Organizations, and the various other "managed care" options, the independent and adventuresome practitioner is forced to discover and invent new professional opportunities. Litigation consulting offers a challenging opportunity to make use of one's professional skills in a real-world, problem-solving environment. It does not offer steady employment, but it does offer lucrative employment, it offers an opportunity to practice as a true scientist-practitioner, and it provides an opportunity to work with professionals outside the human/social services field.

Robert H. Ellis, PhD, is currently Senior Psychologist at The Resource Center in Jamestown, New York. In addition, he maintains a private practice in Fredonia, New York, from which he provides consulting and seminars for attorneys. He is a graduate of the University of California, Santa Barbara, and, before beginning work in the private sector, was on the faculty at Idaho State University in Pocatello, Idaho, and the State University of New York, College at Fredonia. Dr. Ellis may be contacted at 29 East Main, Fredonia, NY 14063.

RESOURCES

Dawes, R. M. (1988). *Rational Choice in an Uncertain World.* San Diego, CA: Harcourt, Brace, Jovanovich.

Dawes, R. M. (1989). Experience and validity of clinical judgment: The illusory correlation. *Behavioral Sciences & The Law, 7,* 457-467.

Dawes, R. M., Faust, D., & Meehl, P. E. (1989). Clinical versus actuarial judgment. *Science, 243,* 1668-1674.

Faust, D., Ziskin, J., & Hiers, J. B., Jr. (1991). *Brain Damage Claims: Coping With Neuropsychological Evidence* (Vols. I & II). Los Angeles, CA: Law and Psychology Press.

Meehl, P. E. (1954). *Clinical Versus Statistical Prediction.* Minneapolis: University of Minnesota Press.

Pope, K. S., Butcher, J. N., & Seelen, J. (1993). *The MMPI, MMPI-2, and MMPI-A in Court: A Practical Guide for Expert Witnesses and Attorneys.* Washington, DC: American Psychological Association.

Rogers, R. (Ed.). (1988). *Clinical Assessment of Malingering and Deception.* New York: Guilford.

Sbordone, R. J. (1991). *Neuropsychology for the Attorney.* Orlando, FL: Paul M. Deutsch.

Ziskin, J., & Faust, D. (1988) *Coping With Psychiatric and Psychological Testimony* (Vols. I-III, 4th ed.). Los Angeles, CA: Law and Psychology Press.

EVALUATION AND TREATMENT OF MOTORISTS CONVICTED OF DRIVING WHILE INTOXICATED

Thomas N. Grant and Mary C. Grant

INTRODUCTION

In recent years, public concern has heightened considerably regarding motorists who drive while intoxicated (DWI), because the numbers have escalated in terms of people injured or killed in alcohol-related accidents. In response to public concern, various states have increased legal penalties considerably. What was 15 years ago the equivalent of a fine similar to speeding now is punishable by jail time, extensive fines, probation, and/or revocation of the DWI motorist's license for as long as 3 years, depending on the number and severity of DWI offenses. Our contribution focuses on the diagnostic issues involved in assessing DWI offenders, evaluation procedures available, and our group psychotherapy program for treating DWI offenders.

The purpose of our treatment program for motorists arrested for driving while intoxicated (DWI) is to help the motorist develop strategies to avoid future DWI arrests within the context of each offender's interpersonal and social situation. Professor Allen Dershowitz, the noted Harvard lawyer who has represented well-known clients appealing their convictions, has stated that the most serious crime in America is drunken driving.

In New York state, the motorist arrested for Driving While Intoxicated (DWI) has a blood alcohol (BAC) level of .10 or greater. Blood alcohol levels between .05 and .09 are considered Driving While Ability Impaired (DWAI), which is a lesser offense. As a general rule, in terms of alcohol content, a 12-ounce beer is the equivalent of a .02 BAC level (Nathan, 1990). The liver breaks down approximately 1 ounce of 90-proof spirits or 12 ounces of beer in 1 hour. Two 12-ounce beers within an hour will result in a BAC of .04 which is below the DWAI level (.05) that would result in arrest. As a basis for comparison, a 12-ounce bottle of beer with 5% volume alcohol is the equivalent of a 5-ounce glass of wine with 12% volume alcohol or 1½ ounces of liquor with a 40% volume of alcohol.

A general rule has been that two drinks per hour will keep one within the legal limits set by New York state. However, as Milam and Ketcham (1981) indicate, a number of factors affect the rate at which the BAC rises and thus the rate at which behaviors are altered. Weight is one factor: the more the drinker weighs, the more water there is in the body to dilute the alcohol and lower the BAC. For example, a 200-pound male might approximate a .15 BAC after drinking eight cans of beer, whereas a 150-pound male drinking at the same rate might have a .20 BAC with the same intake. Gender is another factor that influences the BAC level. Females reach higher BACs more quickly because they have less water in their bodies and more adipose tissue (fat), which is not easily penetrated by alcohol. Hormones affect the BAC level such that women experience the highest BAC premenstrually and the lowest BACs on the first day of the menstrual cycle. Food or lack of it can alter the BAC level in men and women. An empty stomach has no food with which to dilute the alcohol and slow its absorption into the bloodstream. Consequently, the BAC level rises rapidly. High-protein foods such as cheese, meat, and eggs slow absorption rate more effectively than low-protein foods. The type of mixer affects absorption: water and fruit juices slow the process, while carbon dioxide (carbonated mixers) speeds it up. The strength of the drink also affects absorption rate. The higher the concentration of alcohol, the more rapid the absorption. A final effect is that warm alcohol is absorbed more rapidly than cold alcohol. Consequently, the general rule of two drinks per hour does not work for all motorists.

For the nontolerant drinker, impairment of judgment and emotion will start at the .02 BAC level, impairment of coordination at the .04 level, impairment of vision at the .06 level (reduced peripheral vision), and impairment of voluntary movements at the .08 level (New York State Department of Motor Vehicles, 1992). A person's tolerance of alcohol complicates the situation; people with higher tolerance experience less impairment for higher levels of alcohol than the nontolerant drinker. Consequently, a motorist with high tolerance may not feel impaired even though the BAC may be well beyond the .05 level (the New York state legal limit for DWAI). Nathan (1990) states, "characteristics of the drinker that influence intoxication and impairment include the drinker's age, weight, prior experience with alcohol, learned expectations concerning the effects of alcohol and degree of acquired tolerance for alcohol" (p. 113).

National statistics indicate that DWI arrests decrease with increased public service announcements, education of the public by law enforcement agencies, and continued reminders on radio and television regarding the perils of drunk driving, especially at holiday times. National statistics indicate that 24,100 people were killed in 1991 in DWI-related accidents as compared to 23,000 people in 1992 (*Democrat & Chronicle Newspaper*, 1993). Statistically, one person is killed every 26 minutes from DWI-related crashes. For New York state, 705 people were killed in 1990 from such accidents as compared to 603 people in 1991. However, statistics vary not only from state to state but across various counties within each state. For Monroe County in New York state (the location of our treatment program), 1991 statistics indicated 2,980 DWI arrests (83% were men) as compared to 2,849 DWI arrests in 1992. The mean BAC level was .15, with most arrests occurring between 12 p.m. and 3 a.m. on Monday. Presently the New York state legislature is studying a change in law so that the BAC level for DWI would be reduced from .10 to .08. Approximately eight other states have a .08 level for DWI.

DRINKING DRIVER PROGRAMS (DDPs)

Drinking driver programs (DDPs) vary considerably across states as does the amount of control over the DWI motorists' licenses by various state Departments of Motor Vehicles (DMVs). For example, one state DDP requires approximately 6 hours of education which focuses equally on safe driving procedures and on the effects of alcohol. There are no provisions made for evaluation of the DWI motorists or referral for treatment if needed. At the other end of the continuum are states where the DDP is similar to a college course and involves sophisticated information about alcohol, other drugs, stress management, and various factors that influence safe driving. States with more sophisticated programs also control the DWI motorist's license and require evaluations which may result in treatment requirements. The power of these drinking driver programs is that the motorists hold conditional licenses and will have their regular license revoked if they do not comply with the requirements of the drinking driver program. The requirements of the DDP may include an evaluation for alcoholism which in turn may result in recommending treatment. If the motorist does not follow through with the recommendation, the license may be revoked within 30 days.

In New York state a motorist may refuse the Breathalyzer when arrested for DWI. However, refusal of the Breathalyzer implies guilt (admission of the DWI) and results in heavier fines and revocation of license immediately. The motorist who takes the Breathalyzer and is found to be DWI is referred to a New York state DDP and is issued a conditional license (the regular license has been rescinded). Motorists are eligible for the New York state DDP if they have not had a conditional license and a DDP within the past 5 years prior to the most recent conviction. Motorists who successfully complete the DDP receive a completion card that allows them to turn in the conditional license and obtain their regular license. The conditional license during the DDP (7 weeks in New York state) restricts the motorist to driving to work, driving to the DDP, driving to a treatment facility, and 3 personal hours of driving time 1 day each week. Motorists caught driving outside these conditions may have their licenses revoked on the spot, and/or be fined.

The New York state DDP is a 7-week educational course on alcohol, drugs, and safe driving which meets once weekly for 2½-hour sessions. Homework assignments are required, such as bringing in DWI articles from newspapers. Group discussions focus on selected topics related to DWI arrests and safe driving. At the fifth session the instructor meets individually with motorists who require additional evaluation for alcoholism. This is determined by a set of criteria created by the New York state DMV. Drivers are considered at risk and requiring evaluation if they have had more than one DWI or DWAI in the past, refuse the Breathalyzer, or have speeding tickets or other infractions on their driving abstract. Motorists are also referred if they share information in the beginning of the course on questionnaires that indicate prior drinking difficulties. The referred DWI offender has to obtain an evaluation and follow through with subsequent recommendations to maintain the conditional license. Successful completion of the recommendations (i.e., treatment) results in the conditional license being replaced with the regular license. If offenders successfully complete the evaluation, not requiring treatment, they complete the Drinking Driver Program and obtain their regular licenses.

The legal process confuses and antagonizes DWI offenders, because they have little awareness of the procedures involved and the power that the DMV has through the DDP. DWI offenders typically perceive the DDP as the court's final requirement for obtaining their license. They do not realize that the DMV is a separate power that has additional requirements such as successful completion of the DDP which may require an evaluation and possibly treatment. Most motorists are angry and surprised when referred for an alcohol/drug evaluation and may not understand that the conditional license can be revoked if they do not comply. Some clients view the referral situation as a legal problem that can be contested by their attorney and fail to realize that the operator's license is a privilege, not a legal right.

EVALUATION OF DWI OFFENDERS

DWI offenders in an alcoholism evaluation frequently respond with reluctance, anger, and defiance toward the process and attempt to impress on the evaluator that they do not have an alcohol problem. As mentioned previously, one method of determining motorists' need for evaluation is based on the questionnaires they have completed in the DDP. When they come for evaluation, they frequently will not make the same admissions during our professional evaluation. Some offenders become sophisticated and discover that they are allowed a second evaluation if they are not in agreement with the recommendations of the first evaluation. Offenders usually learn what not to disclose as a result of the first evaluation and typically view the evaluation situation as coercive. They frequently confuse evaluation with treatment, feeling that being referred for evaluation means being forced into treatment.

Instruments used in professional alcoholism evaluations for DWI offenders may not always be reliable or valid for a number of reasons. Most alcoholism tests are validated on hospitalized alcoholic groups and rely on self-reports. DWI offenders are typically viewed as falling along a continuum from drinkers who abuse alcohol to those who are alcohol dependent. The more common definition is that someone has abused alcohol if he or she has encountered legal problems because of drinking. By this definition, DWI offenders have abused alcohol in that they drank over the legal limit and were found to be impaired (BAC $\geq$ .05). One line of thinking in the field is that people who drink abusively have a high likelihood of becoming alcohol dependent over a number of years. Consequently, motorists who abuse alcohol may be seen as in danger of becoming alcohol dependent if intervention does not occur. Frequently, problem drinkers are anxious and defiant, and choose to avoid examining past drinking patterns. The more frequent focus is to impress the evaluator that there is no drinking problem.

Psychological research has focused on identifying problem drinkers who wish to remain undetected (Otto et al., 1988) by using more subtle measurements than self-report inventories. This research suggests that subtle measures such as the MacAndrews Alcoholism Scale-Revised (MAC-R) of the Minnesota Multiphasic Personality Inventory-2 (MMPI-2) are effective with extreme groups (inpatient alcoholics) who are being detoxified and are in intensive programs (Graham, 1990). However, drinkers who are not alcoholic but may be problematic frequently score within the normal range. The alternative, namely, self-report inventories, may yield little information, due either to defensiveness on the part of the DWI offender or to intentional withholding of information. Some problematic drinkers are not introspective and are defensive in that they do not acknowledge difficulties because they are unaware of such difficulties or are surrounded by family and friends who drink and have similar experiences. Consequently, they see themselves as "just like everyone else," that is, normal or problem-free. It is not that they withhold information, but that they are not aware of their situation or not aware that they have abused alcohol.

Self-report instruments that are used in assessment number over 180, according to a list distributed by the Alcohol/Drug Abuse and Mental Health Administration in Washington (1992), which currently is attempting to put together an assessment manual listing all available instruments. However, these instruments typically rely on self-awareness and truthfulness of the client responding to the instrument. First-time offenders frequently state that "it will never happen again" and that they have "learned not to drink and drive." This response is also heard from repeat offenders, some of whom have participated in previous treatment interventions. In our experience, DWI offenders are task oriented and action oriented rather than introspective or trying to solve problematic situations. They assume that deciding not to let a DWI arrest happen again will take care of the situation.

Some evaluation and treatment agencies interpret these statements as denial and proof of alcohol dependency. However, this is not helpful in fostering offender participation in the evaluation process or arriving at a valid diagnosis. It would be more helpful to view such statements as indications that the offender is not introspective and has not approached the DWI as a problematic situation that requires strategies to avoid repeating in the future. In terms of treatment, DWI offenders have to be encouraged to be less action oriented and more introspective, and to carefully assess their predicaments and drinking situations that put them at risk. This shift does not occur as a result of an educational program such as the DDP. The estimate frequently given by the New York state DMV is that DWI offenders have driven 200 times DWI prior to their first arrest. This suggests that many motorists are over the .05 BAC level and unaware that they are in violation of the law.

Our assessment attempts to correct for situations that may be mislabeled as denial and, therefore, proof of alcohol dependency. The assessment involves a clinical interview, the Michigan Alcoholism Screening Test (MAST; Selzer, 1971), and the MMPI-2 which includes three addiction scales (Weed et al., 1992). The clinical interview focuses on offender drinking patterns, willingness to disclose information about prior drinking habits and symptoms connected with heavy drinking, the ability to evaluate negative consequences of alcohol, attitude toward the DDP, and awareness of reasons for referral. The MAST, which is administered in the first session of the DDP, is readministered during our assessment as a consistency measure of the client's self-report.

The MAST is a good example of the many self-report inventories available. It contains 25 questions with yes-or-no answers to specific questions that are symptoms of problem drinking. Examples are: "Do you feel you are a normal drinker?" "Can you stop drinking without a struggle after one or two drinks?" "Do you ever feel bad about your drinking?" "Have you ever attended a meeting of Alcoholics Anonymous?" "Have you gotten into fights when drinking?" "Do you drink before noon fairly often?" "Have you ever lost a job because of drinking?" The 25 items yield a score ranging from 0 to 25. Scores of 0 to 2 are interpreted as no problem, scores of 3 to 5 indicate an early or middle problem drinker, and scores above 6 indicate a problem drinker. However, using the MAST as an inventory may not provide an accurate assessment. The items should be discussed carefully with the offender to insure accurate information. For example, answering yes to an item such as "Have you attended a meeting of Alcoholics Anonymous?" may mean that the motorist drove a friend who did not have transportation to Alcoholics Anonymous (AA). Frequently offenders respond to the very first item, "Do you feel you are a normal drinker?," with "No" because they do not drink on a daily basis like many of their friends. However, the answer "No" is interpreted to mean that the offender is an abnormal drinker out of control (typical of an alcoholic). Consequently, each response that is scored "1" should be questioned carefully. Recovered alcoholics or people who have past histories of heavy drinking may have MAST scores well above 8. Other inventories consist of many of these items from the MAST embedded in longer self-report questionnaires. Consequently, without understanding the offender's interpretation of the questions, a total score on such inventories as the MAST may not be meaningful, although many of the items do refer to symptoms experienced by people who abuse alcohol. Clinical interviewing based on the items that the offender has responded to is a more relevant approach to yield accurate information.

Another instrument, the MMPI-2 (Graham, 1990), is currently the most widely used objective personality inventory. The person taking the MMPI-2 sorts out 567 statements into two categories, true or false. The advantage of personality assessment is that other problems may surface that complicate the DWI situation and increase an offender's risk for future DWI arrests. Typical profiles of repeat offenders for DWI arrests include high scores on the psychopathic deviate (Pd), depression (D), and manic (Ma) scales, with scores in the borderline or higher range on the MAC-R (Graham, 1990). Butcher (1990) states that the content of the MAC-R suggests that high-scoring individuals are socially extroverted, self-confident, assertive, and exhibitionistic; enjoy taking risks; show concentration problems; and have a history of acting-out behavior such as school problems. In our experience, some DWI offenders with multiple arrests score well within the normal range on the MAC-R, suggesting that there is an interaction between personality style and alcohol use which may result in DWI arrests rather than strictly an alcohol dependency problem. The MAC-R is an example of an indirect assessment measure and consists of 49 items embedded in the MMPI-2 to which the offender responds true or false. Examples of such items would be, "I am certainly lacking in self-confidence," "I sweat very easily even on cool days," and "I have some habits that are really harmful." Raw scores range from 0 to 49. For males, a raw score of 26 to 28 suggests that alcohol or drug abuse problems are possible; a raw score of 29 to 31 suggests that alcohol or drug abuse problems are likely; and a raw score of 32 or more suggests that alcohol or drug abuse problems are highly probable. For females, a raw score of 23 to 25 suggests that alcohol abuse problems are possible; a raw score of 26 to 29 suggests that alcohol or drug abuse problems are likely; and a raw score of 30 or more suggests that alcohol or drug abuse problems are highly probable. Scores below 24 contraindicate a substance abuse problem. Graham (1990) warns that "incorrect classification of nonabusers as abusers is especially likely to occur for individuals who have the extroverted activity-oriented style commonly found among high MAC-R scorers who do not abuse substances" (p. 153). Persons who previously abused substances but no longer do so tend to obtain high MAC-R scores. Consequently, subtle or indirect measures also have accuracy difficulties. Two new measures on the MMPI-2 are the Addiction Potential Scale (APS) and the Addiction Admission Scale (AAS; Weed et al., 1992). Because alcoholism scales are normed on extreme groups (alcoholics vs. normals), DWI offenders may not score at a level considered problematic. Clinical judgment is necessary to assess the status of an offender's alcohol use and possible need for treatment beyond the educational experience of the DDP.

GROUP PSYCHOTHERAPY PROGRAM FOR DWI OFFENDERS

Our first contact with the DWI offender is an evaluation regarding the need for treatment. If treatment is recommended, the motorist is given a handout on alcohol and stress management

(American Red Cross Office, 1981) which he or she takes home, fills out, and brings back to the initial individual session prior to beginning group. The initial session involves in-depth discussion of past drinking habits based on the alcohol information, review of stress-management materials, and review of goals that are outlined later in this contribution. The DWI offender then begins a 16-week group psychotherapy program which meets once weekly for 90-minute sessions. The group psychotherapy program is followed by an individual session to review the DWI offender's progress and focus on issues that arose in group and are relevant to the client. In our experience, DWI offenders can be quite different from each other in terms of their particular problems, social settings, past drinking patterns, and support systems within the community. They do not score on assessment instruments at a level one would expect in terms of alcoholism, and they present a variety of interpersonal problems that offer a range of situations and strategies for each offender to consider. Group sessions are more effective than individual sessions in that the DWI offender has exposure to a considerable variety of situations that have led to DWI arrests, various strategies that may or may not have worked for others, and varied sentencing outcomes by the legal system for individuals with similar numbers of DWI arrests. Our group is ongoing: new members interact with group members who are halfway through or near completion of the program and thus are exposed to different levels of thinking regarding the DWI situations that brought the offenders into our program.

The typical mind-set of DWI offenders initially starting treatment is that they are being coerced into treatment. They also typically are fearful that they are being seen as alcoholic. This may have been precipitated by the legal process starting with the DWI offender's contact with the courts, DMV, and various treatment agencies. In terms of diagnosis and treatment, the field of alcohol/substance abuse is known for widely different viewpoints and proponents who sometimes become intense about their particular treatment philosophy (Ludwig, 1988). Consequently, DWI offenders may have very different experiences of evaluation and treatment programs depending on the philosophy of the staff. Treatment philosophies range from viewing alcoholism as a genetic disease that ruins one's life physically, psychologically, and socially and for which abstinence is crucial for recovery, to the philosophy that controlled drinking is possible for alcoholics and that the disease model encourages dependency and lack of responsibility for one's drinking behavior. DWI offenders who have not experienced extreme negative consequences from drinking may not relate to the disease approach and may be more concerned about the stigma of being labeled alcoholic because they have been recommended for treatment.

Our program utilizes a cognitive-behavioral approach combined with abstinence during treatment. The role of abstinence is explained as a means of helping offenders experience new behaviors in social situations. We separate abstinence from the disease concept of alcoholism and use abstinence to foster cognitive/behavioral strategies to reduce discomfort, as proposed in rational-emotive therapy (Ellis et al., 1988). For clients who are unable to maintain abstinence, a more intense program is warranted and results in appropriate referral. The initial individual treatment session prior to group psychotherapy focuses on alcohol use, stress, and stress management to enable the DWI offender to evaluate life situations in terms of past abuses of alcohol or other drugs and to assess current life stressors. Specific areas for attitude and behavior change are discussed individually with the DWI offender (Appleton, Barkley, & Katz, 1986) and will then be focused upon in group. These areas are responsibility, insight, feelings, communication skills, identification of needs, experimentation with new behaviors, and restructuring lifestyle to interrupt an established pattern leading to the DWI arrest.

RESPONSIBILITY

DWI offenders are responsible for acknowledging their need to deal with the DWI situation by making personal changes and not viewing their difficulties as a legal problem that an attorney should resolve. Frequently, offenders expect the treatment process to be adversarial based on court experiences, and they expect treatment to be coercive and punitive. They may have had prior contact with other programs with a different philosophy in which confrontation combined with information on alcohol as a disease may have been the main treatment vehicle. DWI offenders have to accept responsibility for their DWI arrest and move beyond the anger of having been caught and punished for breaking the law.

INSIGHT

Offenders have to identify dysfunctional patterns of behavior, which requires increased awareness of situations and friends that have put them at risk to abuse alcohol in the past, whether it was an argument with a significant other, a difficult day at work, frustration or failure with a particular situation, or an attempt to block out unpleasant feelings. Sometimes the offender's dysfunctional behavior is accepted and supported by family members or close associates who drink heavily and see excessive alcohol consumption as normal.

FEELINGS

Many DWI offenders are not feeling oriented or introspective. They have little idea as to how they got their DWI, do not admit to being angry, and may only relate to the frustration with the DMV's requirements to obtain their license. Some offenders, depending on the number of DWI arrests, may be without a license for 3 years and become angry when they visualize finally going to the DMV, standing in line, and being told after waiting for an hour that they do not have the proper paperwork and are required to return. Recounting these situations allows offenders to get in touch with their anger. Other situations are discussed that, in the past, have not been seen as anger provoking but have resulted in the offender being frustrated, annoyed, and triggered to abuse alcohol. Women offenders tend to be more aware of their feelings. However, similarly to male offenders, they typically are unaware of the situations that put them at risk and do not connect unpleasant or negative feelings with an increased urge to abuse alcohol and drink excessively.

COMMUNICATION SKILLS

DWI offenders have poor communication skills; they have difficulty getting in touch with their feelings and prefer to avoid confronting or giving constructive feedback to people who frustrate or anger them. They keep insights to themselves. During group, some offenders express surprise that talking about a past or current stressful situation has allowed them to feel more comfortable and less anxious. There is a lack of awareness that improved communications can lead to improved functioning. Another typical example is that in the final individual session, the offender may share observations about other people in group that are valid and would have been helpful if offered during group. Their initial reaction is to avoid confrontations or communications, expecting that it will not lead to an improved situation.

IDENTIFICATION OF NEEDS

DWI offenders have to assess friends, places, and social situations with whom or in which they have relied on alcohol to feel more comfortable, socialize more easily, or avoid dealing with unpleasant situations. Reviewing friends, places, and social situations allows the offenders to become aware of various needs that they have dealt with through excessive drinking.

EXPERIMENTATION WITH NEW BEHAVIORS

DWI offenders have to be willing to socialize with friends without alcohol. They may be drinking soda and encounter questions from friends about their abstinence. This forces them to learn to respond to such questions. They also notice people around them who are drinking, and they are able to observe changes that occur when people drink excessively over the course of an evening. Offenders who have been in group longer have had experience with family parties or weddings and are able to relate experiences and how they handled questions regarding their abstinence. Group allows offenders to anticipate and prepare to handle social situations they will be encountering. Offenders need to rethink situations and consider strategies for handling questions regarding their DWI arrests. Single males have difficulty socializing if they do not have a license and subsequently meet women whom they would like to date. This involves honesty and assertiveness in communication at the start of a relationship and coping with the anxiety of behaving differently without using alcohol.

RESTRUCTURING LIFESTYLE

Offenders who actively work on the preceding areas restructure their lifestyle in terms of how they relate to friends, the places they go, and the strategies they implement to avoid drinking abusively. These changes in their lives interrupt the established pattern that has led to DWI arrests and allows them to avoid situations that are difficult or nonsatisfying without excessive drinking. Many offenders need to become aware of which situations are enjoyable and which situations are tolerable only with excessive drinking. This is a distinction that becomes more important as offenders focus on improving their life situations through continuous self-evaluation. The earlier framework is one that we use in terms of guiding the group discussions rather than a framework that is given to the DWI offender to implement independently.

THE GROUP PROCESS

The group focus is to develop strategies to avoid future DWI arrests within the context of each offender's interpersonal and social situation. We stress honesty and active exploration of each offender's drinking situation as it pertains to DWI offenses and past abuses of drinking. The group psychotherapy program is ongoing so that there are members at various stages in the program. The advantage of the ongoing group is that we continually have a program available for offenders. They are not asked to wait for 16 weeks until a new psychotherapy group starts. New members interacting with group members already in the program are exposed to different levels of thinking regarding DWI situations. There is greater sharing because the offenders who have been in group have had the benefit of thinking about and using all the structured materials that we distribute during group (see pp. 350-355). This helps the beginning offender to become more quickly integrated into group. Because some treatment groups are extremely confrontative, offenders may be concerned that they are going to be confronted with a particular philosophy and, if they do not agree, will be labeled as "in denial" and recommended for more intensive programing. Our feeling is that labeling offenders or recommending more intensive programing if the offender does not agree with a stated philosophy discourages honesty and thinking analytically about the DWI situation. Some past offenders have attended intensive outpatient groups with strong philosophies regarding alcoholism, learned to say what was expected of them, successfully completed the program, and then received another DWI. Our position is that each offender is an individual who should not be labeled and treated like all other offenders, but may have very different factors accounting for the DWI situation. The offender's responsibility is to look carefully at the situation and not settle for general solutions such as "I'm alcoholic and can't ever drink again." This type of reasoning may close off productive thinking about their abuse of alcohol.

Group topics include labeling and diagnosis, possible causes of alcoholism, family drinking, anger at the legal system and coercive treatment (court mandated). Individual offenders have had from one DWAI to as many as six DWI arrests over a long time span. Approximately 50% of offenders are on probation, and 90% are male between the ages of 20 and 40. The wide range of experiences and recidivism impresses first-time offenders in group. This profile of DWI offenders summarizes our group membership and does not define the ideal range. From our experiences, a more ideal mix would be groups that would have 50% men and 50% women, because women are more in touch with their feelings and help move the group in that direction. The group process that we use is applicable to offenders other than those with this particular profile.

Within the context of each offender's interpersonal and social situation, family drinking patterns are discussed as well as past experiences offenders may have had with more intensive alcoholism programs in which offenders had to regularly admit to being alcoholic and were required to attend Alcoholics Anonymous (AA) four times weekly to complete the program. We found that this type of program has not worked for a number of offenders because they receive subsequent DWI offenses. We believe that such offenders comply externally with program requirements without making internal changes. New movements such as the Secular Organizations for Sobriety (SOS, 1992) and Rational Recovery (RR) groups, which started as alternatives to AA, indicate dissatisfaction with more traditional programs that do not allow for disagreement or flexible ways of looking at drinking problems. In the popular press there have been numerous articles on the plethora of 12-step programs based on AA, citing these movements as fads. The author of the book *I'm Dysfunctional, You're Dysfunctional* (Kaminer, 1992), which confronted the rigidity of the AA philosophy and 12-step programs, mentioned having been threatened physically and receiving death threats from proponents of such programs. We do not think that a fanatical treatment approach allows for the thinking necessary for DWI offenders to make the internal changes that will enable them to avoid future DWI arrests.

THE ABSTINENCE ASSIGNMENT

DWI offenders are encouraged to focus on social situations that they encounter without alcohol and to assess and analyze the differences that they experience due to abstinence. The goal is to develop an awareness socially of what it is like not to drink and to see what other people's behavior is like when people drink reasonably as compared to those who abuse alcohol. Offenders discover that other people frequently assume they are drinking mixed drinks, not soda. Offenders also notice the change in behavior of people who continue to drink excessively. Family weddings and parties are the most difficult and informative situations for abstinent offenders because the offenders have been seen as "partyers" and typically drank heavily in the past with friends and/or family. They now have a different set of behaviors that family and friends have to accept. The offenders also learn to cope with family and friends who may pressure them to drink. Group support is offered to DWI offenders in terms of discussing and role playing the situations while abstinent prior to the actual situation. If offenders encounter difficulty and accept a drink, this is discussed in group in terms of what they might have done differently and what their reactions were at having a drink. Unlike programs that have a rigid philosophy, we do not dismiss offenders who have a drink. We focus on what went wrong with the offender's strategy. If there is repeated difficulty with abstinence and poor control over the urge to drink, referral to a more intensive program is discussed and instituted.

COGNITIVE BEHAVIORAL ASSIGNMENTS

All of the assignments are given during group to focus on specific areas that may be troublesome for the DWI offender (see pp. 350-355). Identifying resources for coping with stress requires assessing the offender's coping skills, physical and emotional strengths, social support systems, intellectual resources, and spiritual strengths. Finally, the offender has to evaluate the present lifestyle as a coping resource (Tubesing, 1981). Offenders are encouraged to generate a list of best stress skills and are given information on various stress-reduction techniques (Yamauchi, 1987; see "Procrastination: Ten Ways to 'Do It Now,' " pp. 350-352). They are encouraged to learn to relax, practice acceptance of their situation, and talk rationally to themselves when in a stressful situation (Ellis et al., 1988). Practicing acceptance, reducing procrastination, and talking rationally to oneself are important skills for offenders to develop because they have to deal with the coercive nature of the mandated treatment process and the requirements of court-ordered probation. Developing methods of correcting "crooked thinking" through rational self-talk, positive self-statements, and avoiding procrastination allows the DWI offender to work toward clear goals (Ellis et al., 1988). Sometimes offenders have been introduced to narrow concepts in prior treatment programs. For example, procrastination may have been interpreted as proof that the offender is alcoholic, because some treatment settings define all dysfunctional behavior as due to alcoholism. The offender may then focus on the label, become defensive, and react in a defiant, nonintrospective manner.

SELF-HELP GROUP ASSIGNMENT

Discussions focus on self-help groups such as AA, RR, and SOS (1992). Offenders are encouraged to attend one of the preceding groups at least once over the course of treatment. Those who have attended AA in the past as a condition of prior treatment or through court sentencing are encouraged to attend RR or SOS as an alternative, because these groups are less dogmatic in their philosophy of recovery.

Typical complaints about AA meetings include AA members labeling newcomers as alcoholic and dismissing disagreement as proof of being in denial. AA groups may focus on "war stories" which can encourage newcomers to compare and distance themselves rather than identify with helpful information. The spiritual emphasis of AA is disturbing to some offenders as is the intense commitment of some AA members for whom AA is the center point of their lives. As counterpoint, there are DWI repeat offenders in our groups who use AA and other groups regularly and have concluded that withdrawing from meetings contributed to their most recent DWI. They offer a balance regarding the positive aspects of self-help groups and usually have less fanaticism to a particular philosophy. For offenders who see themselves as recovering alcoholics, we utilize active approaches that provide building skills necessary for avoiding relapse (Chiauzzi, 1991).

PREVENTION ASSIGNMENT

Another group task involves generation of strategies to reduce risk of future DWI arrests. A typical list of strategies includes (a) have a designated driver; (b) stay the night; (c) use a taxi or bus; (d) don't drive to where you drink; (e) depend on friends to help you either drink in moderation or remain abstinent; (f) don't stop with friends after work; (g) use abstinence; (h) use AA, RR, or SOS; (i) focus more attention on the family; (j) become active and reduce boredom/passivity; and (k) focus on the rewards of your new lifestyle. A related group task is discussing possible personality styles of DWI offenders who will not get another DWI. At the conclusion of the group program, a final individual psychotherapy session focuses on personal strategies that the offender feels will work. Progress during the group as well as concerns or shortcomings that the offender experienced in the program are discussed. The thrust of our program is to foster responsibility, self-awareness, and acceptance of the legal dangers of abusive drinking. An additional goal is to motivate the client to maintain lifestyle changes that foster effective living (Marlatt & Gordon, 1985).

CONCLUSIONS

DWI offenders are a diverse group clinically and not easily diagnosed in terms of alcoholism. The mental health professional must assess each DWI offender as an individual in his or her specific context. Initial reactions of anger, defiance, and confusion about the legal system and the DMV may hinder offenders from focusing realistically on their drinking patterns to assess the extent of their abuse and the need to develop appropriate strategies to avoid future DWI arrests. Diverse philosophies and definitions of alcoholism may prove an additional source of confusion for offenders. The disease model of alcoholism impresses some offenders as authoritarian, confrontative, and belaboring the issue of labels, because acceptance of one's alcoholism is a prerequisite for treatment. Offenders respond defensively by demanding justification for treatment and may conclude that treatment means they are alcoholic. Our philosophy purports that offenders need to understand the legal situation, the DMV's concern, and high-risk factors involved in DWI recidivism. Our group psychotherapy program allows time for attitude and behavior change during a period of abstinence, with the utilization of cognitive-behavioral strategies to improve lifestyle management.

FOLLOW-UP DATA

Our program has been in operation approximately 8 years and has been significantly modified from what was initially an educational program to one that is psychotherapeutic and focuses on behavior change. Follow-up data on our offenders' progress has been obtained by offenders contacting us after 2 to 3 years of probation for an updated evaluation to apply for their operator's license. During the 2- to 3-year interim they have been successful with probation, have remained abstinent, and are considered at that point trustworthy to receive their operator's license. Offenders who have violated probation through failure to maintain abstinence or driving without a license are typically sent back to court for resentencing. In such instances, the offender will contact us and may request an updated evaluation or additional treatment. Another option is that the offender will contact us for referral to a more intensive outpatient program, or we will be requested by that program to forward information. Offenders in our program who are not on probation need a reevaluation when it is time to apply for their license and come back for an updated assessment for the DMV. Should they receive another DWI, they typically receive probation as part of their sentence. In this instance, probation will contact us for recommendations regarding additional treatment. We estimate that approximately 10% of DWI offenders whom we have treated are back in contact with us because of additional DWI arrests. A small percentage of DWI offenders have been referred back to us for additional treatment by the courts.

In our final individual session with the offender, we look for improvement in terms of the offender's self-reports of feeling better, change of friends and socialization patterns, increased hobbies or activities that are not alcohol related, better relationships with spouse and offspring, increased money for leisure activities because they no longer spend money in bars during the week, lack of boredom, and decreased discomfort with free time (which surfaces in the beginning of treatment). Occasionally we receive phone calls from family members during treatment if they are concerned about the offender or if they note improvements in terms of the offender's functioning.

Approximately 70% of our evaluations result in referrals for treatment; this is in agreement with overall statistics from the New York state DMV when all approved evaluation agencies are summarized. However, there is a wide range of evaluation outcomes between agencies; some have had a 98% referral rate for treatment until the DMV intervened, indicating that treatment referral was excessively high, which suggests that the criteria might not be appropriate. DWI statistics are complex and reflect many factors in terms of number of arrests, referral by DDP, evaluations, and subsequent referrals to treatment.

PROCRASTINATION:
TEN WAYS TO "DO IT NOW"*

We've all been plagued by procrastination at one time or another. For some, it's a chronic problem. Others find that it hits only some areas of their lives. The net results, though, are usually the same - wasted time, missed opportunities, poor performance, self-deprecation, or increased stress.

Procrastination is letting the low-priority tasks get in the way of high-priority ones. It's socializing with colleagues when you know that important work project is due soon, watching TV instead of doing your household chores, or talking about superficial things with your partner rather than discussing your relationship concerns.

We all seem to do fine with things we want to do or enjoy doing for fun. But, when we perceive tasks as difficult, inconvenient, or scary, we may shift into our procrastination mode. We have very clever ways of fooling ourselves. See how many of the following excuses hit home for you:

- I'll wait until I'm in the mood to do it.
- It's OK to celebrate . . . besides, I'll start my diet (sobriety) tomorrow.
- My health problem isn't *that* bad. Time will heal this pain.
- There's plenty of time to get it done.
- Why does the boss give us so much to do? It's not fair.
- It's too hard to talk about. I don't know where to begin.
- I work better under pressure so I don't need to do it right now.
- I've got too many other things to do first.

Once exposed, these self-defeating statements don't sound so convincing. But, when we privately tell ourselves these excuses, they seem quite believable. Don't be fooled by how innocent they sound. They get us to postpone important tasks and duties.

CAUSES

Procrastination is a bad habit. Like other habits, there are two general causes. The first is the "crooked thinking" we employ to justify our behavior. The second source is our behavioral patterns.

A closer look at our crooked thinking reveals three major issues in delaying tactics - perfectionism, inadequacy, and discomfort. Those who believe they must turn in the most exemplary report may wait until all available resources have been reviewed or endlessly rewrite draft after draft. Worry over producing the perfect project prevents them from finishing on time. Feelings of inadequacy can also cause delays. Those who "know for a fact" that they are incompetent often believe they will fail and will avoid the unpleasantness of having their skills put to the test. Fear of discomfort is another way of putting a stop to what needs to be done. Yet, the more we delay, the worse the discomforting problem (like a toothache) becomes.

Our behavioral patterns are the second cause. Getting started on an unpleasant or difficult task may seem impossible. Procrastination is likened to the physics concept of inertia - a mass at rest tends to stay at rest. Greater forces are required to start change than to sustain change. Another way of viewing it is that avoiding tasks reinforces procrastination which makes it harder to get things going. A person may be stuck, too, not by the lack of desire, but by not knowing what to do. Here are some things to break the habit. Remember, don't just read them, do them!

---

*Note: From "Procrastination: Ten Ways to 'Do It Now' " by K. T. Yamauchi in *Innovations in Clinical Practice: A Source Book* (Vol. 6, pp. 431-433) by P. A. Keller and S. R. Heyman (Eds.), 1987, Sarasota, FL: Professional Resource Exchange, Inc. Copyright © 1987 by Professional Resource Exchange, Inc. Reprinted by permission.

REMEDIES

CHANGE YOUR CROOKED THINKING

1. **Rational Self-Talk**. Those old excuses really don't hold up to rational inspection. The "two-column technique" will help. Write down all your excuses on one side of a piece of paper. Start challenging the faulty reasoning behind each of the excuses. Write down your realistic thoughts on the opposite side of each excuse. It might look something like this:

EXCUSE (Self-Defeating Thoughts)	SELF-DEFENSE (Realistic Thoughts)
I'm not in the mood right now.	Mood doesn't do my work, actions do. If I wait for the right mood, I may never get it done.
I'm just lazy.	Labeling myself as lazy only brings me down. My work is really separate from who I am as a person. Getting started is the key to finishing.

2. **Positive Self-Statements**. Incorporate a list of self-motivating statements into your repertoire of thoughts. Consider . . .

    - "There's no time like the present."
    - "The sooner I get done, the sooner I can play."
    - "There's no such thing as perfectionism. It's an illusion that keeps me from doing what I have to do right now."
    - "It's cheaper and less painful if I do it now rather than wait until it gets worse."

3. **Don't Catastrophize**. Jumping to the conclusion that you will fail or that you are no good at something will only create a wall of fear that will stop you cold. Recognize that your negative predictions are not facts. Focus on the present and what positive steps you can take toward reaching your goals.

4. **Design Clear Goals**. Think about what you want and what needs to be done. Be specific. If it's getting that work project completed by the deadline, figure out a time table with realistic goals at each step. Keep your sights within reason. Having goals too big can scare you away from starting.

CHANGE YOUR BEHAVIORAL PATTERNS

5. **Set Priorities**. Write down all the things that need to be done in order of their importance. The greater the importance or urgency, the higher their priority. Put "messing around" (distractions) in its proper place - last! Start at the top of the list and work your way down.

6. **Partialize the Tasks**. Big projects feel overwhelming. Break them down into the smallest and most manageable subparts. You'll get more done if you can do it piece by piece. For example, make an outline for a written report before you start composing or do a small portion of the chores rather than all at once. Partializing works especially well with the unpleasant jobs. Most of us can handle duties we dislike as long as they're for a short time and in small increments.

7. **Get Organized**. Have all your materials ready before you begin a task. Use a daily schedule and have it with you all the time. List the tasks of the day or week realistically. Check off the tasks when you have completed them.

8. **Take a Stand**. Commit yourself to doing the task. Write yourself a "contract" and sign it. Better still, tell a friend, partner, or supervisor about your plans.

9. **Use Prompts**. Write reminders to yourself and put them in conspicuous places like on the TV, refrigerator, bathroom mirror, front door, and car dashboard. The more we remember, the greater the likelihood we'll follow through with our plans.

10. **Reward Yourself**. Self-reinforcement has a powerful effect on developing a "do it now" attitude. Celebrate, pat yourself on the back, smile, and let yourself enjoy the completion of even the smallest of tasks. Don't minimize your accomplishments. Remember, you're already that much closer to finishing those things that need to be done. Go ahead, get started . . . NOW!

If you're still faced with a strong procrastination habit after trying the preceding suggestions, you may wish to consult a professional psychologist. Please contact the local office of your state's psychological association or the department of psychology or psychological counseling services at a nearby college or university.

IDENTIFY YOUR RESOURCES*

Generals don't go into battle without knowing the resources at their disposal. Politicians don't go into campaigns without assessing their leverage and personal appeal. Before formulating a plan for working on the troublesome aspects of your life, you need to identify and assess your strengths.

STOP AND REFLECT

Make an inventory of your coping skills.

☐ What do you have going for you physically (energy, strength, agility)?

☐ What are your emotional strengths (self-confidence, calm, empathy)?

☐ What social support systems do you have (family, friends, clubs)?

☐ What are your intellectual resources (creativity, humor, concentration, insight)?

☐ What are your spiritual strengths (prayer, social conscience, hope)?

☐ How is your present lifestyle a coping resource (rituals, habits, hobbies, family traditions)?

☐ What are your best stress skills?

---

*Note: From *Kicking Your Stress Habits: A Do-It-Yourself Guide for Coping With Stress* (p. 172) by D. A. Tubesing, 1981, Duluth, MN: Whole Person Associates. Copyright © 1981 by Whole Person Associates. Reprinted by permission.

GOALS*

On this form describe your goal regarding your use of alcohol *over the next 6 months.*

Do you intend to not drink at all, or to drink but only in certain ways and under certain conditions?

Do not feel tied to any earlier Goal Statement that you filled out as part of this program.

What is your goal now? If your goal mentions drinking, describe what you mean in terms of amount of drinking and circumstances when you would drink.

1. For the next 6 months, my goal is (check either Box A or Box B):

    ☐ A. Not to drink at all.
    If you checked this goal, go on to question 2.

    ☐ B. Only to drink in certain ways.
    If you checked this goal, answer the following questions, using the following definition of one standard drink:

    <u>One standard drink is equal to:</u>

    - 12 ounces of *beer* (5% alcohol)
    - 1½ ounces of hard *liquor* or spirits (e.g., whiskey)
    - 5 ounces of *table wine* (11% to 12%)
    - 3 ounces of *fortified wine* (20%)

    i. On the average when I do drink, I will probably drink about _____ standard drinks during the course of that day.

    ii. I plan to drink no more than _____ standard drinks during the course of any single day. That will be my Upper Limit.

    iii. Over the course of an average week (7 days), I plan to drink on no more than _____ days. (If you plan to drink on less than 1 day per week, check here: ☐)

    iv. Over the course of 1 month (30 days), I plan to drink my Upper Limit of drinks on no more than _____ days. (If you plan to drink to your Upper Limit of drinks less than one time per month, check here: ☐)

    v. I plan to drink *only* under the following conditions:
    _____
    _____
    _____
    _____

    vi. I plan *not to drink at all* under the following conditions:
    _____
    _____
    _____
    _____

Note: From *Problem Drinkers: Guided Self-Change Treatment* (pp. 81-82) by M. B. Sobell and L. C. Sobell, 1993, New York: Guilford. Copyright © 1993 by Guilford Press. Reprinted by permission.

People usually have several things that they would like to change in their lives. Changing their drinking behavior can be one of those things. You have just described your drinking goal for the next 6 months. With regard to that goal, answer the following two questions.

2. At this moment, how important is it that you achieve your stated goal? (How hard are you willing to work, and how much are you willing to do, to achieve your drinking goal?)

   Answer this question by writing a number from 0 to 100 in the designated space below, using the following scale as a guide:

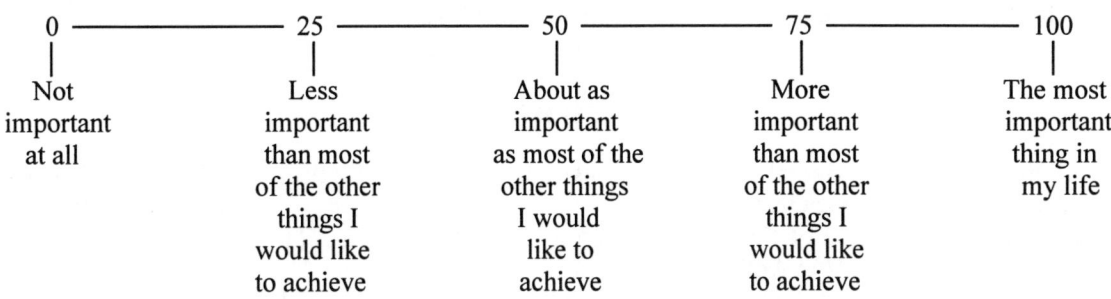

Write your goal importance rating (from 0 to 100) here: _____

3. In the designated space below, indicate how confident you feel at this moment that you will achieve your stated goal. In other words, what is the probability that you will achieve your goal? Use the following scale as a guide:

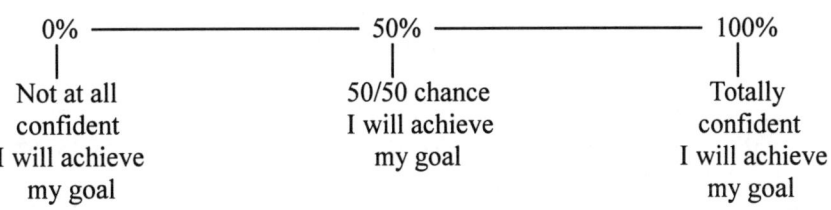

Write your confidence rating (from 0% to 100%) here: ____%

Thomas N. Grant, PhD, is currently in private practice. He taught at St. John's University (New York City) and worked at the Bleuler Psychotherapy Center (New York City) and the Rochester Rehabilitation Center (Rochester, New York). His training is in clinical psychology with special interests in addiction and neuropsychological assessment of profoundly deaf adults. Dr. Grant may be contacted at 1351 Mt. Hope Avenue, Suite 210, Rochester, NY 14620.

Mary C. Grant, PhD, is currently in full-time private practice. Prior to this she was associated with Bellevue Psychiatric Hospital (New York City), Outpatient Mental Health Center, and Bleuler Psychotherapy Center (New York City). Her training has been in clinical psychology with special interest in addictions and women's issues. Dr. Grant may be contacted at 1351 Mt. Hope Avenue, Suite 210, Rochester, NY 14620.

RESOURCES

Alcohol/Drug Abuse and Mental Health Administration. (1992). Rockville, MD: U. S. Department of Health and Human Services.

American Red Cross Office of Personnel Training and Development. (1981, March). *Stress Management*. Alexandria, VA: Author.

Appleton, G., Barkley, K., & Katz, J. (1986). Creative intervention for DWI offenders. *Journal of Alcoholism Treatment Quarterly, Summer, 67*-87.

Butcher, J. N. (1990). *MMPI-2 in Psychological Treatment*. New York: Oxford.

Chiauzzi, E. J. (1991). *Preventing Relapse in the Addictions: A Biopsychosocial Approach*. New York: Pergamon.

Democrat & Chronicle Newspaper. (1993, May 30). Section B, p. 1.

Ellis, A., McInerney, J. F., DiGiuseppe, R., & Yeager, R. J. (1988). *Rational-Emotive Therapy With Alcoholics and Substance Abusers*. New York: Pergamon.

Graham, J. (1990). *MMPI-2: Assessing Personality and Psychopathology*. New York: Oxford University Press.

Kaminer, U. (1992). *I'm Dysfunctional, You're Dysfunctional*. New York: Random House.

Ludwig, A. M. (1988). *Understanding the Alcoholic's Mind: The Nature of Craving and How to Control It*. New York: Oxford University Press.

Marlatt, G. A., & Gordon, J. R. (Eds.). (1985). *Relapse Prevention: Maintenance Strategies in the Treatment of Addictive Behavior*. New York: Guilford.

Milam, J. R., & Ketcham, K. (1981). *Under the Influence*. New York: Bantam.

Nathan, P. (1990). *Residual Effects of Abused Drugs on Behavior* (National Institute on Drug Abuse Research Monograph No. 101). Rockville, MD: U. S. Department of Health and Human Services.

New York State Department of Motor Vehicles. (1992). *DDP-Curriculum Guideline*. Albany, NY: Division of Traffic Safety Services.

Otto, R., Lang, A. R., Megargee, E. I., & Rosenblatt, A. I. (1988). Ability of alcoholics to escape detection by the MMPI. *Journal of Consulting and Clinical Psychology, 56*, 452-457.

Secular Organizations for Sobriety (SOS). (1992). *Save Ourselves: A Reasonable Approach to Recovery*. Buffalo, NY: SOS National Clearinghouse.

Selzer, M. L. (1971). Michigan Alcoholism Screening Test: The quest for a new diagnostic instrument. *American Journal of Psychiatry, 127*, 1653-1658.

Sobell, M. B., & Sobell, L. C. (1993). *Problem Drinkers: Guided Self-Change Treatment*. New York: Guilford.

Tubesing, D. A. (1981). *Kicking Your Stress Habits: A Do-It-Yourself Guide for Coping With Stress*. Duluth, MN: Whole Person Associates.

Weed, N. C., Butcher, J. N., McKenna, T., & Ben-Porath, Y. S. (1992). New measures for assessing alcohol and drug abuse with the MMPI-2: The APS and AAS. *Journal of Personality Assessment, 58*, 389-404.

Yamauchi, K. T. (1987). Procrastination: Ten ways to "do it now." In P. A. Keller & S. R. Heyman (Eds.), *Innovations in Clinical Practice: A Source Book* (Vol. 6, pp. 431-433). Sarasota, FL: Professional Resource Exchange.

INTRODUCTION TO SECTION V: SELECTED TOPICS

This section includes a collection of contributions that address diverse techniques and roles for clinicians in a variety of settings. These contributions represent a sort of potpourri of topics that may not fit neatly into another section of the volume.

Divorce, separation, and chronic marital distress are taking a devastating toll on the well-being of millions of American adults and children. As the public experiences the negative effects of marital distress, more and more couples are seeking both remedial and preventive assistance with their relationships, making marital therapy a burgeoning area of clinical practice. In the first contribution of this section, Richard Magee presents a framework for conducting marital therapy that guides therapists and enables them to check the currency of their clinical practices. The contribution draws heavily on those approaches to marital therapy which have been most objectively and carefully described and for which there is some research foundation regarding outcome.

In the next contribution, Beryce MacLennan reviews the current knowledge and trends that will be useful for clinicians who provide group psychotherapeutic services to adolescents. The increased interest in group psychotherapy with adolescents has been influenced by several factors, including cost-consciousness, the increased range of community problems that affect many adolescents, the changes in the structure of families, and an increased interest in early intervention.

The third contribution, by Michael Perlin, describes the current status of the insanity defense in this country. Written by a leading legal scholar, it describes the history of the insanity plea and discards several myths that appear to influence the public's perception of this defense. In addition, he demonstrates the role of the insanity acquittal of John Hinckley in the reformulation of our contemporary insanity laws. Then, he outlines the role of punishment and other variables in our culture that interact with society's view of insanity. Finally, he offers some conclusions.

Most people have at some time wondered why battered women and children profess to love those who abuse them and elect to stay with those abusers. Edna Rawlings, P. Gail Allen, Dee Graham, and June Peters present a unique perspective on this finding. They describe the Stockholm Syndrome theory to explain such occurrences as well as other situations involving chronic interpersonal abuse. They describe treatment issues and interventions in both individual and group therapy settings for women who have been victims of partner abuse.

Sandra Brodwin, Leo Orange, and Martin Brodwin provide an overview of private practice issues with disabled clients. They describe common reactions to catastrophic injury or illness, family issues that arise when a member is disabled, and suggestions to practitioners when working with clients who have disabilities.

No cure for AIDS is forthcoming in the near future, and behavior change is the only way to slow the spread of AIDS. However, opponents of prevention programs have espoused numerous myths that prevent them from endorsing effective prevention efforts. The contribution by Sam Knapp reviews 12 common myths as they relate to adolescents, sexuality, and AIDS.

A MARITAL THERAPY PROTOCOL*

Richard D. Magee

INTRODUCTION

Divorce, separation, and chronic marital distress are taking a devastating toll on the psychological and physical well-being of millions of American adults and children. With close to half of all marriages ending in divorce, the U.S. now has the highest divorce rate among major industrialized countries (O'Leary & Smith, 1991). Marital distress and disruption have been associated with a number of negative consequences including depression, physical illness, alcoholism, impaired work performance, and conduct disorders in children (Gottman, 1994; O'Leary & Smith, 1991; Renick, Blumberg, & Markman, 1992).

As the public experiences and comes to understand the negative effects of marital distress, more and more couples are seeking both remedial and preventive assistance with their relationships, making marital therapy a burgeoning area of clinical practice. According to O'Leary and Smith (1991), "more individuals seek help in mental health clinics for marital problems than for any other single problem" (p. 192). Therapists of all professional identities need to consider including the assessment and treatment of couples in their clinical armamentarium.

Marital therapy presents special challenges to the therapist and, as a therapeutic modality, may be more difficult to practice than either individual or family therapy. Unlike individual therapy, where the therapist can focus his or her listening and intervention skills on one person, marital therapy requires the therapist to attend and respond to two persons, whose conflicting views make it hard to empathize with one without alienating the other. In contrast to family therapy, where usually at least the adults in the family can be rallied to work together on a child's problem, marital therapy does not provide such a ready-made basis for cooperative effort. One or both partners often see the presenting problem as the fault of the other, thus requiring the therapist to work very hard at the beginning of therapy to create a context in which cooperative work can take place. It cannot be assumed that experience in treating individual adults or families with children automatically transfers to effective clinical work with couples.

Another factor that contributes to the special challenges of marital therapy, while causing consternation among therapists, is the problem of defining therapeutic success. The marital therapist must address both the needs of the relationship and the individual needs of each spouse - which sometimes are best served by disengagement from the relationship. Keeping a couple together is not necessarily a successful outcome, nor is divorce necessarily a therapeutic failure. A cynic

---

*The term "marital therapy" will be used here because of its familiarity and continuing widespread use. It should be understood that this therapeutic modality applies to all couples, including those of the same sex and those who are unmarried. Some authors have chosen to use the terms "couple therapy" or "couples therapy."

could argue that marital therapists are in a "no lose" situation, in that almost any therapeutic outcome could be viewed as favorable, but few people working in the field find comfort in the confusion they frequently encounter in setting therapeutic goals for distressed couples.

A third complicating issue that must be considered in marital therapy concerns gender differences. Men and women differ in communication styles (Tannen, 1990) and physiological responses during arguments (Gottman, 1994). Our social and political context is associated with gender-related power imbalances that affect even the most intimate of relationships. But perhaps the most urgent concern in the practice of marital therapy is the widespread occurrence of the emotional and physical abuse of women by men (Avis, 1992). Marital therapists have the ethical and professional responsibility of securing the knowledge and skills needed to assess for and deal with abuse. Gender sensitivity is a hallmark of competent marital therapy.

The aim of this article is to present a framework for conducting marital therapy that would guide the beginning marital therapist and also provide more experienced therapists with reference points, based on up-to-date theories and research, that would enable them to check the currency of their clinical practices. Fortunately, marital therapy is no longer the neglected orphan of psychotherapy, taking a fourth place behind individual, group, and family approaches. Most significant has been the recent accumulation of studies showing that marital therapy can make a difference in terms of reducing the risk of separation and divorce and also improving marital satisfaction (Alexander, Holtzworth-Munroe, & Jameson, 1994). Moreover, there are emerging marital therapy protocols based, at least in part, on empirically validated procedures that offer guidance to therapists who want to begin couples work or improve the couples work they already are doing (Baucom & Epstein, 1990; Cordova & Jacobson, 1993; Goldman & Greenberg, 1992; Gottman, 1994; Greenberg & Johnson, 1988; Renick et al., 1992; Snyder, Wills, & Grady-Fletcher, 1991). The author will draw heavily on those approaches to marital therapy that have been most objectively and carefully described and for which there is some research foundation regarding outcome.

What follows is a simplified guide to marital therapy that draws on current theory, research, and clinical practice. The purpose is to provide a "big picture" of how one might work with couples from initial assessment through termination. In addition to favoring those approaches with some empirical support, the author admits having a bias toward brief, pragmatic, and problem-focused therapies that rely heavily on client strengths and engage clients as active collaborators in the therapeutic process. The author also favors approaches that reflect current trends in the direction of psychotherapy convergence and integration, wherein, for example, behavioral, cognitive, and affective interventions are combined in a way to match the specific needs of clients (Cordova & Jacobson, 1993; Pinsof, 1994). This brief contribution does not aspire to be one of those "everything you need to know about . . ." encyclopedic treatises. The reader is directed to the following resources for information concerning the treatment of special problems encountered in marital therapy that are not addressed here: depression (Beach, Sandeen, & O'Leary, 1990), divorce (Textor, 1989), domestic violence (Geller, 1992), extramarital affairs (Berman, 1991; Glass & Wright, 1990), sexual dysfunction (Wincze & Carey, 1991), and substance abuse (Treadway, 1989).

ASSESSING AND JOINING WITH THE COUPLE

Haley's admonition, "If therapy is to end properly, it must begin properly" (Haley, 1981, p. 8), should guide all marital therapists. Starting properly in marital work means (a) gathering the information needed to determine if marital therapy is the recommended course of treatment, and, if so, what direction it should take, at least in its beginning phases; and (b) building a working alliance with the couple and each partner. The following steps are recommended as a way of accomplishing these two goals.

INITIAL TELEPHONE CONTACT

The structure of therapy begins to take shape with the very first client contacts. The therapist, if at all possible, should have telephone contact with both partners prior to the initial therapy session. The therapist would use this telephone contact to briefly orient the clients to the logistics of the therapy situation and describe his or her general plans for the first meeting. Several advantages are gained through this early contact: (a) The therapist demonstrates his or her interest in both partners, staking out a position of neutrality; (b) the therapist can make clear the importance of both partners participating in therapy - at least, getting both of them to agree to come to the first meeting as a fallback position; and (c) in requesting a brief description of the presenting problem, the therapist may obtain information about circumstances that would make marital therapy inappropriate at the present time (e.g., ongoing physical abuse, a severe alcohol problem or mental disorder, current involvement with other therapists). If indicated, more appropriate treatment options should be presented to the clients.

BEGINNING THERAPY

The therapist should begin therapy by meeting with the partners together, letting them know that the conjoint meeting would be followed, as a matter of standard practice, with individual meetings to enable the therapist to make a full assessment of the clients' situation. Clients should also be informed that they might be asked to complete questionnaires to assist in the assessment process. After a brief period of social exchange to help the clients feel at ease, the therapist should summarize the information he or she had gathered from one or both of them through telephone contacts - or from other sources, such as from a referral call from another therapist. This is an opportune time to take 5 or 10 minutes to get information to construct a simple two- or three-generational genogram (McGoldrick & Gerson, 1985). The advantage of obtaining the genogram early in therapy is that it enables the therapist (and, perhaps, the clients) to begin seeing the presenting difficulties in a larger context. Moreover, the genogram often reveals information, sometimes overlooked, that might be important for the therapist to have early in therapy - for example, the recent death of a child or parent, or a continuing custody battle with a former spouse.

The next step is to ask each partner to briefly give his or her view of the marital problem, with the therapist explicitly stating that it is to be expected that the views will be different, thus beginning to highlight for the couple the importance of individual perceptions. The therapist should listen reflectively to each spouse, using this as an opportunity to begin modeling good communication skills. The therapist may even want to say something like, "Right now I'm going to work very hard to understand each of your points of view. While I'm listening carefully to one of you, it may be hard for the other to hold back his or her opinion, but each person will have a turn. I'll make sure that both of you have a chance to fully express your views, because I'm interested in what both of you are experiencing." Thus, the first stage of therapy combines assessment with interventions that (a) establish a safe and empathic therapeutic context with the therapist clearly in control, (b) help the therapist join with each partner, and (c) demonstrate cognitive and behavioral skills that the therapist would like the partners to use with each other.

The time taken for problem identification by each spouse should be brief, respecting the need for the clients to tell their stories without allowing themes of anger, blame, and discouragement to dominate the first session. One way to move to a more positive content, while gathering additional information useful in assessment, is to ask the couple to review the history of their relationship. The therapist can guide this process through questions and prompts that shift the focus to the more positive features of their mutual history. For example, the therapist could ask, "When did you first meet? What attracted you to her (him)? How did your parents react to your plans to marry? What was the wedding like? How were the first years of the marriage? How did things change when the first child came? How did you manage a particular problem or stressful situation?" Such a relationship review identifies for the therapist and the couple significant strengths and resources that might be mobilized to deal with present difficulties. The positive focus might also increase the couple's motivation to work on the marriage in therapy. Of course, diagnostically important information is generated if the couple resist the therapist's gentle efforts to have them recall better times (e.g., "For the life of me, I don't know what I ever saw in him!").

Following the relationship review, the therapist should follow his or her stated plan of spending some time alone with each spouse. Depending on time available, this plan could be carried out in a split session during the first or second meeting or in two separate individual meetings. The objectives of the individual sessions would be to make sure the therapist understands the position of each spouse and also to assess for issues that might be of critical importance in the conduct of therapy - and, indeed, in determining whether marital therapy or some other form of treatment is more appropriate. Such issues would include a current extramarital relationship, battering (physical and emotional abuse used by the husband to intimidate the wife), and heavy substance abuse. For these initial individual sessions (and for any others that might come up in the course of therapy), the therapist should make clear to the couple that he or she does not keep secrets, but will handle information carefully, which means in part not revealing any information without first consulting with the informant and not doing anything that would endanger the informant. Enormous demands are placed on the therapist who, at this juncture, must (a) gather information needed for treatment planning, (b) avoid entering into a coalition with either spouse, and (c) respect the position of each spouse and protect each one from harm.

As an alternative to the individual assessment sessions described previously, some marital therapists obtain information from each spouse with questionnaires or inventories administered prior to or in the early stages of therapy. For this purpose, the therapist could use one of the standard inventories, for example the Dyadic Adjustment Scale (Spanier & Filsinger, 1983), the Locke-Wallace Marital Adjustment Scale (Locke & Wallace, 1959), or, to assess for level of violence, the Conflict Tactics Scale (Straus, 1979). Each client's responses should be considered as private communications to the therapist and be treated within the framework of the limited confidentiality provided in the individual assessment sessions.

This first stage of assessment should be followed by the therapist providing feedback to the clients regarding his or her understanding of their difficulties with a recommended program of treatment (Cordova & Jacobson, 1993). The therapist should acknowledge the couple's level of distress and target areas where work has to be done, explaining that the initial focus of treatment would be on the *how* rather than the *what* of their relationship problems. Underlying interactional patterns that impair problem resolution might be identified at this point, with the message that it is not the presence of problems but the way in which they are handled that determines relationship success or failure. Genuine relationship strengths and resources should be highlighted as providing a foundation for work in therapy. The objective here is to establish a positive motivational set for the spouses to cooperate with the therapist and with each other in a program designed to improve the quality of their relationship. It is common for at least one spouse to have doubts about making a commitment to the relationship; what is needed at this juncture is a willingness to engage in the therapeutic process, not an unqualified pledge to remain in the marriage.

THE PROCESS OF THERAPY

Based on the initial assessment, the therapist enters into a collaborative venture with the couple in which the choice and timing of interventions is determined by such things as the couple's severity of distress, degree of commitment to the relationship, and readiness to change. Jacobson and his colleagues (Cordova & Jacobson, 1993) recently proposed a reformulation of behavioral marital therapy that balances the need to press for change with the need to promote emotional acceptance. Some couples (low level of distress, high level of commitment) are primed to respond to interventions aimed at producing immediate and positive changes in relationship patterns; other couples (high level of distress, low level of commitment) would, at least in the beginning phases of therapy, have difficulty complying with such interventions and would gain most from therapeutic efforts aimed at fostering mutual understanding, empathy, and tolerance. All couples probably profit from the complementary needs for change and acceptance being addressed in therapy.

PROMOTING ACCEPTANCE

Several of the currently most influential models of marital therapy, although based on different theoretical perspectives, converge in recommending that a major part of the therapeutic work be directed at expanding what Pinsof (1994) has aptly called "domains of empathy and meaning." Ego Analytic Couples Therapy (Wile, 1981), Emotionally Focused Couples Therapy (Greenberg & Johnson, 1988), Cognitive-Behavioral Marital Therapy (Baucom & Epstein, 1990), Insight-Oriented Marital Therapy (Snyder et al., 1991), and Integrative Behavioral Couple Therapy (Cordova & Jacobson, 1993) all include interventions aimed at modifying the spouses' cognitive and affective responses to each other and to their relationship. Following are two of the most important strategies, adapted primarily from Cordova and Jacobson (1993), for promoting acceptance.

Encouraging the Expression of Softer Emotions. The therapist engages each client in discussion about a relationship problem or troublesome episode in a way that encourages the client to move beyond expressions of the hard emotions (e.g., anger, criticism, blame) to the soft emotions (e.g., pain, insecurity, loneliness). Facilitating the expression of the soft emotions is a challenging therapeutic task, requiring the therapist to make use of client-centered and emotionally evocative interviewing skills, as he or she essentially conducts individual counseling with one spouse in the presence of the other. Spouses are thus given the opportunity to explore their own thoughts and feelings without the immediate threat of attack or rebuttal - and the opportunity of hearing the other spouse talk about the relationship in a less defensive and more vulnerable way. As the discussion evolves, the therapist encourages the spouses to speak directly to each other, while continuing to provide the coaching and modeling needed to prevent the eruption of attacks and counterattacks. Thorough descriptions of this therapeutic strategy can be found in Greenberg and Johnson (1988) and Cordova and Jacobson (1993). For a clinically sensitive treatment of the role of the therapist in carrying out this kind of work see Wachtel (1993).

Putting the Problem in New Perspective. Another useful method of promoting acceptance is to assist the couple in viewing their difficulty as an external problem, an "it," which is "bigger than both of them." One useful "it" is the predictable patterns of negative interaction in which they become ensnared. Through tracking sequences of reported or observed interactions, the therapist can usually identify one or more patterns (e.g., pursue/withdraw, symmetrical escalations of anger) that repeatedly surface in the relationship. Such sequences typically are experienced by the couple as discrete spontaneous episodes for which they blame each other. When the therapist maps these sequences and demonstrates the steps taken by each partner in the "dance," the couple often gain a shared perspective on their problem which diminishes blame, increases empathy, and may lead to new behaviors ("dance steps"). Other useful "its" are relationship themes or hidden agendas (e.g., conflict avoidance) and differences programmed by their families of origin (e.g., emotionally expressive vs. emotionally distant). For more complete information about these strategies, see Wile, (1981), Greenberg and Johnson (1988), White (1989), Goldman and Greenberg (1992), and Cordova and Jacobson (1993).

PROMOTING CHANGE

The methods of marital therapy that have received the strongest empirical support are the behavioral interventions aimed at increasing positive interactions and improving skills in communication and conflict management (Alexander et al., 1994; Gottman, 1994). These methods can be employed early in therapy when spouses are ready to collaborate with each other in working to improve their relationship (Cordova & Jacobson, 1993) or introduced later in therapy after some degree of acceptance has been achieved.

Increasing Positive Exchanges. Marriages suffer when partners don't do those everyday things for each other that contribute to relationship satisfaction (P. H. Bornstein & M. T. Bornstein, 1986). Gottman (1994) recently has reported that marital satisfaction is associated with a five to one ratio of positive to negative exchanges, whereas marital dissatisfaction was associated with a ratio of less than one to one. It is no surprise that one of most commonly practiced interventions in behavioral marital therapy is a straightforward attempt to increase the number of positive exchanges in a couple's daily life (Jacobson & Margolin, 1979; Stuart, 1980). Of the many versions of this intervention (commonly labeled Behavior Exchange or BE), the approach recommended by Cordova and Jacobson (1993) fits best within the therapeutic framework presented here.

The first step in this procedure is to have each partner identify those actions that he or she could take that would increase the other's satisfaction with the marriage and would not be too personally difficult to carry out. The second step is to coach the couple to introduce these actions into their everyday life. Typically, a list of potentially partner-pleasing behaviors (e.g., make coffee in the morning, carry out a particular household chore) would be generated by each spouse either in session or as homework. Each partner is then given the general directive of carrying out one or more of these activities during the coming week. In subsequent sessions, the couple would discuss whether the desired results of pleasing the partner were achieved, and, if necessary, adjustments could be made to make the assignment more successful. The focus of this intervention is the good faith effort of the "giver" to change his or her behavior for the sake of the marriage.

Cordova and Jacobson (1993) point out that increasing positive exchanges has several beneficial effects, including an immediate boost to marital satisfaction, a shift of focus from negative to positive events, and a demonstration to the couple of their ability to improve their relationship. Difficulty in carrying out this assignment is diagnostically useful, and should guide the therapist to do more to promote acceptance before making further attempts to promote change. One caveat: Increasing positive exchanges, although bringing rapid improvement in the relationships of many couples, is not a complete marital therapy; continued progress depends on combining this intervention with training in communication and problem-solving skills (Holtzworth-Munroe & Jacobson, 1991).

Improving Skills in Communication and Problem Solving. An impressive body of longitudinal research has shown that the most powerful predictors of marital success or failure are the ways in which couples communicate and manage their differences (Gottman, 1994; Markman, 1984). Approximately 90% of distressed couples identify communication problems as their major difficulty (P. H. Bornstein & M. T. Bornstein, 1986). Escalating negative interactions marked by what Gottman (1994) has labeled "the four horsemen of the apocalypse" - criticism, defensiveness, contempt, and stonewalling - can destroy a relationship. ("Stonewalling" refers to emotional or physical withdrawal and is primarily a male response to conflict. Gottman [1984] has found that men become more physiologically upset at the onset of conflict than women, and remain upset for a longer period of time. Withdrawal or shutting down may be a way for men to avoid or escape from physiological distress. Stonewalling is strongly aversive to women and contributes to the pursuer-distancer pattern common to many distressed marital relationships. Current methods of communication training address this gender difference [Markman, Stanley, & Blumberg, 1992]). Communication skills can help couples handle disagreements in a more constructive manner and also provide avenues for developing greater understanding and intimacy (Cordova & Jacobson, 1993). Training in communication is a component of almost all approaches to marital therapy, and its usefulness in improving marital relationships has received strong empirical support (Gottman, 1994; Jacobson & Holtzworth-Munroe, 1986).

Several comprehensive and detailed guides to the practice of communication training for couples are available for the clinician (e.g., Guerney, 1977; Jacobson & Margolin, 1979; Stuart, 1980). In addition, two excellent books can be recommended for client use: the classic *A Couple's Guide to Communication* (Gottman et al., 1976) and the recently published *We Can Work It Out: Making Sense Out of Marital Conflict* (Notarius & Markman, 1993). Also highly recommended for client use are the audio- and videotapes entitled *Fighting for Your Marriage,* featuring the Prevention and Relationship Enhancement Program (PREP) developed at the University of Denver by Markman, Stanley, and Blumberg (1992).

What follows is a brief overview of communication and problem-solving training based primarily on the latest formulations of Gottman (1994), Jacobson and his associates (Cordova & Jacobson, 1993), and Markman, Blumberg, and Stanley (1992). Because the characteristics of couples and the specific problems they present vary considerably, the effective marital therapist must exercise sensitivity and flexibility in applying any standardized protocol. The framework for changing patterns of communication outlined here should be followed in a way that matches the idiosyncratic needs of the client and, as noted previously, should be balanced with continuing efforts to promote understanding, empathy, and tolerance.

The three major components of communication training are (a) instruction and modeling, (b) practice, and (c) feedback. The therapist instructs the couple regarding the elements of good communication, including the importance of nonprovocative speaking and nondefensive listening. Couples are taught methods of mutual validation and the usefulness of paraphrasing to slow down potentially troublesome exchanges and to make sure that the intent of the speaker equals the impact on the listener (Gottman et al., 1976). Given the corrosive effects of negative escalations, couples should also be given "ground rules" (Markman, Stanley, & Blumberg, 1992) for keeping their discussions under control. These "ground rules" would include an agreement that "time out" would be called when either spouse began to experience emotional discomfort. Gottman (1994) believes that the most important entry-level skills to be taught to distressed couples are "exiting" from hostile interactions and the "soothing" or calming of intense emotional states.

The subsequent steps in communication training involve having the couple practice these communication skills in session with feedback provided by the therapist. Topics should be chosen that are important to the couple, but not highly toxic. The therapist, in the beginning, may need to actively coach and continue to demonstrate the correct use of the skills. Couples should be advised that these new ways of talking to each other may seem awkward and stilted, but that they will become more natural with practice. The therapist's ongoing coaching and feedback should, of course, include large doses of positive reinforcement. Practice in communication could continue for several sessions, and not until the skills have been mastered in session should they be assigned as homework (Cordova & Jacobson, 1993).

Training in problem solving can be introduced after the couple have made progress mastering the basic communication skills - although this additional training may not be needed. The practice of clear communication and the experience of mutual validation often lead to the spontaneous generation of solutions and the settlement of disagreements. When training in formal problem solving is required - and often it is best introduced in response to a current problem that has surfaced in the everyday life of the couple - the clinician can once more use established protocols that are fully described in the marital therapy literature (e.g., Cordova & Jacobson, 1993). The most important consideration in problem solving is to clearly separate discussion focused on defining the problem from discussion aimed at solving it. Many couples rush prematurely into suggesting solutions before they have come to full agreement on the nature of the problem. Once the problem is defined, it becomes externalized, an "it" about which they can collaborate to find a mutually satisfactory solution. The remaining steps in formal problem solving are brainstorming, deciding on a plan of action, and, finally, carrying out the plan with a review of the results. As with communication training, problem solving should be mastered in session with the guidance of the therapist before being tried at home.

THERAPEUTIC CLOSURE AND OUTCOME

Therapy progresses as the therapist and the couple collaborate within the framework outlined earlier to reach the goals of treatment. Communication and problem-solving skills are applied in session to difficult relationship issues, and the therapist helps the couple implement these skills at home. Throughout therapy, the therapist continues to balance direct work on behavior change with the development of a greater degree of mutual understanding, empathy, and acceptance.

The therapy models on which this framework is based are all relatively brief, ranging in duration from 8 to 15 sessions for Emotionally Focused Couples Therapy (Greenberg & Johnson, 1988) to approximately 20 sessions for the behavioral approaches (Jacobson & Holtzworth-Munroe, 1986). Although weekly sessions are typical, the collaborative model is best honored by moving from frequent meetings at the onset of therapy (when the therapist is building a therapeutic alliance and creating a therapeutic context) to less frequent, even intermittent, meetings toward the end of therapy (when the clients have learned the skills to work on relationship issues on their own).

How successful is marital therapy? Despite the debate over whether saving the marriage always constitutes a success, marital therapy has been almost always evaluated by its effectiveness in improving marital satisfaction and/or preventing divorce. In the most recent comprehensive review of marital therapy outcomes, it is reported that "virtually all the marital therapy approaches investigated to date . . . are effective relative to no-treatment control groups (Alexander et al., 1994, p. 605). The most systematic research, using very stringent criteria of improvement, suggests that about two-thirds of couples treated with behavioral approaches significantly improve by the end of therapy. After 2 years, however, approximately one-third of the improved clients have relapsed, yielding an overall long-term improvement rate of only 50% (Holtzworth-Munroe & Jacobson, 1991).

Concern over the substantial number of couples who either don't improve or eventually relapse has resulted in (a) the revision of behavioral marital therapy, noted previously, to include interventions aimed at promoting emotional acceptance as well as behavioral change (Cordova & Jacobson, 1993), (b) recommendations for a "family dentistry" model of marital therapy that would incorporate periodic check-up or booster sessions to prevent relapse (Holtzworth-Munroe & Jacobson, 1991), and (c) suggestions for the practice of a "minimal marital therapy" that would focus exclusively on the thorough mastery (i.e., overlearning) of the basic skills required to control the negative emotional escalations so destructive of relationships (Gottman, 1994).

Marital therapy has become a dynamic, challenging, and significant area of clinical specialization. Those of us who work with couples have the professional responsibility to be informed and guided by the rapidly growing body of empirical research relevant to our practice.

Richard D. Magee, PhD, is Professor of Psychology at the Indiana University of Pennsylvania where he directs the Center for Applied Psychology and the Family Clinic. His work involves family therapy supervision and community consultation. He is an Approved Supervisor of the American Association for Marriage and Family Therapy. Dr. Magee may be contacted at the Center for Applied Psychology, Indiana University of Pennsylvania, Indiana, PA 15705.

RESOURCES

Alexander, J. F., Holtzworth-Munroe, A., & Jameson, P. (1994). The process and outcome of marital and family therapy: Research review and evaluation. In A. E. Bergin & S. L. Garfield (Eds.), *Handbook of Psychotherapy and Behavior Change* (4th ed., pp. 595-630). New York: Wiley.

Avis, J. (1992). Where are all the family therapists? Abuse and violence within families and family therapy's response. *Journal of Marital and Family Therapy, 18,* 225-232.

Baucom, D. H., & Epstein, N. (1990). *Cognitive Behavioral Marital Therapy.* New York: Brunner/Mazel.

Beach, S. R. H., Sandeen, E. E., & O'Leary, K. D. (1990). *Depression in Marriage: A Model for Etiology and Treatment.* New York: Guilford.

Berman, E. M. (1991). *Patterns of Infidelity and Their Treatment.* New York: Brunner/Mazel.

Bornstein, P. H., & Bornstein, M. T. (1986). *Marital Therapy: A Behavioral-Communications Approach.* New York: Pergamon.

Cordova, J. V., & Jacobson, N. S. (1993). Couple distress. In D. Barlow (Ed.), *Clinical Handbook of Psychological Disorders* (2nd ed., pp. 481-512). New York: Guilford.

Geller, J. A. (1992). *Breaking Destructive Patterns: Multiple Strategies of Treating Partner Abuse.* New York: The Free Press.

Glass, S. H., & Wright, T. L. (Presenters). (1990). *Reconstructing After Extramarital Involvement* [Videotape #V502]. Washington, DC: American Association for Marriage and Family Therapy.

Goldman, A., & Greenberg, L. S. (1992). Comparison of integrated systemic and emotionally focused approaches to couples therapy. *Journal of Consulting and Clinical Psychology, 60,* 962-969.

Gottman, J. M. (1994). *What Predicts Divorce?* Hillsdale, NJ: Lawrence Erlbaum.

Gottman, J. M., Notarius, C., Gonso, J., & Markman, H. J. (1976). *A Couple's Guide to Communication.* Champaign, IL: Research Press.

Greenberg, L. S., & Johnson, S. M. (1988). *Emotionally Focused Therapy for Couples.* New York: Guilford.

Guerney, B. G. (1977). *Relationship Enhancement.* San Francisco: Jossey-Bass.

Haley, J. (1981). *Problem-Solving Therapy* (2nd. ed.). San Francisco: Jossey-Bass.

Holtzworth-Munroe, A., & Jacobson, N. S. (1991). Behavioral marital therapy. In A. S. Gurman & D. P. Kniskern (Eds.), *Handbook of Family Therapy, Vol. II* (pp. 96-133). New York: Brunner/Mazel.

Jacobson, N. S., & Holtzworth-Munroe, A. (1986). Marital therapy: A social learning/cognitive perspective. In N. S. Jacobson & A. S. Gurman (Eds.), *Clinical Handbook of Marital Therapy* (pp. 29-70). New York: Guilford.

Jacobson, N. S., & Margolin, G. (1979). *Marital Therapy: Strategies Based on Social Learning and Behavior Exchange Principles.* New York: Brunner/Mazel.

Locke, H. J., & Wallace, K. M. (1959). Short marital-adjustment and prediction tests: Their reliability and validity. *Marriage and Family Living, 21,* 251-255.

Markman, H. J. (1984). The longitudinal study of couples' interactions: Implications for understanding and predicting marital distress. In K. Hahlweg & N. S. Jacobson (Eds.), *Marital Interaction: Analysis and Modification* (pp. 253-381). New York: Guilford.

Markman, H. J., Blumberg, S. L., & Stanley, S. M. (1992). *PREP Leader's Manual.* Denver, CO: PREP.

Markman, H. J., Stanley, S. M., & Blumberg, S. L. (Producers and Speakers). (1992). *Fighting for Your Marriage* [Audio- and Videotapes]. Denver, CO: PREP Educational Videos.

McGoldrick, M., & Gerson, R. (1985). *Genograms in Family Assessment.* New York: Norton.

Notarius, C., & Markman, H. J. (1993). *We Can Work It Out: Making Sense Out of Marital Conflict.* New York: Putnam.

O'Leary, K. D., & Smith, D. A. (1991). Marital interactions. *Annual Review of Psychology, 42,* 191-212.

Pinsof, W. M. (1994, March). *Angry Couples: A Progressive Treatment Model.* Workshop presented at Family Therapy Network Symposium, Washington, DC.

Renick, M. J., Blumberg, S. L., & Markman, H. J. (1992). The prevention and relationship enhancement program (PREP): An empirically based preventive intervention program for couples. *Family Relations, 41,* 141-147.

Snyder, D. K., Wills, R. M., & Grady-Fletcher, A. (1991). Long-term effectiveness of behavioral versus insight-oriented marital therapy. *Journal of Consulting and Clinical Psychology, 59,* 138-141.

Spanier, G. B., & Filsinger, E. E. (1983). The Dyadic Adjustment Scale. In E. E. Filsinger (Ed.), *Marriage and Family Assessment: A Source Book for Family Therapy* (pp. 155-168). Beverly Hills, CA: Sage.

Straus, M. A. (1979). Measuring intrafamily conflict and violence: The Conflict Tactics (CT) Scales. *Journal of Marriage and the Family, 41,* 75-88.

Stuart, R. B. (1980). *Helping Couples Change: A Social Learning Approach to Marital Therapy.* New York: Guilford.

Tannen, D. (1990). *You Just Don't Understand: Women and Men in Conversation.* New York: Ballantine.

Textor, M. (Ed.). (1989). *The Divorce and Divorce Therapy Handbook.* Northvale, NJ: Aronson.

Treadway, D. C. (1989). *Before It's Too Late: Working With Substance Abuse in the Family.* New York: Norton.

Wachtel, E. F. (1993). Postscript: Therapeutic communication with couples. In P. L. Wachtel (Ed.), *Therapeutic Communication: Principles and Effective Practice* (pp. 273-293). New York: Guilford.

White, M. (1989). *Selected Papers.* Adelaide, Australia: Dulwich Center Publications.

Wile, D. B. (1981). *Couples Therapy: A Nontraditional Approach.* New York: Wiley.

Wincze, J. P., & Carey, M. P. (1991). *Sexual Dysfunction: A Guide for Assessment and Treatment.* New York: Guilford.

CONTEMPORARY ISSUES IN ADOLESCENT GROUP PSYCHOTHERAPY

Beryce W. MacLennan

Group psychotherapy with adolescents has received increased attention over the last 10 years. Theoretical advances have expanded our understanding of adolescent problems, and practical advances have added to treatment options including problem-specific group interventions. This contribution will review current understandings and trends that may be useful for the clinician when conducting group psychotherapy with adolescents.

In the 1980s, training guidelines for group psychotherapists working with adolescents were drafted by the American Group Psychotherapy Association. These guidelines stated that therapists working with adolescent psychotherapy groups should have received basic training in group theories and methods, undergone a group experience themselves, and led groups under supervision. They should be familiar with adolescent development and with the habits, values, and language of the teenage subculture to which their group members belong. Unfortunately, these guidelines were not formally adopted by the Association, and many therapists are still required to lead groups without any specialized training.

The increased interest in group psychotherapy with adolescents has been influenced by five major factors. First, health and mental health cost containment reforms have resulted in shorter stays in hospital and residential treatment programs. Short-term problem-specific interventions are becoming the norm, and group therapy is being seen as a potentially cost-effective alternative to individual, long-term treatment.

Second, teenage environments have become more stressful and dangerous in the last 10 years. Teenagers are currently faced with many major obstacles in their journeys to adulthood. A substantial number of teenagers live in poverty-stricken, drug-ridden, and violent neighborhoods. All teenagers must confront the tasks of sexual development during this time period. However, normal stresses are multiplied by the spread of sexually transmitted diseases and Acquired Immunodeficiency Syndrome (AIDS), the frequency of teenage parenthood, and the dangers of sexual assault and incest. Substance abuse, suicide, homicide, depression, and eating disorders continue to gain in their influence on teenagers. Group therapy can be a major tool in counteracting the negative effects of stressful environments.

Third, the family framework in the United States continues to experience widespread change. Over a quarter of the households with children under 18 are single-parent families, and at least a million couples divorce each year (Bureau of the Census, 1991). Many of these parents marry again, creating reconstituted families in which all members must redefine their roles. A recent phenomenon is that many families have had to give up or have been ejected from their homes, resulting in large numbers of homeless families. This may in part be due to regional economic depressions that affect not only the lives of many families with teenagers but also whole communities reliant on industries such as oil production, automobile manufacturing, high-tech operations, and farming.

Fourth, although racial and ethnic tension has always been a part of American life, there is a trend toward multigroup separatism that seems to have heightened racial and ethnic rivalries (Hodgekinson, 1989). Moreover, the United States has recently experienced a large influx of immigrant and refugee families with teenagers and young children. These trends require group therapists to be culturally sensitive in their work with teenagers.

Fifth, interest in prevention and early intervention group programs is increasing among professionals and society at large. Psychoeducational groups and groups that teach social skills and the management of transitions and life crises can prepare teenagers to face the tough decisions they will encounter in today's society and to make better life choices. This, it is hoped, will result in the reduction of the high costs to society of maladaptive behaviors and mental breakdown.

In this contribution, I discuss some of the advances in theory and practice that have affected adolescent group psychotherapy and describe some of the problem-specific group interventions that have been designed to treat teenagers. Additional summaries can be found in the American Group Psychotherapy Association monograph edited by Azima and Richmond (1989), the updated edition of *Group Counseling and Psychotherapy With Adolescents* by MacLennan and Dies (1992), and "Group Psychotherapy With Girls in Early Adolescence: Then and Now" (MacLennan, 1991).

TRENDS IN THEORY AND PRACTICE

Four trends in theory and practice have evolved from our increased understanding of group psychotherapy with adolescents. These factors are the use of well-defined contracts; a greater understanding of stages in group development and its implications for group management; the exploration of different "curative factors" such as information giving and catharsis in teenage group therapy; and the effects of the race, sex, age, and personality of the therapist on the capacity of teenagers from different subgroups and environments to identify with their leader.

USE OF CONTRACTS

Teenagers have been notoriously difficult both to engage in treatment and to keep involved. Consequently, groups are frequently conducted in settings where teenagers are naturally found. This can reduce the hassle of insuring transportation and some of the initial difficulties in dealing with poorly motivated teenagers and preoccupied parents. Although groups are still run in traditional mental health settings such as outpatient psychiatric and youth counseling clinics, many are now conducted in schools, public health clinics, and recreation centers.

Because group psychotherapy for teenagers is moving out of traditional settings where therapy is the primary function of the institution, it is particularly important that the program be fully accepted and endorsed by the institution. The relationship between the therapist, the group, and the institution should be clearly spelled out in a contract, each party having a full understanding of who has what authority, where responsibilities lie, and to what extent the therapist and the group members are bound to abide by the rules of the institutions. Elements of the contract include who will select the members for the group, who will prepare them, and who will insure that they come to the group. Without an adequate contract, therapists may arrive at a school prepared to run a group, only to find that the youths have gone off for the day on a field trip. Similarly, when they go to a hospital, they may find that doctors' appointments have been scheduled for members of the group at the time the group meets. The therapist tries to insure, through the contract, that the basic necessities for holding a group are available: a room of reasonable size and suitable furnishings set aside at a regular time, privacy, supplies for activities on hand, and a place to store them. With no contract, one may be obliged to run groups in a different room every week, in a corridor, or in an enormous high school cafeteria with staff clearing away the meals. All professionals associated with the youth must also be aware of what they can expect in terms of feedback about what goes on in the group. Referring teachers, principals, counselors, probation officers, and nurses may want to know exactly what goes on in the group, so that the parameters of confidentiality must be spelled out and agreement reached. Staff may hope for immediate improvement, and they need to know that this is not likely in most cases.

In psychiatric and youth counseling settings, contracting with youth and their parents is also common practice. Therapists often work with parents and youth to establish specific treatment goals for each member in the group. Very frequently, both parents and teenager will sign off on the treatment goal statement and participate in reviewing progress made. In other settings, goals for individual members may not have been preset. The teenagers may have been given a general invitation to participate in the group. Although state laws and regulations are applicable, in most cases if the teenager is under legal age, written permission must be obtained from the parents and the parents must be given some understanding of what they can expect from the group and offered the opportunity for periodic feedback.

The development of a contract with the group as a whole can be an important therapeutic tool, particularly with youth who are impulsive and have poor social skills. Such a contract is usually established at the first session. The contract generally consists of two parts: the focus and goals for the group and the rules for acceptable behavior in the group. As they negotiate the contract, members discuss together what they want to get out of the group and often reveal some of the problems that bring them to the group. Sometimes, with poorly motivated or reluctant members, the goals may be very general, such as "having a place to talk," "having someone to depend on," or even just "having a place to have fun." When members are fearful or embarrassed to reveal their problems initially, some therapists allow members to write their problems and goals in their own private book which only they and the therapist see.

Teenagers need to have a part in setting the rules and in discussing what should be done if the rules are broken. Rules usually include some or all of the following:

- Members should be concerned for and try to help each other.
- Only one person should speak at once while the others should try to listen without interrupting.
- There should be no name calling, pushing each other, or physical fighting.
- If games are played, members should keep to the rules.
- If members meet each other outside the group, they are expected to discuss their relationships with the other group members.
- Members are expected to attend regularly and be on time and if they cannot they must let the other members know the reason why.

Conditions for feedback to parents and confidentiality are also established. At this time the therapist does not reveal the details of what goes on in the group. However, parents or other persons of importance in the members' lives may require some general statement from time to time about the members' progress. Some therapists reserve sessions periodically for members to discuss what shall be reported. Also, the therapist must take whatever action is necessary if a member is going to hurt himself or herself or others, and is legally obligated to report any child abuse. These exceptions are explained in the first session so that, if the therapist has to supersede the general rule of confidentiality, it comes as no surprise to the group members. Group members are also expected to keep confidential what happens and what they learn about each other in the group. This is particularly important in schools and residential settings where the members are part of a common community.

Obviously, learning how to keep to the rules is one of the tasks in most adolescent groups. Therapists vary in how they achieve this. Behavioral therapists frequently employ tokens signifying rewards for keeping the rules and penalties for breaking them. Others require members who get out of control to sit outside the group circle or to leave the group for the rest of the session. This decision can be made by the therapist alone or together with the group members. Sometimes, the group merely spends time discussing how and why the particular problem has occurred in the group. The author prefers to encourage the group members to take maximum responsibility for their own behavior and to decide how to deal with problems in the group. For instance, in a group where the boys were living in a violent environment and did not know how to control the violence, learning how to cope with aggressive behavior in the group was very important. Early in the group sessions, they poked and teased each other, got into physical fights, called each other names, got up and marched around the room singing rap songs, and made many racist remarks. They felt that they were discriminated against, could not trust anyone, and believed that they would not be able to survive through adolescence in their inner city ghetto. They practiced different ways of avoiding and resolving conflicts through role playing, they learned about the dynamic interaction in the group, and they played *The Anger Control Game* (Berg, 1988), a board game that suggests alternative ways for dealing with physical and verbal aggression. By the end of the school year, they felt much more competent to manage their lives and to survive the stresses of adolescence.

STAGES OF GROUP DEVELOPMENT

It has been recognized at least since 1940 that psychotherapy groups pass through identifiable stages of development. Members start by exploring the nature of the group and its fit with their needs as individuals. They then proceed to explore the norms and boundaries of the group and test the strength of the therapist. They vie for position in the group and form tentative relationships. Members gradually develop greater trust in each other and the leader and work on individual tasks and problems together. In the final stage of the group, they review their progress and come to terms with the ending of the group and the need for members to proceed independently with their own lives. Tuchman and Jensen's model (1977) of "forming," "storming," "norming," "performing," and "adjourning" is probably the best known of these. Dies (1991) has renamed these stages and applied them to adolescent group psychotherapy, identifying some of the tasks that therapists need to perform at each stage of group development.

Dies' first stage is "initial relatedness." In this stage the members begin to learn about each other and to understand what is expected from them in the group. The leader is fairly active in controlling the level of self-revelation and in modeling how the group should function. The group contract is developed and affirmed. Her second stage is "testing the limits" and her third "resolving authority issues." In these two stages the members test the strength of the leader and establish their positions in the group. In the third stage, members establish a level of trust in each other and in the leader so that they can move to deeper levels of self-revelation. During these three stages, the leader is active in helping the group members move toward taking more responsibility for themselves and the group. In the fourth stage, "working on self," the members gain greater understanding of their issues and work on resolving their problems. Dies names the final stage "moving on," during which the members review and evaluate what has happened to them in the group and work on separation and forming stronger ties in their lives outside the group. As those of us who work with adolescents have recognized, group therapists working with adolescents need to make clear to the group members what kind of person they are and what they stand for. Therapists in adolescent groups must be fairly active and firm, particularly in the early stages of the group. These stages are present in groups even if they are designed to be quite structured. Members still have to settle issues regarding what kind of group they are in, what the leader is like, what position they will have in the group, and test out whether it will meet their needs, before they can really use the group effectively. Work on the group contract is particularly important for members who are impulsive, hyperactive, or defiant and enraged, and is a useful tool in moving the group to its more productive stages. As most writers have noted, progressing from one stage to another is not a smooth process; groups swing back and forth from one stage to another when anxiety is high or when the composition of the group changes.

The development of the group and the group dynamics vary greatly depending on whether the group is a short-term closed group; whether it is an intermediate or long-term semiclosed group with occasional changes in membership; or whether it is an open-ended group with revolving membership. Short-term crisis and inpatient groups are frequently of this last type, and each meeting may have a slightly different membership although the ways of working and the group norms may be carried on by a core of "older" members. In a "revolving group," each session may go through the stages of group development in an abbreviated form, clarifying the purposes and norms of the group, testing the leader and other members, working on particular issues, and then terminating for that session.

CURATIVE FACTORS

Experiences within groups that appear to have therapeutic value for the members have been named "curative factors" (Yalom, 1975). Writers on group psychotherapy with adolescents, such as MacLennan and Felsenfeld (1968), identified group therapy as a treatment of choice for adolescents because groups reduce the sense of isolation and uniqueness from which troubled teenagers suffer. Corder, Whiteside, and Haizlip (1981) asked the adolescent members of their groups to rank "curative factors" and found group cohesion, catharsis, and interpersonal learning as most valuable and insight interpretation as the least helpful. Group emphasis may vary depending on the problems of the members and goals of the group. Poorly socialized youth who must learn to control their impulses and emotional outbursts will probably find that the development of interpersonal skills through practice in the group will be most helpful. In contrast, severely traumatized youth may need to reexperience and reinterpret repressed memories in order to put them to rest.

CHOICE OF THERAPIST

There is a general consensus that group therapists working with adolescents need to like to work with this population. They must be able to be active, firm, expressive, and caring as need arises. They should be secure in their capacity to deal with their own issues which may be stirred up in the group. MacLennan and Dies (1992) also emphasize that the leader must be knowledgeable about the adolescent members' subcultures and interests. In the 1990s, when many minority groups are competing for their place in American society, the appearance and life experiences of the therapists may play an important part in the adolescent group's acceptance of the therapist as a leader. Young adolescents between the ages of 12 and 16 are often particularly affected by external factors such as the therapist's gender, age, appearance, race, ethnic group, and economic background, and differences may influence the capacity of the group members to identify with the leader and see him or her as relevant for them. For example, MacLennan and Rosen (1963) found that boys when they reached puberty identified more easily with male therapists than female therapists although younger boys had no such difficulty. Sue (1990) provides an interesting discussion of racial and ethnic choice of therapist in relation to the self-identifications of the members. Teenagers who are still adhering to the old "assimilation model" of American society, in which immigrants adopt the values of the larger society, may prefer leaders who typify the ideal American. Others, however, may be struggling to retain their racial and ethnic heritage and may reject leaders who are not like them and who have not undergone similar experiences. For example, in a recent group of the author's, one member, an inner city teenager living in a violent, impoverished environment, was not able to accept that any therapist who had not undergone similar experiences could be helpful to him. He finally decided to leave the group. Sue also identifies a third group for whom ethnic and racial issues seem less important and for whom the personal style of the therapist is critical. MacLennan (1975), in a paper on the personalities of group therapists, describes the employment of youth drawn from a similar background to work as group counselors with impoverished inner-city children.

Language may also be a limiting factor, even though most teenagers in the United States speak English as a first or second language. In any group of teenagers, group therapists must understand the special vocabulary and expressions currently used by them if they are to be effective. However, if they are working with groups drawn from specific ethnic cultures, then a leader who does not understand the language and customs may be severely handicapped. Statistically, our American population is divided into Caucasian, Afro-American, Hispanic, Asian, Native American, and other ethnic groups. However, Asians such as Japanese, Vietnamese, Hmong, and Korean are all very different culturally and linguistically. African-Americans from the Caribbean and from Africa have different values, backgrounds, and language than those from the southern United States; and Hispanics may speak many different dialects depending on the country and class from which they come. Even if therapists learn the language, they may not be sufficiently fluent to catch all the nuances. Using an interpreter even in individual therapy has its own problems because we must take into consideration the relationships between interpreters and clients. Interpreters are not really satisfactory in a group as they slow down and inhibit the group interaction so greatly. Because of the paucity of therapists from many cultural groups, there is currently no truly satisfactory solution. However, therapists can encourage group members who are bilingual to let them know if they do not fully understand what is being said.

PROBLEM-SPECIFIC GROUP INTERVENTIONS

Problem-specific groups focus on one particular issue, and all the members in the group are affected by that problem. This may be the only criterion for selection into the group. However, other criteria may also be important, such as the developmental age of the teenagers, their lifestyles, and their economic and cultural backgrounds. There may be little opportunity for choice of group members in a short-term psychiatric unit where the teenagers are concerned with how they came to be hospitalized, how they can retain a grasp of reality and control of their impulses while in the hospital, and what tasks they will have to face upon returning to life in the community. However, in other groups where perhaps the youth are transitioning from elementary to junior high school or from high school to work or college, age must be taken into consideration because, although the element of transition is common to each situation, the contexts of the problems are quite different. Although predelivery teenage mothers' groups may not need to be age specific, age is important once the mother and infant return home from the hospital. Groups for older teenagers who are caring for their children on their own have much less relevance for the young teenager who is still living with her parents or foster parents and going to school. In this section, current practice in teenage groups related to divorce and remarriage; traumatic experiences such as disasters, sexual assault, and sexual abuse; teenage parenting; substance abuse; and groups for delinquent youth will be discussed.

DIVORCE AND REMARRIAGE

Adolescents, similarly to parents, experience different stages in the breakup of a marriage: parental conflict, separation, divorce, living in a single-parent family or switching from one parent to another, and then possibly having to adapt to a reconstituted family if one or both parents remarry. In conflicted marital situations, the youth are often drawn into the conflict, pressured to take sides, and made to feel responsible for the breakup of the marriage. Short-term groups have been designed to help children get through these periods of separation and divorce (Pedro-Carroll & Cowen, 1985). These groups aim to provide a place where members can talk about the situation, express their feelings, recognize that other teenagers are facing the same problems, and work through their anger and grief in adjusting to their new life. A psychoeducational component may explain and allow rehearsal of court and custody issues, explain choice options, teach adolescents about responsibilities for self and family, or explore viewpoints on both sides of the conflict. These problem-focused groups are usually short, lasting perhaps 6 to 12 sessions. They may take place in schools, mental health clinics, recreation programs, or sometimes even in private practice. They are often age specific and may be composed of one or both sexes. On occasion, more severe difficulties such as depression, difficulty concentrating, poor academic performance, or acting out through aggression, sexuality, or substance abuse may develop. The therapist should then determine if additional therapeutic action is necessary.

Another form these groups can take involves the reconstituted family in therapy. Sometimes, two or three such families, consisting of each living unit (usually there will be the couple from each family and the children from each of the former marriages who are living with them), may meet together as a group. The focus is on how each unit can develop into a cohesive family. In a reconstituted marriage, members of the two or more families now made one have had different ways of functioning and different values. Parents have set different limits on the children and members have had different ways of resolving problems and expressing their feelings. These issues have to be worked out before the new unit can function well. Group members share how they have encountered and solved these difficulties.

A third format occurs when a team of therapists brings together all the actors in the reconstituted marital situation (Serrano, 1989). This could include three or four different households and several generations. Often these meetings will extend over a day or even a weekend, with team members working with selected individuals, couples, small groups, or all the participants together to resolve their issues. The focus is on solving whatever problems are experienced by the members and in defining their new roles. Members are often asked to role play how they would interact and deal with different situations.

POST-TRAUMATIC STRESS DISORDER AND SEXUAL ABUSE

Post-Traumatic Stress Disorder (PTSD) became an official psychiatric diagnosis only in 1979 when it was included in *DSM-III,* but since that time many practitioners have specialized in its treatment, and groups have been developed for disaster survivors including adolescents, Vietnam veterans, victims of terrorism, and survivors of incest and sexual assault. All these traumatic experiences may have some elements in common. Similar symptoms may include numbing, dissociation, repression, denial, nightmares, flashbacks, self-medication with drugs and alcohol, or acting out the rage and despair sexually or violently.

However, groups are usually formed on the basis of a similar type of trauma. The time frame is also important. Some groups may be formed immediately after the traumatic event, when the aim is to work through the trauma and return the individuals to their prior level of functioning. Other groups include members who are dealing with chronic trauma or experiences from a distant past. These members may have developed dysfunctional habits and coping mechanisms which have become ingrained.

POST-DISASTER GROUPS

In this section, post-disaster groups and groups for teenagers who have experienced violent death in their schools and neighborhoods will be discussed.

Groups held immediately after disasters are often held in shelters where the survivors are being cared for, warmed, fed, and encouraged to get enough rest. They are then quite heterogeneous in composition. Alternatively, they may be specifically designed for children and adolescents and held in the schools. In either case, the focus is on helping to desensitize the experiences through sharing the memories and reexperiencing the feelings and through imaging different outcomes. Members in these groups are encouraged to express their grief and recognize the irrationality of feeling guilty because one has survived when others have died, and to express their anger that they experienced losses when others may have survived without any injury to themselves or damage to their property. They learn to face up to their problems in remaking their lives and to cope with them effectively. They rehearse how they would behave if a similar disaster were to recur. Sometimes these groups are repeated on the anniversary of the disaster for several years. Preventive groups, which prepare for disasters through training inhabitants of disaster-prone areas in how to cope, are also commonly held in school and can be helpful in reducing injury and death, increasing self-confidence, and preventing fear and confusion.

In recent years, particularly in poverty-stricken inner-city neighborhoods, there has been a pandemic of violent death, and many teenagers are afraid for their lives. They have seen friends, neighbors, and family gunned down before them and may themselves have been caught in the middle of a battle. When such an event occurs, brief trauma groups are often held in schools to help students and staff deal with the grief and shock. These groups are designed to encourage members to ventilate their emotions, their sense of loss, their anxieties about dying, and their guilt at surviving or perhaps at having disliked the victims.

In some inner cities, violence may be an everyday occurrence. Additionally, many of the youth live in chaotic families in which they have never learned how to develop effective, caring interpersonal relationships. Under these circumstances, longer term groups are necessary to help the youth feel differently about themselves and others. They need to learn new skills in how to avoid getting into fights and how to mediate conflict. The members also play games such as *The Anger Control Game* (Berg, 1988), which teaches different options for dealing with conflict. Sometimes, members role play scenes, make up plays, or create videos about their dilemmas.

GROUPS FOR VICTIMS OF SEXUAL ASSAULT

Sexual assault is a devastating experience for the victims. They are not only violated and feel despoiled but they have almost always been afraid that they are going to die. They no longer feel safe anywhere and have lost their trust in others. Although stranger rape is terrifying, in some ways acquaintance rape can be even worse in that the victims question their own judgment and possible complicity. Many victims have difficulty enduring any medical examination or going to the dentist. They may find it intolerable to allow anyone to touch them, let alone have sexual relations. All these problems have to be worked through if members are to live normal lives again. For some victims of assault, the experiences revive memories of earlier traumas, which must also be processed before they can recover. The reactions of their families, friends, and cultural group are all extremely important in recovery. If everyone is supportive, then recovery is much easier, but if they are blamed or disbelieved, it is hard for them to recover their self-esteem. If the perpetrator can be confronted and punished, members can feel vindicated. Traditionally, groups have focused on adult rape survivors to which teenagers have been added. However, teenage groups are now becoming much more common. Groups are usually comprised of one sex only and have one or two therapists of the same sex. Often cotherapists are employed to provide support because the groups are emotionally draining for the therapists as well as the members. Consultation or supervision is advisable. Most of these groups are short, 10 or 20 sessions, although sometimes they may continue for a year. Groups are usually quite intense. Members experience much abreaction and catharsis. They relive and desensitize their experiences and support each other in combating the "blame the victim" syndrome. They also learn to cope with concrete situations such as deciding whom to tell or testifying in court through discussion and rehearsal. They learn how to protect themselves in the future and to trust again.

Most frequently members are also in individual treatment either with the same or a different therapist, and there is considerable interaction between the two forms of treatment.

GROUPS FOR INCEST SURVIVORS

Although all teenage victims of incest have in common that they have been sexually molested by a family member or caregiver, the extent of the trauma varies greatly. Some teenagers may have been molested from early childhood, while others have had only one experience. Nonabusing parents may provide warm support or have connived with the perpetrator and may blame, denounce, and reject the teenager. Teenagers may have very mixed feelings of love and hate toward the perpetrator, who may have been a one-time caregiver or a close family member. Generally speaking, the longer the abuse has lasted, the earlier the experience, the more entangled the emotional relationships, the more terrifying the experience, and the more rejecting or disbelieving the family, the more destructive the experience will have been for the teenager. Incest that has commenced in early childhood may have arrested the individual's development. If the incest did not occur until early adolescence, the girl or boy may have developed quite normally up until that time. Consequently, reactions to the trauma vary greatly. Some teenagers become fearful and withdrawn, others attempt to medicate themselves with alcohol or drugs, and others act out their rage and despair through destructive sexual promiscuity or self-mutilation.

Recent reviews of the incest literature (Kitchur & Bell, 1989; MacLennan 1993) have identified a number of groups for teenagers of varying duration, focus, and structure. Some are educational and cognitively focused and others are more psychodynamic, but all are influenced by feminist theories related to assertiveness, eliminating learned helplessness, and resisting society's tendency to blame the victim. Almost all groups have been composed of members of one sex and are generally led by therapists of the same sex. Groups are usually held in addition to individual therapy. Some have been very brief, quite structured, essentially an orientation to the issues with some attempt to reduce the sense of isolation, shame, and guilt. Others have lasted for 2 or more years with much broader goals, helping members to reduce their dissociation, recover, relive and desensitize repressed memories, restore their self-esteem, learn how to trust appropriately, confront their perpetrators, and develop satisfying relationships Such groups have usually been eclectic theoretically, building on a psychodynamic base but using desensitization techniques, cognitive restructuring imagery, and relaxation.

GROUPS FOR TEENAGE MOTHERS

As early as the 1950s, groups were being held in shelters for unmarried mothers awaiting the delivery of their babies (Slavson & MacLennan, 1956). The members were mainly Caucasian between the ages of 14 and 35. These included many teenagers, as the peak ages for reported unwed pregnancy was between the ages of 15 and 16 years. It was quite rare in those days to find pregnant girls below the age of 14. Many girls and young women spent the last 4 months of their pregnancy in shelters away from home, and the groups were designed to help them decide what they wanted to do about their babies - whether to keep them, place them in foster homes, or give them up for adoption. The girls also talked about the fathers of their children and what role they might play in bringing up the child. A major concern was the pregnancy itself and the delivery of the baby. These groups were ongoing "revolving" groups with most members attending for about 12 sessions. Usually about 12 members attended the groups. Some attempt was made to conduct groups for the mothers who kept their babies, but attendance was sporadic, and it was hard to keep a group going. There were almost no programs for the young mothers who had to cope on their own.

In recent years, teenage pregnancy has become much more frequent, with about 1 million pregnancies a year and about half of these being brought to term (Simons, Finlay, & Yang, 1991). These young mothers and the fathers, if available, are encouraged to attend prenatal and well-baby clinics. Some comprehensive programs for teenage mothers returning to school include infant and early child care, counseling, and health care as well as the regular educational program. Some mothers and their infants require foster home placement as they are underage and have no relative to live with. The most successful groups are generally those attached to the school programs, because there are fewer problems with attendance and transportation. Some groups have been run in foster group homes where several teenage mothers are placed with their children, and some are conducted in conjunction with well-baby clinic attendance. It has been much harder to persuade teenage mothers and fathers to attend groups at mental health clinics or family service agencies.

The focus of these groups has been either on parenting or on the teenagers' own needs. In the first type of group, parents have generally brought their infants. They learn how to have pleasurable experiences with their babies and how to bond and to care for them. They are also taught the sequence of child development. Similar groups have also been conducted for mentally disturbed mothers and mothers in treatment for drug addiction. The second type of group focuses on the parents' own futures and what they want for themselves. They explore what careers they want to have, their relationships with their partners or other intimates, and their emotional and sexual development. These groups may be run as couples groups or for mothers or fathers only. All the groups help these teenagers understand how to protect themselves from sexually transmitted diseases and unplanned pregnancies. Some of these teenagers are already infected with AIDS, and special groups are formed for this population which can, over time, become long-term support groups.

Groups for the prevention of unwanted teenage pregnancy and the contraction of sexually transmitted diseases are conducted in many school systems. These groups are generally held in the classroom, last for one or two semesters, and are conducted by either counselors or the school nurse. Sometimes this material is included in courses on human growth and development and may be taught by a psychologist. The format is usually instructional with extensive use of audiovisual aids and some small group discussion. Depending on the capacities of the staff, the program will be more or less formal. In some school systems, sex education is combined with social skills development and with drug prevention.

TEENAGE SUBSTANCE ABUSE GROUPS

Alcoholics Anonymous (AA) groups represented the first systematic treatment of alcoholics in groups, and for over 30 years, groups have formed a major part of drug abuse treatment. These have included milieu groups, 12-step groups, and therapy groups. Since the mid-1980s, relapse prevention groups have become common (Marlatt & Gordon, 1985). However, there were almost no drug abuse programs for teenagers until the 1970s (Bratter, 1989). In the last 10 years there has been an increase in treatment for teenagers, but mainly for boys. Programs for girls or even programs that include girls are still in very short supply. Alcohol has always been the major substance of abuse for teenagers, followed by tobacco, marijuana, and cocaine. The 1985 National Household Survey on Drug Abuse (National Institute of Drug Abuse, 1988) indicated that 12.4% of boys and 11.2% of girls between the ages of 12 and 17 smoked cigarettes; 55.8% of boys and 23.5% of girls drank alcohol; 6.1% and 6.7% respectively smoked marijuana, and .9% and 1.4% respectively used cocaine (primarily crack). The percentages increased with age. Eating disorders, such as anorexia and bulimia, have largely been the domain of teenage girls and young women.

Residential programs for substance abusers include a variety of groups, such as educational and community groups, 12-step groups, and psychotherapy groups. Psychotherapy groups have been mainly based on confrontational, transactional, and reality therapy models. Most groups include role playing to help members understand how they interact with others and to train them through rehearsal to cope with everyday problems. Some programs, based on feminist theory, teach assertiveness and self-responsibility. Outpatient therapy groups have followed the same models, and Alateen groups have provided support both for those who have problems with drinking and drug addiction and for those who are members of families in which the parents are addicted. Some residential and outpatient programs have included survival wilderness groups to boost self-reliance, self-confidence, and self-esteem.

In relapse-prevention groups, addiction is viewed as a chronic disease; an occasional lapse is expected and is not considered to be a disaster. The groups concentrate on helping members understand the nature of addictive thinking so that they can identify changes before a relapse actually occurs. For instance, overconfidence is a major problem for addicts. They start to believe that they can go back to their old life, consort with users, and visit places where they drank or took drugs without actually indulging. They may start to believe that they can manage one drink or two without getting out of control. Relapse-prevention group members help each other become aware of these changes in thinking. A major change among teenage girls is the high percentage who now smoke, which follows the trend for women in general. This is of great concern both because of the likelihood of increased lung cancer among women and because of the danger of passive-smoke exposure for young children. It has been difficult to get teenagers into smoking cessation programs, and success rates are not very high (Flay, 1985). Groups employ behavior-modification techniques such as developing a reward system and desensitization taught to help deal with the craving; the group members provide each other with social supports which are particularly important for teenagers who may otherwise succumb to peer pressure.

During the 1980s, the federal government funded a number of alcohol and drug abuse prevention programs which included educating children and youth about the nature of addiction, teaching them resistance skills, and counseling them on the development of social skills which would enable them to develop more satisfying relationships and help keep them out of trouble. Researchers have concluded that a combination of all three techniques is necessary to be effective (Sussman et al., 1993).

GROUPS FOR EATING DISORDERS

Anorexia was common among young women in the 19th century and became prominent again in the 1980s. Teenage girls adopt an ideal of thinness and develop a delusion that even when they are starving they are still fat. If the disease is not treated, they are likely to die of starvation. These girls seem to have very low self-esteem and to come from perfectionistic families where nothing they do is ever good enough. In its severest form anorexia may require hospitalization and forced feeding. Groups are helpful (both in and outside the hospital), encouraging the girls to share their experiences, to dispel their delusions, and to eat more sensibly.

Bulimia is a disease in which individuals alternately gorge themselves and then vomit up the food. It is associated with depression, low self-esteem, generalized anxiety, and social phobia. Specialized groups can be helpful and generally incorporate a mixture of cognitive restructuring, behavior modification reward systems, and relationship therapy. Self-psychology and assertiveness training have also proved helpful in increasing self-esteem and self-confidence.

GROUP THERAPY WITH JUVENILE DELINQUENTS

Groups have always been used extensively with juvenile delinquents in and out of training schools to help them control their impulses, change their self-identifications, and adopt a socially acceptable way of life. Different approaches have been used to develop therapeutic milieus, including transactional analysis groups and token economies. Ferrara (1991) describes three different types of groups in a residential program to teach youth how to deal with crises and learn social skills and problem solving. The first type is "called" groups, in which everyone involved in a dispute is called together to discuss the situation. Protagonists are required to stay together until the dispute is resolved. The second type is daily groups, which are held to teach problem-solving techniques. The third is personal problem-solving groups, in which members work on understanding how and why they got themselves into trouble and learn to empathize with their victims. Many offenders have been victims themselves in physically or sexually abusive families and need to resolve their fear and anger as well as control their impulses. We have come to realize that many youth who become batterers or rapists have themselves been abused, and their acceptance of their own trauma is an essential component in gaining empathy for their victims. Like substance abusers, juvenile delinquents use denial, projection, and the shifting of responsibility for their behavior onto others as major defenses, so that groups are particularly helpful in assisting delinquents to become aware of the games they play. In these groups, particularly in residential settings, therapists often have some control over the lives of the members and thus combine authoritative and therapeutic roles. Bratter (1989) and MacLennan and Dies (1992) discuss the value of this combination of roles in working with members who have uncertain motivation and who tend to deny their problems.

Substance abusers and juvenile delinquents have usually lived in disturbed social environments, thus it is extremely important that they be helped to build a socially supportive world when they return to the community. Treatment alone is not sufficient to help the youth maintain the gains they have made if their social environment and peer pressure push them back into the old antisocial and dysfunctional ways. The poverty programs in the 1960s, which were successful, included treatment, training for jobs and careers, and assistance in creating a positive social network. Today, social support groups are assisting youth to maintain their therapeutic gains and to prevent them from returning to the antisocial environments that got them into trouble.

STRUCTURED MATERIALS IN PROBLEM-SPECIFIC GROUPS

A major development which has followed the proliferation of problem-specific groups has been the creation of a wide range of materials directed toward the treatment of different problems (Schaefer & Reid, 1986). These have included manuals, questionnaires, games, storybooks, and videotapes. There are now publishing houses that specialize in the production and sale of these materials. In a few instances, the materials have been tested in research programs, such as those published by the Research Press in Champaign, Illinois. However, at this time there is still very little in the literature that discusses the relationship between the management of the groups and the use of structured materials. For instance, the first task with impulsive and poorly socialized youth is to develop a working group. The group contract is a critical tool. Before games can be played or orderly discussion engaged in, the members have to learn to take turns and listen to each other. A manual is a guide that can serve only as a framework. Specific situations must rely on clinical judgment. The youths' attachment to the group becomes critical in helping them keep to the contract and interact effectively. A balance must be maintained between content and process. A strict classroom format inhibits intragroup interaction between members, while overly permissive group management with poorly socialized youth may create chaos and confusion and make it difficult to use the structured materials.

SUMMARY

In this contribution I have described recent changes in the treatment of adolescents with a range of problems. Progress has been made in understanding the stages of group development and the role of the therapist in creating an effective group. Some factors that have curative value for adolescents have been identified. There has been increased emphasis on the use of contracting with the youth, with their parents, with institutional authorities, with staff, and in the group itself in order to define the goals and boundaries of the treatment, set limits, and improve communication. The personality and characteristics of the therapist have also come under greater scrutiny as we become increasingly aware of the importance of multicultural sensitivity.

A major trend has been toward short-term problem-focused groups, which are often quite structured and use materials that have been written for the particular problem. Therapists use different theoretical approaches such as cognitive restructuring, relaxation therapy, and imaging as well as older psychodynamic methods, transactional analysis, experiential groups, rational-emotive therapy, behavior modification, and desensitization. Choice of theoretical methods does not rest only on the predilections and training of the therapists but also on the demands of the problem and the type of defenses that are typically used by the adolescents. Early traumas are often reacted to with repression and dissociation, which may require regression and reliving of the experiences in order to reduce their power, whereas substance abusers and delinquents need to develop social skills, learn to accept responsibility for their actions, and control their emotions and impulses in the here and now. All programs with teenagers have a component that aims to increase the adolescent's self-esteem.

Although training for therapists to lead groups for adolescents with different types of problems has become quite widespread, formal training standards have not been adopted, and many therapists are still required to run groups without any specialized training. Progress still needs to be made in the validation of approaches for different populations, personality types, and problems. Azima and Dies reviewed the research literature in 1989 and made some recommendations for practitioners who are interested in undertaking clinical research. In the 1990s it is hoped that more therapists will evaluate their adolescent groups.

Beryce W. MacLennan, PhD, FAPA, is a Distinguished Fellow of the American Group Psychotherapy Association. She is currently in private practice in Bethesda, Maryland; Clinical Professor, Psychology, in the Department of Psychiatry and Behavioral Sciences, George Washington University; Group Therapy Consultant, Child and Adolescent Training Program, DC Mental Health Commission and Coordinator, School Treatment Program for the DC Psychological Association's volunteer Community Initiative. She is coauthor with Felsenfeld (1968) and Dies (1992), of *Group Counseling and Psychotherapy With Adolescents* and many other publications and presentations. Dr. MacLennan may be contacted at 6307 Crathie Lane, Bethesda, MD 20816.

RESOURCES

Azima, F. J. C., & Dies, K. R. (1989). Clinical research in adolescent group psychotherapy: Status, guidelines and directions. In F. J. C. Azima & K. R. Dies (Eds.), *Adolescent Group Psychotherapy* (pp. 193-224). Madison, CT: International Universities Press.

Azima, F. J. C., & Richmond, L. H. (Eds.). (1989). *Adolescent Group Psychotherapy.* Madison, CT: International Universities Press.

Berg, B. (1988). *The Anger Control Game.* Dayton, OH: Cognitive Counseling Resources.

Bratter, T. E. (1989). Group psychotherapy with alcohol and drug addicted adolescents. In F. J. C. Azima & K. R. Dies (Eds.), *Adolescent Group Psychotherapy* (pp. 163-193). Madison, CT: International Universities Press.

Bureau of the Census. (1991). Statistical Abstract of the U.S. (111th ed.). *Marriages and Divorces 1960-1987* (86 No. 128). Washington DC: U.S. Government Printing Office.

Corder, B. F., Whiteside, L., & Haizlip, T. M. (1981). A study of curative factors in group psychotherapy with adolescents. *International Journal of Group Psychotherapy, 31,* 345-354.

Dies, K. R. (1991). A model for adolescent group psychotherapy. *Journal of Child and Adolescent Group Therapy 1,* 59-70.

Ferrara, M. L. (1991). *Group Counseling With Juvenile Delinquents: The Limit and Lead Approach.* Newbury Park, CA: Sage.

Flay, B. R. (1985). Psychosocial approaches to smoking prevention: A review of the findings. *Health Psychology, 4,* 449-488

Hodgekinson, H. L. (1989). *The Same Client: The Demographics of Education and Service Delivery Systems.* Washington, DC: Center for Demographic Policy.

Kitchur, M., & Bell, R. (1989). Group psychotherapy with preadolescent sexual abuse victims: Literature review and description of an inner-city group. *International Journal of Group Psychotherapy, 39,* 285-310.

Klein, W. L., & MacLennan, B. W. (1965). Utilization of groups in job training for the socially deprived. *International Journal of Group Psychotherapy, 15,* 424-433.

MacLennan, B. W. (1975). The personalities of group leaders: Implications for selection and training. *International Journal of Group Psychotherapy, 25,* 177-185.

MacLennan, B. W. (1991). Group psychotherapy with girls in early adolescence: Then and now. *Journal of Child and Adolescent Group Therapy, 1,* 25-41.

MacLennan, B. W. (1993). Group treatment after child and adolescent sexual abuse: Introduction [Special issue]. *Journal of Child and Adolescent Group Therapy, 3,* 3-11.

MacLennan, B. W., & Dies, K. R. (1992). *Group Counseling and Psychotherapy With Adolescents* (2nd ed.). New York: Columbia University Press.

MacLennan, B. W., & Felsenfeld, N. (1968). *Group Counseling and Psychotherapy With Adolescents* (1st ed.). New York: International Universities Press.

MacLennan, B. W., & Rosen, B. (1963). Female therapists in activity group group psychotherapy with boys in latency. *International Journal of Group Psychotherapy, 13,* 34-42.

Marlatt, G. A., & Gordon, J. R. (Eds.). (1985). *Relapse Prevention: Maintenance Strategies in Behavior Change.* New York: Guilford.

National Institute of Drug Abuse. (1988). National Household Survey 1985 (DHHS Publication No. ADM 88-1586). Washington, DC: U.S. Government Printing Office.

Pedro-Carroll, J. L., & Cowen E. L. (1985). The children of divorce intervention program: An investigation of the efficacy of a school-based prevention program. *Journal of Counseling and Clinical Psychology 53,* 603-611.

Schaefer, C. E., & Reid, S. E. (Eds.). (1986). *Game Play: Therapeutic Use of Childhood Games.* New York: Wiley.

Serrano, A. (1989, October). *Group Therapy With the Reconstituted Family.* Workshop presented at the Mid-Atlantic Group Therapy Society Meeting, Berkeley Springs, WV.

Simons, J. M., Finlay, B., & Yang, A. (1991). Births to adolescent and young women Table No. 6.10. *The Adolescent and Young Adult Fact Book.* Washington, DC: The Children's Defense Fund p. 137.

Slavson, S. R., & MacLennan, B. W. (1956). Group therapy with unmarried mothers. In S. R. Slavson (Ed.), *Fields of Group Psychotherapy.* New York: International Universities Press.

Sue, D. (1990). *Counselling the Culturally Different* (2nd ed.). New York: Wiley.

Sussman, S., Dent, C. W., Stacy, A. W., Sun, P., Craig, S., Simon, T. R., Burton, S., & Flay, B. R. (1993). Project toward no tobacco use: 1-year behavior outcomes. *American Journal of Public Health, 3,* 1245-1250.

Tuchman, B., & Jensen, M. (1977). Stages of small group development revisited. *Group and Organizational Studies, 2,* 419-427.

Yalom, I. D. (1975). *Theory and Practice of Group Psychotherapy* (1st ed.). New York: Basic Books.

THE CURRENT STATUS OF THE INSANITY DEFENSE*

Michael L. Perlin

Our insanity defense jurisprudence is incoherent. It reflects the public's episodic outrage at apparently unreasonable forgiveness of obviously "guilty" acts, the legislatures' pandering responses to constituency cries, and the judiciary's desperate ambivalence about having to decide hard cases involving mentally disabled criminal defendants (English, 1988; Perlin, 1992a, 1993). Although we are beginning to come to grips with the multitude of scientific, biological, neurological, and psychological factors that play a role in the commission of some otherwise-inexplicable crimes, we are simultaneously narrowing and limiting the substance of the insanity defense and the procedures used in these court cases and postacquittal commitment hearings (Callahan, Mayer, & Steadman, 1987).

The jurisprudence's incoherence is important because of its social impact. First, through a series of legislative "reform" measures, it sanctions the criminal punishment of a significant number of individuals who, by any substantive standard, are not "responsible" for their "criminal acts." In addition to its evident punitive and damaging impact on these defendants, this outcome also makes prisons more chaotic and dangerous places for other inmates and for correctional staff.

Second, it allows us, and perhaps even forces us, to deplete our intellectual and emotional resources and our creative energies by endlessly debating issues that are fundamentally irrelevant to the real-life impact of the defense (e.g., whether there should be a volitional as well as a cognitive standard employed) and that lead, at best, to illusory change. At the same time, it allows us - perhaps *encourages* us - to ignore empirical evidence, scientific study, and moral reasoning that could shed light on the underlying issues.

Third, it leads us to spend money in counterproductive ways. Recent reforms will lead to more individuals being institutionalized for longer periods of time in more punitive facilities, at precisely the same time that community resources are becoming scarcer. If the insanity defense is successful only in a fraction of 1% of all cases, why do we devote such time and capital to this question, and why do we exaggerate the impact that these cases have on the operation of our criminal justice system?

Fourth, it leads us to avoid consideration of the single most important issue in mental disability law: Why do we feel the way we do about "these people," and how do these feelings control our legislative, judicial, and administrative policies? The answer to this question is the "wild card" here, and it is essential that we see its role in the incoherence of the policies I am discussing.

---

*The author wishes to thank Janet Abisch and Dave Scott for their extraordinary editing assistance, and Lori Kranczer for her excellent research assistance.

This contribution is adapted from *The Jurisprudence of the Insanity Defense* (pp. 13-133) by M. L. Perlin, 1994, Durham, NC: Carolina Academic Press. Copyright © 1994 by Carolina Academic Press.

No aspect of the criminal justice system is more controversial than the insanity defense. Nowhere else does the successful employment of a defense regularly bring about cries for its abolition. When the defense is successful in a high-level publicity case (especially when it involves a defendant whose "factual guilt" is clear), the acquittal triggers public outrage and serves vividly as a screen upon which each relevant interest group can project its fears and concerns.

Our fixation on the insanity defense has evolved into a familiar story. The insanity defense, so common wisdom goes, encourages the factually (and morally) guilty to seek refuge in an excuse premised upon pseudoscience, shaky rehabilitation theory, and faintly duplicitous legal *legerdemain*. The defense, allegedly, is used frequently (mostly in abusive ways), is generally successful, and often results in brief slap-on-the-wrist periods of confinements in loosely supervised settings. Because it is basically a no-risk maneuver, the story continues, even when it fails, the defendant will suffer no harm. Purportedly, the defense is used disproportionately in death penalty cases (often involving garish multiple homicides) and inevitably results in trials in which high-priced experts do battle in front of befuddled jurors who are inevitably unable to make sense of contradictory, highly abstract, and speculative testimony. Finally, the insanity defense is seen as being subject to the worst sort of malingering or feigning, and it is assumed that, through this gambit, clever defendants can "con" gullible, "soft" experts into accepting a fraudulent defense.

The largely unseen counterworlds of empirical reality, behavioral advance, scientific discovery, and philosophical inquiry paint quite a different picture. Empirically, the insanity defense is rarely used, is less frequently successful, and generally results in lengthy stays in maximum security facilities (often far more restrictive than many prisons or reformatories) for far longer periods of time than the defendants would have been subject to had they been sentenced criminally (Perlin, 1989-1990).

Defendants who plead it unsuccessfully and are convicted are often sentenced to significantly longer penal terms than defendants found guilty in similar cases in which the defense is never raised. The defense is most frequently pled in cases *not* involving a victim's death and is often raised in cases involving minor property crimes. The vast majority of cases are so-called "walkthroughs" (i.e., where both state and defense experts agree both as to the severity of the defendant's mental illness and his or her lack of responsibility). Feigned insanity is rare; successfully feigned insanity even rarer. It is far more likely for a jury to convict in a case in which the defendant meets the relevant substantive insanity criteria than to acquit where the defendant does not (Perlin, 1989-1990).

As a result of these myths, we demand legislative "reform." This reform leads to a variety of changes in insanity defense statutes - in substantive standards, in burdens of proof, in standards of proof, in the creation of "hybrid" verdicts such as "guilty but mentally ill," even, in a few instances, in supposed "abolition" of the defense itself. No matter what their final reform, these reforms stem from one primary source: "the public's overwhelming fear of the future acts of [released insanity] acquittees" (Steadman et al., 1993, p. 39).

Behaviorally, researchers are beginning to develop sophisticated assessment tools that can translate insanity concepts into quantifiable variables that appear to easily meet the traditional legal standard of "reasonable scientific certainty" (Rodriguez, LeWinn, & Perlin, 1983). Scientifically, the development of "hard science" diagnostic tools (such as CT scanning or Magnetic Resonance Imaging) has helped determine the presence and severity of certain neurological illnesses that may be causally related to some forms of criminal behavior (Garber et al., 1988). Finally, moral philosophers are increasingly trying - with some measure of success - to clarify such difficult underlying issues as the contextual meaning of terms such as "causation," "responsibility," and "rationality" (Moore, 1984).

Yet, these discoveries and developments have had virtually no impact on the basic debate. They are ignored, trivialized, and denied. Why is this? What is there about the insanity defense that allows for (perhaps encourages) such a discontinuity between firmly held belief and statistical reality? Why, most importantly, do we continue to ignore the most fundamental and core question - Why do we feel the way we do about "these people"? - and why, when we engage in our endless debates and incessant retinkering with insanity defense doctrine do we not seriously consider our answer to this question?

I believe that our insanity defense jurisprudence is a prisoner of a combination of these empirical myths and related social metamyths. The legal system is a prisoner of these myths and of the concomitant powerful symbols that permeate any criminal trial (especially any highly visible criminal trial) at which a nonresponsibility defense is raised. It rejects psychodynamic explanations of human motivation and behavior, and remains intensely suspicious of concepts of mental health and disability, of mental health professionals, and of the ability of such professionals to assess or ameliorate mental disability (Perlin, 1987, 1992a, 1993; Perlin & Dorfman, 1993). As a result, it remains most comfortable with all-or-nothing tests of mental illness (*Johnson v. State*, 1982 ["For the purposes of guilt determination, an offender is either wholly sane or wholly insane," p. 52]), and demands that nonresponsible defendants match visual images of "deranged madmen" who, indisputably, "look crazy" (*Battalino v. People*, 1948 [finding no evidence of defendant exhibiting "paleness, wild eyes and trembling," p. 901]). Again, it does this in utter disregard of the past 150 years of scientific and behavioral learning.

The remainder of this contribution will proceed in this manner. First, I will trace the development of the doctrine of the insanity defense and show how the public has always demanded a rigid all-or-nothing construct of criminal responsibility. Secondly, I will demonstrate the role of the insanity acquittal of John W. Hinckley, Jr., in the reformulation of our contemporary insanity defense laws. Third, I will examine the role of punishment and demonstrate how our "culture of punishment" is dominated by the obsessive fear that a responsible defendant will "beat the rap." Fourth, I will discuss the role of "externalities" in the formulation of the insanity defense. Finally, I will offer some modest conclusions.

THE DEVELOPMENT OF INSANITY DEFENSE DOCTRINE

PRE-*M'NAGHTEN* HISTORY

The development of the insanity defense prior to the mid-19th century tracked both the prevailing scientific and the popular concepts of mental illness, "craziness," responsibility, and blameworthiness (Perlin, 1989-1990). In existence since at least the 12th century, the insanity defense has always aroused more discussion than any other topic of criminal law, despite the fact that there were few insanity pleas entered prior to the mid-18th century (Eigen, 1984). Prior to *M'Naghten* (1843), the insanity defense went through three significant stages: the "good and evil" test, the "wild beast" test, and the "right and wrong" test.

"Good and Evil" Test. The "good and evil" test, which apparently first appeared in a 1313 case involving the capacity of an infant under the age of 7, reflected the "moral dogmata reflected in [the medieval] theological literature" (Platt & Diamond, 1966, p. 1231). The insane, like children, were incapable of "sin[ning] against [their] will" since man's freedom "is restrained in children, in fools, and in the witless who do not have reason whereby they can choose the good from the evil" (Platt & Diamond, 1966, p. 1233).

During the 14th through 16th centuries, this test, the source of which was most likely biblical, remained constant in English law, and, by the end of that time (coinciding with the reign of Elizabeth I), insane persons who met this test were treated as "nonpersons" not fit subjects for punishment, "since they did not comprehend the moral implications of their harmful acts." This test was transfigured in 1724 to the "wild beast" test.

"Wild Beast" Test. Under this formulation, in *Rex. v. Arnold* (Howell, 1812), a 1724 case in which the defendant had shot and wounded a British Lord in a homicide attempt, Judge Tracy instructed the jury that it should acquit by reason of insanity:

a mad man . . . must be a man that is totally deprived of his understanding and memory, and doth not know what he is doing, no more than *a brute, or a wild beast,* such a one is never the object of punishment. (p. 695)

In short, the emphasis was on lack of *intellectual ability,* rather than the violently wild, ravenous beast image that the phrase calls to mind; the test continued to be used until at least 1840 (Platt & Diamond, 1966).

"Right and Wrong" Test. The following step, the "right and wrong" test (the true forerunner of *M'Naghten*), emerged in two 1812 cases; in the second of the two, the jury was charged that it must decide whether the defendant "had sufficient understanding to distinguish good from evil, right from wrong . . ." (Lewinstein, 1969, p. 279, discussing *Bellingham's Case*). It was finally expanded upon in 1840 in *Regina v. Oxford,* in which Lord Denman charged the jury that it must determine whether the defendant, "from the effect of a diseased mind," knew that the act was wrong, and that the question that must thus be answered was whether "he was quite unaware of the nature, character, and consequences of the act he was committing" (p. 525).

Even with these rigid tests in place, the public's perceptions of abuse of the insanity defense differed little from its reactions in the aftermath of the Hinckley acquittal nearly a century and a half later. The public's representatives demanded an "all or nothing" sort of insanity, a conceptualization that has been "peculiarly foreign" to psychiatry since at least the middle of the 19th century (Diamond, 1961, p. 62). Similarly, the "demonological" concept of mental illness retained its power centuries after it became clear that such a view was never supported by scientific data.

THE *M'NAGHTEN* RULE

In 1843, the most significant case in the history of the insanity defense in England arose out of the shooting by Daniel M'Naghten of Edward Drummond, the secretary of the man he mistook for his intended victim: Prime Minister Robert Peel. After nine medical witnesses testified that M'Naghten was insane, and after the jury was informed that an insanity acquittal would lead to the defendant's commitment to a psychiatric hospital, M'Naghten was found not guilty by reason of insanity (NGRI) (Hermann & Sor, 1983; *M'Naghten,* 1843; Moran, 1981).

Enraged by the verdict, Queen Victoria questioned why the law was of "no avail," since everybody is morally convinced that [the] malefactor . . . [was] perfectly conscious and aware of what he did," and demanded that the legislature "lay down the rule" so as to protect the public "from the wrath of madmen who they feared could now kill with impunity" (Eule, 1978, p. 644). In response, the House of Lords asked the Supreme Court of Judicature to answer five questions regarding the insanity law, and the judges' answers to two of these five became the *M'Naghten* test:

> The jurors ought to be told in all cases that every man is presumed to be sane, and to possess a sufficient degree of reason to be responsible for his crimes, until the contrary be proved to their satisfaction; and that to establish a defence on the ground of insanity, it must be clearly proved that, at the time of the committing of the act, the party accused was labouring under such a defect of reason, from disease of the mind, as not to know the nature and quality of the act he was doing; or, if he did know it, that he did not know he was doing what was wrong. (*M'Naghten,* 1843, p. 722)

This rigid, cognitive-only responsibility test, established under royal pressure, reflected "the prevailing intellectual and scientific ideas of the times" and stemmed from an "immutable philosophical and moral concept which assumes an inherent capacity in man to distinguish right from wrong and to make necessary moral decisions" (Hovenkamp, 1981, p. 551).

The M'Naghten rules reflected a theory of responsibility that was outmoded far prior to its adoption, and which bore little resemblance to what was known about the human mind, even at the time of their promulgation. Nonetheless, with almost no exceptions, they were held as sacrosanct by American courts that eagerly embraced this formulation and codified it as the standard test with little modification in virtually all jurisdictions until the middle of the 20th century (Callahan et al., 1987).

POST-*M'NAGHTEN* DEVELOPMENTS

Irresistible Impulse. Although there was some interest in the post-*M'Naghten* years in the so-called "irresistible impulse" exception - allowing for the acquittal of a defendant if his mental disorder caused him to experience an "irresistible and uncontrollable impulse to commit the offense, even if he remained able to understand the nature of the offense and its wrongfulness" - this formulation was no more than a transitory detour in the development of an insanity jurisprudence (Dix, 1986, p. 7).

Durham. The first important theoretical alternative to *M'Naghten* emerged in the District of Columbia in the 1954 case of *Durham v. United States*. Writing for the court, Judge David Bazelon rejected both *M'Naghten* and the irresistible impulse tests on the theory that the mind of man was a functional unit, and that a far broader test would be appropriate. *Durham* thus held that an accused would not be criminally responsible if his "unlawful act was the product of mental disease or mental defect" (pp. 874-875). This test would provide for the broadest range of psychiatric expert testimony, "unbound by narrow or psychologically inapposite legal questions" (Weiner, 1985, p. 710). Further, it reiterated the jury's function in such a case:

> Juries will continue to make moral judgments, operating under the fundamental precept that "Our collective conscience does not allow punishment where it cannot impose blame." But in making such judgments, they will be guided by wider horizons of knowledge concerning mental life. The question will be simply whether the accused acted because of a mental disorder, and not whether he displayed particular symptoms which medical science has long recognized do not necessarily or even typically, accompany even the most serious disorder. (*Durham*, 1954, p. 876)

Durham was the first modern, major break from the *M'Naghten* approach and created a "feeling of ferment" as the District of Columbia "became a veritable laboratory for consideration of the details of insanity, in its fullest substantive and procedural ramifications" (Goldstein, 1967, p. 83). Within a few years, however, *Durham* was judicially criticized, modified, and ultimately dismantled by the District of Columbia Circuit (*Frigillana v. United States*, 1962; *McDonald v. United States*, 1962), its burial being completed by the 1972 decision in *United States v. Brawner* (1972) to adopt the Model Penal Code/American Law Institute (ALI-Model Penal Code) test.

United States v. Brawner. *Brawner* (1972) discarded *Durham's* "product" test but added a volitional question to *M'Naghten's* cognitive inquiry. Under this test:

> A defendant would not be responsible for his criminal conduct if, as a result of mental disease or defect, he "lack[ed] substantial capacity either to appreciate the criminality of his conduct or to conform his conduct to the requirements of law." (Model Penal Code § 4.01, 1955; *United States v. Brawner*, 1972, p. 973)

Although the test was rooted in *M'Naghten*, there were several significant differences. First, its use of the word "substantial" was meant to respond to caselaw developments which had required a showing of total impairment for exculpation from criminal responsibility. Second, the substitution of the word "appreciate" for the word "know" showed that "a sane offender must be emotionally as well as intellectually aware of the significance of his conduct," and "mere intellectual awareness that conduct is wrongful when divorced from an appreciation or understanding of the moral or legal import of behavior, can have little significance." Third, by using broader language of mental impairment than had *M'Naghten*, the test "capture[d] both the cognitive and affective aspects of impaired mental understanding." Fourth, its substitution in the final proposed official draft of the word "wrongfulness" for "criminality" reflected the position that the insanity defense dealt with "an impaired moral sense rather than an impaired sense of legal wrong" (Goldstein, 1967, p. 87).

It was assumed that the spreading adoption of *Brawner* would augur the death of *M'Naghten*. That assumption, of course, has proven to be mortally inaccurate (Insanity Defense Reform Act of 1984, 1988). *Brawner*, did, however, serve as the final burial for the *Durham* experiment (Diamond, 1973).

Guilty But Mentally Ill (GBMI). Perhaps the most important development in substantive insanity defense formulations in the 20 years post-*Brawner* has been the adoption in over a dozen jurisdictions of the hybrid "guilty but mentally ill" (GBMI) verdict (McGraw, Farthing-Capowich, & Keilitz, 1985). It received its initial recent impetus in 1975 in Michigan as a reflection of legislative dissatisfaction with and public outcry over a state Supreme Court decision that prohibited automatic commitment of insanity acquittees (Mickenberg, 1987; *People v. McQuillan*, 1974). The GBMI statute was adopted to "protect the public from violence inflicted by persons with mental ailments who slipped through the cracks of the criminal justice system" (*People v. Seefeld*, 1980, p. 124).

The rationale for the passage of GBMI legislation was that the implementation of such a verdict would decrease the number of persons acquitted by reason of insanity and would assure treatment of those who were GBMI within a correctional setting (*People v. Smith*, 1984). A GBMI defendant would purportedly be evaluated upon entry to the correctional system and be provided appropriate mental health services either on an inpatient basis as part of a definite prison term or, in specific cases, as a parolee or as an element of probation (Weiner, 1985).

Practice under GBMI statutes reveals that the verdict does little or nothing to insure effective treatment for mentally disabled offenders. As most statutes vest discretion in the director of the state correctional or mental health facility to provide a GBMI prisoner with such treatment as he or she "determines necessary," the GBMI prisoner is not insured treatment "beyond that available to other offenders" (Slobogin, 1985, p. 513). A comprehensive study of the operation of the GBMI verdict in Georgia revealed that only 3 of the 150 defendants who were found GBMI during the period in question were being treated in hospitals (Steadman et al., 1993).

HINCKLEY AND ITS AFTERMATH

The acquittal of John W. Hinckley galvanized the American public in a way that led directly to the reversal of 150 years of study and understanding of the complexities of psychological behavior and the relationship between mental illness and certain violent acts (Caplan, 1984; Perlin, 1989-1990). The public's outrage over a jurisprudential system that could allow a defendant who shot an American president on national television to plead "not guilty" (for *any* reason) became a "river of fury" after the jury's verdict was announced (Perlin, 1985, p. 859).

Sensational trials such as Hinckley's consume the hearts and minds of the American public. They reflect our basic dissatisfaction with the perceived incompatibility of the due process and crime control models of criminal law, and with the notion that psychiatric "excuses" can allow a "guilty" defendant to "beat a rap" and escape punishment (Fentiman, 1985; Sendor, 1986). Such dissatisfaction leads to a predictable response, especially when the defendant, like Hinckley, is perceived as one *not* sufficiently "like us" so as to warrant empathy or sympathy. As Roth has suggested, when a "wrong verdict" is entered in a sensational trial, the American public may simply be nothing more than a "bad loser" (Roth, 1986-1987, p. 91).

Members of Congress responded quickly to the public's outpouring of outrage by introducing 26 separate pieces of legislation designed to limit, modify, severely shrink, or abolish the insanity defense; the debate on these bills illuminates with clarity the character of the legislative decision-making process (Perlin, 1985, 1989-1990). Statements by legislators introducing these bills or by Reagan administration spokespersons supporting them reflected the fears and superstitions that have traditionally animated the insanity debate, as well as the public's core ambivalence about mentally disabled criminal defendants (Mickenberg, 1987; Perlin, 1985, 1989-1990).

THE INSANITY DEFENSE REFORM ACT (IDRA).

The Reagan administration originally had called loudly for the abolition of the insanity defense (Perlin, 1985, p. 860). However, in the face of a nearly unified front presented by most of the relevant professional organizations and trade associations, it eventually quietly dropped its loud public call for abolition and supported the IDRA as a "reform compromise" (Perlin, 1989, Vol. 3, pp. 398-399). This quiet change in position, of course, insured that the symbolic call for abolition would be the lasting public image. The legislation ultimately enacted by Congress, legislation that closely comported with the public's moral feelings, returned the insanity defense to "*status quo ante* 1843: the year of . . . *M'Naghten*" (Perlin, 1985, p. 862).

Besides relocating the burden of proof in insanity trials to defendants (18 U.S.C. § 17), establishing strict procedures for the hospitalization and release of defendants found not guilty by reason of insanity (18 U.S.C. § 4243 et seq.), and severely limiting the scope of expert testimony in insanity cases (Federal Rules of Evidence 704 (b)), the IDRA discarded the ALI-Model Penal Code test and adopted a more restrictive version of *M'Naghten* by specifying that the level of mental disease or defect that must be shown to qualify be "severe" (18 U.S.C. § 17(a)).

The states quickly followed the lead of the federal government. Two-thirds of all states reevaluated the defense; as a result, 12 states adopted the guilty but mentally ill (GBMI) test, 7 narrowed the substantive test, 16 shifted the burden of proof, and 25 tightened release provisions in the cases of those defendants found to be NGRI. Three states adopted legislation that purported to abolish the defense, but actually retained a mens rea exception in which the defendant must demonstrate a "guilty mind" to be held responsible (Callahan et al., 1987; Steadman et al., 1993).

POST-*HINCKLEY* DEBATE

The debate over the future of the insanity defense that followed John Hinckley's insanity acquittal was utterly predictable. State and federal legislators and federal prosecutors repeated discredited and outdated myths based on ancient superstitions and then conceded that their actions were driven by myth, not reality. Their statements went unchallenged; the empirical evidence refuting them went unnoticed. Had a mid-19th century member of parliament stumbled into one of the legislative arenas during this debate, he would have felt, correctly, that we had learned nothing in the 140 years that had passed since the *M'Naghten* rules were articulated.

Congress responded directly and swiftly to public perceptions of a system run amok, one that, purportedly, allowed uncountable numbers of dangerous defendants to escape punishment through the meretricious loophole of the insanity defense ("Insanity Defense," 1990). Even though Congress knew full well that this perception was a myth, it responded as it did to assuage these fears and to persuade the voters that it was "doing something" by laudably enhancing public protection values. In short, it participated knowingly and openly in a massive legislative charade.

CONCLUSION

All of this had the ultimate effect of returning to a test that compelled the law to "do its punitive worst," that had "the rigidity of an army cot and the flexibility of a Procrustean bed," and that was, simply, "bad psychiatry and bad law" (Sadoff, 1986, p. 20; English, 1988, p. 47).

THE ROLE OF PUNISHMENT

Courts and legislators have traditionally feared that acceptance of psychodynamic principles, allegedly characterized by the mental health professionals' perceived peculiar tolerant attitude toward criminal behavior and perceived urge to replace the negative pattern of fear and repression which has dominated penology, would wrongly undermine the powerful force of punishment in the criminal justice process. This fear is mirrored in President Reagan's campaign rhetoric on behalf of conservative Republican Senate candidates whom he could count on to support his efforts to appoint "tough" federal judges ("We don't need a bunch of sociology majors on the bench") (Krisberg, 1991, p. 141). Although we know that these fears are inaccurate, perhaps even irrational, they help explain, as much as any other source, the incoherence of our insanity defense jurisprudence (Perlin, 1989-1990, 1990; Perlin & Dorfman, 1993).

THE SOCIAL ROLE OF PUNISHMENT

Punishment "has been the main device for enforcing laws ever since the mists of prehistory lifted" (van den Haag, 1975, p. 4). At least five major aims of punishment have been identified by criminologists and philosophers: restraint, general deterrence, individual deterrence, rehabilitation, and desert (Andenaes, 1956, 1971; R. J. Rychlak, 1990; R. J. Rychlak & J. F. Rychlak, 1990). As recently as 1974, Schulhofer noted that most American jurisdictions exclude retaliation from the legitimate goals of the criminal law, that legal theorists "[we]re virtually unanimous in applauding the judgment" (pp. 1510-1511), and that the idea of punishment was "giving way" to the idea of treatment (Devlin, 1963). Yet, the notion of *desert* has since regained prominence as the most important contemporary justification for and aim of punishment (Gaylin & Rothman, 1976). The Supreme Court's recent decision upholding a first offender's sentence of life imprisonment without parole for a cocaine possession conviction specifically invokes retribution as one of the acceptable rationales for such a penalty (*Harmelin v. Michigan*, 1991, p. 2706).

PUNISHMENT AS RITUAL

Punishment was originally needed to "remove the evil spirit thought to cause an individual to transgress against society" ("The Modern Day Scarlet Letter," 1989, p. 1360). It is also a "ritualistic device" conveying "moral condemnation," inflicting humiliation, and dramatizing evil through a public "degradation ceremony" (Boldt, 1986, p. 1004). By nurturing emotions of vengeance, the punishment of criminals "furthers social solidarity and protects against the terrifying anxiety that the forces of good might not triumph against the forces of evil after all" (Diamond, 1973, p. 110). It does this through the context of a trial process that is a "moral parable [with] a religious meaning essential as a public exercise in which the prevailing moral ideals are dramatized and reaffirmed" (Roche, 1958, p. 245). The celebration of "punishment as *punishment*" legitimatized the institutional "infliction of suffering" in much the same way as disease was seen as having to be "completely suffered" as a way of insuring that one's soul would find purification (Pillsbury, 1989, p. 773).

More than mere disapproval, punishment expresses "a kind of vindictive resentment" as a "way of getting back at the criminal" (Feinberg, 1970, p. 98). This may be the reason that "the moment . . . rehabilitative impulses emerge into expressions, the legal system is doomed to encounter contradiction, confusion and frequent public criticism" (Watson, 1958, p. 622). This symbolic function explains "why even those sophisticated persons who abjure resentment of criminals and look with small favor generally on the penal law are likely to demand that certain kinds of conduct be punished when or if the law lets them go by" (Feinberg, 1970, p. 102).

One underlying theme throughout the centuries of insanity defense test formulation has been the question of the extent to which externalities such as empirical research, scientific advances, political confrontations, and teachings of moral philosophers have had a significant impact on the actual structuring of the substantive legal formula for responsibility.

If we now understand so much more about science, human behavior, and empiricism than we did at the time of, say, the *M'Naghten* verdict, why have we shrunken our insanity defense to the point where it now approximates but is even *more* restrictive than what was scientifically, empirically, and morally out of date 145 years ago?

The insanity defense is, to a significant majority of the American public, counterintuitive. We are generally uncomfortable with the entire notion of "excuse" defenses (putting aside self-defense); the use of the others (duress, choice of evils, etc.), however, does not appear to imperil the operation of the criminal justice system (as the insanity defense appears to do).

EMPIRICAL DATA AND MYTHS

In the wake of the *Hinckley* verdict, commentators began to examine carefully the "myths" that had developed about the insanity defense in an effort to determine the extent "to which this issue has been distorted in the public eye" (Rodriguez et al., 1983, p. 400). The research shows that (a) the insanity defense opens only a "small window of nonculpability" (Jeffrey, Pasewark, & Bieber, 1988, p. 39), (b) defendants who successfully use the NGRI plea "do not beat the rap" (Pogrebin, Regoli, & Perry, 1986, p. 240), and, perhaps more importantly, (c) the "tenacity of these [false] beliefs in the face of contrary data is profound" (Rogers, 1987a, p. 840).

Myth #1: The Insanity Defense Is Overused. All empirical analyses have been consistent: The public at large and the legal profession (especially legislators) dramatically and grossly overestimate both the frequency and the success rate of the insanity plea, an error which is abetted by the media's bizarre depictions, distortions, and inaccuracies in portraying mentally ill individuals charged with crimes (Rodriguez et al., 1983). The most recent research reveals, for instance, that the insanity defense is used in only about 1% of all felony cases and is successful just about one-quarter of the time (Steadman et al., 1993). What is as startling as any other fact unearthed by empiricists is the realization that, as recently as 1985, directors of forensic services in only 10 of the 50 states could even provide researchers with baseline information regarding the frequency of the insanity plea and its success, and that officials in 20 states could provide no information whatsoever about the use of the plea (Pasewark & McGinley, 1985).

Myth #2: Use of the Insanity Defense Is Limited to Murder Cases. In one jurisdiction where the data have been closely studied, contrary to expectations, slightly less than one-third of the successful insanity pleas entered over an 8-year period were reached in cases involving a victim's death (Rodriguez et al., 1983). Further, individuals who plead insanity in murder cases are no more successful in being found NGRI than persons charged with other crimes (Steadman et al, 1983).

Myth #3: There Is No Risk to the Defendant Who Pleads Insanity. Defendants who asserted an insanity defense at trial, and who were ultimately found guilty of their charges, served significantly longer sentences than defendants tried on similar charges who did not assert the insanity defense. The same ratio is found when only homicide cases are considered (Rodriguez et al., 1983).

Myth #4: NGRI Acquittees Are Quickly Released from Custody. Of the entire universe of individuals found NGRI over an 8-year period in one jurisdiction, only 15% had been released from all restraints; 35% remained in full custody, and 47% were under partial court restraint following conditional release (Rodriguez et al., 1983). A comprehensive study of California practice showed that only 1% of insanity acquittees were released following their NGRI verdict and that another 4% were placed on conditional release, the remaining 95% being hospitalized (Steadman et al., 1993). In other recent research, Golding and his colleagues discovered, in their study of all persons found NGRI in the Canadian province of British Columbia over a 9-year period, that the average time spent in secure hospitalization or supervision was slightly over 9½ years (Golding, Eaves, & Kowaz, 1989).

Myth #5: NGRI Acquittees Spend Much Less Time in Custody Than Do Defendants Convicted of the Same Offenses. Contrarily, NGRI acquittees spend almost *double* the amount of time that defendants convicted of similar charges spend in prison settings, and often face a lifetime of post-release judicial oversight (Rodriguez et al., 1983). In California, while the length of confinement for individuals acquitted by reason of insanity on murder charges was less than for those convicted, defendants found NGRI for other violent crimes were confined twice as long as those found guilty of such charges, and those found NGRI of nonviolent crimes were confined for periods over nine times as long (Steadman et al., 1993).

Myth #6: Criminal Defendants Who Plead Insanity Are Usually Faking. This is perhaps the oldest of the insanity defense myths, and is one that has bedeviled American jurisprudence since the mid-19th century (Ray, 1853, § 247). Of the 141 individuals found NGRI in one jurisdiction over an 8-year period, there was no dispute that 115 were schizophrenic (including 38 of the 46 cases involving a victim's death), and in only three cases was the diagnostician unwilling or unable to specify the nature of the patient's mental illness (Rodriguez et al., 1983). Also, most studies show that a large number of NGRI defendants have significant histories of prior hospitalizations (Hawkins & Pasewark, 1983).

Myth #7: Most Insanity Defense Trials Feature "Battles of the Experts." The public's false perception of the circus-like "battle of the experts" is one of the most telling reasons for the rejection of psychodynamic principles by the legal system. A dramatic case such as the *Hinckley* trial thus reinforced the public's perception that the insanity defense is characterized by battles of experts who overwhelm the jury, engendering judicial and public skepticism as to the ability of psychiatrists to actually come to reasoned and reasonable judgments in cases involving mentally disabled individuals charged with crime (Anchor, 1982; "The Right to a Partisan," 1986).

The empirical reality is quite different. In a Hawaii survey, there was examiner congruence on insanity in 92% of all cases; in Oregon, prosecutors agreed to insanity verdicts in 80% of all cases (Fukunaga et al., 1981; Rogers, Bloom, & Manson, 1984). Most importantly, these are not recent developments: over 25 years ago, a study of the impact of the *Durham* decision in Washington, DC, found that between two-thirds and three-quarters of all insanity defense acquittals were uncontested (Acheson, 1963). In short, the empirical evidence refuting this myth has been available to judges, legislators, and scholars since almost a decade *prior* to the adoption of the ALI-Model Penal Code test in *Brawner*.

Myth #8: Criminal Defense Attorneys Employ the Insanity Defense Plea Solely to "Beat the Rap." Attorneys representing mentally disabled defendants have been routinely criticized for "seeking refuge" in the insanity defense as a means of technically avoiding a deserved conviction (Kavanagh, 1928, p. 90). In reality, the facts are quite different. First, the level of representation afforded to mentally disabled defendants is frequently substandard (Perlin, 1992b). Second, the few studies that have been done paint an entirely different picture: Lawyers often enter an insanity plea to obtain immediate mental health treatment of their client, as a plea-bargaining device to insure that their client ultimately receives mandatory mental health care, and to avoid malpractice litigation (Pasewark & Craig, 1980). Third, the best available research suggests that jury biases exist relatively independent of lawyer functioning and are generally not induced by attorneys (J. Tanford & S. Tanford, 1988).

THE SIGNIFICANCE OF SCIENTIFIC EVIDENCE

Although it might be assumed that, as our data base of the etiology, epidemiology, pathology, and physiology of mental disability increases, our construct of mental responsibility will become increasingly more sophisticated, especially in light of the recent attention being paid by legal commentators to the scientific method and its implications for the law, to date this has not happened.

Development of insanity defense jurisprudence has proceeded with extreme indifference to new scientific discoveries. If anything, the retrenchment of the cognitive-only test (as reflected in the *M'Naghten* rules and the even more restrictive IDRA) may have reflected a conscious decision on the part of legal decision makers to ignore the Freudian revolution and its aftermath.

Scientific Measures of Responsibility. Through the use of such instruments as the Mental State at the Time of the Offense Screening Evaluation (MSO; Slobogin, Melton, & Showalter, 1984), the Schedule of Affective Disorders and Schizophrenia (SADS; Rogers & Cavanaugh, 1981), the Research Diagnostic Criteria (RDC; Spitzer, Endicott, & Robins, 1978), and the Rogers Criminal Responsibility Assessment Scales (R-CRAS; Rogers, Seman, & Clark, 1986), mental health practitioners have focused on the provision of standardized and empirically based approaches to criminal responsibility (Rogers, Cavanaugh, et al., 1984). These instruments were designed to translate legal insanity concepts into quantifiable variables that will meet the standard of reasonable scientific certainty (Golding & Roesch, 1987).

In a series of studies, R-CRAS has been validated for the ALI-Model Penal Code standard, and for M'Naghten and GBMI as well (Rogers, 1987b; Rogers & Cavanaugh, 1981; Rogers, Dolmetsch, & Cavanaugh, 1981; Rogers, Seman, & Wasyliw, 1983; Rogers, Wasyliw, & Cavanaugh, 1984). The instrument tellingly revealed that malingering was not associated in criminal defendants either with severe psychopathology or expert opinion regarding sanity (Rogers et al., 1981; Rogers, Gillis, & Bagby, 1990). These tools remain, however, virtually irrelevant both to the policy debate over the future of the insanity defense and to the substantive and procedural contours of the defense itself (English, 1988).

The Relevance of Scientific Studies. In this light, it is especially ironic that the key common denominator between law and science is a central emphasis on "the critical method of hypothesis formulation and empirical testing" ("The Scientific," 1987, p. 1981). For it is here that one of the great ironies of insanity defense jurisprudence - the ultimate *irrelevance* to decision makers of the results of empirical testing (Tancredi & Volkow, 1988) - glares at us: Even where we are made aware of the inaccuracy of the myths that form the underpinning of that jurisprudence, we continue, via a process known as attribution theory (Bersoff, 1993; Perlin, 1990), to ignore overwhelming and virtually uncontradicted evidence and, instead, to adhere to the persistent myths. Just as we have demurred to uncontested empirical evidence, so do we demur, in large part, to "interpretive and contextual" scientific explanations of mentally disordered criminal behavior (Kaplan & Rinella, 1988, p. 226).

Although science continues to offer "new insights and techniques applicable to the law and to all aspects of human understanding," it is not at all clear that society is prepared to accept these insights and expand its base of understanding. If the number of criminal defendants who are "not responsible" goes beyond some abstract "pressure point," new dilemmas for society are created. The empirical reality is that few defendants plead insanity and fewer are successful. Yet, if we integrate new scientific evidence into our jurisprudence, we would then have to deal with an insanity defense system which has a potentially significant impact on the judicial system and the criminal process. That might plausibly lead to new pressure to abolish the defense because its legitimate use would, for the first time in history, actually have an operational impact on the crime control model of criminal law (S. Brehm & J. Brehm, 1981).

In short, where science does appear to inform us of ways in which the criminal justice system is operating unfairly, we choose to reject it rather than to confront the underlying issues that are raised.

THE ABOLITIONIST MOVEMENT

The Contemporary Revival. Although the movement to abolish the insanity defense dates to the turn of the century (Perlin, 1989, Vol. 3), its contemporaneous revival can be traced to the Nixon administration's unsuccessful attempts to "gut the [insanity] defense" by limiting it to cases where the defendant, by mental disease or defect, "lacked the state of mind required as an element of the offense charged" (Wales, 1976, p. 687). This proposed limitation has been characterized as the "lemon squeezer" exception: The defense would apply only where the defendant thought the strangulation-victim's head was a lemon (American Law Institute, 1956, p. 156).

Actual Results of Abolition. Steadman and his colleagues are now beginning to publish data giving us some inklings as to what actually *happens* when abolition is attempted (Steadman et al., 1993). Their research reveals that, basically, "abolition" in Montana was a pretext. First, abolition had no meaningful statistical impact on the number of defendants pleading NGRI. Defendants continued to allege that they lacked the requisite mens rea for criminal responsibility (Steadman et al., 1993).

Second, defendants who previously would have been found NGRI are now found incompetent to stand trial. Two-thirds of these were subsequently committed indefinitely to state hospitals where they were frequently treated on the same units as patients who had been found NGRI prior to abolition "reform." In short, "the insanity statutes were reformed, but the detention system was not" (Steadman et al., 1993, pp. 136-137). It is certainly possible that some of the postabolition pleas were the result of defense counsel wanting to "flag" for the court that the defendants were seriously mentally ill and in need of psychiatric hospitalization. This is precisely the same strategy often employed by counsel in jurisdictions where the defense has not been abolished.

It is not yet clear what impact Steadman's empirical breakthrough will have on politically motivated abolitionist measures. If the Montana experience is a representative one, then the full measure of the abolition charade is clear. The defense is abolished in name, but the plea is entered for pretextual reasons. Severely mentally ill criminal defendants are treated in the same wards of the same forensic hospitals to which they would have been sent had they been found NGRI. This suggests the meretriciousness of much of the politically based abolition movement: Voters are being told that their representatives are "doing something" about the crime problem, but only the labels describing the patients' forensic status change.

In short, the "abolition movement" is a textbook example of the way that insanity defense mythology and opportunistic politicians have helped corrupt our jurisprudence. Empiricism, science, and philosophy are subverted; old shibboleths are repeated, and little changes.

CONCLUSION

It is impossible to understand the current state of insanity defense jurisprudence without reflecting on the links between mental illness and sin, criminal law and theology, and the impact of medievalism on our conscious and unconscious social attitudes. Despite the development of dynamic psychology and psychiatry, we have regularly rejected psychodynamic explanations for behavior because such explanations were cognitively dissonant with our need to punish: We choose to reinterpret information and experience that conflicts with our internally accepted beliefs to avoid the unpleasant state that such inconsistency produces (Perlin, 1991). As a result, our jurisprudence has developed out of consciousness.

The development of the insanity defense has tracked the tension between psychodynamics and punishment, and reflects our most profound ambivalence about both. On one hand, we are especially punitive toward the mentally disabled, "the most despised and feared group in society" (Scott, Zonana, & Getz, 1989, p. 982); on the other, we recognize that in some narrow and carefully circumscribed circumstances, exculpation is - and historically has been - proper and necessary. This ambivalence infects a host of criminal justice policy issues that involve mentally disabled criminal defendants beyond insanity defense decision making: issues of expert testimony, of mental disability as a mitigating (or aggravating) factor at sentencing and in death penalty cases, and of the creation of a "compromise" GBMI verdict.

The post-*Hinckley* debate revealed the fragility of our insanity defense policies and demonstrated that there was simply not enough "tensile strength" in the criminal justice system to withstand the public's dysfunctionally heightened arousal (Wexler, 1985, p. 537) that followed the jury verdict. In spite of doctrinal changes and judicial glosses, the public remains wed to the "wild beast" test of 1724 (Roberts, Golding, & Fincham, 1987). It should thus be no surprise that, when Congress chose to replace the ALI-Model Penal Code insanity test with a stricter version of *M'Naghten*, that decision was seen as a victory by insanity defense supporters (Milner, 1984).

These dissonances, tensions, and ambivalences - again, rooted in medieval thought - continue to control the public's psyche. They reflect the extent of the gap between academic discourse and social values and the "deeply rooted moral and religious tension" that surrounds responsible decision making (Golding, 1990). Ours is a culture of punishment. Only when we acknowledge that psychic and physical reality can we expect to make sense of the underlying jurisprudence.

Michael L. Perlin is Professor of Law at New York Law School. Formerly the Director of the Division of Mental Health Advocacy in the New Jersey Department of the Public Advocate, and Deputy Public Defender in charge of the Mercer County (Trenton) New Jersey Office of the Public Defender, he now serves on the National Advisory Board of the Institute of Mental Disability and Law of the National Center for State Courts, and on the Board of Directors of the International Academy of Law and Mental Health. His three-volume treatise, *Mental Disability Law: Civil and Criminal*, won the 1990 Walter Jeffords Writing Prize. His most recent books, *The Jurisprudence of the Insanity Defense* and *Law and Mental Disability*, were published earlier this year. Professor Perlin may be contacted at New York Law School, 57 Worth Street, New York, NY 10013.

RESOURCES

18 U.S.C. § 4243 et seq. (1988).

Acheson, D. (1963). *McDonald v. United States*: The *Durham* rule redefined. *Georgetown Law Journal, 51,* 580-591.

American Law Institute. (1956). Comments to *Model Penal Code* § 4.01.

Anchor, K. (1982). Expert witness testimony in the John Hinckley trial. *American Journal of Trial Advocacy, 6,* 153-162.

Andenaes, J. (1956). Determinism and criminal law. *Journal of Criminal Law, Criminology & Police Science, 47,* 406-413.

Andenaes, J. (1971). The moral or educative influence of criminal law. *Journal of Social Issues, 27,* 17-31.

Battalino v. People, 118 Colo. 587, P.2d 897 (1948).

Bersoff, D. (1993). Judicial deference to nonlegal decisionmakers: Imposing simplistic solutions on problems of cognitive complexity in mental disability law. *Southern Methodist University Law Review, 46,* 329-372.

Boldt, R. (1986). Restitution, criminal law, and the ideology of individuality. *Journal of Criminal Law and Criminology, 77,* 969-1022.

Brehm, S., & Brehm, J. (1981). *Psychological Reactance: A Theory of Freedom and Control.* New York: Academic Press.

Callahan, L., Mayer, C., & Steadman, H. (1987). Insanity defense reform in the United States -- Post-Hinckley. *Mental & Physical Disability Law Reporter, 11,* 54-59.

Caplan, L. (1984). *The Insanity Defense and Trial of John W. Hinckley, Jr.* Boston: D. R. Godine.

Devlin, P. (1963). Mental abnormality and the criminal law. In R. S. MacDonald (Ed.), *Changing Legal Objectives* (p. 71). Toronto: University of Toronto Press.

Diamond, B. (1961). Criminal responsibility of the mentally ill. *Stanford Law Review, 14,* 59-86.

Diamond, B. (1973). From *Durham* to *Brawner*, a futile journey. *Washington University Law Quarterly, 1973,* 109-154.

Dix, G. (1986). Criminal responsibility and mental impairment in American criminal law: Responses to the Hinckley acquittal in historical perspective. In D. Weisstub (Ed.), *Law and Mental Health: International Perspectives* (pp. 1-44). New York: Pergamon.

Durham v. United States, 214 F. 2d 862 (D.C. Cir. 1954), overruled in *United States v. Brawner,* 471 F. 2d 969 (D.C. Cir. 1972).

Eigen, J. P. (1984). Historical developments in psychiatric forensic evidence: The British experience. *International Journal of Law and Psychiatry, 6,* 423-429.

English, J. (1988). The light between twilight and dusk: Federal criminal law and the volitional insanity defense. *Hastings Law Journal, 40*(1), 1-52.

Eule, J. (1978). The presumption of sanity: Bursting the bubble. *University of California at Los Angeles Law Review, 25,* 637-699.

Federal Rules of Evidence 704(b).

Feinberg, J. (1970). *Doing and Deserving: Essays in the Theory of Responsibility.* Princeton, NJ: Princeton University Press.

Fentiman, L. (1985). "Guilty but mentally ill": The real verdict is guilty. *Boston College Law Review, 26,* 601-653.

Frigillana v. United States, 307 F. 2d 665 (D.C. Cir. 1962).

Fukunaga, K. K., Pasewark, R. A., Hawkins, M., & Gudeman, H. (1981). Insanity plea: Interexaminer agreement in concordance of psychiatric opinion and court verdict. *Law and Human Behavior, 5,* 325-328.

Garber, H., Weilburg, J., Buonanno, F., Manschreck, T., & New, P. (1988). Use of Magnetic Resonance Imaging in psychiatry. *American Journal of Psychiatry, 145,* 164-171.

Gaylin, W., & Rothman, D. (1976). Introduction. In A. von Hirsch (Ed.), *Doing Justice: The Choice of Punishments.* Boston: Northeastern University Press.

Golding, S. (1990). Mental health professionals and the courts: The ethics of expertise. *International Journal of Law and Psychiatry, 13,* 281-307.

Golding, S, Eaves, D., & Kowaz, A. (1989). The assessment, treatment and community outcome of insanity acquittees. *International Journal of Law and Psychiatry, 12,* 149-179.

Golding, S., & Roesch, R. (1987). The assessment of criminal responsibility: A historical approach to a current controversy. In I. Weiner & A. Hess (Eds.), *Handbook of Forensic Psychology* (pp. 395-436). New York: John Wiley.

Goldstein, A. (1967). *The Insanity Defense.* New Haven, CT: Yale University Press.

Harmelin v. Michigan, 111 S. Ct. 2680, 2706 (1991) (Kennedy, J., concurring in part & concurring in judgment).

Hawkins, M. R., & Pasewark, R. A. (1983). Characteristics of persons utilizing the insanity plea. *Psychological Reports, 53,* 191-195.

Hermann, D., & Sor, Y. (1983). Convicting or confining? Alternative directions in insanity law reform: Guilty but mentally ill versus new rules for release of insanity acquittees. *Brigham Young University Law Review, 1983,* 499-638.

Hovenkamp, H. (1981). Insanity and responsibility in progressive America. *North Dakota Law Review, 57,* 541-575.

Howell, T. B. (Ed.). (1812). *A Complete Collection of State Trials.*

Insanity Defense Reform Act of 1984, 18 U.S.C. § 17 (1988).

Insanity defense: Should the shock of the *Hayes* verdict compel North Carolina to fix what "ain't broke"? (1990). *Wake Forest Law Review, 25,* 547-589.

Jeffrey, R. W., Pasewark, R. S., & Bieber, S. (1988). Insanity plea: Predicting not guilty by reason of insanity adjudications. *Bulletin of the American Academy of Psychiatry and Law, 16,* 35-39.

Johnson v. State, 292 Md. 405, 439 A. 2d 542 (1982).

Kaplan, L., & Rinella, V. (1988). Jurisprudence and the appropriation of the psychoanalytic: A study in ideology and power. *International Journal of Law and Psychiatry, 11,* 215-248.

Kavanagh, M. (1928). *The Criminal and His Allies.* Indianapolis: Bobbs-Merrill.

Krisberg, B. (1991). Are you now or have you ever been a sociologist? *Journal of Criminal Law and Criminology, 82,* 141-155.

Lewinstein, S. (1969). The historical development of insanity as a defense in criminal actions, Part I. *Journal of Forensic Sciences, 14,* 275-293.

Livermore, J., & Meehl, P. (1967). The virtues of *M'Naghten. Minnesota Law Review, 51,* 789-856.

McDonald v. United States, 312 F. 2d 847 (D.C. Cir. 1962).

McGraw, B., Farthing-Capowich, D., & Keilitz, I. (1985). The "guilty but mentally ill" plea and verdict: Current state of the knowledge. *Villanova Law Review, 30,* 117-191.

Mickenberg, I. (1987). A pleasant surprise: The guilty but mentally ill verdict has succeeded in its own right and successfully preserved the insanity defense. *University of Cincinnati Law Review, 55,* 943-996.

Milner, N. (1984). What's old and new about the insanity plea. *Judicature, 67,* 499-509.

M'Naghten's Case, 8 Eng. Rep. 718 (1843).

Model Penal Code (1955 Tent. Draft No.4), § 4.01.

The modern day scarlet letter: A critical analysis of modern probation conditions. (1989). *Duke Law Journal, 1989,* 1357-1385.

Moore, M. (1984). *Law and Psychiatry: Rethinking the Relationship.* New York: Cambridge University Press.

Moran, R. (1981). *Knowing Right from Wrong: The Insanity Defense of Daniel M'Naghten.* New York: The Free Press.

Pasewark, R., & Craig, P. (1980). Insanity plea: Defense attorneys' view. *Journal of Psychiatry and Law, 8,* 413-441.

Pasewark, R., & McGinley, H. (1985). Insanity plea: National survey of frequency and success. *Journal of Psychiatry and Law, 13,* 101-108.

People v. McQuillan, 392 Mich. 511, 221 N.W. 2d 569 (1974).

People v. Seefeld, 95 Mich. App. 197, 290 N.W. 2d 123 (App. 1980).

People v. Smith, 124 Ill. App. 3d 805, 465 N.E. 2d 101 (1984).

Perlin, M. L. (1985). "The things we do for love": John Hinckley's trial and the future of the insanity defense in the federal courts [book review]. *New York Law School Law Review, 30,* 857-875.

Perlin, M. L. (1987). The Supreme Court, the mentally disabled criminal defendant, and symbolic values: Random decisions, hidden rationales, or "doctrinal abyss"? *Arizona Law Review, 29*(1), 1-98.

Perlin, M. L. (1989). *Mental Disability Law: Civil and Criminal.* Charlottesville, VA: The Michie Co.

Perlin, M. L. (1989-1990). Unpacking the myths: The symbolism mythology of insanity defense jurisprudence. *Case Western Reserve Law Review, 40,* 599-731.

Perlin, M. L. (1990). Psychodynamics and the insanity defense: "Ordinary common sense" and heuristic reasoning. *Nebraska Law Review, 69,* 3-70.

Perlin, M. L. (1991). Morality and pretextuality, psychiatry and law: Of "ordinary common sense," heuristic reasoning, and cognitive dissonance. *Bulletin of the American Academy of Psychiatry and Law, 19,* 131-150.

Perlin, M. L. (1992a). On "sanism." *Southern Methodist University Law Review, 46,* 373-407.

Perlin, M. L. (1992b). Fatal assumption: A critical evaluation of the role of counsel in mental disability cases. *Law and Human Behavior, 16,* 39-59.

Perlin, M. L. (1993). Pretexts and mental disability law: The case of competency. *University of Miami Law Review, 47,* 625-688.

Perlin, M. L., & Dorfman, D. A. (1993). Sanism, social science, and the development of mental disability law jurisprudence. *Behavioral Sciences and the Law, 11,* 47-66.

Pillsbury, S. (1989). Understanding penal reform: The dynamics of change. *Journal of Criminal Law and Criminology, 80,* 726-780.

Platt, A., & Diamond, B. (1966). The origins of the "right and wrong" test of criminal responsibility and its subsequent development in the United States: An historical survey. *California Law Review, 54,* 1227-1260.

Pogrebin, M., Regoli, R., & Perry, K. (1986). Not guilty by reason of insanity: A research note. *International Journal of Law and Psychiatry, 8,* 237-241.

Ray, I. (1853). *Medical Jurisprudence of Insanity* (3rd ed.). Boston: Little & Brown.

Regina v. Oxford, 9 Carr. & P. 525 (1840).

The right to a partisan psychiatric expert: Might indigency preclude insanity? (1986). *New York University Law Review, 61,* 703-707.

Roberts, C. F., Golding, S. L., & Fincham, F. D. (1987). Implicit theories of criminal responsibility decision making and the insanity defense. *Law and Human Behavior, 11,* 202-232.

Roche, P. (1958). *The Criminal Mind.* Westport, CT: Greenwood.

Rodriguez, J. H., LeWinn, L. M., & Perlin, M. L. (1983). The insanity defense under siege: Legislative assaults and legal rejoinders. *Rutgers Law Journal, 14,* 397-430.

Rogers, R. (1987a). APA's position on the insanity defense: Empiricism versus emotionalism. *American Psychologist, 42,* 840-848.

Rogers, R. (1987b). Assessment of criminal responsibility: Empirical advances and unanswered questions. *Journal of Psychiatry and Law, 15,* 73-82.

Rogers, J. L., Bloom, J. D., & Manson, S. M. (1984). Insanity defense: Contested or conceded? *American Journal of Psychiatry, 141,* 885-888.

Rogers, R., & Cavanaugh, J. (1981). Application of the SADS diagnostic interview to forensic psychiatry. *Journal of Psychiatry and Law, 9,* 329-344.

Rogers, R., Cavanaugh, J. L., Seman, W., & Harris, M. (1984). Legal outcome and clinical findings: A study of insanity evaluations. *Bulletin of the American Academy of Psychiatry and Law, 12,* 75-83.

Rogers, R., Dolmetsch, R., & Cavanaugh, J. (1981). An empirical approach to insanity evaluations. *Journal of Clinical Psychology, 37,* 683-687.

Rogers, R., Gillis, J. R., & Bagby, R. M. (1990). The SIRS as a measure of malingering: A validation study with a correctional sample. *Behavioral Sciences and the Law, 8,* 85-92.

Rogers, R., Seman, W., & Clark, C. R. (1986). Assessment of criminal responsibility: Initial validation of the R-CRAS with the M'Naghten and GBMI standards. *International Journal of Law and Psychiatry, 9,* 67-75.

Rogers, R., Seman, W., & Wasyliw, O. (1983). The R-CRAS and legal insanity: A cross validation study. *Journal of Clinical Psychology, 39,* 554-559.

Rogers, R., Wasyliw, O., & Cavanaugh, J. (1984). Evaluating insanity: A study of construct validity. *Law and Human Behavior, 8,* 293-303.

Romanucci-Ross, L., & Tancredi, L. (1986). Psychiatry, the law, and cultural determinants of behavior. *International Journal of Law and Psychiatry, 9,* 265-293.

Roth, L. (1986-1987). Preserve but limit the insanity defense. *Psychiatric Quarterly, 58,* 91-105.

Rychlak, R. J. (1990). Society's right to punish: A further exploration of the denunciation theory of punishment. *Tulane Law Review, 65,* 299-338.

Rychlak, R. J., & Rychlak, J. F. (1990). The insanity defense and the question of human agency. *New Ideas in Psychology, 8,* 3-24.

Sadoff, R. L. (1986, September 10). *Insanity: Evolution of a Medicolegal Concept.* Paper presented at College Night, The College of Physicians of Philadelphia, PA.

Schulhofer, S. (1974). Harm and punishment: A critique of emphasis on the results of conduct in the criminal law. *University of Pennsylvania Law Review, 122,* 1497-1607.

The scientific model in law. (1987). *Georgetown Law Journal, 75,* 1968-2003.

Scott, D., Zonana, H., & Getz, M. (1989). Monitoring insanity acquittees: Connecticut's Psychiatric Review Board. *Hospital and Community Psychiatry, 41,* 980-984.

Sendor, B. (1986). Crime as communication: An interpretative theory of the insanity defense and the mental elements of crime. *Georgetown Law Journal, 74,* 1371-1434.

Slobogin, C. (1985). The guilty but mentally ill verdict: An idea whose time should not have come. *George Washington Law Review, 53,* 494-527.

Slobogin, C., Melton, G., & Showalter, C. (1984). The feasibility of a brief evaluation of mental state at the time of the offense. *Law and Human Behavior, 8,* 305-320.

Spitzer, R. L., Endicott, J., & Robins, E. (1978). Research diagnostic criteria: Rationale and reliability. *Archives of General Psychiatry, 35,* 773-782.

Steadman, H., McGreevy, M., Morrisey, J., Callahan, L., Robbins, P., & Cirincione, C. (1993). *Before and After Hinckley: Evaluating Insanity Defense Reform.* New York: Guilford.

Steadman, H., Keitner, L., Braff, J., & Arvanites, T. M. (1983). Factors associated with a successful insanity plea. *American Journal of Psychiatry, 140,* 401-405.

Tancredi, L., & Volkow, N. (1988). Neural substrates of violent behavior: Implications for law and public policy. *International Journal of Law and Psychiatry, 11,* 13-49.

Tanford, J., & Tanford, S. (1988). Better trials through science: A defense of psychologist-lawyer collaboration. *North Carolina Law Review, 66,* 741-780.

United States v. Brawner, 471 F. 2d 969 (D.C. Cir. 1972).

van den Haag, E. (1975). *Punishing Criminals.* New York: Basic Books.

Wales, H. (1976). An analysis of the proposal to "abolish" the insanity defense in S.1: Squeezing a lemon. *University of Pennsylvania Law Review, 124,* 687-712.

Watson, A. (1958). A critique of the legal approach to crime and correction. *Law and Contemporary Problems, 23,* 611-632.

Weiner, B. (1985). Mental disability and criminal law. In S. Brakel, J. Parry, & B. Weiner (Eds.), *The Mentally Disabled and the Law* (pp. 693-801). Chicago: American Bar Foundation Press.

Wexler, D. (1985). Redefining the insanity problem. *George Washington Law Review, 53,* 528-561.

CHINKS IN THE PRISON WALL: APPLYING GRAHAM'S STOCKHOLM SYNDROME THEORY TO THE TREATMENT OF BATTERED WOMEN

*Edna I. Rawlings, P. Gail Allen,
Dee L. R. Graham, and June Peters*

Most people have at some time wondered why battered women and children alike profess to love those who abuse them and do whatever they can to stay with those abusers. Most mental health professionals who have worked with battered women can recall cases in which women who came to them for help denied, minimized, or excused the abuse they received at the hands of their partners. Often, these women prematurely leave treatment rather than face the reality and implications of their abuse. Even as we write this contribution, a case is appearing in newspapers across the country about a woman whose boyfriend allegedly caused her to lose an arm, a leg, and a pregnancy, but who asked the judge to drop charges against him ("My Fault," 1993). Graham (Graham & Rawlings, 1991; Graham, Rawlings, & Rigsby, 1994) has proposed an innovative theory, which is called Graham's Stockholm Syndrome theory, to help explain such occurrences as well as other situations involving chronic interpersonal abuse (e.g., cult members' idolization of abusive leaders).

In this contribution we will describe treatment issues and therapeutic interventions in both individual and group therapy settings for women who have been victims of intimate partner abuse (in courtship or marital situations). Before discussing the clinical implications, we will briefly describe the major tenets of the theory, because most readers will not be familiar with it.

GRAHAM'S STOCKHOLM SYNDROME THEORY

Bonding to one's captor is a survival strategy for victims that has been observed in a variety of hostage-taking situations. This strategy was labeled *Stockholm Syndrome* following a hostage-taking situation in a bank robbery in Stockholm, Sweden, in 1973 (see Lang [1974] for a description of this event). After examining psychological literatures of nine hostage or hostagelike groups (hostages, concentration camp prisoners, cult members, prisoners of war, civilians in Chinese Communist prisons, procured prostitutes, incest victims, physically and/or emotionally abused children, and battered women), Graham (1987) concluded that, under certain conditions, bonding with an abuser may be a survival strategy for victims of chronic interpersonal abuse. Graham uses the terms "captor" and "abuser," and "victim" and "hostage," synonymously, for an abuser has to hold a victim captive or the victim would not stay to be abused again, and a captor, by simply holding another against her or his will is, minimally, psychologically abusive. Similarly, an abuse victim who does not perceive a way to escape is a captive.

In the nine literatures surveyed, Graham identified four situational factors that she hypothesized to be precursors to the Stockholm Syndrome: (a) perceived threat to one's physical or psychological survival and the belief that the captor (abuser) would carry out the threat, (b) perceived kindness from the captor to the captive (victim); (c) isolation from perspectives other than those of the captor, and (d) perceived inability to escape. The presence and extent of these four conditions determine whether a victim/captive develops Stockholm Syndrome and the extent of the syndrome.

The psychodynamics of the Stockholm Syndrome as hypothesized by Graham (Graham & Rawlings, 1991) are as follows. An abuser/captor traumatizes a victim (who cannot escape) with a threat to the victim's survival. The traumatized victim, who is isolated from outsiders who could provide nurturance and protection, must look to the abuser to meet those needs. If the abuser shows the victim some kindness, however small, the victim bonds to the positive side of the abuser, denying the side of the abuser that produced the terror. The victim begins to work to see the world from the abuser's perspective so that she or he will know what keeps the abuser happy, thus helping to insure survival. As a result, the victim becomes hypervigilant to the abuser's needs and unaware of her or his own needs. The victim comes to see the world from the abuser's perspective, losing touch with her or his own perspective, which is unimportant or even counterproductive to survival. With denial of the violent side of the abuser and, thus, denial of danger, the victim finds it difficult to psychologically separate from the abuser. Other mechanisms that make it difficult for the victim to psychologically separate from the abuser include fear of losing both the only positive relationship available to her or him - due to isolation - and the only identity that remains - her/his self seen through the abuser's eyes (which, in the case of the adult victim of chronic abuse, has replaced any previous sense of self).

Based on her survey of the nine literatures cited previously, Graham has postulated 66 aspects of Stockholm Syndrome which are typically found in persons who have developed the syndrome. (See Graham et al., [1994] for a list of these aspects.) Empirical tests of the aspects have been carried out on the following populations: battered women (Graham, Ott, & Rawlings, 1990), women in dating relationships (Graham et al., 1993), adults who were abused as children (Naber-Morris, 1990), and female incest survivors (Gervers, 1994). For brevity of description, Graham has reduced these aspects to the following nine major indicators of Stockholm Syndrome:

- A bi-directional bond between victim and abuser.
- Intense gratitude for kindnesses, however small, shown by the abuser.
- Denial or rationalization of violence; denial of anger toward the abuser.
- Hypervigilance to the abuser's needs.
- Perceives the world from only the abuser's perspective.
- Perceives authorities trying to win her release as the "bad guys" and the abuser as the "good guy."
- Finds it difficult to leave the abuser even after release is won.
- Fears the abuser will come back to get her even after her release is won, even if the abuser is dead or is in prison.
- Symptoms of Post-Traumatic Stress Disorder (PTSD). (Graham et al., 1994; Graham & Rawlings, 1991)

In order for bonding to an abuser to occur, certain cognitive distortions are necessary. These reduce terror and permit the victim to perceive the abuser as someone other than the source of her or his terror. Still other cognitive and perceptual distortions aid the victim in coping with the abuse. Graham and associates (Graham et al., 1993; Graham, Ott, & Rawlings, 1990) have examined the cognitive distortions associated with Stockholm Syndrome that are observed in battered women and women in dating relationships. Cognitive distortions used to help reduce terror include splitting off cognitions from emotions; self-blame, as this helps the victim feel she can prevent future abuse; denial that she is being abused; rationalizing the partner's abuse of her; and minimizing his abuse of her.

Cognitive distortions used by battered women and women in dating relationships to help create and maintain bonding with their abusive partners include the belief that they must win their abusers' love to survive; gratitude that their abusers have not yet killed them; seeing their abusers as victims; seeing their abusers as good and themselves as bad; seeing their abusers as the "good guys" and those trying to help them as the "bad guys"; believing that their abusers are not responsible for their abuse of them; seeing abuse as a sign of their abusers' love; the belief that if they give enough love, their abusers will let them live and/or stop abusing them; the belief that they are the only ones who can help their abusers; seeing small kindnesses as huge, which also serves to help maintain hope and thus to reduce their terror; seeing their relationships with their partners as perfect were it not for the abuse; and the belief that they love their abusers. The victim's belief that she loves the abuser may actually be a misattribution that love, not terror, is responsible for her high arousal level and her behavior: her compliance with the abuser's commands and even her anticipating his needs and taking care of them before he even knows he has them (cf. Schachter & Singer, 1962). Readers interested in additional information about this phenomenon can consult Dutton and Aron (1974), Walster (1971), and Walster and Berscheid (1971).

Other distortions serving as coping strategies for battered women are, for example, their narrowing of perceptions so that they focus on surviving in the here and now, their taking their abusers' perspective, and their seeing their abusers as omnipotent, which encourages their compliance. Readers interested in further discussion of cognitive distortions associated with Stockholm Syndrome are referred to Graham et al. (1994).

ALLEN'S UNBONDING CONTINUUM: INDIVIDUAL TREATMENT MODEL FOR ABUSED WOMEN WITH STOCKHOLM SYNDROME

In this section we describe research findings by Allen (1991), interpreted in terms of Graham's Stockholm Syndrome theory, and an individual treatment model growing out of that interpretation. Allen's research findings suggest that battered women go through an "unbonding process" in working toward disengagement from the battering partner. This unbonding process is described by four stages (described on pp. 404-406). Treatment interventions are tailored to the individual client's current stage, or position along this unbonding pathway.

Fifty percent of all abused women who leave their batterers return (Ferraro & Johnson, 1983; Strube, 1988). On average, battered women leave their partners and return six times before leaving permanently (Walker, 1979; see also Okun, 1986). Allen (1991) hypothesized that each time a woman goes to a shelter, even though she may return to the abuser, she is actually mastering some aspect of the separation process. Eventually, a sufficient number of aspects are mastered for separation to occur. Although it is not clear what enables women to move through stages of the unbonding process, it is likely that situational factors related to the abuse (e.g., the precursor conditions giving rise to Stockholm Syndrome) and internal factors (such as loss of self) drive the process. Because disengagement from the abusive partner is herein viewed as a *process*, rather than an event, the woman who leaves but returns to her abusive partner is not viewed as a treatment "failure" but as a survivor actively working toward separation.

In Allen's research, 249 battered women staying in 27 different shelters or attending shelter support groups throughout three states were asked to prioritize the psychological issues on which they felt they needed to work. In particular, the women were asked to indicate the priority they placed on working on each of 50 issues, using the response options: (a) "I would like to work on this issue and place the *highest* priority on it"; (b) "I would like to work on this issue but it is not as important as the issues I would put in category [a]"; (c) "I recognize that this is an issue for me, but it has low priority for me now"; (d) I have *already* dealt with this issue"; and (e) "This issue has never been a problem for me so I do not need to work on it." Using a factor analysis with varimax rotation, Allen found four distinct groupings of issues, or factors. Only items with factor loadings of at least .40 were retained. The percentage of common variance accounted for by this

4-factor solution was 71%. Individually, Factor 1 accounted for 20% of the variance; Factor 2, 19%; Factor 3, 16%; and Factor 4, 15%. Cronbach Alphas for each factor were: Factor 1, .86; Factor 2, .84; Factor 3, .84; and Factor 4, .81. These factors were interpreted to represent four stages through which battered women move as they unbond from their abusive partners.

THE UNBONDING PATHWAY

Two key constructs - attachment to partner and sense of self - describe differences in the four stages. In general, at the beginning of the hypothesized unbonding continuum, there is a strong attachment to the partner and an absence of self. Movement through the stages is characterized by a lessening of the attachment and an increase in sense of self. The following discussion of the four stages and certain common profiles of women along the stages will address these tasks.

STAGES OF UNBONDING

First, we will describe the psychological issues on which battered women reported it was most important for them to work at each stage of unbonding. We will discuss what their prioritization of the particular issues suggests they thought and felt about their partners, their relationships, and themselves. While reading about each stage, or factor, of unbonding described next, the reader may find it helpful to refer to Table 1 (pp. 405-406), which describes the issues associated with each.

It is important to recognize that the stages appear to be continuous, not discrete. For example, a client might work on issues primarily associated with Stage 3 while continuing to struggle with issues related to Stage 2. Although the stages are ordered in a linear path from enmeshment to disengagement with partner, it is likely that an individual woman's movement along the pathway may not be fully linear. Rather, the process may involve the repetition of stages and the reworking of issues from earlier stages. As yet, research has not been conducted to illuminate this question.

Following the descriptions of the stages, we will present a typology of battered women, based on the stages. As a caveat, we note that although the stages and typology presented here are empirically based, this work is in an early phase of empirical investigation. We invite you to compare your clinical experience with the model presented here, and we welcome feedback.

Stage 1. Immersion With Partner. The title, "Immersion With Partner," underscores the seeming strength of the bond at this stage. The particular issues that women at this stage chose as most important on which to work (refer to Factor 3 of Table 1 for items comprising this factor) address both an enmeshment with the partner (see Items 10, 28, 35, and 45 and even Items 8 and 47) and a questioning or concern regarding this enmeshment (Why do I love someone who hurts me? Item 50). Their focus is on the partner. Even those items about her feelings or needs are in relation to him. Of the four stages, this stage reflects the most Stockholm Syndrome, the most enmeshment, and the least sense of self.

Stage 2. Awakening to the Consequences of Loss of Self. The stage titled, "Awakening to the Consequences of Loss of Self" (Factor 4 in Table 1) indicates endorsers are aware of being trapped: They do not know if they can make it on their own (Items 1 and 2), appear to feel isolated from persons other than the partner (Item 20), yet also do not know how to prevent their partner's abusiveness (Items 42 and 48). They also appear to be suffering from a loss of self, as revealed by their dependence on their partner (Item 39).

Stages 1 and 2 are closely related, both showing a high degree of enmeshment with the abuser and a loss of self. In contrast with Stage 1 items, Stage 2 items reflect the women having considered permanently leaving their partner, though having not as yet figured out how to do so. Stage 1 items reflect feeling badly for having left their partner to go to a shelter, presumably to escape his recent abuse. In sum, Stage 2 items exhibit a high degree of Stockholm Syndrome, though less than that reflected in Stage 1 items.

TABLE 1: ITEMS COMPRISING FACTORS AND STAGES (AND ITEM FACTOR LOADINGS)

Factor 3. (Stage 1. Immersion With Partner)

35. How to get my partner to forgive me for leaving him. (.62)
45. To deal with my feeling of guilt for leaving (or thinking about leaving) my partner. (.61)
41. To understand how I can both love and fear my partner. (.60)
34. To understand how I can feel both anger at and love for my partner. (.55)
50. To understand how I can love someone who treats me so badly. (.45)
28. Why it seems that my happiness is dependent upon my partner's happiness. (.45)
10. How bad I feel knowing that my leaving has (will) hurt my partner. (.44)
8. To figure out how I can get my partner to seek psychological help. (.41)
47. To figure out how I can help my partner who mistreats me only because he has been mistreated himself. (.47)

Factor 4. (Stage 2. Awakening to the Consequences of Loss of Self)

1. My fear that I will not be able to make it on my own without my partner. (.66)
2. Proving to myself that I can take care of myself apart from my partner. (.64)
42. To figure out what I can do to keep my partner happy. (.51)
48. To figure out how I can stop making my partner so angry at me. (.50)
20. To examine my fear that if I leave my partner no one else will want me. (.44)
39. To deal with my feelings that I don't want to live unless my partner loves me. (.41)

Factor 1. (Stage 3. Emergence of an Observing Self)

22. To identify early signs that my partner is getting angry and to make an escape plan that I can use to avoid being the target of his anger. (.70)
17. My confusion over how my partner can be both kind and abusive to me. (.60)
25. Why I don't feel angry with my partner for the way he treats me. (.63)
18. Why it is I know more about how my partner feels than how I feel. (.60)
19. My feelings about how hard it is to admit to myself that my partner abuses me; that I am an abused woman. (.57)
21. To figure out the reasons my partner abuses me. (.56)
26. To stop worrying about how my partner is feeling and to start being more concerned with how I feel. (.52)
15. To deal with the feeling that I don't know who I am apart from my partner. (.49)
16. To deal with the emptiness and loss that I feel when I am away from my partner. (.48)
24. To figure out how to end my isolation from persons other than my partner. (.48)
27. To understand how my isolation has made me less effective in dealing with my partner's abuse. (.46)

Factor 2. (Stage 4. Reclaiming the Self)

7. To build my self-esteem. (.59)
29. To discuss the difficulty I have trusting others, even those who are supportive of me and nonabusive. (.58)
46. To deal with the hurt I feel. (.58)
32. My anger at myself for putting up with my partner's mistreatment of me for so long. (.55)
3. To figure out who is safe to trust and who is not. (.52)
38. Finding a sense of myself that is not influenced by my partner's feelings about me. (.48)
11. To identify ways that my partner has isolated me from others. (.47)
31. To understand how I got into this abusive relationship. (.46)

Factor 2. (Stage 4. Reclaiming the Self) *(Continued)*

13. To discover the strength and power within me. (.43)
23. To deal with the nightmares and/or flashbacks I have. (.42)
37. Why I feel like it is my fault that my partner abuses me even though I know it isn't. (.41)

Stage 3. Emergence of an Observing Self. The third stage, "Emergence of an Observing Self" (Factor 1 in Table 1) is characterized by the woman's new-found ability to observe her relationship more objectively. The items comprising it suggest that, for the first time, the women's denial of their partner's abuse is crumbling, evidenced by their desire to figure out how to identify early signs that abuse is imminent and to make plans for escaping impending abuse (Item 22). Further indication that they are aware of their partner's abusive side is their stated confusion as to how their partner can be both kind and abusive to them (Item 17) and their desire to figure out *why* their partner abuses them (Item 21). That they have gained some psychological distance from the abuse is indicated by their desire to understand why they do not feel angry with their partner for abusing them (Item 25) and their acknowledged difficulty in admitting to themselves that their partner abuses them and that they are abused women (Item 19). They appear to be coming to some awareness of their loss of self, suggested by recognition and confusion that they know more about how their partner feels than how they feel (Item 18), that they do not know who they are apart from their partner (Item 15), and that they feel empty when away from their partner (Item 16).

Items 15, 16, and 26 are worded in a way that indicates willingness to deal with the consequences of loss of self. Many of the items characterizing this stage indicate confusion regarding the paradoxical behavior that is characteristic of Stockholm Syndrome (e.g., Item 25). This expressed confusion is a healthy sign that old behavior patterns are breaking up and that the woman is less enmeshed in the relationship; hence the title, "Emergence of an Observing Self."

Stage 4. Reclaiming the Self. Finally, Stage 4, titled "Reclaiming the Self" (Factor 2 in Table 1), describes women focused on acquiring their own selves apart from their partner's feelings about them (Item 38). The issues of highest priority for women at this stage reflect less bonding with the abuser than those of highest priority in the other four stages. This pattern suggests that these women have had Stockholm Syndrome and are breaking out of it. The women appear to be struggling with self-blame - one of the major cognitive distortions associated with Stockholm Syndrome. Items indicate these women are struggling with both anger at themselves for putting up with the abuse (Item 32) and, at the same time, feelings that the abuse was their fault, even though they know it was not (Item 37).

Women at this stage desire healing and self-nurturance (Items 46 and 13). They know the path to healing includes finding a self of their own (Item 38) and building self-esteem (Item 7). These women look forward to the future, but with realism and caution, and a healthy need for self-protection. They desire new relationships with persons who will be supportive and nonabusive. They are cognizant of the fact that they need to understand what has happened to them in their abusive relationship so as to help insure that their new relationships will be nonabusive (Items 31, 11, and 29).

TREATMENT INTERVENTIONS GUIDED BY TYPOLOGY

Cluster analysis of women's factor scores revealed five clusters of women. All but two of the 249 women in the study were included in one of five clusters. Using a Stepwise Discriminant Analysis, it was found that the variable "number of instances of physical abuse" in which the responses ranged from "1" to "more than 50" failed to discriminate among the five clusters of subjects. However, what constituted an "instance" of abuse may have differed for the women and for the clusters. Only 5% of the women in the sample reported that the most recent assault had been the first. Twenty-seven percent (the modal response) reported they had been assaulted by their partners more than 50 times.

Three of the clusters clearly reflect varying positions along the unbonding pathway. These three clusters of women are described below in terms of the degree of Stockholm Syndrome that appears to have been present. We suggest specific treatment interventions for women in these three clusters. In so doing, we are assuming that these three clusters have external validity for battered women as a population.

Two additional clusters emerged, appearing to represent women for whom other issues such as denial or traumatic anxiety must first be addressed before their place along the unbonding continuum can be assessed. Women in one of these two clusters - labeled the "Acute Trauma Group" - equally endorsed items for all stages, suggesting an inability to focus and discriminate, possibly due to high anxiety. Women in the second of these two clusters - labeled "Deniers" - had a low endorsement rate of all items, indicating the items had low relevancy to them or that they had already worked through them, though they were currently in a shelter. Allen is currently conducting research to further assess the issues of women in these groups. For this reason, these two clusters will not be discussed further in this contribution.

Although the three clusters or groups described next are presented as a typology, the groups are probably fluid. As women work through the issues relevant to them, they presumably move into a new group, thereby proceeding along the unbonding pathway, where new treatment issues present themselves.

Application of this model to therapy is premised on the presumptions that identification of a particular client's primary stage can guide effective intervention, helping clinicians to meet the current individual needs of the client; that knowledge of the unbonding pathway can aid shelters in providing more pertinent and useful assistance to individual women; that an understanding of separation as a process can help therapists or counselors adjust their expectations for clients to fit their clients' readiness; and that sharing the model with battered women can help them see their movement, thus empowering them.

Core Stockholm Syndrome Group. Women making up the "Core Stockholm Syndrome" group reported that Stages 1 (Factor 3), "Immersion With Partner," and 2 (Factor 4), "Awakening to the Consequence of Loss of Self," had the most current relevance for them. In other words, they placed the highest priority on the issues describing the first two stages. They described issues in Stages 3, "Emergence of an Observing Self," and 4, "Reclaiming the Self," as least relevant to them. Their responses suggest that these women had a high degree of Stockholm Syndrome, that is, they were strongly bonded to their partners and displayed a loss of sense of self. Denial of the abuse appeared to be strong. The higher degree of attachment, higher degree of loss of self, and greater denial of abuse suggest that women in this group were unlikely to be able to remain separated from their partners. In fact, discriminant analysis revealed that the women comprising this cluster reported the shortest period of separation from their partners and were most likely to report that they intended to return to their partners after leaving the shelter.

When working with women resembling those from this group, a therapist should refrain from prematurely expecting, or particularly urging, the women to leave their batterers. Any separation is likely to be short-lived, and the therapist's urging may jeopardize the therapeutic relationship. Instead, the primary focus of therapy should be on eliminating the conditions that produce Stockholm Syndrome - the four precursors described earlier - and on strengthening the women's sense of self.

Helping the battered woman to reduce her isolation and to develop alternate sources of nurturance and caring are appropriate therapeutic goals for working with women at this stage. Another important therapeutic goal for a woman in this group is acknowledgment of the polarities of love and terror the woman feels toward her partner. Helping the client integrate both the terrorizing and the loving sides of the abuser will assist her in giving up her dream that the relationship will become the type of relationship she had hoped it would be. This integration requires that the therapist validate both the positive and negative parts of the abuser and encourage the client to express both her anger and love for him.

Although one of the primary tasks for women in this group is breaking through the strong denial of the abuse and its effects, direct confrontation of the denial by the therapist is generally counterproductive. We recommend that the Core Stockholm Syndrome woman continually be reminded of the abuse, but in ways that do not make the therapist responsible for the reminder. An example of this type of subtle confrontation is to request the client to keep a journal or write an autobiography of the relationship years. In this way she will confront herself with the abuse. Because of the strength of the denial and the importance of the isolation in maintaining denial, we recommend the use of group work as an adjunct to individual treatment, or as the primary mode of treatment if individual therapy cannot be accommodated. A group setting, using exercises such as those described by Peters (1993; discussed later in this contribution), permits more direct confrontation of the woman's denial of her abuse than does individual therapy. It also has the potential to reduce women's isolation more than does individual therapy.

Because it is less likely that a woman from this group will be able to remain separated from the abusive partner, it is extremely important that the therapist work with her to develop an escape route. Although the woman's denial may impede this process, persistent insistence of such a plan will signal the woman of the therapist's refusal to enter into the denial even as the therapist is empathic to the contradictory feelings the woman has for her abuser.

Breaking Out of Stockholm Syndrome Group. Issues involved in "Reclaiming the Self," Stage 4, were of highest priority for these women. They also reported concern with many of the issues at Stage 3, "Emergence of an Observing Self," suggesting that they had not yet completed the work at this stage. Women in this group reported low relevancy for issues at Stages 1 and 2, suggesting that they had already accomplished most of the tasks of these earlier stages. In short, women in this group, while still grappling with making sense of their abusive relationship and its consequences, desired to heal the psychological wounds created by that abusive relationship (e.g., a loss of sense of self, distrust of others). Discriminant analysis indicated that the women in this group were less likely than the women in the "Core Stockholm Syndrome Group" to state an intention to return to their abusive partners.

We see the primary task for the therapist of a battered woman at this stage as helping her to understand the survival functions of her responses to her abusive partner, as well as the conditions that led to the development of Stockholm Syndrome. Sharing a description of Stockholm Syndrome theory with this woman can help her understand why she has split her partner's good and bad sides, why she has taken on his perspective, and why she often does not know how she feels. Then she can begin to integrate the splits and work on reframing the cognitive distortions she has been maintaining. This will help her to realize the severity of the wounds she has suffered so that she will feel empathy for herself. This understanding has the potential to empower her with the strength to continue the work of mending and reclaiming her self.

Clients resembling the women in this group, having come out of the denial of the abuse, should be assisted in redirecting the anger toward the abuser. As seen from Item 32 (see Factor 2 or Stage 4 in Table 1), at present, their anger at the abuser - anger that was previously split off and repressed for survival reasons - may be misdirected toward themselves. As women at this place on the unbonding continuum give up their denial of the abuse, they are likely to experience grief over the lost dreams of the relationship. They will also likely require assistance with mourning the loss of that dream.

Broken Out of Stockholm Syndrome Group. Women in this group reported the issues at Stage 4 (Factor 2), "Reclaiming the Self," to be the most relevant for them and indicated low relevancy for the issues of Stages 1, 2, and 3, suggesting they had already dealt with those issues. Women in this group were hypothesized to be the most likely to separate successfully from their partners, as they displayed the least degree of attachment to their abusive partners and sought to recover the psychological losses - for example, of self-esteem, trust, and strength and power -

created by the abuse. Empirically, women in the "Broken Out of Stockholm Syndrome Group" were the least likely to state an intention to return to their partners and were the most likely to have contacted an attorney to explore their legal options. They were also the group that had maintained the longest separation from their abusive partners.

Helping clients resembling the women in this cluster to experience empathy for themselves, to express their needs and respond by nurturing themselves, and to find mutually responsive relationships are appropriate therapeutic goals. Another important therapy task for women "Broken Out of Stockholm Syndrome" is understanding the precursor conditions that the abuser used to make and keep the women captive in their relationships. For example, these women need to understand the role their isolation played in their bond with their abuser and to begin setting up a supportive network to guard against future isolation. For these women, too, group work would be a particularly appropriate mode of therapy. In a group they could focus on interpersonal issues such as trust and intimacy with people other than their abusers. In the subsequent section, we will discuss a group therapy model for battered women.

PETERS' PHOENIX PROGRAM: GROUP TREATMENT MODEL FOR ABUSED WOMEN WITH STOCKHOLM SYNDROME

Peters (1993) has developed a highly structured group for battered women which she calls the Phoenix Program. This program contains exercises that address the precursors and the psychodynamics of the Stockholm Syndrome as well as the unbonding process described by Allen (1991).

PARAMETERS OF THE PHOENIX PROGRAM

The Phoenix Program is comprised of 16 structured group exercises. It is designed for groups of 8 to 10 women who are, or have recently been, in battering relationships. The group, which meets for 1½ hours per week for 12 weeks, can be used as a primary treatment modality or as an adjunct to individual therapy. Ideally, participants are heterogeneous not only in terms of age, race, social class, and so on, but also in terms of their places on the unbonding continuum described previously.

Mixing women from different stages of the unbonding process facilitates rapid movement along the unbonding continuum. This is because women who are at earlier stages in this process have models of women who have successfully mastered some of the tasks essential for psychologically separating from their abusive partners, giving them hope. Women who have separated and/or taken legal action can serve as role models for women who are still enmeshed with an abuser. Women who are further along the continuum are reminded of their progress by the women who are just beginning the journey, thereby empowering them.

PROGRAM GOALS

Grounded in Stockholm Syndrome theory, the Phoenix Program benefits battered women in the following ways:

1. *Stockholm Syndrome Theory Helps Women Focus on the Social Contexts of their Symptoms.* In one of the early sessions of the Phoenix Program, group members are introduced to Stockholm Syndrome theory and are asked to compare their own symptoms with indicators of Stockholm Syndrome. Understanding the Stockholm Syndrome reduces self-blame and enhances self-esteem as women come to understand that their symptoms are coping strategies for dealing with unhealthy environments. In the group setting women are able to see how the experiences of other women fit into the precursors and indicators of the Stockholm Syndrome, "normalizing" their psychological reactions to abuse.

2. *Stockholm Precursors - Isolation and Dependence on Abuser's Kindness - Are Diminished by the Bonds That Develop Among Group Participants.* Although women in all women's groups experience communication and understanding from other group members and begin to form positive bonds, in the Phoenix Program, group members are actively encouraged to maintain close contact within and outside of the group. They are encouraged to call each other between sessions if possible and to communicate immediately after the weekly sessions (Peters, 1993).

   Ideological and physical isolation are highly correlated with physical and psychological abuse for battered women (Graham et al., 1990). Even a woman who has a network of friends, family members, and coworkers is isolated if these others are unaware of her being abused, are unsympathetic to her feelings, or are even frankly supportive of her being abused. The most effective way to alleviate isolation is to actually deal with abuse directly in the presence of an ongoing, empathic, nonblaming audience.

   The Stockholm Syndrome precursors are highly correlated (Graham et al., 1990, 1993). Reducing one precursor tends to reduce others. To use a metaphor, one need not destroy an entire prison wall to escape, but dismantle only enough bricks to create a hole large enough to crawl out (Rimini, 1988). Having the support of other group members, besides reducing isolation, diminishes the women's emotional dependence on kindness from their abusers.

3. *The Stockholm Syndrome Precursor, "Perceived Inability to Escape" is Weakened by Women Affirming Each Other's Strengths.* In the Phoenix Program, battered women can begin to recognize the behaviors of abuse victims that signal psychological strength and healthiness but are labeled by others, including abusers and the mental health system, as "sick." The Stockholm Syndrome precursor - perceived inability to escape - begins to crumble when women recognize that they can use their survival strengths (e.g., the ability to form relationships, sensitivity to danger) not just to cope with abuse, but to create a new life for themselves apart from abusive partners.

4. *Denial of Abuse is Diminished as Women Explore and Share the Commonalities of Their Abusive Experiences.* Group cohesiveness increases members' tolerance for intense negative feelings, allowing the therapist to introduce exercises to break down denial much earlier in the therapeutic process than could be done in individual therapy. As women share their experiences, they learn both to recognize abuse so that they can identify it the moment it begins and to understand what the abusive interaction is really about (namely, control). Recognition and understanding are gained first in relation to abuse in the lives of other group members and then in relation to abuse in their own lives.

   Additionally, through sharing their experiences, the women learn that abusive men tend to say and do the same things. They develop empathy for other group members before they learn to extend such empathy to themselves. As they realize that other group members do not deserve abuse, they begin to question whether they themselves deserve it. Once a battered women realizes that the other women, whom she knows are not stupid, are being called stupid, she begins to disbelieve the abuser, to question his perception of her stupidity, and consequently to question his perception of herself, her relationship with him, and his perception of the world. This recognition and understanding of abuse helps break down the denial of abuse which is a key defense mechanism at the heart of the Stockholm Syndrome. Breaking down denial is *sine qua non* to the unbonding process. Consequently, women sharing their experiences of abuse lessens the impact of the abuse as their interpretations of the meaning of it changes.

   In addition, the group serves a memory function when the woman herself is in the honeymoon stage of the cycle of violence. In other words, when the abuse temporarily dissipates, it is quite difficult for the victim to go into a state of denial in the presence of group members if the abuse itself has effectively become a part of the shared group experiences.

5. *Unbonding Is Facilitated as Women Are Encouraged to Focus on Their Unique Identity Apart from Their Abusive Partner.* Exercises within the Phoenix Program further help

women strengthen their autonomous sense of self, weakening their sense of self seen through their abusers' eyes. This enables battered women to begin and continue the process of unbonding described previously by Allen.

One of the major reasons that abused women appear difficult to treat is that they are enmeshed with - including being emotionally dependent on and hypervigilant to - their partners (Graham & Rawlings, 1991). Therapists can misinterpret this enmeshment in various ways, from an extreme form of codependency to different types of personality disorders (Peters, 1993). In contrast, we view this enmeshment as created by chronic, inescapable abuse, interspersed with kindness, and as indicative of the Stockholm Syndrome (Graham & Rawlings, 1991). Subjected to chronic abuse, the woman loses her observing self or ego function and begins to live in a moment-to-moment survival mode. This survival mode consists of a vigilant struggle to please her abusive partner in order to avoid future abuse. A group format can effectively alleviate narrowed perceptions and enmeshment in two ways. First, the group aids women in seeing the overall picture of abusive relationships. Second, the group can be structured to assist women in restoring their separate identity, one that preceded and will extend beyond the abuse.

6. *Post-Traumatic Stress Symptoms Are Healed as Women Allow Dissociated and Numbed Feelings to Surface.* Feelings of anger, connected to feelings of terror, have been dissociated ("numbed out") because expressing anger at their abuser can have dire consequences. In a battered women's group, when women begin to feel safe they often recover the feelings of terror, followed by anger and, later, loss and grief. Because women in the group are at difference places in the healing process, it becomes apparent that healing *is* a process and that one need not remain stuck in a particular phase (e.g., terror, anger, or grief) forever. As the women realize that these feelings are created by the abuse, they realize that the feelings signify "healthiness" and "healing," not "craziness."

SAMPLE EXERCISES

In this section we will describe two sample exercises from the Phoenix Program, identifying specific ways in which certain of the preceding goals are implemented. The following exercise on verbal abuse is a technique for breaking down denial that one has been abused (Goal 4).

Exercise on Verbal Abuse. This is an emotionally difficult exercise for battered women. However, it is one of the most important exercises in this program because it is designed to break down their denial of being abused. It also improves their understanding of what constitutes abuse. The focus of blame is shifted from the women's behavior to the abusers' behavior. This exercise can reduce not only battered women's shame about being abused, but also the intimidation generated by the strong, derogatory language of verbal abuse.

In order for a battered woman to heal, she needs to realize that the abuse has nothing to do with her, and she needs to be free to be angry and sad about what she has experienced. She needs to face the reality of what she has experienced and separate it from her identity as a person. Therefore, the therapist needs to reframe the woman's experiences and to validate her feelings. The therapist needs to feel comfortable looking at and talking about very graphic and offensive words before undertaking this exercise. The first few times the therapist uses this exercise, he or she may feel shocked or overwhelmed at the amount of abuse.

> *Directions:* Take a blank sheet of paper and write down every name your partner has ever called you and every incidence of verbal abuse, including subtle things. Words like "slut" are obvious, but some batterers are more covert and say things implying you can't cook or drive, and so on. Next to each word or phrase, estimate how many times your partner has said it. So if he has said it 4 times a week for 5 years, multiply 4 x 52(weeks in a year) x 5(years). If he has said it 4 times a month, multiply 4 x 12(months) x 5(years). Then, calculate the total number of

times he has verbally abused you. I understand that this is painful to do, but it is important for you to see the amount of verbal abuse to which you are being subjected.

Some women in the group may object to this exercise by saying they cannot remember, don't know, or don't want to do this. The therapist needs to insist that they should just do the best they can and estimate the number of times they have experienced verbal abuse by their partners. The therapist should make every effort to be empathic to the women's concerns and reactions. It can also be helpful to point that they live with this abuse and that it affects virtually every aspect of their lives.

Table 2 is a sample of what the therapist can expect in this exercise (Peters, 1993, p. 50). The hypothetical person whose responses are shown in Table 2 has been with her partner for 1,460 days (4 years). On average, she has had her self-image and self-esteem attacked 3.5 times a day for the last 4 years. One would expect this woman to be experiencing some serious symptoms. If a woman has been called stupid 624 times, she is likely to feel stupid, to believe she is stupid, and to feel alone in her experience. At this point it is useful to discuss psychological symptoms produced by abuse.

After calculating frequencies, all the women record on the blackboard the names they have been called and the put-downs they have experienced. Names and put-downs used against more than one woman are underlined, one underline for each additional woman. Each woman is then asked how she thinks and feels about what she has recorded and about the composite record. Women typically get upset and cry or get angry. The therapist needs to point out to participants that the more intense their emotional reactions, the greater the healing. Toward the end of the exercise, the women typically begin to laugh as they realize that their partners are basically saying the same things about them, leading the members to comment that they all must be married to the same man. Such laughter is healthy, for it signals psychological distancing from the abusive experience and from the abuser.

TABLE 2: A TYPICAL EXAMPLE SHOWING CALCULATION OF ESTIMATE OF INSTANCES OF VERBAL ABUSE BY ABUSIVE PARTNER

Description	#/day x Wks x Yrs	Total
slut	4 x 52 x 4	832
bitch	5 x 52 x 4	1040
a bad mother	2 x 12 x 4	96
stupid	3 x 52 x 4	624
fat ass	1 x 52 x 4	208
slob	3 x 52 x 4	624
crazy	1 x 52 x 4	208
ugly	2 x 52 x 4	416
you're worth nothing	1 x 52 x 4	48
fucking whore	2 x 52 x 4	416
dumb	2 x 12 x 4	96
can't drive	2 x 52 x 4	416
can't cook	1 x 52 x 4	208
TOTAL		5,232

One of the reasons many therapists fail to effectively treat abused women is because they unwittingly collude in the woman's denial system. This exercise helps both the therapist and client avoid this pitfall by having the client establish a clear, concrete picture of one type of abuse (verbal, as illustrated previously) which she then shares with an empathic group or therapist. Similar exercises can be done with physical, psychological, and sexual abuse. These exercises can be conducted in both group and individual therapy. However, they are more effective in a group context because the women can recognize commonalities in their responses.

Exercise on the Abusive Interaction. This exercise was designed to provide the women with a microscopic analysis of the dynamics of abuse. Ideally, they should leave the group with the ability to identify even subtly abusive interactions. This analysis empowers the women to look for deeper messages than the surface content in a conversation. It reduces their psychological isolation by permitting them to share their trauma with an empathic group, and can help to reduce cognitive distortions associated with Stockholm Syndrome (e.g., self-blame).

Because every woman in the group should write one or more verbal interactions with her abuser on the blackboard, it may take a few sessions to complete this exercise. If a woman comes to group tearful or upset about an interaction with her partner, the group can empathize with her and proceed to this type of analysis. So the technique can be used anytime, once the group has been introduced to it.

Sometimes, during these sessions, members of the group will begin to laugh as they recognize the absurdity of their interactions. This laughter can be healing.

The therapist should have two different colors of chalk: one for the actual conversation and one for its underlying meaning. Large spaces should be left between lines of dialogue for the therapist to later insert the underlying meaning. In the first interaction analyzed in the group, the therapist can take the lead, but the women should do much of the interpretation of subsequent interactions.

Introduction to the exercise: "In this exercise, we are going to analyze actual conversations. I want you to give an example of an interaction with your partner that is relatively short, but that made you feel upset."

During this process, the therapist should ask members of the group what they think about (a) what is really going on in the interaction, (b) when the abuse started (see line 2 in the following example), (c) when he turned the tables and started trying to make her responsible for his behavior, (d) the implied meaning of each line he is saying and what he is doing, and (e) how she is demonstrating Stockholm Syndrome. It is also important that the therapist focus on how the woman felt during each of these interactions.

The following typical sample of a hypothetical dialogue, which would be written on the blackboard, is an interaction from the beginning stages of an abusive relationship (Peters, 1993, p. 55). (Sue and Ted are at a shopping mall. Sue is engaged to Ted.)

Sue: I'd like to buy that rug.
Ted: Go ahead. Spend all our money. You don't have any sense with money.

Here is where the abuse begins. He attacks her self-esteem.

Sue: Well, I work. I pay all my bills. I think I do O.K. with money.

Sue begins a process of self-defense, trying to convince him she is O.K.

(Sue does not buy the rug. They go home.)

She disregards her own feelings and is too intimidated to deal with the real problem: his abusiveness.

Sue: You know, I would really like that rug. I think we can afford it.

Ted: You are such a dumb bitch. You'll probably get fired. Don't you care what I think? This really pisses me off. You can't buy that without me. I'll probably have to pay for it.

His real message here is: Don't cross me. What I want is more important than what you want. I want control.

Sue: Of course I care what you think. I'll buy it with my own money.

Ted: (Turning red) You inconsiderate slut. You are using me for my money. Well, I've got your number. I'll kill you if you buy that rug.

Here he's saying he'll do anything for control, even kill her to maintain his power. He is trying to turn the tables here and blame her for his abusiveness, that is, saying he's abusive because of her attitude.

Sue: You think I'm using you? It's just a rug. I want it.

(He hits her. She goes upstairs and cries. A few hours later. . . .)

Ted: Listen, I'm sorry I hit you. But, we're getting married and need to make decisions together. You can't buy things on your own, without asking me.

Here he blames her for his behavior and minimizes the gravity of his abuse.

Sue: Well, I don't really care about the rug. I guess I should have asked your opinion. I can't believe you hit me.

Sue is trying to placate him but is in shock over his hitting her. Here we see the seeds of Stockholm Syndrome: She begins to adjust her perceptions to fit his as she denies that she wants the rug.

Ted: Don't start again. Let's make up. (He kisses her)

Here his message is twofold: (a) If you cross me, I'll hit you again, and (b) I'm blaming <u>you</u> for <u>my</u> abusive behavior.

A central point of this exercise is that there is *no way* for a victim to ever convince an abuser either to act nonabusively or that, because she is on his side, he does not need to abuse her. These examples expose that his abuse of her has nothing to do with her as a person; he will abuse whomever he is with.

Therapists can make a variety of therapeutic interventions using these conversations. The conversations can be linked to the indicators and psychodynamics of the Stockholm Syndrome. In addition, they can be used to illustrate the cycle of violence (Walker, 1979).

OUTCOME DATA

An outcome pilot study involving over-the-phone interviews was conducted by Peters with about 30 former group members and a small subset (five) of individual therapists of former group members. Findings indicated that about 93% of the women who had completed the Phoenix Program had either separated from their abuser and not returned or otherwise stopped the abuse and not been victimized by other partners. Peters had had some concern that the results would be poorer with time and that many women would return or be victimized by another man. However, she found that the reverse occurred and that the results appeared to improve with time. This delayed improvement suggests once again that separation is a process. In addition, a number of women who left the group prematurely returned months later to complete the program.

Additional research is needed to determine whether Peters' high success rate is due to her personal style or can be replicable by anyone using her program. If replicable by others, the Phoenix Program will be a real boon for practitioners providing managed care, with its emphasis on providing more for less. Therapists interested in the Phoenix Program are invited to contact Quinco Behavioral Health Systems, Lifework Products, Columbus, IN 47202-0628 (Phone: 812-379-2341).

CONCLUSION

Those of us who work in the area of woman abuse must walk a fine line. On the one hand, we must vigilantly guard against this widespread tendency to account for battered women's situations in terms of internal characteristics of the women. Such blame-the-victim attributions have devastating consequences for battered women: They promote the criminal justice system's deafness to the plight of these women and create the belief among battered women that the problem lies in them and thus would remain even if they managed to escape their abusive partners, so why try?

On the other hand, we must guard against taking all control out of the hands of the women. To argue that they do what they do - for example, ask that charges be dropped, stay with the abuser - because the abuser is likely to kill them if they leave can take virtually all control out of the hands of the women. The only choice that may remain is whether to leave the abuser and very likely be killed in the short run or to stay and very likely be killed in the long run.

What does this mean to us as mental health professionals? Although we must recognize the very real situational variables controlling battered women's behavior - including such behaviors as their bonding with their abusers and their pleading with judges to drop the charges against their abusers - we can also recognize those areas within battered women's lives wherein movement is possible.

So where is movement possible? Psychological and physical abuse steadily whittles away at its victims' self. Mental health providers can help women abused by their partners to rebuild their selves. Doing so can help the women to function more independently of their abusers, to oppose their abusers during those times when doing so *might* stop the abuse (e.g., in court), and to develop or redevelop boundaries that might shield them from becoming involved with future abusers.

Violence and threats of violence are often used by abusers to both isolate their victims and to prevent escape. Mental health providers can help reduce that isolation, through both individual and, more particularly, group therapy. Reducing a woman's isolation can help her to maintain or find her own perspective, enabling her to psychologically and emotionally disengage from her abuser. The alternative perspective provided by the therapist and other battered women can enable the woman to see that the abuser, not her own deficiencies, is the reason she is being battered. In other words, there is no way that mental health professions can "save" battered women by causing the abuse to end - only the abuser or the criminal justice system can do that. We *can* help the women prepare psychologically so that they can take maximum advantage of any opportunities afforded them, eventually creating a large enough chink in the prison wall to climb out.

Edna I. Rawlings, PhD, is a professor of Psychology at the University of Cincinnati. She is a clinical psychologist and supervisor at the university's Psychological Services Center and maintains a small private practice. Dr. Rawlings may be contacted at the Psychological Services Center, M.L. 34, University of Cincinnati, Cincinnati, OH 45221-3434.

P. Gail Allen, MA, JP, Distinguished Dissertation Fellow at the University of Cincinnati, is currently collecting data for her dissertation in clinical psychology - a follow-up study of her master's thesis findings reported here. Ms. Allen can be contacted at the Department of Psychology, University of Cincinnati, M.L. 376, Cincinnati, OH 45221-0376.

Dee L. R. Graham, PhD, is an Associate Professor of Psychology at the University of Cincinnati. Dr. Graham may be contacted at the Psychology Department, University of Cincinnati, M.L. 376, Cincinnati, OH 45221-0376.

June Peters, PhD, is a clinical psychologist currently in private practice at the Princeton Adult and Child Center, Cincinnati, Ohio. She specializes in the treatment of abused women and abusive men. Dr. Peters developed the Phoenix Program while she was Supervisor and Director of the Domestic Violence Program at the Clermont Counseling Center, Clermont County, Ohio, between 1989 and 1992. Dr. Peters can be contacted at Princeton Adult and Child Center, 1 Triangle Park, Suite 101, Cincinnati, OH 45246.

RESOURCES

Allen, P. G. (1991). *Separation Issues of Battered Women.* Unpublished master's thesis, University of Cincinnati, Cincinnati, OH.

Dutton, D. G., & Aron, A. P. (1974). Some evidence for heightened sexual attraction under conditions of high anxiety. *Journal of Personality and Social Psychology, 30,* 510-517.

Dutton, D., & Painter, S. L. (1981). Traumatic bonding: The development of emotional attachments in battered women and other relationships of intermittent abuse. *Victimology, 6,* 139-155.

Ferraro, K. J., & Johnson, J. M. (1983). How women experience battering: The process of victimization. *Social Problems, 30,* 325-339.

Gervers, S. (1994). *A Study of the Stockholm Syndrome in Father-Daughter Relationships.* Unpublished master's thesis, University of Cincinnati, Cincinnati, OH.

Graham, D. L. R. (1987). *Loving to Survive: Men and Women as Hostages.* Unpublished manuscript.

Graham, D. L. R., Ihms, K., Rawlings, E. I., Foliano, J., Latimer, D., Thompson, A., Suttman, K., & Farrington, M. (1993). *Stockholm Syndrome in Young Women's Dating Relationships: Factor Structure, Reliability and Concurrent Validity.* Unpublished manuscript, University of Cincinnati, Cincinnati, OH.

Graham, D. L. R., Ott, B., & Rawlings, E. I. (1990). *Stockholm Syndrome and Battered Women: A Test of the Validity of Graham's Stockholm Syndrome Theory.* Unpublished manuscript, University of Cincinnati, Cincinnati, OH.

Graham, D. L. R., & Rawlings, E. I. (1991). Bonding with abusive dating partners: Dynamics of Stockholm Syndrome. In B. Levy (Ed.), *Dating Violence: Young Women in Danger* (pp. 119-135). Seattle, WA: Seal Press.

Graham, D. L. R., Rawlings, E. I., & Rigsby, R. (1994). *Loving to Survive: Sexual Terror, Men's Violence, and Women's Lives.* New York: New York University Press.

Graham, D. L. R., Rawlings, E. I., & Rimini, N. (1988). Survivors of terror: Battered women, hostages and the Stockholm Syndrome. In K. Yllo & M. Bograd (Eds.), *Feminist Perspectives on Wife Abuse* (pp. 217-233). Beverly Hills: Sage.

Kemp, A. (1991). *Incidence and Correlates of Post-Trauma Responses in Battered Women.* Unpublished doctoral thesis, University of Cincinnati, Cincinnati, OH.

Kemp, A., Rawlings, E. I., & Green, B. (1991). Post-traumatic stress disorder (PTSD) in battered women: A shelter sample. *Journal of Traumatic Stress, 4,* 137-148.

Lang, D. (1974, November 25). A reporter at large: The bank drama. *New Yorker,* pp. 56-126.

"My fault, maimed woman says." (1993, November 13). *The Cincinnati Post,* p. A2.

Naber-Morris, A. (1990). *Stockholm Syndrome in Adult Abused Children: A Scale Validation Project.* Unpublished doctoral dissertation, University of Cincinnati, Cincinnati, OH.

Okun, L. (1986). *Woman Abuse: Facts Replacing Myths.* New York: State University of New York Press.

Peters, J. (1993). *The Phoenix Program: Healing Therapy for Abused Women.* Columbus, IN: Quinco Behavioral Health Systems, Lifework Products.

Rimini, N. (1988, February). *The Stockholm Syndrome in Victims of Domestic Violence: Practical Implications.* Paper presented at the Butler County Domestic Violence Coalition, Hamilton, OH.

Schachter, S., & Singer, J. E. (1962). Cognitive, social, and physiological components of the emotional state. *Psychological Review, 69,* 379-399.

Strube, M. J. (1988). The decision to leave an abusive relationship: Empirical evidence and theoretical issues. *Psychological Bulletin, 104,* 236-250.

Walker, L. E. (1979). *The Battered Woman.* New York: Harper & Row.

Walster, E. (1971). Passionate love. In B. I Murstein (Ed.), *Theories of Attraction and Love* (pp. 85-99). New York: Springer.

Walster, E., & Berscheid, E. (1971, June). Adrenaline makes the heart grow fonder. *Psychology Today, 5,* 46-50, 62.

DISABLED CLIENTS: WHAT EVERY THERAPIST NEEDS TO KNOW

Sandra K. Brodwin, Leo M. Orange, and Martin G. Brodwin

People with disabilities represent a large section of our population. It is estimated that there are more than 43 million people who have disabilities and disabling conditions in the United States (West, 1991). The recent passage of the Americans With Disabilities Act (ADA; Public Law 101-336, 1990) is providing increased opportunities for these individuals. The ADA is antidiscrimination legislation that covers the following areas: employment, public services, accessibility, transportation, and telecommunications. Its intent is to allow people with disabilities full access and equal opportunities in all phases of life. According to Kay and Glatz (1992), the provisions of the ADA have two major purposes: (a) to decrease attitudinal barriers in society and (b) to decrease physical (architectural) barriers.

This contribution is composed of four sections. The first section, "Issues of Clients With Disabilities," discusses the following subjects: reactions to a catastrophic injury or a chronic illness; social, emotional, and physical restrictions; locus of control as related to disability; and self-efficacy of clients with disabilities. The second section discusses terminology and language regarding persons with disabilities and the effects of negative societal attitudes. "Implications in the Counseling Process," Section 3, provides concepts for practitioners in the areas of counseling skills, individual and family counseling issues, and the impact of disability. The final section offers suggestions to practitioners when working with clients who have disabilities.

ISSUES OF CLIENTS WITH DISABILITIES

REACTIONS TO CATASTROPHIC INJURY (LOSS) OR CHRONIC ILLNESS

A catastrophic injury or loss or a chronic illness causes a crisis in the life of the individual which extends to his or her support network. It is a crisis in that the coping mechanisms typically used do not effectively help the person deal with the situation. The "process of adaptation" (Beardmore, 1993; Shontz, 1975) involves the various phases an individual may go through in coping with catastrophic illness or injury. The three primary stages of emotional responses are (a) the pre-impact stage, (b) the impact stage, and (c) the post-impact stage. Within each of these phases are several substages. Not every person will encounter each phase or go through the same sequence of phases.

Pre-Impact Phase. This is the initial phase. It involves the prelude and warning substages (Shontz, 1975). Persons with chronic, progressive illnesses typically experience this particular phase. During the prelude substage, the client attempts to use current coping mechanisms to explain the first signs of a serious illness. The warning substage is a time when the client is vacillating among denial of the seriousness of the illness, rationalization of the symptoms, and accepting the diagnosis. At this time the client attempts to modify prior coping strategies to fit the current crisis, which produces a high level of tension.

The practitioner can be of assistance during the pre-impact phase by aiding the client in identifying coping mechanisms. Also useful at this time is the clinician's ability to be empathic and understanding. As the client shifts among denial, rationalization, and acceptance, the clinician can encourage the client to identify these reactions. Given this identification, and the ensuing tension, the clinician assists the client in developing additional coping strategies.

Impact Phase. The impact phase (Shontz, 1975) is the time when there is a definite diagnosis of a chronic illness or the onset of a catastrophic injury. This phase consists of the shock and encounter substages. Typically, shock occurs when there is no prolonged onset of illness, such as in the crisis of a traumatic injury. During the shock substage, the practitioner needs to be listening in an active and involved manner in order to establish rapport necessary for a professional relationship to develop. During the encounter substage, the client begins to acknowledge the reality of the injury or illness. Feelings that the client may experience during this substage include anxiety, depression, panic, disorganization, helplessness, anger, and loss of control. The role of the practitioner during this time is to demonstrate empathy and understanding, allowing the client the opportunity to display each of the emotions being experienced, as this is part of the healing process.

Post-Impact Phase. The third phase, post-impact, consists of two substages, defensive retreat and adaptation (Shontz, 1975). In the first substage, defensive retreat, the individual may withdraw. This is a sign that the realization of the consequences of the serious illness or injury are more than can be dealt with at this time. By withdrawing, the client avoids feeling overwhelmed, and is denying or avoiding the reality of the situation. The practitioner may best assist the client to face reality by being empathic, understanding, and accepting of the presenting emotions. The second substage of the post-impact phase is acknowledgment. It is during this time that the client begins to understand the illness or injury and the resulting limitations. As these limitations become apparent, some clients experience depression. Symptoms that may indicate the client is experiencing depression include loss of energy, insomnia, loss of appetite, loss of interest in activities, poor attention and concentration, and loss of sexual desire. The practitioner must be cautious not to confuse this depression with lack of motivation so as not to confound treatment.

The symptoms of depression during this stage may present as suicidal ideation and intent. Suicidal ideation is fairly common among persons who have severe disabilities. However, there is a considerable distinction between suicidal ideation and suicide intent. The practitioner needs to ask the client direct questions to determine if there is a plan for suicide and if the client has the means to carry it out. If it is determined that the client is seriously considering suicide, it is necessary for the practitioner to immediately take appropriate action (VandeCreek & Knapp, 1993). There are occasions when the appropriate mental health professional will be the practitioner. However, if the practitioner is not fully qualified to address the issues raised once a diagnosis of depression has been made, it is in the client's best interest to be referred to a mental health professional. If there is no plan of suicide, it is necessary for the practitioner to discuss the client's feelings, to show understanding and empathy and assist the client in establishing short-term goals that can be accomplished and will provide the client with successful experiences and a sense of control.

The final stage of the "process of adaptation" (Beardmore, 1993) is the adaptation stage. This occurs when the client is able to focus on abilities that can be used to function at full potential. This is where the practitioner can empower the client to determine realistic goals for daily living and possible employment.

Practitioners must be cognizant of these phases and substages in order to provide individual services that address the needs of clients with severe disabilities at any particular point in the adaptation process. If the mental and intellectual needs of the client are not addressed during the adaptation process, permanent social and emotional restrictions may occur as a result of physical or mental restrictions brought on by chronic illness or catastrophic, traumatic injury.

SOCIAL, EMOTIONAL, AND PHYSICAL RESTRICTIONS

The following factors relate to the adjustment process of a person with permanent limitations from a chronic illness or catastrophic injury: (a) the number and length of hospitalizations; (b) symptoms that limit mobility; (c) feelings of being alone, alienated, and isolated; (d) excessive feelings of anger, anxiety, and depression; (e) use of mechanical or assistive devices; (f) change of roles within relationships due to the disability; and (g) changes in financial, family, vocational, and sexual functioning (Buckelew, Baumstark, & Frank, 1990). Also, social rejection and avoidance from others as well as isolation caused by the disability may cause the person with a disability to reject offers of help that place demands on others for support and assistance. Practitioners may view this as a lack of motivation and discontinue assisting these clients in their efforts to adapt to the disabling condition (Elliott et al., 1990).

Issues affecting life satisfaction involve a combination of age, health, education, marriage, and employment. In ranking feelings of life satisfaction, persons with disabilities who felt they were unable to be involved in daily activities or seek gainful employment reported the lowest level of life satisfaction. Those persons who felt limited in the amount or type of work or daily activities in which they could be involved noted the second lowest life satisfaction. Third lowest life satisfaction was noted by the group of persons who were limited in sports, social and community life, and family life. Persons who needed to rely on assistance from others for activities of daily living such as bathing, dressing, getting in and out of bed, or doing household chores also reported low life satisfaction, as did persons needing mechanical or assistive devices for going outside or walking. Persons with disabilities who were gainfully employed reported the highest life satisfaction (Mehnert et al., 1990).

LOCUS OF CONTROL

An individual's perception of disability affects his or her locus of control. Fourteen percent of working-age African-Americans have disabilities; of those, only 16% are employed (Belgrave & Walker, 1991). Self-concept and confidence are critical factors for employment success of persons with disabilities. Persons with disabilities whose locus of control is seen as external (such as when they interface with the medical system) view the outcome as being determined by luck, fate, or other people's influence. This may lead the client to assume no responsibility and give up. When the client is actively involved (internal locus of control), the outcome is thought to be owned by the client. This means the client is sanctioned to assume responsibility for the recovery and employment. It must be understood that the client may choose not to assume locus of control.

A facilitative role by physicians, family members, practitioners, and the community helps the client internalize the locus of control. This type of support is a key factor in favorable employment and life satisfaction of persons with disabilities. The Americans With Disabilities Act (ADA), passed in 1990, provides for accessibility of public transportation for persons with disabilities. Inaccessible transportation has been reported as one of the main reasons why persons with disabilities have not entered the labor force.

CLIENT SELF-EFFICACY

What Is Self-Efficacy? Efficacy expectations concern a person's beliefs about his or her ability to undertake given tasks. Outcome expectations are concerned with a person's beliefs about whether the outcomes of effort will be beneficial or not. Both efficacy and outcome expectations must be high for persons to attempt tasks toward rehabilitation during chronic illness or after catastrophic injury or loss. Self-efficacy consists of four essential elements as discussed below (Bandura, 1982; M. G. Brodwin & S. K. Brodwin, 1993; Mitchell, M. G. Brodwin, & Benoit, 1990).

Elements of Self-Efficacy. First, self-efficacy is enhanced when a person is aware of the behavior required to produce a given outcome (the person knows what to do and how to do it). The practitioner can help by explaining what a client can do to improve an aspect of life and how to go about it. We often assume individuals with chronic illness or catastrophic injury or loss know the "how to," but this is not always the case. It appears that more time spent working with clients on the steps of "how to" is often needed.

Mental health practitioners, counselors, and medical professionals are all part of the overall rehabilitation team that needs to assist in this process of helping the client understand the "what and how to" of recovery. One method of achieving this is through having the client identify behavioral objectives with the assistance of the practitioner. Behavioral objectives may help the client in realizing the necessary steps to take toward adaptation to the disability. As practitioners, we frequently assume the individual knows what will happen next and we are often incorrect. When clients fail in achieving one of the steps toward recovery, we may assume, correctly or incorrectly, that they are not motivated.

The second element of self-efficacy is that clients appraise their capabilities and develop confidence in their ability to do particular tasks. Members of the health-care team work with the practitioner and the client in establishing these behavioral goals. When the client participates in the identification of goals and setting the pace of achieving these goals, he or she is involved in the outcome expectations. This, in turn, increases the client's self-efficacy.

An increase of self-efficacy reinforces a client's level of confidence. To accomplish this element of self-efficacy, the practitioner must be skilled at breaking complicated behavior into small-enough segments so that the client's confidence is strengthened at critical points. Breaking seemingly impossible tasks into small, easily achieved units effectively builds an individual's level of confidence. If an individual will not act, or has ceased to act, even with adequate incentives and outcome expectancies, this loss of confidence can most likely be attributed to the perception of excessive task difficulty or loss of self-image due to the perceived functional limitations. The task must then be analyzed and reduced to manageable units.

The third element of self-efficacy is that the client perceives a functional relationship between behavior (taking action) and the attainability of the outcome (the individual believes that what he or she does will have an impact on how things turn out). The practitioner needs to stress the functional relationship between the locus of control process and successful adaptation to disability. Active involvement of the client in the early stages will help facilitate this process. The individual needs to see the connection between positive actions and attainability of control. The client with a disability is not just a passive recipient, but an active participant in determining outcome. "Locus of control" is within the client, not the practitioner, medical system, insurance system, or family system.

The fourth element of self-efficacy states that the outcome needs to be of sufficient importance to the client that he or she will actually seek it (the individual wants what the outcome will provide). This directly relates to the adaptation stage, when the client is focusing on abilities, not limitations.

This element also points out the importance of client choice in planning the rehabilitation goals and objectives. The client must be involved in the decision-making process in order to accomplish the process of adaptation. The eventual goal, of course, needs to be a joint decision between practitioner and client. If the client does not feel the proposed rehabilitation program is at least partially his or her choice, however, efforts to succeed may be less than optimal.

Interaffective Effects. Figure 1 (p. 423; Bandura, 1982) presents a grid which is useful in exploring various self-efficacy configurations and their corresponding patterns of behavior. In

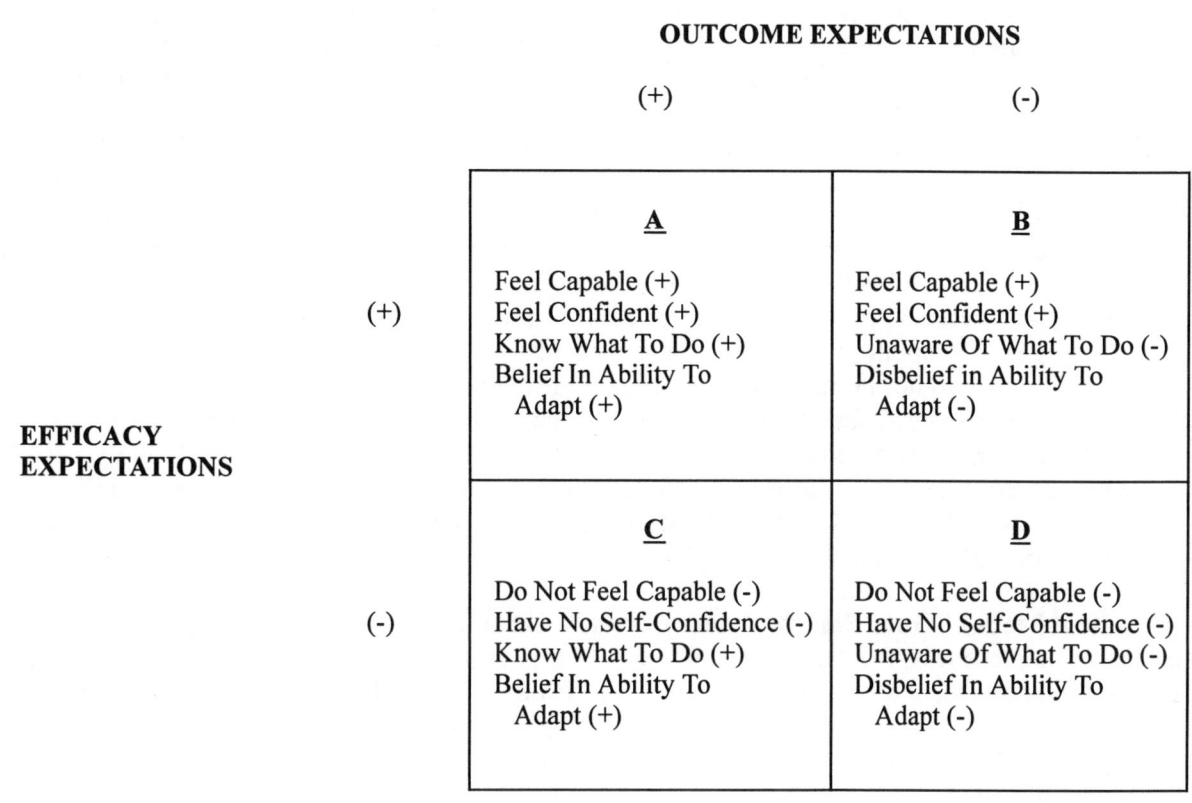

Figure 1. Interactive effects of efficacy ratings
and outcome expectations (adapted from Bandura, 1982).

Figure 1, all possible combinations of high (+) and low (-) efficacy and outcome expectations are presented.

It is our contention, based on the preceding matrix, that unless individuals with disabilities have both high efficacy and high outcome expectations, they are not likely to complete the adaptation process or benefit fully from all services provided. However, counseling services would be beneficial in that these services can help move a client from one of the three nondesirable expectations (Squares B, C, and D of Figure 1) to a desirable expectation (Square A).

Case Study. How does an individual with a severe disability lose self-efficacy? A client, Ms. Deborah Swilie,* was involved in a motorcycle accident and seriously injured her lower extremities. At the time, she was employed by ABC Electric Company as a journeyman electrician. It appeared that Ms. Swilie would not be able to walk without the use of an assistive device. She was hospitalized for 2 weeks and is still receiving medical treatment, physical therapy, and rehabilitation. Her young children frequently ask her when she will be able to do the activities with them she did before the occurrence of the accident. Ms. Swilie's husband, supportive at first, gradually begins to express doubt and concern because of their deteriorating finances and the impact of this situation, especially on the children. Further diminishing of efficacy occurs as this client remains unemployed and no professional is assigned to discuss the possibilities of returning to work. She begins to lose confidence in her abilities and gradually loses skills and abilities the longer she remains away from active employment, socialization, and family interactions.

---

*Names and all identifying characteristics of persons in all case examples have been disguised thoroughly to protect privacy.

This client's outcome expectations are diminished as the insurance company providing disability benefits views her case from a disability standpoint, rather than an ability perspective. The treating and evaluating physicians place physical and emotional limitations on her. These limitations include the inability to walk without the use of a cane, the inability to lift and carry more than 15 pounds, and moderately severe anxiety and depression. Ms. Swilie's functional skills and abilities are further eroded, and her confidence is further reduced. To resolve cognitive dissonance, the client begins to tell herself and others, "See how disabled I really am."

The client is finally assigned to a clinical practitioner. By now, the adjectives in both Square C and Square D of Figure 1 may be appropriate. Many clients who have been diagnosed with chronic illness or severe disability show signs and symptoms of loss of self-image, helplessness, feelings of incompetence, giving up locus of control, unwillingness to try, and depression during the initial stages of adaptation. They do not feel capable or confident, are unaware of what can be done to adjust, and do not believe psychological adjustment is possible. Occasionally, practitioners see clients in Square A (see Figure 1), who feel capable, are confident, know what to do, and believe in the possibility of adapting to the disabilities. These individuals are relatively easy to work with and are likely to succeed. The client who has developed low self-efficacy, on the other hand, may be difficult to work with and the chances for a successful outcome are greatly diminished (Bandura, 1982; Mitchell et al., 1990).

Medical Model Versus Self-Sufficiency Model. Disability has often been considered synonymous with helplessness; the "handicapped role" in this country has been viewed as one of helplessness, dependence, and passivity (Fine & Asch, 1988). The tendency "has been to view people with disabilities as (a) victimized by a disability condition and (b) in need of treatment - not of rights" (Biklen, 1988, p. 128). This is based, in part, on the fact that people with disabilities have received treatment under the medical model instead of a self-sufficiency model, which involves focusing on the client's abilities to achieve maximum productivity and mainstreaming into the social environment. The medical model sees the physician as the expert and the primary decision maker in the care of the person. The patient is to assume the "sick" role. This exempts the client from assuming responsibility (loss of locus of control) and prevents normal social activities. Individuals learn to accept dependency under the sick role and give up assuming responsibility for their own needs (Nosek, 1992).

TERMINOLOGY, LANGUAGE, AND ATTITUDES

NONDISABLING LANGUAGE

Practitioners need to use "nondisabling language" when referring to people with disabilities. More than a decade of rehabilitation literature has called attention to the use of imprecise, stereotypical, and devaluing language when discussing people with disabilities and disabling conditions (Bowe, 1978; Hadley & M. G. Brodwin, 1988; Kailes, 1985; LaForge, 1991; Patterson, 1988). Language should be precise and convey a person's intended meaning in an exact and unambiguous manner. "Wheelchair-bound" and "confined to a wheelchair" are examples of imprecise and devaluing language. A person is not "bound" or "confined" to a wheelchair; rather, the wheelchair serves as the individual's source of mobility. In fact, the wheelchair provides a very positive service. Affirmative terminology in this case would be "a person who uses a wheelchair." The use of imprecise language can give one the feeling of decreased capability and diminished power (Hadley & M. G. Brodwin, 1988).

Words such as "victim" and "sufferer" should not be used because of the negative innuendoes and passive connotations of these and similar words. Although it is true that the issue of terminology is partially the choice of the client, the practitioner is the professional. This person can set the tone of the working relationship by the language used in addressing the client. Although the exact relationship between language terminology and attitudes is still unclear (LaForge, 1991), the Americans With Disabilities Act of 1990 strongly encourages the use of language that places the person first and the disability second.

ATTITUDES

In the past, persons with disabilities were referred to as "handicapped." This label has many negative connotations and portrays people as weak, ineffective, and powerless. "Disabled person" was the terminology that replaced handicapped; it was felt that the term "disabled" was less negative. Recently, the recommended terminology has changed from referring to people as disabled to calling them "persons with disabilities." In this way, the emphasis is on the person, rather than on the disability. The person is seen as an individual with various characteristics (many of them positive), rather than simply as a disabled person. "A person with mental retardation" is preferred terminology over "mentally retarded"; "a person with an amputation" is preferred over "amputee."

Misunderstandings between nondisabled people and people with disabilities frequently occur in everyday social interactions. Practitioners need to do their best to minimize the chances of misunderstandings occurring between their clients and themselves. According to Makas (1988), persons with disabilities and nondisabled people differed significantly in their perceptions of what is the most positive attitude toward persons with disabilities.

In this research study, respondents with disabilities felt that positive attitudes involved either totally dispensing with the category of disability or in promoting the rights of persons with disabilities. Respondents without disabilities felt that positive attitudes involved a desire to be nice, to be helpful, and ultimately to place the person with a disability in a "needy" situation. Although the respondents without disabilities felt they were doing their best to be helpful, persons with disabilities often took these actions and attitudes as offensive. Two examples cited by Makas (1988) are illustrative.

> Doris goes to her friend's house for a game of Trivial Pursuit. Much to Doris' surprise, she finds that one member of the group, Suzanne, is blind. Determined to show Suzanne that she is not prejudiced against people with disabilities, when Suzanne mistakenly names Portland as the capital of Maine, Doris insists that Suzanne be given another chance. Suzanne responds angrily that she can do well in the game without Doris' help, and that Doris should mind her own business. Doris decides that she will never again try to be polite to people who have disabilities.
>
> Mike learns that Rick, the new employee hired by his company, has a physical disability. He stops by Rick's office to welcome him. He tells Rick that he is looking forward to getting to know him, since he has always considered disabled people to be easy-going and very courageous. Rick tells Mike to get out of his office and slams the door behind him. Mike decides that disabled people are not so nice after all. (pp. 49-50)

Learning occurs through communication. Communications between people often become distorted. As in the examples cited previously, a person may be attempting to openly communicate a particular feeling, but the recipient perceives this communication in a different way, based upon certain needs, feelings, past history, and opinions about the other person. There are possibilities for misperceptions at any point in the communication. The person wants to be seen as friendly, open, and caring, but is instead perceived as unfriendly, hostile, and aggressive.

Makas (1988) suggested that people without disabilities need to be educated about areas in which their behaviors offend persons with disabilities. Persons with disabilities also need to work with nondisabled people in correcting, but not overreacting to, those statements and accompanying behaviors. Overall, persons with disabilities want equality through civil rights, not special treatment afforded because of disability.

IMPLICATIONS IN THE COUNSELING PROCESS

COUNSELING SKILLS

Clinicians use counseling skills and techniques daily when working with clients. It should be emphasized that these same abilities and techniques are effective when counseling clients with disabilities. When counseling a person who has a disability, if the disability is not related to the subject matter at hand, it is usually not discussed. Persons with disabilities seek counseling for many problem areas that are unrelated to their disability.

A practitioner may need to assist a client in "owning" management of personal issues. This may be necessary when a disability seems to be controlling the client, rather than the client maintaining control of the disability. People with disabilities learn to control and manage their disabling conditions just as all people need to learn management over the many issues in their lives.

Sympathy involves sharing common feelings or mutual understanding. It also may involve feelings or expressions of pity or charity, therefore, it is inappropriate in the counseling context. Empathy, however, is the identification with and understanding of another's situation, feelings, or motives. Further, it means participating in the inner world of another while remaining yourself (Berenson & Carkhuff, 1967). "The empathic interviewer explores with the interviewee the latter's internal world of thought and feeling so that the interviewee may come close to his own world, his own self" (Benjamin, 1981, p. 50).

To understand a client's world, the practitioner must get in contact with that world. "If attending and listening are the skills that enable helpers to get in touch with the world of the client, then empathy is the skill that enables them to communicate their understanding of this world" (Egan, 1990, p. 126). It is of utmost importance that, when counseling clients with disabilities, the practitioner remember the differences between sympathy and empathy. Expressions of empathy typically are accepted by clients and are beneficial; feelings of sympathy are often inappropriate and are rejected.

Some clients with disabilities will need help in surmounting environmental barriers. The Americans With Disabilities Act requires that all new building construction and alterations to existing facilities be fully accessible. This includes public transportation services, as well as social programs, recreational facilities, and employment sites. It also requires that telecommunications systems be accessible to people with hearing and speech impairments. Telephone companies must provide telecommunication relay services for hearing-impaired and speech-impaired persons 24 hours a day. Clinicians who are cognizant of the provisions of the Americans With Disabilities Act can provide guidance to their clients. They also can furnish resources to the client for assistance in obtaining services within the provisions of the Act. One such service is provided by the Job Accommodation Network (JAN). This is a resource facility which will answer questions regarding accommodations in the workplace. The telephone number for JAN is (800) 526-7234. This is a free service providing information about employment issues to employers, practitioners, and people with disabilities.

INDIVIDUAL AND FAMILY COUNSELING ISSUES

The family has been defined as the most important institution in society. This is particularly apparent for persons with disabilities as the patterns of development, self-identity, and ability are often influenced by the family environment. Family concerns are crucial because families, like individuals, have different coping capabilities. Nagler (1990) reported that the attitude and adjustment of the family to the disability is often instrumental in providing the family member with a disability insulation from social barriers (discrimination) that will be encountered in society.

Many families can maintain a state of positive adjustment and equilibrium with the support and understanding of skilled professionals to cope with the difficulties associated with disability status.

Many authors comment on the importance of the family in determining the outcome of rehabilitation efforts. Harris et al., (1973) believe that the family helps determine the reaction and eventual adjustment of the patient to the disability. The quality of the interpersonal relationships within the family can be as important as the disability itself. If the family communicates positive attitudes of worth to the person with a disability, a positive self-concept can be reinforced. This increases the likelihood that the individual will participate in the rehabilitation process. If rehabilitation efforts fail for no apparent reason, it is suggested that dynamics within the family be thoroughly examined (Lowe & Carroll, 1985).

Vargo (1984) and Vargo and Stewin (1984) studied the wives of males with spinal-cord injuries regarding the process of coping with their husbands' disabilities. The information provided from this research identified recurrent themes indicative of the process of coping and adapting. Initially, there was fear, primarily involving images of the husband's potential death. During the early months after onset, interpersonal support from family and friends was of critical importance to these women. It was during this time that the wives felt that they had to be controlled and emotionally strong when interacting with their husbands who were involved in their own emotional coping processes; this was often encouraged by hospital personnel. However, these women were often denied their own emotional needs. This points out the importance of involving family members in the counseling process. Practitioners may want to make sure that family members who need help in coping mechanisms are not neglected when addressing the issues of disability with the client.

IMPACT OF DISABILITY

DeLoach and Greer (1981) reported that the onset of a physical disability imposes a series of lifestyle adjustments on the family. One of these adjustments involves the pace of life. The person with a physical disability will require more time to perform many of the basic activities of life; this may become frustrating to the other family members. A tendency to assist the person with the disability "just so we can get ready faster" can ultimately add to the disability by undermining the individual's progress toward independence (Trieschmann, 1988).

Another impact of the disability is the allocation of income. Life with a disability can impose a financial burden on the individual and the family. Persons with disabilities show higher rates of unemployment and underemployment when compared to persons without disabilities. Furthermore, the family often experiences a decline in social and leisure-time activities. Initially, after the onset of disability, some friends tend to drift away because they cannot handle the disability. Thus, the individual, couple, or family members may find themselves eliminated from their former social circle because of the reaction of others to the disability.

Living with a physical disability assaults one's personal identity and the lives of others in the support group. The individual with a disability and family members do not necessarily have to be happy with the disability, but they do need to feel they have the power to direct their lives. One of the processes of coping with a disability involves adaptation to disability. One of the family's most important functions in the rehabilitation process is supporting the social adjustment of the individual with the disability in dealing with avocational or recreational issues. The family can help the individual with the disability learn to use leisure time productively. Having hobbies or returning to social activities helps in the adjustment to a normal life (Crewe & Krause, 1987; Orange, M. G. Brodwin, & Johnson, 1993; Trieschmann, 1988; Vash, 1981).

SUGGESTIONS FOR PRACTITIONERS

1. Always use nondisabling language when referring to people with disabilities, whether the discussion is with someone who has a disability or with nondisabled people.

2. Negative attitudes pose one of the most significant barriers for persons who have disabilities. A practitioner's positive attitudes and behavior can be a model for other professionals and for society at large.
3. Although initial attitudes toward persons with disabilities are often influenced by disability-related characteristics, after interaction with a person who has a disability, the disability characteristics become less important and personal characteristics become more important (Yuker, 1992).
4. When counseling a person with a disability, if the disability is not related to the subject matter, it need not be discussed, unless the practitioner needs a clearer understanding of the condition to provide appropriate services to the client.
5. A person who has a disability usually feels comfortable discussing the disability and related issues. However, not everyone with a disability is at ease discussing it. If a question related to the disability arises, a practitioner should use professional judgment in addressing the issue. The practitioner, however, does want the client to feel that he or she is comfortable addressing issues related to the disability.
6. Focus on what the client can do, not on what he or she cannot do. One needs to emphasize an individual's capabilities, not his or her limitations.
7. Make sure your offices are fully accessible to persons with disabilities. If not, attempt to have physical (architectural) barriers removed or modified. The Americans With Disabilities Act requires that accommodations be provided, including removal of architectural barriers, so that persons with disabilities can participate fully in all phases of society and life. This includes access to the offices of practitioners in private practice.
8. Practitioners involved in helping persons with disabilities to secure employment need to be aware that research (Yuker, 1992) has shown that employers value employees who have job skills, have social skills, and are dependable. Employers who have had experiences with employees who have disabilities usually have positive attitudes, particularly toward the disability types with which they are familiar.
9. If unsure about a particular issue regarding disability, a practitioner may want to consult a rehabilitation psychologist or counselor familiar with that disability or disability-related issue. It is suggested the practitioner also utilize information from the client relating to the disability; the person with the disability often has the most extensive information.
10. The practitioner may want to become more familiar with the recently enacted Americans With Disabilities Act. One may do this by attending professional workshops or by obtaining one of the many available published resources on the subject (see "Resources").
11. The practitioner must be sensitive to attitudinal barriers. These barriers will be observed in the manner in which the public interacts with a person with a disability. Attitudinal barriers are encountered when meeting with an employer in an attempt to return a person with a disability to work when the employer has had no experience in working with people with disabilities. The practitioner can provide flexible and innovative services addressing these attitudinal barriers.

Sandra K. Brodwin, MS, CRC, CCCC, has a Master of Science Degree in education from Drake University in Des Moines, Iowa, and a Master of Science Degree in counseling from California State University, Los Angeles. She was certified as a rehabilitation counselor (CRC) in 1981, and as a community college counselor (CCCC) in 1990. Ms. Brodwin currently is the Assessment Center Manager in the Job Training Partnership Act (JTPA) program with the cities of Glendale, LaCañada, and Burbank, California, where she works with individuals who have multiple barriers to employment. She is also a vocational expert for the Social Security Administration and a part-time lecturer in the rehabilitation services program at California State University. Ms. Brodwin may be contacted at 9181 E. Arcadia Avenue, San Gabriel, CA 91775.

Leo M. Orange, MS, is a rehabilitation counselor with Liebman and Associates in Northridge, California. He received his Master of Science Degree in rehabilitation counseling from California State University, Los Angeles. His areas of specialization include workers' compensation injuries, long-term disability, and consultation on the Americans With Disabilities Act. Mr. Orange received a pre-doctoral scholarship from California State University, Los Angeles, and will be attending doctoral studies in counseling/educational psychology. Mr. Orange can be contacted at 2870 White Ridge Place, #13, Thousand Oaks, CA 91362.

Martin G. Brodwin, PhD, CRC, is an Associate Professor and Coordinator of the Rehabilitation Education Programs at California State University, Los Angeles. He received his PhD in rehabilitation counseling from Michigan State University in East Lansing, Michigan, and became a certified rehabilitation counselor (CRC) in 1975. He currently serves on the Commission on Standards and Accreditation of the Council on Rehabilitation Education (CORE) and as a vocational expert for the Social Security Administration. Dr. Brodwin may be contacted at California State University, Division of Administration and Counseling, 5151 State University Drive, Los Angeles, CA 90032.

RESOURCES

CITED RESOURCES

Bandura, A. (1982). Self-efficacy mechanism in human agencies. *American Psychologist, 37*, 122-147.

Beardmore, C. (1993). Coping with physical disability - A biopsychosocial approach. In M. G. Brodwin, F. A. Tellez, & S. K. Brodwin (Eds.), *Medical, Psychosocial and Vocational Aspects of Disability* (pp. 107-111). Athens, GA: Elliott & Fitzpatrick.

Belgrave, F. Z., & Walker, S. (1991). Predictors of employment outcome of Black persons with disabilities. *Rehabilitation Psychology, 36*, 111-119.

Benjamin, A. (1981). *The Helping Interview* (3rd ed.). Boston: Houghton Mifflin.

Berenson, B., & Carkhuff, R. (1967). *Beyond Counseling and Psychotherapy.* New York: Holt, Rinehart, and Winston.

Biklen, D. (1988). The myth of clinical judgment. *Journal of Social Issues, 44*, 127-140.

Bowe, F. (1978). *Handicapping America: Barriers to Disabled People.* New York: Harper & Row.

Brodwin, M. G., & Brodwin, S. K. (1993). Rehabilitation: A case study approach. In M. G. Brodwin, F. A. Tellez, & S. K. Brodwin (Eds.), *Medical, Psychosocial and Vocational Aspects of Disability* (pp. 1-19). Athens, GA: Elliott & Fitzpatrick.

Buckelew, S. P., Baumstark, K. E., & Frank, R. G. (1990). Adjustment following spinal cord injury. *Rehabilitation Psychology, 35*, 101-109.

Crewe, N., & Krause, J. S. (1987). Spinal cord injury: Psychological aspects. In B. Caplan (Ed.), *Rehabilitation Psychology Desk Reference* (pp. 3-35). Rockville, MD: Aspen.

DeLoach, C., & Greer, B. (1981). *Adjustment to Severe Disability: A Metamorphosis.* New York: McGraw Hill.

Egan, G. (1990). *The Skilled Helper: A Systematic Approach to Effective Helping* (4th ed.). Pacific Grove, CA: Brooks/Cole.

Elliott, T. R., Frank, R. G., Corcoran, J., Beardon, L., & Byrd, E. K. (1990). Previous personal experience and reactions to depression and physical disability. *Rehabilitation Psychology, 35*, 111-119.

Fine, M., & Asch, A. (1988). Disability beyond stigma: Social interaction, discrimination, and activism. *Journal of Social Issues, 44*, 3-21.

Hadley, R. G., & Brodwin, M. G. (1988). Language about people with disabilities. *Journal of Counseling and Development, 67*, 147-149.

Harris, P., Patel, S., Greer, W., & Naughton, J. (1973). Psychological and social reactions to acute spinal paralysis. *Journal of Paraplegia, 11*, 132-136.

Kailes, J. (1985). Watch your language, please! *Journal of Rehabilitation, 51*, 68-69.

Kay, C., & Glatz, W. (Producers). (1992). *Americans With Disabilities Act: Facts and Fears* [Videotape]. Grand Rapids, MI: Cynthia Kay/Wayne Glatz Film & Video.

LaForge, J. (1991). Preferred language practice in professional rehabilitation journals. *Journal of Rehabilitation, 57*, 49-51.

Lowe, J., & Carroll, D. (1985). The effects of spinal injury on the intensity of emotional experience. *Journal of Clinical Psychology, 24*, 135-136.

Makas, E. (1988). Positive attitudes toward disabled people: Disabled and non-disabled persons' perspectives. *Journal of Social Issues, 44*, 49-61.

Mehnert, T., Krauss, H. H., Nadler, R., & Boyd, M. (1990). Correlates of life satisfaction in those with disabling conditions. *Rehabilitation Psychology, 35*, 3-17.

Mitchell, L. K., Brodwin, M. G., & Benoit, R. B. (1990). Strengthening the workers' compensation system by increasing client efficacy. *Journal of Applied Rehabilitation Counseling, 21*, 22-26.

Nagler, M. (1990). *Perspectives on Disability.* Palo Alto, CA: Health Market Research.

Nosek, M. A. (1992). Independent living. In R. M. Parker & E. M. Szymanski (Eds.), *Rehabilitation Counseling: Basics and Beyond* (2nd ed., pp. 103-133). Austin, TX: Pro-ed.

Orange, L. M., Brodwin, M. G., & Johnson, S. (1993). Early intervention to facilitate employment of persons with spinal cord injury. *California Association for Counseling and Development Journal, 13*, 9-15.

Patterson, J. B. (1988). Disabling language: Fact or fiction? *Journal of Applied Rehabilitation Counseling, 19*, 30-32.

Shontz, F. C. (1975). *The Psychological Aspects of Physical Illness and Disability.* New York: Macmillan.

Trieschmann, R. B. (1988). *Spinal Cord Injury: The Psychological, Social, and Vocational Rehabilitation* (2nd ed.). New York: Demos.

VandeCreek, L., & Knapp, S. (1993). *Tarasoff and Beyond: Legal and Clinical Considerations in the Treatment of Life-Endangering Patients* (rev. ed.). Sarasota, FL: Professional Resource Press.

Vargo, F. A. (1984). Adaptation to disability by the wives of spinal cord-injured males: A phenomenological approach. *Journal of Applied Rehabilitation Counseling, 15*, 28-32.

Vargo, F. A., & Stewin, L. L. (1984). Spousal adaptation to disability: Ramifications and implications for counseling. *International Journal of Advanced Counseling, 7*, 253-260.

Vash, C. (1981). *The Psychology of Disability.* New York: Springer.

West, J. (Ed). (1991). *The Americans With Disabilities Act: From Policy to Practice.* New York: Milbank Memorial Fund.

Yuker, H. E. (1992). Attitudes toward persons with disabilities: Conclusions from the data. *Rehabilitation Psychology News, 19*, 17-18.

RESOURCES CONCERNING THE AMERICANS WITH DISABILITIES ACT

Bureau of National Affairs. (1990). *The Americans With Disabilities Act: A Practice and Legal Guide to Impact, Enforcement and Compliance.* Washington, DC: Author.

Kay, C., & Glatz, W. (Producers). (1992). *Americans With Disabilities Act (ADA): Facts and Fears* [Videotape]. Grand Rapids, MI: Cynthia Kay/Wayne Glatz Film & Video.

Lotito, M. J., Alvarez, F. R, & Pimentel, R. (1992). *The Americans With Disabilities Act: Making the ADA Work for You* (2nd ed.). Northridge, CA: Milt Wright and Associates.

Pimentel, R., Bissonnette, D., & Lotito, M. J. (1992). *What Managers and Supervisors Need to Know About the ADA.* Northridge, CA: Milt Wright and Associates.

Public Law 101-336. (1990). *Americans With Disabilities Act of 1990.* [104, 42 U.S.C.] § 12101. Washington, DC: U.S. Government Printing Office.

West, J. (Ed.). (1991). *The Americans With Disabilities Act: From Policy to Practice.* New York: Milbank Memorial Fund.

TWELVE MYTHS ABOUT ADOLESCENTS, SEXUALITY, AND AIDS*

Samuel Knapp

No vaccine or cure for AIDS is forthcoming in the near future, and behavior change is the only way to slow the spread of AIDS. However, opponents of prevention programs have espoused numerous myths that prevent them from endorsing effective prevention efforts. This contribution will review 12 common myths as they relate to adolescents, sexuality, and AIDS. These myths limit the acceptance of prevention as a viable means to deal with the challenge of AIDS or, when prevention programs are accepted, lead to the development of programs that are less than optimally effective.

MYTH #1: HETEROSEXUAL ADOLESCENTS NEED NOT WORRY ABOUT HIV/AIDS

Although adolescents still represent only a minority of HIV-infected persons, the number of infected adolescents has increased 77% in the last 2 years. Among adolescents, half of the cases of transmission of the virus occur through heterosexual intercourse (Goldsmith, 1993). Throughout the world, more persons have contracted AIDS through heterosexual contact than through all other means combined. Within the United States, the number of persons who are contracting AIDS through heterosexual contact is rapidly increasing (Ehrhardt, 1992).

AIDS is the number-one cause of death for men 25 to 44. Most of those who died from AIDS in their 20s acquired the infection in their teens (Selik, Chu, & Buehler, 1993).

The exact prevalence of HIV infection among adolescents is not known (Gardner & Wilcox, 1993). However, available information about HIV prevalence from volunteers for military service, Job Corps applicants, shelters for runaways, sexually transmitted disease (STD) clinics, and other sources shows that HIV rates among adolescents have been increasing rapidly in recent years (Hein, 1992).

Because data on the prevalence of HIV among adolescents is limited to a few specific populations, estimates of its spread may be obtained by looking at the rate of STDs, because many behaviors that put adolescents at risk for STDs (such as failure to use condoms or having sex with multiple partners) also put them at risk for HIV infection. Furthermore, infection with an STD increases the likelihood of contracting an HIV infection because the genital lesions commonly found with STDs increase the likelihood that HIV will be transmitted through sexual contact.

---

*The views expressed do not necessarily represent those of the Pennsylvania Psychological Association.

The data are not encouraging. Each year 1 in 7 teenagers contracts an STD (Hein, 1989). One-fourth of adolescents will have an STD before graduating from high school. The rate of STDs among adolescents is twice that of persons in their 20s.

MYTH #2: SCIENTISTS WILL SOON DISCOVER A VACCINE OR CURE FOR HIV/AIDS

Some people denigrate prevention efforts because they assume scientists will discover a vaccine or cure in the near future. Nevertheless, no vaccine for HIV or cure for AIDS appears on the horizon. Although HIV is the most intensively studied virus in history, scientists lack a clear understanding of how it replicates or attacks the immune system (Greene, 1993). All of the claims in the popular press of breakthroughs in finding a cure for AIDS have proven to be illusory.

Even if a vaccine or cure for laboratory HIV strains were found, the "vaccine" or "cure" may not be effective with actual cases. HIV mutates so rapidly that a single person may have several different HIV strains over the course of the infection (Caldwell, 1993).

On a more fundamental level, the focus on a vaccine or cure for AIDS ignores the fact that cures for diseases presume that a person is already infected. Even if effective treatments could lower its prevalence, many people who contract HIV/AIDS will suffer physically as a consequence of the infection before they seek the cure. Many HIV-infected persons do not get tested for AIDS until they have contracted the opportunistic infections associated with a suppressed immune system.

MYTH #3: MOST ADOLESCENTS DON'T HAVE SEX (AT LEAST NOT MY ADOLESCENT)

Most adolescents do have sex, although the frequency, demographics, and correlates vary considerably. Sixty percent of youths between the ages of 15 and 19 are sexually active (Ehrhardt, 1992). The percentage of adolescents who have had sexual intercourse increases with age. Oswalt and Matsen (1993) found that 79% of undergraduate college students had engaged in sexual intercourse. It is not clear if the overall percentage of adolescents having intercourse is increasing or decreasing. However, the age of first intercourse is getting younger.

Hein (1989) placed adolescents into no-risk, middle-risk, and high-risk groups according to behaviors that place them at risk for HIV infection. The following section will describe these three groups according to probable size, demographics, and other characteristics.

NO-RISK ADOLESCENTS

Hein's first group consists of adolescents who are not at risk because they are virgins and do not use drugs. The size of this group varies according to the age and sex of the adolescent. About 70% of 15-year-old males and 20% of college females fall into this category.

MIDDLE-RISK ADOLESCENTS

Hein's second group includes adolescents who are heterosexually active, but who use discretion, often engaging in serial monogamy. J. Fisher and Misovich (1990) found that 68% of college males and 80% of college females had an intimate relationship at any given time. Many were involved in a series of exclusive (albeit sequential or short-term) intimate relationships. J. Fisher and Misovich also found that the frequency of sexual intercourse and the number of college students having multiple sexual partners has been increasing in recent years. Although the risks to these students are low in some parts of the country, they will increase as HIV becomes more prevalent, even if adolescents increase their use of condoms.

HIGH-RISK TEENAGERS

The third group consists of sexually adventurous teenagers at high risk. Ku, Sonenstein, and Pleck (1992) classified 10% of adolescent males as high risk because they had multiple sexual partners, had homosexual contact, had sex with prostitutes, or used IV drugs. Also, between 125,000 and 200,000 adolescents (less than 1%) are involved in prostitution every year (Prothrow-Smith, 1989). Often these are runaways or street youth who engage in sex for economic survival.

No national data exist on the rate of anal intercourse among adolescents (Gardner & Wilcox, 1993). However, Oswalt and Matsen (1993) found that 10% of college students had engaged in anal intercourse. Of those, 90% failed to use a condom during anal intercourse. Hein (1992) reported that 26% of adolescents who attended STD clinics in New York City practiced anal intercourse (of those, 70% never used condoms during anal intercourse) and 21% of female adolescents attending an outpatient clinic in San Francisco reported engaging in anal intercourse.

Certain adolescents constitute a bridge group between those who are currently infected and the rest of the adolescent population. These adolescents may, for example, belong to the middle-risk group but have a one-time or occasional sexual contact with an adolescent in the high-risk group.

Although frequency varies according to age and sex, most adolescents will engage in sexual activity. A minority of adolescents are at high risk of developing AIDS because they have multiple sexual partners, practice anal intercourse, or use intravenous drugs.

MYTH #4: PREVENTION DOES NOT WORK

Health education efforts have a well-documented background of failure. For example, during the syphilis epidemics in the early part of this century, the American government launched very extensive public scare campaigns to encourage soldiers and civilians to change their sexual habits, including the slogan used with American soldiers during World War I: "A whore is as deadly as a German bullet." They were, however, unable to stop the spread of syphilis (Brandt, 1988).

Initially, behavior change campaigns with AIDS followed a similar path with equally disappointing results. Educators again naïvely believed they just needed to tell people to stop engaging in highly risky sexual behavior or stop using intravenous drugs. The naïve optimism about the ease with which change would occur was followed by a sweeping cynical pessimism that "prevention doesn't work."

A more accurate reading of the prevention literature shows that poorly designed and conducted programs are ineffective. Nevertheless, properly conducted programs can substantially reduce the frequency of high-risk behaviors (see reviews in DiClemente, 1992b). However, behavior change is difficult and requires effort to maintain.

Of course, even effective programs do not produce improvements in behavior for all participants. Many adolescents will not improve their behavior at all, other adolescents may show sporadic or inconsistent improvement, and still others who do improve will show relapses. Still, the elimination of risk for one adolescent means that at least one life will be saved (perhaps more if the number of potentially infected future partners is considered).

MYTH #5: SEXUAL DRIVES CANNOT BE MODIFIED

Some argue that prevention programs cannot work because they run contrary to the instinctual drive to have sex. This statement ignores the richness and diversity of human experiences and fails to note that societies vary considerably in their degree of sexual constraint. At one time, for example, American society demonstrated far more sexual restraint than has been exercised in recent years.

Why do adolescents have sex? It is naïve to believe that sexual behavior occurs only because of its intrinsic pleasures. Sexual behavior has many causes. For prostitutes and street youths, sex is a means of survival. Even recreational sex is deeply intertwined with social (not just physiological) motives. Prieur (1990) found that the most important factor that distinguished high-risk from low-risk behaviors among gay men was the lack of a supportive social support group. "Sexuality then becomes the main way to get close contact with others, and this makes them dread changing, and makes them deny the anxiety they feel" (p. 109). Sex holds an exaggerated place of importance for persons with poor ties to a community because it compensates for loneliness and acts as a substitute for lasting, loving relationships. According to Prieur (1990), "Sex is more than actions and positions. Actions carry meanings . . . ways of showing devotion and belonging" (p. 109).

Similarly, Quadland and Shattls (1987) claimed that loneliness, inadequacy, and anxiety (not just genital gratification) cause much ego-dystonic sexual behavior. Although teenagers may claim that the contemporary parental norms about sexual activity are oppressive, Quadland and Shattls noted that people can oppress themselves if they use sex to divert themselves from unmet emotional needs. "Freedom of sexual expression is accomplished when individuals are not oppressed by their own, as well as society's perceived needs, but rather when they are free to make choices about their sexual lives" (p. 293).

Many high-risk behaviors occur in the context of depression or loneliness. The development of friendships and alternative ways to reduce loneliness will reduce the frequency of high-risk behaviors. Effective programs consider how the undesired sexual behavior often comes out of unmet emotional needs and include relationship-building skills. The optimal program should then help adolescents meet their emotional needs rather than merely attempt to reduce or eliminate risky sexual behaviors.

MYTH #6: HIGH-RISK BEHAVIOR AMONG ADOLESCENTS IS INEVITABLE

A widely held belief is that all adolescents will go through a "stormy decade" of intense emotional turmoil or "developmental insanity." During these times of inevitable emotional turmoil, it is argued, adolescents will be moody, disobedient, and experiment with high-risk behaviors.

This is not true. Offer (1969) found that most adolescents do not experience serious or continuous turmoil. Furthermore, in reviewing the subjective well-being of adolescents, Myers (1992) found that adolescents were no more nor less happy than persons in other age groups. No doubt, some adolescents find the particular challenges of this developmental stage stressful. However, angry rebellion and persistent turmoil are not inevitable.

Instead, healthy or unhealthy behaviors are correlated with certain demographic, attitudinal, and family variables. Durant and Sanders (1989) found that teenagers with safe, or safer, behaviors were more likely to perceive themselves susceptible to infection, to have self-efficacy, to know more about HIV/AIDS, and to have social support for their healthy lifestyles. Teenage girls who abstained from sex were more likely to attend church frequently.

The parental correlates of healthy behavior include an authoritative parenting style (neither permissive nor too authoritarian). The positive quality of the mother-daughter relationship was most associated with less sexual experience. The more mothers communicated with (not talked at) their daughters about sex, the less likely the daughters were to engage in sex. High-risk adolescents were also likely to come from families with histories of chronic conflict and to have relatives who engage in high-risk behaviors (Durant & Sanders, 1989).

Adolescents with high-risk sexual behaviors were likely to have other difficulties as well, such as aggression, juvenile delinquency, substance abuse, academic failure, and mental illness (Brown, DiClemente, & Beausoleil, 1992; Kazdin, 1993; Stiffman et al., 1992). The disinhibiting effects of alcohol or other drugs may partially explain this relationship with sexual activity. However, the multiple problem behaviors may all serve similar functions, such as providing peer acceptance or demonstrating autonomy from parents.

MYTH #7: PREVENTION PROGRAMS DO NOT WORK BECAUSE ADOLESCENTS BELIEVE THEMSELVES TO BE INVULNERABLE TO HARM

Some health care professionals believe that adolescents have an innate sense of invulnerability that cannot be modified. Adolescents believe they are invulnerable to illness or accidents, the argument goes, so they will not modify their behaviors in response to informational or preventive programs.

The empirical literature does not support this concept. Among all persons there is a general "tendency for people to underestimate their own health risks compared to those of others. This is a robust phenomenon that appears to apply to a wide range of specific health outcomes ranging from drug addiction to senility" (Jeffrey, 1989, p. 1195). Adolescents are no more likely to underestimate their risks than persons from any other age group (Quadrel, Fischhoff, & Davis, 1993).

There is no reason to believe that education or prevention programs with adolescents would be any less successful than with any other age group. Adolescents will modify their behavior if they are educated properly about the risks and taught alternative ways to meet their social and developmental needs.

MYTH #8: EDUCATION ALONE WILL CHANGE BEHAVIOR

Educational information about AIDS, HIV infection, and transmission is important, but not sufficient for change. Effective programs contain several components, of which education is only one.

The educational component of a prevention program for older teenagers should include all of the relevant information on HIV and AIDS that is given to adults. The educational program should contain information on transmission, incubation, the spectrum of diseases related to the HIV infection, the risks of specific sexual practices, testing, and proper use of condoms. Messages may need to be repeated from many different sources in order to have the desired impact.

CORRECTING MISCONCEPTIONS

Not only must the participants learn the basic facts about AIDS, they must also unlearn misconceptions about AIDS. Many adolescents do not understand how AIDS is spread, and many more believe in unsubstantiated alternative means of casual transmission.

These misunderstandings may be caused by adolescents' reliance on unreliable sources of information about HIV/AIDS. Ford and Norris (1991) found that 78% of African-American adolescents talked with friends, siblings, or classmates about AIDS while only 3% talked to teachers and counselors.

Misconceptions are often difficult to dispel, and the simple presentation of accurate information is not always sufficient. For some adolescents, their ego-involvement about the issue may lead them to minimize the hazards of transmission through their preferred mode of sexual activity.

SCARE TACTICS

Much of the original AIDS education focused on fear and the dire consequences of contracting an HIV infection. For example, the fear motive was clear in the name of Australia's public information campaign, the "Grim Reaper." On the other hand, it is impossible to give accurate information about HIV/AIDS without arousing a certain amount of fear and discomfort.

Fear, however, does not facilitate long-term lifestyle change. Furthermore, it can lead to discouragement in reforming behavior, low morale, antigay hysteria, or AIDS phobia. Effective programs focus on emotionally and physically healthy activities. "Playing it safe" measures can focus on freedom from fear, positive health, secure and stable relationships, and positive self-esteem.

BEYOND GIVING INFORMATION

Although information is a first step, most individuals need more substantive and intensive efforts to modify high-risk behaviors. Knowledge about the dangers of high-risk sexual behavior does not automatically lead to behavior change. Too often people who choose celibacy end up losing their resolve and engaging in binges of high-risk behavior. Problems with adherence are especially problematic for highly pleasurable activities such as sexual intercourse. This is similar to the experiences in treating overeating or smoking, which also show that simply providing more information will not necessarily produce behavior change. Nevertheless, properly conducted programs that combine educational and psychological formats can produce higher and more consistent levels of change.

A multifaceted behavior change program attempts to intervene on educational, behavioral, affective, cognitive, and environmental levels. Assertive behaviors can be used to counter unwanted sexual advances or intrusions. Unpleasant emotions can be expressed to a loved one instead of denied or diverted into sexual behavior. Unproductive cognitions can be challenged and replaced with more productive thoughts. The identification of objective or subjective precipitants of high-risk behavior is important. High-risk behavior is more likely to occur immediately after drinking or in response to emotional turmoil. The overlap between the different components is obvious. The expression of emotion may utilize many behavioral (e.g., communication) skills. The identification of unmet psychological needs such as loneliness, inadequacy, or anxiety would overlap with the cognitive skills.

A group format is extremely important so that peers can reinforce appropriate behaviors. Often the group members become friends after the termination of the group and can use each other for support, such as is the case with Alcoholics Anonymous, Recovery Incorporated, or other self-help groups.

As may be inferred, these multicomponent programs take time to work, and relapse among some should be expected. Short-term programs are unlikely to produce lasting changes. Repeated contacts are necessary to establish social support and change behaviors.

MYTH #9: PREVENTION PROGRAMS SHOULD FOCUS PRIMARILY ON USING CONDOMS

Condoms, if properly used, can substantially reduce the risk of infection. However, some HIV/AIDS education programs limit their discussion of condoms to the homily "use condoms." They assume everyone knows how to use condoms properly and that condom use will protect the adolescent. Both these assumptions are faulty.

Condom use is a form of "safer" sex because it greatly reduces the likelihood of infection. However, it should not be promoted as "safe" sex because condoms are not always effective. Condom use is a complex phenomenon that requires both information and social skills.

Condom failure is almost always due to user failure. The Food and Drug Administration evaluates condoms carefully for manufacturers' failures ("Can You Rely on Condoms," 1989). Proper use of condoms means that water-based lubricants alone should be used, condoms should be stored in a dry, cool place (not in a wallet or back pocket), and the base of the condom should be held while removing the penis from the partner's rectum or vagina. If at all possible, it is best to remove the penis from the rectum or vagina prior to ejaculation. Only latex condoms (not animal fiber condoms) should be used.

Even if persons understand how to use condoms properly, their actual use depends on the social context and power differential in the sexual relationship. Girls are not always equal partners in the negotiations. For many girls, sex is their only asset in maintaining a relationship, and failure to maintain the relationship may result in physical abuse or loss of financial support. Furthermore, about 7% of girls have their first sexual contact as the result of actual or threatened force (Voydanoff & Donnelly, 1990). These girls have little say about the use of condoms. Additionally, boys and girls are not at equal risk of contracting the virus. For a variety of reasons, girls have a much higher chance of getting the virus.

Frequency of condom use is also related to the age of the sexual partners. The wider the difference in age, the less likely that condoms will be used. Male partners of adolescent male partners tend to be 7 years older, while male partners of female partners tend to be 2 to 3 years older.

Even in noncoercive relationships, girls may be less likely to assert themselves and insist on the use of condoms. Some girls lack the skills to insist on condom use. For reasons that are not clear, boys (but not girls) who consume alcohol before sex are less likely to use condoms (DiClemente, 1992a). These data suggest that girls may need to negotiate the use of condoms before drinking starts.

Couples who communicate openly about sexual matters are more likely to use contraceptives regularly. The failure to use barrier contraceptives is a special problem with "regular" or "primary" relationships. Some partners may use condoms with brief acquaintances, but feel reluctant to use them with steady lovers.

Although effective programs should discuss condom use and its advantages, they should not focus exclusively on condom use and ignore other aspects of HIV prevention such as monogamy (or at least reducing the number of sexual partners), getting to know one's partners well, and using safe sexual techniques such as mutual masturbation.

MYTH #10: PREVENTIVE PROGRAMS SHOULD FOCUS PRIMARILY ON ABSTINENCE

Some advocates believe that effective programs should focus only on abstinence. They believe that discussion of "safer sex" or the option of condoms encourages riskier behaviors.

AIDS prevention programs should include information on the benefits of monogamy or abstinence. However, many adolescents will engage in behavior that is not universally accepted, such as premarital sex or unprotected anal intercourse. Consequently, programs should provide information on "safer" practices such as the use of condoms.

Abstinence or an exclusive relationship with a seronegative person is the only real form of safe sex. However, it is more important to focus on the positive aspects of lasting relationships than to focus only on abstinence from brief sexual encounters. The ability to develop positive relationships with one person requires skills such as expressing thoughts and feelings in an acceptable manner and listening with empathy and understanding. Often people seek multiple sexual partners because they do not know how to maintain a single relationship over time. Learning to improve relationships should reduce the likelihood of seeking multiple sexual partners.

MYTH #11: ONE EFFECTIVE INTERVENTION PROGRAM WORKS FOR ALL ADOLESCENTS

Not all programs work equally well for all audiences. AIDS is best considered as a series of "subepidemics" as opposed to one epidemic. Psychotherapists have been cautioned against the "uniformity myth" when selecting psychotherapy treatments for patients. Similarly, they must also be cautioned against a "uniformity myth" when it comes to changing high-risk behaviors.

The unique aspects of the teenage experience with HIV and AIDS must be considered when conducting intervention programs. Proportionally more teenagers acquire HIV through heterosexual transmission, and a higher percentage are currently asymptomatic (Centers for Disease Control, 1992). Furthermore, the testing of minors involves special legal issues. Teenagers have a subculture that differs from adults, and teenage mothers have special problems concerning access to health care.

Effective programs vary according to the age, gender, culture, and credibility of the messenger and the vernacular of the target audience. Adolescents are not a homogeneous group. The cognitive development and needs of a 13-year-old differ from those of a 19-year-old. In addition, the needs and experiences of girls differ considerably from boys.

Adolescents come from many subcultures with a wide range of individuals with cognitive, socioeconomic, cultural, and geographic differences. For example, materials in Spanish, Black English, and so on, must go beyond the use of the vernacular and consider the culture of the audience. It is erroneous, for example, to speak of Hispanic and Black populations as if they were homogeneous. The cultural differences between a New York Puerto Rican, a Miami Cuban, and a second-generation Mexican-American from Los Angeles can be quite substantial.

The messenger can be as important as the message. The messengers must be able to listen and understand the teenagers. Often peer counselors are effective with teenagers.

Effective programs use language that the intended audience understands. Materials that talk about the need to avoid "exchanging bodily fluids" may have little meaning to certain audiences, whereas explicit street language may convey the meaning more clearly.

Examples of misunderstanding of terminology abound. When cautioned against "multiple partners," some women believed that it referred to more than one partner at a time. Others believed that a series of exclusive sexual relationships constituted monogamy. One young girl denied being sexually active, even though she was pregnant. In all seriousness, she responded that during sex she just lay there and let her boyfriend be active.

The street language may, however, offend a middle-class audience. Although explicit educational materials appear to communicate information more effectively, consideration needs to be shown to the social convention that disapproves of the use of sexual terms in public.

MYTH 12: OUTCOME STUDIES ARE NOT NEEDED

Although HIV/AIDS prevention programs can be successful, we need to know more. Even successful programs may have many adolescents who do not change their behavior or who relapse quickly. Furthermore, often researchers establish dependent variables, such as frequency of condom use, which are not optimal in measuring program effectiveness. Alternate dependent variables could include number of sexual partners, degree of knowledge about sexual partners, and the frequency of the proper use of condoms.

Researchers with HIV/AIDS prevention programs have to consider many of the same problems and issues as researchers with psychotherapy outcome studies. Researchers need to look at the content and length of the program, the match between audience and interveners, the long-term follow-up, the relapse rates, and other factors. As the data base develops, we can develop more effective programs and seek additional funding for these programs.

CONCLUSIONS

Regrettably, past predictions about the rapidity of the spread of AIDS have come true. The first "AIDS generation" (those who were born after the HIV infection first came to the attention of health care providers in the late 1970s) is living in an era of great personal risk. With no cure or vaccine in sight, AIDS prevention programs are vitally needed.

Although effective AIDS prevention programs have been developed in recent years and several have been referenced here, they are often resisted by persons who are ill-informed about HIV and AIDS. Researchers have developed effective (albeit imperfect) programs. Effective programs are time intensive and require knowledge of AIDS and of the target audience. They should emphasize the development of quality relationships and self-control over sexual behavior. Programs should not focus too much on just the use of condoms or the benefits of abstinence. Instead, effective programs help adolescents find safe ways to meet their legitimate developmental and social needs.

Data gathered from outcome studies will help refine future programs. It is hoped that programs in the future will lead to a higher success and lower relapse rate for participants.

Samuel Knapp, EdD, is currently the Professional Affairs Officer of the Pennsylvania Psychological Association. He is the author or co-author of 14 books and numerous articles in psychology. His interests include issues affecting professional psychology, public mental health, and psychopathology. Dr. Knapp may be contacted at 2801 Rumson Drive, Harrisburg, PA 17104.

RESOURCES

Adib, S. M., Joseph, J., Ostrow, D., & James, S. (1990). Predictors of relapse in sexual practices among homosexual men. *Aids Education and Prevention, 3,* 293-304.

Bandura, A. (1992). A social cognitive approach to the exercise of control over AIDS infection. In R. DiClemente (Ed.), *Adolescents and AIDS: A Generation in Jeopardy* (pp. 89-116). Newbury Park, CA: Sage.

Basen-Engquist, K. (1992). Psychosocial predictors of "safer sex" behaviors in young adults. *AIDS Education and Prevention, 4,* 120-134.

Becker, M., & Joseph, J. (1988). AIDS and behavioral change to reduce risk: A review. *American Journal of Public Health, 78,* 394-410.

Brandt, A. (1988). AIDS in historical perspective: Four lessons from the history of sexually transmitted diseases. *American Journal of Public Health, 78,* 367-371.

Brooks-Gunn, J., Boyer, C., & Hein, K. (1988). Preventing HIV infection and AIDS in children and adolescents: Behavioral research and intervention strategies. *American Psychologist, 43,* 958-964.

Brown, L., DiClemente, R., & Beausoleil, N. (1992). Comparison of Human Immunodeficiency Virus related knowledge, attitudes, intentions, and behaviors among sexually active and abstinent young adolescents. *Journal of Adolescent Health Care, 13,* 140-145.

Caldwell, M. (1993). The long shot. *Discover, 14,* 60-69.

Can you rely on condoms? (1989, March). *Consumer Reports, 54,* 135-141.

Centers for Disease Control. (1992, March). *HIV/AIDS Surveillance* (newsletter). Atlanta, GA: Author.

Coates, T. (1990). Strategies for modifying sexual behavior for primary and secondary prevention of HIV disease. *Journal of Clinical and Consulting Psychology, 58,* 57-69.

DiClemente, R. (1992a, August). *HIV Prevention Programs With Adolescents.* Paper presented at the Annual Meeting of the American Psychological Association, San Francisco, CA.

DiClemente, R. (1992b). Psychosocial determinants of condom use among adolescents. In R. DiClemente (Ed.), *Adolescents and AIDS: A Generation in Jeopardy* (pp. 34-52). Newbury Park, CA: Sage.

DiClemente, R., Forrest, K., & Mickler, S. (1990). College students' knowledge of attitudes about AIDS and changes in HIV-preventive behaviors. *AIDS Education and Prevention, 2,* 201-212.

Durant, R., & Sanders, J. (1989). Sexual behavior and contraceptive risk taking among adolescent females. *Journal of Adolescent Health Care, 10,* 1-9.

Ehrhardt, A. (1992). Trends in sexual behavior and the AIDS pandemic. *American Journal of Public Health, 82,* 1459-1461.

Fisher, J., & Fisher, W. (1992). Changing AIDS-risk behavior. *Psychological Bulletin, 111,* 455-474.

Fisher, J., & Misovich, S. (1990). Evolution of college students' AIDS-related behavioral responses, attitudes, knowledge, and fear. *AIDS Education and Prevention, 2,* 322-337.

Flora, J., & Thoresen, C. (1988). Reducing the risk of AIDS in adolescents. *American Psychologist, 43,* 965-970.

Ford, K., & Norris, A. (1991). Urban African-American and Hispanic adolescents and young adults: Who do they talk to about AIDS and condoms? What are they learning? *AIDS Education and Prevention, 3,* 197-206.

Gardner, W., & Wilcox, B. (1993). Political intervention in scientific peer review: Research on adolescent sexual behavior. *American Psychologist, 48,* 972-983.

Goldsmith, M. (1993). "Invisible" epidemic now becoming visible as HIV/AIDS pandemic reaches adolescents. *Journal of the American Medical Association, 270,* 14-19.

Greene, W. (1993). AIDS and the immune system. *Scientific American, 269,* 98-105.

Hein, K. (1989). AIDS in adolescence. *Journal of Adolescent Health Care, 10,* 195-355.

Hein, K. (1992). Adolescents at risk for HIV infection. In R. DiClemente (Ed.), *Adolescents and AIDS: A Generation in Jeopardy* (pp. 3-16). Newbury Park, CA: Sage.

Jeffrey, R. (1989). Risk behaviors and health: Contrasting individual and population perspectives. *American Psychologist, 44,* 1194-1202.

Kasen, S., Vaugn, R., & Walter, H. (1992). Self-efficacy for AIDS preventive behaviors among tenth grade students. *Health Education Quarterly, 19,* 187-202.

Kazdin, A. (1993). Adolescent mental health: Prevention and treatment programs. *American Psychologist, 48,* 127-141.

Kelly, J., & Murphy, D. (1992). Psychological interventions with AIDS and HIV: Prevention and treatment. *Journal of Consulting and Clinical Psychology, 60,* 576-585.

Kelly, J., St. Lawrence, J., Betts, R., Brasfield, T., & Hood, H. (1990). A skills-training group intervention model to assist persons in reducing risk behaviors for HIV infection. *AIDS Education and Prevention, 2,* 24-35.

Kelly, J., St. Lawrence, J., & Brasfield, T. (1991). Predictors of vulnerability of AIDS risk behavior relapse. *Journal of Consulting and Clinical Psychology, 59,* 163-166.

Kelly, J., St. Lawrence, J., Hood, H., & Brasfield, T. (1989). Behavioral intervention to reduce AIDS risk activities. *Journal of Consulting and Clinical Psychology, 57,* 60-67.

Knapp, S., & VandeCreek, L. (1989). *What Every Therapist Should Know About AIDS.* Sarasota, FL: Professional Resource Exchange.

Ku, L., Sonenstein, F., & Pleck, J. (1992). Patterns of HIV risk and preventive behaviors among teenage men. *Public Health Reports, 107,* 131-138.

McKirnan, D. (1989, June). *Tension Reduction Expectancies Underlie the Effect of Alcohol Use on AIDS-Risk Behavior Among Homosexual Males.* Paper presented at the Fifth International Conference on AIDS, Montreal.

Morris, R., Baker, C., & Huscroft, S. (1992). Incarcerated youth at risk for HIV infection. In R. DiClemente (Ed.), *Adolescents and AIDS: A Generation in Jeopardy* (pp. 52-70). Newbury Park, CA: Sage.

Myers, D. (1992). *The Pursuit of Happiness.* New York: Morrow.

Nelking, V., & Oliva, G. (1989). AIDS policies on youth: Recommendations of the work group. *Journal of Adolescent Health Care, 10,* 505-515.

Offer, D. (1969). *The Psychological World of the Teenager.* New Haven: Yale.

Oswalt, R., & Matsen, K. (1993). Sex, AIDS, and the use of condoms: A survey of compliance in college students. *Psychological Reports, 72,* 764-766.

Pennbridge, J., Freese, T., & MacKenzie, R. (1992). High risk behaviors among male street youth in Hollywood, California. *AIDS Prevention and Education, 4*(Suppl.), 24-33.

Prieur, A. (1990). Norwegian gay men: Reasons for continued practice of unsafe sex. *AIDS Education and Prevention, 2,* 109-115.

Prothrow-Smith, D. (1989). Excerpts from address. *Journal of Adolescent Health Care, 10,* 55-75.

Quadland, M., & Shattls, W. (1987). AIDS, sexuality, and sexual control. *Journal of Homosexuality, 14,* 287-298.

Quadrel, M., Fischhoff, B., & Davis, W. (1993). Adolescent (in)vulnerability. *American Psychologist, 48,* 102-116.

Ricert, V., Jay, S., & Gottlieb, A. (1991). Effects of a peer-counselor AIDS education program on knowledge, attitudes, and satisfaction of adolescents. *Journal of Adolescent Health, 12,* 28-43.

Rotheram-Borus, M. J., & Koopman, C. (1991). Sexual risk behaviors, AIDS knowledge, and beliefs about AIDS among runaways. *American Journal of Public Health, 81,* 206-208.

Rotheram-Borus, M. J., Koopman, C., & Ehrhardt, A. (1991). Homeless youths and HIV infection. *American Psychologist, 46,* 1188-1197.

Selik, R., Chu, S., & Buehler, J. (1993). HIV infection as leading cause of death among young adults in U.S. cities and states. *Journal of the American Medical Association, 269,* 2991-2994.

Sy, F., Richter, D., & Copello, G. (1989). Innovative education strategies and recommendations for AIDS prevention and control. *AIDS Education and Prevention, 1,* 53-56.

Stiffman, A. R., Dore, P., Earls, F., & Cunningham, R. (1992). The influence of mental health problems on AIDS-related risk behaviors in young adults. *The Journal of Nervous and Mental Disease, 180,* 314-320.

Vermund, S. (1993). Rising HIV-related mortality among young Americans. *Journal of the American Medical Association, 269,* 3034-3035.

Voydanoff, P., & Donnelly, B. (1990). *Adolescent Sexuality and Pregnancy.* Newbury Park, CA: Sage.

INTRODUCTION TO THE CLIENT HANDOUTS

Two client handouts are included in this section of Volume 13. The handouts in each volume are designed so that they may be photocopied and distributed to your clients. It should be noted that other handout materials are included with contributions throughout the volume and may be located by referring to "Handouts for Clients" in the subject index at the back of the volume.

Controlling Anger - Before It Controls You was written by Chi Chi Sileo and produced by the Office of Public Affairs of the American Psychological Association.

Plain Talk About Depression, is adapted from a brochure produced by the Office of Scientific Information of National Institute of Mental Health.

CONTROLLING ANGER - BEFORE IT CONTROLS YOU*

We all know what anger is, and we've all felt it: whether as a fleeting annoyance or as a full-fledged rage.

Anger is a completely normal, usually healthy, human emotion. But when it gets out of control and turns destructive, it can lead to problems: problems at work, in your personal relationships, and in the overall quality of your life. And it can make you feel as though you're at the mercy of an unpredictable and powerful emotion. This handout is meant to help you to understand and get a handle on handling anger.

WHAT IS ANGER?

THE NATURE OF ANGER

Anger is "an emotional state that varies in intensity from mild irritation to intense fury and rage," according to Charles Spielberger, PhD, a psychologist who specializes in the study of anger. Like other emotions, it is accompanied by physiological and biological changes: When you get angry, your heart rate and blood pressure go up, as does the level of your energy hormones, adrenalin, and nonadrenalin.

Anger can be caused by both external and internal events. You could be angry at a specific person (such as a coworker or supervisor) or event (a traffic jam, a canceled flight), or your anger could be caused by worrying or brooding about your personal problems. Memories of traumatic or enraging events can also trigger angry feelings.

EXPRESSING ANGER

The intrinsic, natural way to express anger is to respond aggressively. Anger is a natural, adaptive response to threats; it inspires powerful, often aggressive, feelings and behaviors, which allow us to fight and to defend ourselves when we are attacked. A certain amount of anger, therefore, is necessary to our survival.

On the other hand, we can't physically lash out at every person or object that irritates or annoys us; laws, social norms, and common sense place limits on how far our anger can take us.

People use a variety of both conscious and unconscious processes to deal with their angry feelings. The three main approaches are *expressing, suppressing,* and *calming.*

---

*Reproduced from *Psychology and You: Controlling Anger - Before It Controls You,* a pamphlet produced by the Public Affairs Office of the American Psychological Association (APA).

The following APA members assisted in the production of the brochure: Jerry Deffenbacher, PhD, Colorado State University and Charles D. Spielberger, PhD, University of South Florida. This brochure was written by Chi Chi Sileo.

Expressing your angry feelings in an assertive - not aggressive - manner is the healthiest way to express anger. To do this, you have to learn how to make clear what your needs are and how to get them met without hurting others. Being assertive doesn't mean being pushy or demanding; it means being respectful of yourself and others.

Anger can be *suppressed*, and then converted or redirected. This happens when you hold in your anger, stop thinking about it, and focus on something positive. The aim is to inhibit or suppress your anger and convert it into more constructive behavior. The danger in this type of response is that if it isn't allowed outward expression, your anger can turn inward - on yourself. Anger turned inward may cause hypertension, high blood pressure, or depression.

Unexpressed anger can create other problems. It can lead to pathological expressions of anger, such as passive-aggressive behavior (getting back at people indirectly, without telling them why, rather than confronting them head-on) or a personality that seems perpetually cynical and hostile. People who are constantly putting others down, criticizing everything, and making cynical comments haven't learned how to constructively express their anger. Not surprisingly, they aren't likely to have many successful relationships.

Finally, you can *calm down inside*. This means not just controlling your outward behavior but also controlling your internal responses, taking steps to lower your heart rate, calm yourself down, and let the feelings subside.

As Dr. Spielberger notes, "when none of these three techniques work, that's when someone - or something - is going to get hurt."

ANGER MANAGEMENT

The goal of anger management is to reduce both your emotional feelings and the physiological arousal that anger causes. You can't get rid of, or avoid, the things or the people that enrage you, nor can you change them, but you can learn to control your reactions.

ARE YOU TOO ANGRY?

There are psychological tests that measure the intensity of angry feelings, how prone to anger you are, and how well you handle it. But chances are good that if you do have a problem with anger, you already know it. If you find yourself acting in ways that seem out of control and frightening, you might need help finding better ways to deal with this emotion.

WHY ARE SOME PEOPLE MORE ANGRY THAN OTHERS?

According to Jerry Deffenbacher, PhD, a psychologist who specializes in anger management, some people really are more "hotheaded" than others; they get angry more easily and more intensely than the average person. There are also those who don't show their anger in loud spectacular ways but are chronically irritable and grumpy. Easily angered people don't always curse and throw things; sometimes they withdraw socially, sulk, or get physically ill.

People who are easily angered generally have what some psychologists call a *low tolerance for frustration,* meaning simply that they feel that they should not have to be subjected to frustration, inconvenience, or annoyance. They can't take things in stride, and they're particularly infuriated if the situation seems somehow unjust; for example, being corrected for a minor mistake.

What makes these people this way? A number of things. One cause may be genetic or physiological; there is evidence that some children are born irritable, touchy, and easily angered, and that these signs are present from a very early age. Another may be sociocultural. Anger is often regarded as negative; we're taught that it's all right to express anxiety, depression, or other emotions but not to express anger. As a result, we don't learn how to handle it or channel it constructively.

Research has also found that family background plays a role. Typically, people who are easily angered come from families that are disruptive, chaotic, and not skilled at emotional communications.

IS IT GOOD TO "LET IT ALL HANG OUT"?

Psychologists now say that this is a dangerous myth. Some people use this theory as a license to hurt others. Research has found that "letting it rip" with anger actually escalates anger and aggression and does nothing to help you (or the person you're angry with) resolve the situation.

It's best to find out what it is that triggers your anger and then to develop strategies to keep those triggers from tipping you over the edge.

WHAT STRATEGIES CAN YOU USE TO KEEP ANGER AT BAY?

RELAXATION

Simple relaxation tools such as deep breathing and relaxing imagery can help calm down angry feelings. There are books and courses that can teach you relaxation techniques, and once you learn them you can call upon them in any situation. If you are involved in a relationship where both partners are hot-tempered, it might be a good idea for both of you to learn these techniques.

Some simple steps you can try:

- Breathe deeply, from your diaphragm; breathing from your chest won't relax you. Picture your breath coming up from your "gut."
- Slowly repeat a calm word or phrase such as "relax," "take it easy." Repeat it to yourself while breathing deeply.
- Use imagery; visualize a relaxing experience from either your memory or your imagination.
- Nonstrenuous, slow, yogalike exercises can relax your muscles and make you feel much calmer.

Practice these techniques daily. Learn to use them automatically when you're in a tense situation.

COGNITIVE RESTRUCTURING

Simply put, this means changing the way you think. Angry people tend to curse, swear, or speak in highly colorful terms that reflect their inner thoughts. When you're angry, your thinking can get very exaggerated and overly dramatic. Try replacing these thoughts with more rational ones. For instance, instead of telling yourself, "oh, it's awful, it's terrible, everything's ruined," tell yourself, "it's frustrating, and it's understandable that I'm upset about it, but it's not the end of the world and getting angry is not going to fix it anyhow."

Be careful of words like "never" and "always" when talking about yourself or someone else. "This !&*%@ machine never works," or "You're always forgetting things" are not just inaccurate, they also serve to make you feel that your anger is justified and that there's no way to solve the problem. They also alienate and humiliate people who might otherwise be willing to work with you on a solution.

For example, you have a friend who is constantly late when you make plans to meet. Don't go on the attack; think instead about the *goal* you want to accomplish (that is, getting you and your friend there at about the same time). So avoid saying things like, "You're always late! You're the most irresponsible, inconsiderate person I've ever met!" The only goal that accomplishes is hurting and angering your friend.

State what the problem is and try to find a solution that works for both of you; or take matters into your own hands by, for instance, setting your meeting time a half-hour earlier so that your friend will, in fact, get there on time, even if you have to trick him or her into doing it! Either way, the problem is solved and the friendship isn't damaged.

Remind yourself that getting angry is not going to fix anything, that it won't make you feel better (and may actually make you feel worse).

Logic defeats anger, because anger, even when it's justified, can quickly become irrational. So use cold hard logic on yourself. Remind yourself that the world is "not out to get you," you're just experiencing some of the rough spots of daily life. Do this each time you feel anger getting the best of you, and it'll help you get a more balanced perspective.

Angry people tend to demand things: fairness, appreciation, agreement, willingness to do things their way. Everyone wants these things, and we are all hurt and disappointed when we don't get them, but angry people *demand* them, and when their demands aren't met their disappointment becomes anger. As part of their cognitive restructuring, angry people need to become aware of their demanding nature and translate their expectations into desires. In other words, saying "I would like" something is healthier than saying "I demand" or "I must have" something. When you're unable to get what you want, you will experience the normal reactions - frustration, disappointment, hurt - but not anger. Some angry people use this anger as a way to avoid feeling hurt, but that doesn't mean the hurt goes away.

PROBLEM SOLVING

Sometimes, our anger and frustration are caused by very real and inescapable problems in our lives. Not all anger is misplaced, and often it's a healthy, natural response to these difficulties. There is also a cultural belief that every problem has a solution, and it adds to our frustration to find out that this isn't always the case. The best attitude to bring to such a situation, then, is not to focus on finding the solution but rather on how you handle and face the problem.

Make a plan, and check your progress along the way. (People who have trouble with planning might find a good guide to organizing or time management helpful.) Resolve to give it your best, but also not to punish yourself if an answer doesn't come right away. If you can approach it with your best intentions and efforts, and make a serious attempt to face it head-on, you will be less likely to lose patience and fall into all-or-nothing thinking, even if the problem does not get solved right away.

BETTER COMMUNICATION

Angry people tend to jump to - and act on - conclusions, and some of those conclusions can be pretty wild. The first thing to do, if you're in a heated discussion, is to slow down and think through your responses. Don't say the first thing that comes into your head, but slow down and think carefully about what you want to say. At the same time, listen carefully to what the other person is saying and take your time before answering.

Listen, too, to what is underlying the anger. For instance, you like a certain amount of freedom and personal space, and your "significant other" wants more connection and closeness. If he or she starts complaining about your activities, don't retaliate by painting your partner as a jailer, a warden, or an albatross around your neck.

It's natural to get defensive when you're criticized, but don't fight back. Instead, listen to what's underlying the words: the message that this person might feel neglected and unloved. It may take a lot of patient questioning on your part, and it may require some breathing space, but don't let your anger - or a partner's anger - let a discussion spin out of control. Keeping your cool can keep the situation from becoming a disastrous one.

USING HUMOR

"Silly humor" can help diffuse rage in a number of ways. For one thing, it can help you get a more balanced perspective. When you get angry and call someone a name or refer to them in some imaginative phrase, stop and picture what that word would literally look like. If you're at work and you think of a coworker as a "dirtbag" or a "single-cell life form," for example, picture a large bag full of dirt (or an amoeba) sitting at your colleague's desk, talking on the phone, going to meetings. Do this whenever a name comes into your head about another person. If you can, draw a picture of what the actual thing might look like. This will take a lot of the edge off your fury; and humor can always be relied on to help unknot a tense situation.

The underlying message of highly angry people, Dr. Deffenbacher says, is *"things oughta go my way!"* Angry people tend to feel that they are morally right, that any blocking or changing of their plans is an unbearable indignity, and that they should NOT have to suffer this way. Maybe other people do, but not them!

When you feel that urge, he suggests, picture yourself as a god or goddess, a supreme ruler who owns the streets and stores and office space, striding alone and having your way in all situations while others defer to you. The more detail you can get into your imaginary scenes, the more chances you have to realize that maybe you are being a little unreasonable; you'll also realize how unimportant the things you're angry about really are.

There are two cautions in using humor. First, don't try to just "laugh off" your problems; rather, use humor to help yourself face them more constructively. Second, don't give in to harsh, sarcastic humor; that's just another form of unhealthy anger expression.

What these techniques have in common is a refusal to take yourself too seriously. Anger is a serious emotion, but it's often accompanied by ideas that, if examined, can make you laugh.

CHANGING YOUR ENVIRONMENT

Sometimes it's our immediate surroundings that give us cause for irritation and fury. Problems and responsibilities can weigh on you and make you feel angry at the "trap" you seem to have fallen into and all the people and things that form that trap.

Give yourself a break. Make sure you have some "personal time" scheduled for times of the day that you know are particularly stressful. One example is the working mother who has a standing rule that when she comes home from work, for the first 15 minutes "nobody talks to Mom unless the house is on fire." After this brief quiet time, she feels better prepared to handle demands from her kids without blowing up at them.

Some other tips for easing up on yourself follow.

Timing. If you and your spouse tend to fight when you discuss things at night - perhaps you're tired, or distracted, or maybe it's just habit - try changing the times when you talk about important matters so these talks don't turn into arguments.

Avoidance. If your child's chaotic room makes you furious every time you walk by it, shut the door. Don't make yourself look at what infuriates you. Don't say "well, my child should clean up the room so I won't have to be angry!" That's not the point. The point is to keep yourself calm.

Finding Alternatives. If your daily commute through traffic leaves you in a state of rage and frustration, give yourself a project - learn or map out a different route, one that's less congested or more scenic. Or find another alternative, such as a bus or commuter train.

DO YOU NEED COUNSELING?

If you feel that your anger is really out of control, if it is having an impact on your relationships and on important parts of your life, you might consider counseling to learn how to handle it better. A psychologist or other licensed mental health professional can work with you in developing a range of techniques for changing your thinking and your behavior.

When you talk to a prospective therapist, tell him or her that you have problems with anger that you want to work on, and ask about his or her approach to anger management. Make sure this isn't only a course of action designed to "put you in touch with your feelings and express them" - that may be precisely what your problem is.

With counseling, psychologists say, a highly angry person can move closer to a middle range of anger in about 8 to 10 weeks, depending on circumstances and the techniques used.

WHAT ABOUT ASSERTIVENESS TRAINING?

It's true that angry people need to learn to become assertive (rather than aggressive), but most books and courses on developing assertiveness are aimed at people who don't feel *enough* anger. These people are more passive and acquiescent than the average person; they tend to let others walk over all them. That isn't something most angry people do. Still, these books can contain some useful tactics to use in frustrating situations.

Remember, you can't eliminate anger - and it wouldn't be a good idea if you could. In spite of all your efforts, things will always happen that will cause you anger; and sometimes it will be justifiable anger. Life will always be filled with frustration, pain, loss, and the unpredictable actions of others. You can't change that; but you can change the way you let such events affect you. Controlling your angry responses can keep them from making you even more unhappy in the long run.

PLAIN TALK ABOUT DEPRESSION*

During any 6-month period, 9 million American adults suffer from a depressive illness. The cost in human suffering cannot be estimated. Depressive illnesses often interfere with normal functioning and cause pain and suffering not only to those who have a disorder, but also to those who care about them. Serious depression can destroy family life as well as the life of the ill person.

Possibly the saddest fact about depression is that much of this suffering is unnecessary. Most people with a depressive illness do not seek treatment, although the great majority - even those with the severest disorders - can be helped. Thanks to years of fruitful research, the medications and psychosocial therapies that ease the pain of depression are at hand.

Unfortunately, many people do not recognize that they have a treatable illness. Read this handout to see if you are one of the many undiagnosed depressed people in this country or if you know someone who is. The information briefly presented here may help you take the steps that may save your own or someone else's life.

WHAT IS A DEPRESSIVE DISORDER?

A depressive disorder is a "whole-body" illness, involving your body, mood, and thoughts. It affects the way you eat and sleep, the way you feel about yourself, and the way you think about things. A depressive disorder is *not* the same as a passing blue mood. It is *not* a sign of personal weakness or a condition that can be willed or wished away. People with a depressive illness cannot merely "pull themselves together" and get better. Without treatment, symptoms can last for weeks, months, or years. Appropriate treatment, however, can help most people who suffer from depression.

---

*Modified from *Plain Talk About . . . Depression*, a brochure produced by the Office of Scientific Information of National Institute of Mental Health. The writer was Marilyn Sargent.

TYPES OF DEPRESSION

Depressive disorders come in different forms, just as do other illnesses, such as heart disease. This handout briefly describes three of the most prevalent types of depressive disorders. However, within these types there are variations in the number of symptoms, their severity, and their persistence.

Major depression is manifested by a combination of symptoms (see symptom list) that interfere with the ability to work, sleep, eat, and enjoy once pleasurable activities. These disabling episodes of depression can occur once, twice, or several times in a lifetime.

A less severe type of depression, *dysthymia,* involves long-term, chronic symptoms that do not disable, but keep you from functioning at "full steam" or from feeling good. Sometimes people with dysthymia also experience major depressive episodes.

Another type is *bipolar disorder,* formerly called manic-depressive illness. Not nearly as prevalent as other forms of depressive disorders, bipolar disorder involves cycles of depression and elation or mania. Sometimes the mood switches are dramatic and rapid, but most often they are gradual. When in the depressed cycle, you can have any or all of the symptoms of a depressive disorder. When in the manic cycle, any or all symptoms listed under mania may be experienced. Mania often affects thinking, judgment, and social behavior in ways that cause serious problems and embarrassment. For example, unwise business or financial decisions may be made when an individual is in a manic phase. Bipolar disorder is often a chronic recurring condition.

SYMPTOMS OF DEPRESSION AND MANIA

Not everyone who is depressed or manic experiences every symptom. Some people experience a few symptoms, some many. Also, severity of symptoms varies with individuals.

Depression

- Persistent sad, anxious, or "empty" mood
- Feelings of hopelessness, pessimism
- Feelings of guilt, worthlessness, helplessness
- Loss of interest or pleasure in hobbies and activities that were once enjoyed, including sex
- Insomnia, early-morning awakening, or oversleeping
- Appetite and/or weight loss or overeating and weight gain
- Decreased energy, fatigue, being "slowed down"
- Thoughts of death or suicide; suicide attempts
- Restlessness, irritability
- Difficulty concentrating, remembering, making decisions
- Persistent physical symptoms that do not respond to treatment, such as headaches, digestive disorders, and chronic pain

Mania

- Inappropriate elation
- Inappropriate irritability
- Severe insomnia
- Grandiose notions
- Increased talking
- Disconnected and racing thoughts
- Increased sexual desire
- Markedly increased energy
- Poor judgment
- Inappropriate social behavior

CAUSES OF DEPRESSION

Some types of depression run in families, indicating that a biological vulnerability can be inherited. This seems to be the case with bipolar. Studies of families, in which members of each generation develop bipolar disorder, found that those with the illness have a somewhat different genetic makeup than those who do not get ill. However, the reverse is not true: Not everybody with the genetic makeup that causes vulnerability to bipolar disorder has the illness. Apparently additional factors, possibly a stressful environment, are involved in its onset.

Major depression also seems to occur, generation after generation, in some families. However, it can also occur in people who have no family history of depression.

Psychological makeup also plays a role in vulnerability to depression. People who have low self-esteem, who consistently view themselves and the world with pessimism, or who are readily overwhelmed by stress are prone to depression.

A serious loss, chronic illness, difficult relationship, financial problem, or any unwelcome change in life patterns can also trigger a depressive episode. Very often, a combination of genetic, psychological, and environmental factors is involved in the onset of a depressive disorder.

DIAGNOSTIC EVALUATION AND TREATMENT

The first step to getting appropriate treatment is a complete physical and psychological evaluation to determine whether you have a depressive disorder, and if so what type you have. Certain medications as well as some medical conditions can cause symptoms of depression and the examining clinician should rule out these possibilities.

A good diagnostic evaluation also will include a complete history of your symptoms, that is, when they started, how long they have lasted, how severe they are, whether you've had them before and, if so, whether you were treated and what treatment you received. You will be asked about alcohol and drug use, and if you have thoughts about death or suicide. Further, a history should include questions about whether other family members have had a depressive illness and if treated, what treatments they may have received and which were effective.

Last, a diagnostic evaluation will include a mental status examination to determine if your speech or thought patterns or memory have been affected, as often happens in the case of a depressive or manic-depressive illness.

Treatment choice will depend on the outcome of the evaluation. There are a variety of psychotherapies and antidepressant medications that can be used to treat depressive disorders. Some people do well with psychotherapy, some with antidepressants. Some do best with combined treatment: medication to gain relatively quick symptom relief and psychotherapy to learn more effective ways to deal with life's problems. Depending on your diagnosis and severity of symptoms, you may be prescribed medication and/or treated with one of the several forms of psychotherapy that have proven effective for depression.

ANTIDEPRESSANT MEDICATIONS

There are several different types of medications used to treat depressive disorders. Sometimes your doctor will try a variety of antidepressants before finding the medication or combination of medications most effective for you. Sometimes the dosage must be increased to be effective. Also, new types of antidepressants are being developed all the time, and one of these may be the best for you.

Antidepressant drugs are not habit-forming, so you need not be concerned about that. However, as is the case with any type of medication prescribed for more than a few days, antidepressants have to be carefully monitored to see if you are getting the correct dosage. Your doctor will want to check the dosage and its effectiveness regularly.

Antianxiety drugs, such as Valium, are *not* antidepressants. They are sometimes prescribed along with antidepressants; however, they should not be taken alone for a depressive disorder. Sleeping pills and stimulants, such as amphetamines, are also inappropriate.

PSYCHOTHERAPIES

There are many forms of psychotherapy effectively used to help depressed individuals, including some short-term (10-20 weeks) therapies. "Talking" therapies help patients gain insight into and resolve their problems through verbal "give-and-take" with the therapist. "Behavioral" therapists help patients learn how to obtain more satisfaction and rewards through their own actions and how to unlearn the behavioral patterns that contribute to their depression.

Two of the short-term psychotherapies that research has shown helpful for some forms of depression are Interpersonal and Cognitive/Behavioral therapies. Interpersonal therapists focus on the patient's disturbed personal relationships that both cause and exacerbate the depression. Cognitive/behavioral therapists help patients change the negative styles of thinking and behaving often associated with depression.

Psychodynamic therapies, sometimes used to treat depression, focus on resolving the patient's internal psychological conflicts that are typically thought to be rooted in childhood.

The severe depressive illnesses, particularly those that are recurrent, may require medication along with psychotherapy for the best outcome.

HELPING YOURSELF

Depressive disorders make you feel exhausted, worthless, helpless, and hopeless. Such negative thoughts and feelings make some people feel like giving up. It is important to realize that these negative views are part of the depression and typically do not accurately reflect your situation. Negative thinking fades as treatment begins to take effect. In the meantime:

- Do not set yourself difficult goals or take on a great deal of responsibility.
- Break large tasks into small ones, set some priorities, and do what you can as you can.
- Do not expect too much from yourself too soon as this will only increase feelings of failure.
- Try to be with other people; it is usually better than being alone.
- Participate in activities that may make you feel better.
- You might try mild exercise, going to a movie, a ballgame, or participating in religious or social activities.
- Don't overdo it or get upset if your mood is not greatly improved right away. Feeling better takes time.
- Do not make major life decisions, such as changing jobs, getting married, or getting divorced, without consulting others who know you well and who have a more objective view of your situation. In any case, it is advisable to postpone important decisions until your depression has lifted.
- Do not expect to snap out of your depression. People rarely do. Help yourself as much as you can, and do not blame yourself for not being up to par.
- *Remember,* do not accept your negative thinking. It is part of the depression and will disappear as your depression responds to treatment.

FAMILY AND FRIENDS CAN HELP

Since depression can make you feel exhausted and helpless, you will want and probably need help from others. However, people who have never had a depressive disorder may not fully understand its effect. They won't mean to hurt you, but they may say and do things that do. It may help to share this handout with those you most care about so they can better understand and help you.

HELPING THE DEPRESSED PERSON

The most important thing anyone can do for the depressed person is to help him or her get appropriate diagnosis and treatment. This may involve encouraging the individual to stay with treatment until symptoms begin to abate (several weeks), or to seek different treatment if no improvement occurs. On occasion, it may require making an appointment and accompanying the depressed person to the doctor. It may also mean monitoring whether the depressed person is taking medication.

The second most important thing is to offer emotional support. This involves understanding, patience, affection, and encouragement. Engage the depressed person in conversation and listen carefully. Do not disparage feelings expressed, but point out realities and offer hope. Do not ignore remarks about suicide. Always report them to the depressed person's therapist.

Invite the depressed person for walks, for outings, to the movies, and to other activities. Be gently insistent if your invitation is refused. Encourage participation in some activities that once gave pleasure, such as hobbies, sports, or religious or cultural activities, but do not push the depressed person to undertake too much too soon. The depressed person needs diversion and company, but too many demands can increase feelings of failure.

Do not accuse the depressed person of faking illness or of laziness, or expect him or her to "snap out of it." Eventually, with treatment, most depressed people do get better. Keep that in mind, and keep reassuring the depressed person that, with time and help, he or she will feel better.

WHERE TO GET HELP

A complete physical and psychological diagnostic evaluation will help you decide the type of treatment that might be best for you. Listed below are the types of people and places that will make a referral to, or provide, diagnostic and treatment services. Check the *Yellow Pages* under "mental health," "psychologist," "health," "social services," "suicide prevention," "hospitals," or "physicians" for phone numbers and addresses.

- Family doctors
- Mental health specialists, such as psychiatrists, psychologists, social workers, or mental health counselors
- Health maintenance organizations
- Community mental health centers
- Hospital psychiatry or psychology departments and outpatient clinics
- University- affiliated programs or medical school-affiliated programs
- State hospital outpatient clinics
- Family service/social agencies
- Private clinics and facilities
- Employee assistance programs
- Local medical and/or psychiatric societies

SUBJECT INDEX TO VOLUMES 11, 12, AND 13

A complete subject index for Volumes 1 through 5 is contained in Volume 5. A complete subject index for Volumes 6 through 10 is contained in Volume 10. A cumulative index for all 13 volumes is also available from the publisher.

A

Abuse,
    child, 11: 315-324, 12: 15-34
    Child Abuse Blame Scale, 11: 315-324
    physical, 11: 315-324
    ritualistic, 11: 189-191, 193, 195-196
    sexual,
        in adolescents, 13: 375-376
        assessing allegations of, in custody disputes, 12: 15-34
        in correctional centers, 11: 413-423
        hypnosis and, 12: 519-527
        imagery rescripting for, 13: 73-85
        possibility therapy for, 12: 99-113
        of preteen girls, 11: 109-122
        validation with anatomically correct dolls, 12: 505-518
    wife, 11: 123-138
        community intervention, 11: 124
        prevalence of, 11: 123
        Stockholm Syndrome theory, Graham's, and, 13: 401-417
        treatment alternatives, 11: 124-127
Addiction,
    to alcohol, 11: 75-85
    to nicotine, 12-Step program for, 12: 455-474
    object relations therapy for, 11: 63-74
    to over-the-counter drugs, 11: 53-61
    to prescription drugs, 11: 53-61
ADHD (*see* Attention-Deficit/Hyperactivity Disorder)
Adolescents,
    and AIDS, myths about, 13: 431-441
    group psychotherapy for, 13: 369-382
        problem-specific group interventions, 13: 374-380
        trends in theory and practice, 13: 370-374
    substance abuse treatment with, 13: 97-121
Adoption workbook, 12: 363-376

Affairs, secret, 12: 133-145
    ancient affairs, 12: 138
    denial, 12: 138-139
    preparation for revealing, 12: 139-142
    revelation session, 12: 142-144
    therapist concerns, 12: 134-136, 144
    when not to reveal an affair, 12: 136-138
African-American assessment style, 11: 457
African-Americans, interventions for, 12: 295-310
    Africentric worldview, 12: 296-297
    clients' ethnic socialization and identification, 12: 297-301
        Africentric approaches, 12: 300
        developmental approaches, 12: 299-300
        group-based approaches, 12: 300
        measures of ethnic stereotyping, 12: 300
    issues concerning therapists, 12: 304-307
        attendance and participation, 12: 304-305
        communication, 12: 306
        termination, 12: 306-307
    sensitivity and competence, 12: 295-296
Aging, normal effects versus organic mental disorders, 12: 209-226
    changes, normal, 12: 210-216
        cognitive, 12: 210, 211-216
        physiological, 12: 210-211, 214-216
    clinical issues, 12: 216-219
        age-specific norms, 12: 217-218
        comprehensive mental status screening tests, 12: 218-219
        short mental status screening tests, 12: 218
    language function, 12: 213-214
    organic mental syndromes and disorders, 12: 219-223
        delirium, 12: 220-222, 479
        dementia, 12: 221-222, 479-480
        pseudodementia, 12: 222-223
Agoraphobic Cognitions Questionnaire, 12: 77

AIDS,
- myths about, concerning adolescents, 13: 431-441
- and substance abuse, 11: 541-552

Alcoholism and anxiety, 11: 75-85
- diagnosis, 11: 79
- family studies, 11: 80
- prevalence, 11: 75-79
- theoretical considerations, 11: 82
- treatment, 11: 80-82

American Indians (*see* Native Americans)

Amnesia,
- detection of malingered, 12: 9-10
- syndrome, 12: 574

Anatomically correct dolls, 12: 505-518

Anger,
- children's, 12: 337-362
    - assessment, 12: 337-338
    - Children's Anger Response Checklist, 12: 349-360
- Controlling Anger Before It Controls You, 13: 445-450

Anxiety,
- and alcoholism, 11: 75-85
- medical disorders and, 13: 170
- scales for assessment of, 13: 167-178
    - for adults, 13: 169-172
    - for children and adolescents, 13: 172-174

Anxiety disorders, 12: 65-83 (*see also* Panic attack disorder)
- brief dynamic therapies, 12: 71-75
    - Davanloo's Intensive Short-Term Psychotherapy, 12: 71-72
    - Luborsky's Short-Term Supportive-Expressive Psychoanalytic Psychotherapy, 12: 73-74
    - Sifneos' Short-Term Anxiety-Provoking Psychotherapy, 12: 73
    - Strupp's Time-Limited Dynamic Psychotherapy, 12: 75
- differential diagnosis, 12: 65-70
    - generalized anxiety disorder, 12: 70
    - obsessive compulsive disorder, 12: 69
    - panic attack disorder, 12: 65-67
    - post-traumatic stress disorder, 12: 69-70
    - simple phobia, 12: 68-69
    - social phobia, 12: 67-68
- pharmacology interventions, 12: 75-76

Anxiety Disorders Interview Schedule-Revised (ADIS-R), 12: 78-80

Asian-American assessment style, 11: 458

Assertiveness training, 11: 112-115

Assessment, forms for, 12: 313-328

Assessment in rehabilitation counseling, 11: 351-362

Attention-Deficit/Hyperactivity Disorder (ADHD), 13: 123-138
- comorbidity and medical intervention, 13: 132-135
- definition, 13: 123-125
- etiology, 13: 125-126
- identification, 13: 126-128
- prevalence, 13: 125
- school-based interventions and services, 13: 128-132
- special education eligibility, 13: 128

Attorneys, agreements with psychologists, 13: 255-262
- conflict, sources of, 13: 255-257
- statement of principles, 13: 257-261

Avoidant personality disorder, 11: 5-22
- cognitive-interpersonal integration, 11: 5-7
- intervention, 11: 13-20
    - awareness of cognitive-interpersonal patterns, 11: 15-18
    - behavioral experimentation, 11: 19-20
    - cognitive reevaluation, 11: 19-20
    - increasing interest in new strategies, 11: 18-19
    - treatment goals, 11: 13
    - treatment process issues, 11: 13-15
- patterns of avoidant patients, 11: 7-13

B

Battered women, Stockholm theory and, 13: 401-417
- Allen's unbonding continuum, 13: 403-409
- Graham's Stockholm Syndrome theory, 13: 401-403
- Peters' Phoenix Program, 13: 409-415

Behavior therapy for,
- acute pain in children, 12: 193-208
- children's nighttime fears, 11: 139-155
- panic disorder, 12: 115-133

Biofeedback, in chronic pain management, 13: 62-63

Borderline personality, 12: 49-64

Bravery tokens (for children's nighttime fears), 11: 145, 152

Brief dynamic therapies, 12: 71-75

C

Cancer pain patients, adjunctive treatment for, 12: 431-436
- guidelines, 12: 433-435
    - application, 12: 435
    - skill acquisition, 12: 434
- overview, 12: 432

Case management for seriously mentally ill persons, 11: 505-519
- definition of case management, 11: 505-506
- history and clientele, 11: 506-507
- skills, 11: 507-515
    - advocacy, 11: 512
    - counseling and psychoeducation, 11: 514
    - crisis prevention, 11: 512-513
    - diagnosis, 11: 507-508
    - ethical issues and boundary problems, 11: 514-515
    - families, 11: 509-510
    - functional assessment, 11: 508
    - hospitalization, 11: 513-514
    - legal issues, 11: 510
    - liaison with other providers, 11: 511-512
    - medication, 11: 509
    - poverty, 11: 510-511

Challenging Beliefs Worksheet (for crime victims), 11: 36

Challenging Questions Sheet (for crime victims), 11: 34

CHAMPUS, 11: 233

Child Abuse Blame Scale, 11: 315-324

Child abuse, ritualistic, 11: 189-191, 195-196

Child and adolescent forensic assessment, 11: 335-349

Child sexual abuse,
- assessing allegations of, in custody disputes, 12: 15-34
- use of anatomically correct dolls for validation of, 12: 505-518

Children,
- acute pain, behavioral treatment for, 12: 193-208
- Attention-Deficit/Hyperactivity Disorder (ADHD) in, 13: 123-138
- chronic pain, behavioral treatment for, 13: 55-72
- conduct problems, behavior inventories for, 11: 261-270
- filial therapy for chronically ill, 11: 87-97
- manipulative, 12: 601-602
- memory of, for witnessed events, 12: 35-47
- with traumatic brain injury, 12: 581-594

Children's Anger Response Checklist, 12: 337-362

Children's Apperceptive Story-Telling Test (CAST), 11: 271-283
- case study, 11: 276-282
- dynamic versus static assessment, 11: 271-272
- nature of apperception, 11: 275-276

Children's nighttime fears, 11: 139-155
- bravery tokens, 11: 145, 152
- Daily Monitoring, 11: 152

Children's nighttime fears *(Continued)*
    evaluation of treatment programs, 11: 140
    fear of the dark program, 11: 140-155
        assessment, 11: 141-143
        child training, 11: 145-146
        parent training, 11: 143-145
        treatment, 11: 143-147
    fear versus compliance, 11: 140
    Interview with Child, 11: 150-151
    Interview with Parents, 11: 148-149
Chronic illness in children, family issues with, 11: 87-97
Chronic pain,
    in children, 13: 55-72
        assessment of, 13: 57-61
        definition of, 13: 56
        sources of, 13: 56
        treatment of, 13: 61-66
        types of referrals, 13: 57
    cognitive-behavioral management for, 12: 169-191
        cognitive variables, 12: 170-171
        coping strategies for pain, 12: 171-175
            catastrophizing, 12: 173-174
        features, 12: 170
        goal setting, 12: 177-179
        Inventory of Negative Thoughts in Response to Pain, 12: 183-185
        memory for pain, 12: 179-182
            influence of affect and cognitive appraisal, 12: 179-180
            influence of assessment technique, 12: 180-181
            pain diary, 12: 181, 188, 13: 61, 69
        pain beliefs, 12: 175-177
        Pain Beliefs and Perceptions Inventory, 12: 175-176, 186-187
Chronic problems, brief therapy for, 12: 85-97
Client Satisfaction Survey, 13: 293-297
Clinical and Administrative Management Checklist, 13: 299-305
Cognitive-behavioral therapy for,
    adolescent substance abusers, 13: 97-121
    chronic pain management, 12: 169-191
    depression in elderly, 13: 155
    driving while intoxicated (DWI) offenders, 13: 339-356
    families of head-injured patients, 11: 173-185
    marital violence, 13: 8-12
    satanism, 11: 193-199
    victims of crime, 11: 23-38
    withdrawal, 11: 59-60
Cognitive-behavioral treatment for panic disorder, 12: 133-145
Cognitive processing therapy, 11: 23-38
Cognitive therapy for,
    avoidant personality disorder, 11: 5-22
Comorbidity, alcoholism and anxiety, 11: 75-85
Comprehensive Forensic Data Organization Sheet: Adult Version, 12: 387-402
Comprehensive Forensic Data Organization Sheet: Child and Adolescent Version, 11: 335-349
Computerized psychological assessment,
    computer-based test and interpretation (CBTI) guidelines, 11: 252-256
    liability issues, 11: 251-257
    test developer responsibilities, 11: 252
    test user/administrator responsibilities, 11: 252-255
Conduct problems in children, behavior inventories for, 11: 261-270
Contracts with adolescent groups, 13: 370-371
Contract with the Group (for men who batter), 11: 134-135
Controlling Anger Before It Controls You, 13: 445-450
Conversion Disorder, 12: 8-9
Coping Strategies Questionnaire, 12: 172

Corrections facilities,
    sexual abuse prevention program, 11: 413-423
    suicide prevention program, 11: 467-480
Countertransference, 12: 49-64, 13: 49-51, 158
Crime, victims of, 11: 23-38
    cognitive processing therapy, 11: 26-33
    prolonged exposure, 11: 24-25
    stress inoculation training, 11: 25-26
Crisis stabilization, inpatient, 12: 417-429
    admission process, 12: 418
    intervention strategy, 12: 422-427
    systems management, 12: 427-428
    target symptoms, 12: 418-422
Cults, satanic, 11: 187-201
Cultural competence (*see* Multicultural competence in assessment)
Custody disputes, sexual abuse allegations in, 12: 15-34
Custody evaluations, ethical issues in, 12: 257-262
    abuse, handling allegations of, 12: 260-261
    avoiding dual relationships, 12: 259-260
    documentation, 12: 261
    financial arrangements, 12: 258
    informing parents, 12: 259
    mediation versus litigation, 12: 258
    using appropriate techniques, 12: 261

D

Davanloo's Intensive Short-Term Psychotherapy, 12: 71-72
Deaf clients,
    causes of deafness, 11: 100-101
    deaf culture, 11: 99-100
    education, 11: 102
    family issues, 11: 101-102, 105
    psychosocial issues, 11: 102-103
    psychotherapy for, 11: 99-107
        personality factors, 11: 104
        psychotherapeutic difficulties, 11: 104
        use of interpreter, 11: 104-105
Deception (*see* Malingering)
Delirium, 12: 220-222, 479
Dementia, 12: 221-222, 479-480
Dementia-related illness, 12: 574-576
Dependency in patients, 13: 139-150
    assessment of, 13: 140-141
    effective psychotherapy for, 13: 145-148
    research on, 13: 141-144
Depression,
    and anxiety, 13: 168
    Attention-Deficit/Hyperactivity Disorder (ADHD) and, in children, 13: 134
    and dependency, 13: 142
    in elderly, 12: 222-223, 13: 151-166
    and memory performance, 12: 576-578
    Plain Talk About Depression, 13: 451-455
    postpartum, 11: 39-51
Disabled clients, 13: 419-430
    counseling process, 13: 426-427
    issues of disabled clients, 13: 419-424
    suggestions for practitioners, 13: 427-428
    terminology, language, attitudes, 13: 424-426
Disaster response, 11: 403-411
    general treatment issues, 11: 408-409
        antiburnout measures, 11: 409
        therapist flexibility, 11: 409
        timing, 11: 408
        touch, 11: 408
        triage, 11: 408

Disaster response *(Continued)*
    loss and bereavement, 11: 407-408
        intervention techniques, 11: 407-408
        knowledge base/background, 11: 407
    post-disaster groups for adolescents, 13: 375-376
    training issues, 11: 409
    working with survivors, 11: 404-407
        intervention techniques, 11: 405-407
        knowledge base/background, 11: 404-405
Discrimination, sexual, 12: 263-276
Dissociative disorders, incest and, 13: 37-54
Distraction, in chronic pain management, 13: 64
Divorce, *(see also* Therapy, marital)
    adolescents and, 13: 374-375
    affairs and, 12: 137
    custody disputes regarding sexual abuse, 12: 15-34
    predivorce stage, group treatment for, 13: 309-322
Dolls, anatomically correct, why not to use, 12: 505-518
Domestic Violence Blame Scale (DVBS), 13: 265-278
    applications, 13: 270-271
    development of, 13: 268-269
    scoring, 13: 269-270
    theoretical perspective, 13: 267-268
Drug abuse, over-the-counter and prescription, 11: 53-61
    characteristics of abuser, 11: 53-54
    commonly abused medications, 11: 54-57
        analgesics, 11: 56
        ergots, 11: 56-57
        nonsteroidal drugs, 11: 56
        psychoactive medications, 11: 54-55
        steroids and human growth hormone, 11: 55-56
        stimulants, 11: 55
    in elderly, 12: 477-496
    relapse prevention, 11: 60
    role of mental health professional, 11: 58-60
    withdrawal, 11: 57-59
DSM-IV, 12: 497-504
    childhood disorders, 12: 502-503
    clinically significant problems, 12: 503
    cognitive impairment disorders, 12: 499
    mood disorders, 12: 501
    new categories, 12: 503
    personality disorders, 12: 501-502
    psychotic disorders, 12: 500-501
    substance-related disorders, 12: 500
Dual relationships, nonsexual, 11: 443-454
    causes, 11: 448-452
        decreased role distance, 11: 451-452
        denial or rationalization by therapist, 11: 451
        emotional vulnerability, 11: 449-450
    definition, 11: 443-444
    types of, 11: 444-448
        accepting gifts or favors, 11: 446-447
        accepting significant other referrals, 11: 447
        business transactions with clients, 11: 445
        dual role hazards in small communities, 11: 448
        entering new relationships with former clients, 11: 447-448
        psychotherapy with employees, 11: 445
        psychotherapy with friends and family, 11: 444-445
        psychotherapy with students or supervisees, 11: 445-446
        service bartering, 11: 446
        socializing with current clients, 11: 447
DWI (driving while intoxicated) offenders, evaluation and treatment of, 13: 339-356
    drinking driver programs, 13: 340
    evaluation of offenders, 13: 341-343
    group process, 13: 346-348
    group psychotherapy program, 13: 343-346

E

Eating disorders,
    adolescent groups for, 13: 379
    dependent patients and, 13: 143
Elderly
    depression and loss, 13: 151-166
        assessment and diagnosis, 13: 152-154
        techniques for addressing loss, 13: 158-161
        treatment strategies, 13: 154-158
    and substance abuse, 12: 477-496
ERISA, 11: 234
Ethical issues
    in case management for seriously ill clients, 11: 514-515
    in child custody evaluations, 12: 257-262
    in custody disputes involving sexual abuse allegations, 12: 30
    in family mediation, 12: 413
    in insurance reimbursement, 11: 234-236
    with managed-care patients, 11: 481-493
        assumptions, 11: 481-482
        competence, 11: 485-486
        professional relationships, 11: 490-492
        screening, initial assessment, and referral, 11: 486-487
        standards of care, 11: 485-490
        termination, 11: 489
        testing and evaluation, 11: 487-488
        treatment, 11: 488-489
    in multicultural assessment, 11: 463-464
    with Native Americans, 12: 448
    in therapy involving exercise, 12: 165-166
    welfare of the consumer, and, 11: 482-485
        confidentiality, 11: 482-483
        conflict of interest, 11: 484-485
        documentation, 11: 489-490
        informed consent, 11: 483-484
Exercise in psychotherapy, 12: 155-168
    case examples, 12: 159-164
    contraindications, 12: 165
    ethical, legal, and process considerations, 12: 165-166
    involvement in therapy, 12: 156-159
    role of therapist, 12: 156-158
    suggestions and recommendations, 12: 164-166
Expert witness, cross-examination of, 13: 323-338
Eyberg Child Behavior Inventory, 11: 261-267

F

Factitious disorder, 12: 7-8
Families of seriously mentally ill, 11: 389-402
    a competence paradigm, 11: 390-391
    familial reality, 11: 392-394
        coping and adaptation, 11: 392-393
        family burden, 11: 392
        family needs and need satisfaction, 11: 392
        lifespan, subsystem, and spousal concerns, 11: 394
    family-professional relationships, 11: 389-390
    intervention strategies, 11: 394-398
        clinical, 11: 396-398
        nonclinical, 11: 394-396
    release of information form, 11: 399
Families, storytelling and, 12: 147-154
Family issues with head injury patients, 11: 173-185
    acceptance and reintegration, 11: 183-184
    case examples, 11: 179-183

Family issues with head injury patients *(Continued)*
   family impact, 11: 175-176
      denial, 11: 176-177
      detachment, 11: 178
      overprotectiveness, 11: 177
      unrealistic expectations, 11: 177
   mechanisms of brain damage, 11: 173-174
   therapy models, 11: 178-179
Family mediation, 12: 405-415
   applications, 12: 408-411
      divorce, 12: 408-409
      elder care, 12: 409-410
      marital, 12: 409
      parent-child, 12: 409
   definition, 12: 405-407
      distinguishing mediation from psychotherapy, 12: 406-407
   ethical issues, 12: 413
   training, 12: 411-413
Family Survival Sheet (for homeless), 11: 170
Family therapy for, depression in elderly, 13: 156-157
Faulty Thinking Patterns (for crime victims), 11: 35
Fear, children's nighttime fears, 11: 139-155
Fear of the dark program, 11: 141-147
Federal Employees Health Benefits Program, 11: 233
Fees in psychotherapy, 13: 223-235
   patients' roles, 13: 227-230
   policies, 13: 230-234
   therapists' roles, 13: 223-227
Filial therapy and chronic childhood illness, 11: 87-97
   case examples, 11: 94-96
   developmental issues, 11: 90
   family stresses and needs, 11: 87-90
      affective, 11: 89
      informational-cognitive, 11: 88-89
      social-interpersonal, 11: 89-90
   intervention, 11: 90-91
      parent training, 11: 92-93
      play sessions, 11: 92-94
Flooding *(see* Prolonged exposure treatment)
Forensic assessment,
   adult, 12: 387-402
   child and adolescent, 11: 335-349
   malingering, detection of, 12: 5-13
Forms and instruments,
   Adoption Workbook, 12: 363-376
   Agoraphobic Cognitions Questionnaire, 12: 77
   Answers to Your Questions About Panic Disorder, 12: 597-600
   Anxiety Disorders Interview Schedule-Revised (ADIS R), 12: 78-80
   Bravery Tokens (for children's nighttime fears), 11: 152
   Case Assessment Forms in Rehabilitation Counseling, 11: 353-361
   Child Abuse Blame Scale, 11: 320-322
   Children's Anger Response Checklist, 12: 338-362
   Children's Apperceptive Story-Telling Test (CAST), 11: 271-283
   Client Satisfaction Survey, 13: 294-295
   Clinical and Administrative Management Checklist, 13: 300-304
   Comprehensive Forensic Data Organization Sheet: Adult Version, 12: 392-401
   Comprehensive Forensic Data Organization Sheet: Child and Adolescent Version, 11: 339-348
   Consumer Satisfaction Measures (parent training programs), 12: 377-382

Forms and instruments *(Continued)*
   Contract with the Group (for men who batter), 11: 134-135
   Daily Monitoring (for children's nighttime fears), 11: 152
   Daily Rating System (for pain management), 11: 535-536
   Daily Record of Dysfunctional Thoughts, 12: 81
   Developmental History, 12: 316
   Domestic Violence Blame Scale, 13: 272-274
   Drug and Alcohol Abuse History, 12: 322-323
   Eyberg Child Behavior Inventory, 11: 267
   Family History, 12: 318
   Family Survival Sheet (for homeless), 11: 170
   Geriatric Depression Scale, 13: 162
   Group Therapy Needs Assessment Survey, 12: 383-386
   Hamilton Anxiety Rating Scale, 13: 175
   HOMELESS Assessment Interview, 11: 164-167
   Impact of Event Scale (for rape victims), 11: 331
   Informed Consent Form, 13: 296
   Intake Checklist (for men who batter), 11: 132-133
   Interoceptive Exposure Forms (for panic disorder), 12: 332-335
   Interview with Child (for children's nighttime fears), 11: 150-151
   Interview with Parents (for children's nighttime fears), 11: 148-149
   Inventory of Negative Thoughts in Response to Pain, 12: 183-185
   Job Analysis (for rehabilitation), 11: 366-373
   Legal History, 12: 328
   Leisure Interests Checklists, 12: 553-555, 560-561
   Life Stressors, 12: 325
   Marital History, 12: 319-320
   McGill Pain Questionnaire, 11: 290
   Medication Record (for pain management), 11: 534
   Notice to Medicare Patients, 11: 237
   Occupational History, 12: 326-327
   Pain Beliefs and Perceptions Inventory, 12: 175-176, 186-187
   Pain Diary, 11: 533, 12: 188, 13: 69
   Parental History, 12: 317
   Patient Contract (for pain management), 11: 532
   Physical History, 12: 324
   Release of Information Form (for families of seriously mentally ill), 11: 399
   Scale of Feelings and Behavior of Love, 11: 309-312
   Scale of Marriage Problems, 11: 299-300
   Sleep Diary, 13: 193
   Stress Job Analysis (for rehabilitation), 11: 374-384
   Suicidal Ideation History, 12: 321
   Sutter-Eyberg Student Behavior Inventory, 11: 268
   Techniques to Manipulate Parents, 12: 602
   Therapy Attitude Inventory, 12: 377-380
   Therapy History, 12: 315
   TMJ Interview Points, 11: 215
   Violence Attitudes Scale, 13: 285-288
   Wharton Scale (for TMJ patients), 11: 214
   Workshop Attitude Inventory, 12: 377-379, 381

G

Generalized anxiety disorder, 12: 70
Graham's Stockholm Syndrome theory, 13: 401-417
Grief, therapy for unresolved, 11: 495-503
   tasks of therapy, 11: 500-501
Group Therapy Needs Assessment Survey, 12: 383-386
Group treatment for,
   adolescents, 13: 369-382
   battered women, 13: 10

Group treatment for *(Continued)*
    depression in elderly, 13: 156
    driving while intoxicated (DWI) offenders, 13: 339-356
    men who batter, 11: 123-138, 13: 10
        format, 11: 130-131
        rationale, 11: 125-126
        referral and intake, 11: 127-130
        structure and organization, 11: 126-127
    separated couples, 13: 309-322
    sexually abused preteen girls, 11: 109-122
        exercises, 11: 110-121
        organization, 11: 109-110
        phases, 11: 110
        termination, 11: 121
Guided imagery, in management of chronic pain, 13: 64-65

H

Handouts for clients,
    Answers to Your Questions About Panic Disorder, 12: 597-600
    Challenging Beliefs Worksheet, 11: 36
    Challenging Questions Sheet, 11: 34
    Controlling Anger Before It Controls You, 13: 445-450
    Family Survival Sheet (for homeless), 11: 170
    Faulty Thinking Patterns, 11: 35
    Goals (DWI offenders), 13: 354-355
    How to Deal With Manipulative Children, 12: 602
    Identify Your Resources, 13: 353
    Plain Talk About Depression, 13: 451-455
    Remedies (DWI offenders), 13: 351-352
Harassment, sexual, 12: 263-276, 13: 237-253
Head injury, family issues, 11: 173-185 *(see also* Traumatic brain injury [TBI])
Headache, rebound, 11: 57-58
Health care reform, 12: 241-256
Hispanic-American assessment style, 11: 458
Homeless families, assessment and treatment, 11: 157-172
    compared to housed poor families, 11: 158
        Family Survival Sheet, 11: 170
    HOMELESS Assessment Interview, 11: 161-167
    sample family assessment report, 11: 168-169
    therapeutic intervention, 11: 159-161
        church-shelter consultations, 11: 160-161
        health care access, 11: 160
        private space, 11: 159-160
        support groups, 11: 160
        time out, 11: 160
        use of volunteers, 11: 159
Hypnosis and suggestions of abuse, 12: 519-527

I

Imagery, guided, in chronic pain management, 13: 64-65
Imagery rescripting for childhood sexual abuse survivors, 13: 73-85
    traumatic memory, 13: 74-75
    treatment outline, 13: 75-81
Impact of Event Scale (for rape victims), 11: 325-333
Incest, treatment of, 13: 37-54
    adolescent groups for, 13: 376-377
    complex dissociative post-traumatic stress reactions, 13: 39-41
    damage potential of incest, 13: 37-39
    treatment model for, 13: 41-51
Informed Consent Form, 13: 297

Insanity defense, 13: 383-399
    abolitionist movement, 13: 394
    development of, 13: 385-389
    myths, 13: 391-392
    role of punishment, 13: 390-391
    scientific evidence, 13: 393
Insomnia, 13: 179-195
    assessment, 13: 182-184
    causes, 13: 180-181
    natural history, 13: 181-182
    overview, 13: 179-180
    treatment protocol, 13: 184-192
Insurance reimbursement, 11: 227-237
    ethical and legal issues, 11: 234-236
        abandonment, 11: 234-235
        assistants and supervisees, 11: 235-236
        waiving co-payments, 11: 235
    freedom of choice and mandated coverage, 11: 233-234
        ERISA, 11: 234
    insurance concept, 11: 227-228
    Medicare, 11: 228-232
        "incident to" services, 11: 230
        physician consultation, 11: 230
        procedure codes, 11: 229-230
        OBRA-89 definitions, 11: 228-229
        other changes, 11: 232
        reimbursement, 11: 231
        resource based relative value scale, 11: 231-232
    other government programs, 11: 232-233
        CHAMPUS, 11: 233
        Federal Employees Health Benefits Program, 11: 233
        Medicaid, 11: 232-233
Intake Checklist (for men who batter), 11: 132-133
Intellectual tests, malingering on, 12: 11
Intelligence, in aging process, 12: 211-212
Interoceptive exposure in treatment of panic disorder, 12: 329-336

J

Job analyses in rehabilitation counseling, 11: 363-386
    sample job analysis, 11: 366-373
    sample stress job analysis, 11: 374-384
    stress factors, 11: 365
Job-finding firms *(see* Outplacement firms, consultation to)
Juvenile delinquents, groups for, 13: 379-380

L

Language function, in aging, 12: 213-214
Law, psychology and, 13: 255-262
Learning disabilities, and Attention-Deficit/Hyperactivity Disorder (ADHD), 13: 134-135
Learning disorders, neuropsychological evaluation of, 12: 227-238
    goals, 12: 228-229
    methods, 12: 230-233
        assessing the neuropsychology of learning, 12: 231-233
        evaluating learning and attention disorders, 12: 230
Leisure Interests Checklists, 12: 545-563
    distraction and stress reduction, 12: 548-561
    rumination and vicious cycles, 12: 547-548
    stress and preoccupation with self, 12: 545-546
Liability,
    in computerized psychological assessment, 11: 251-257
    regarding subpoenas, 11: 224-225

Litigation,
    against practitioner, 11: 223
    consulting, as to cross-examination of neuropsychologists, 13: 323-338
    involving clients, 11: 222-223
Loss and bereavement, 11: 407-408
    and depression in the elderly, 13: 151-166
Luborsky's Short-Term Supportive-Expressive Psychoanalytic Psychotherapy, 12: 73-74

M

Malingering, 12: 5-13
    expert testimony on, 12: 12
    specific disorders, 12: 7-10
    testing for, 12: 10-12
Malpractice,
    in computerized testing, 11: 251-257
    subpoenas, 11: 223
Managed care, 11: 241-250, 12: 241-256, 13: 199-221
    compensation, 11: 245
    confidentiality, 11: 246
    contract terms, 11: 245
    co-payments, 11: 245
    cost containment, 12: 243
    covered services, 11: 246
    definition, 11: 241-242
    ethical and legal issues, 11: 247-248
    ethical practice with managed-care patients, 11: 481-493
    fees, 13: 230-234
    financial risk, 11: 245, 246
    group therapy models, 12: 251-252
    initiation fees, 11: 245
    language of, 12: 245-247
    limit of sessions, 11: 245
    market analysis, 13: 203-204
    marketing, 11: 244
    mental health care, 12: 241-256
    models of psychotherapy, 12: 250-253, 13: 206-210
    quality control, 12: 243
    research relevant to mental health treatment, 12: 247-249
    treatment effectiveness, 12: 243-244
    trends, 11: 249, 13: 202-203
    types, 11: 242-243, 12: 245-246
        Exclusive Provider Organizations (EPOs), 11: 243
        Health Maintenance Organizations (HMOs), 11: 242-244
        Preferred Provider Organizations (PPOs), 11: 243-244
    utilization review, 11: 246, 247
Manipulative children, 12: 601-602
A marital therapy protocol, 13: 359-368
    assessing and joining with the couple, 13: 360-362
    therapeutic closure and outcome, 13: 365-366
    therapy process, 13: 362-365
Marital violence (see Violence, marital)
Marriage,
    Scale of Feelings and Behavior of Love, 11: 303-314
    Scale of Marriage Problems, 11: 293-302
McGill Pain Questionnaire, 11: 285-291
Medicaid, 11: 232-233
Medicare, 11: 228-232
    Notice to Medicare Patients, 11: 237
Medication,
    and depression in elderly, 13: 153, 157-158
    and insomnia, 13: 189-190
Meditative breathing, in chronic pain management, 13: 63

Memory,
    in aging process, 12: 212-213
    children's, for witnessed events, 12: 35-47
        deficiencies in, 12: 41-42
        demonstrating, 12: 38-41
        influencing factors, 12: 42-44
        memory processes, 12: 36-38
        strategies for, 12: 41-42
    and hypnosis, 12: 519-527
Memory Assessment Scales, 12: 565-580
    clinical validity studies, 12: 571-572
    development and validation, 12: 568-570
    interpretation, 12: 572-574
    normative studies, 12: 570
    reliability studies, 12: 571
    representative syndromes, 12: 574-578
    test materials and use, 12: 566-567
Men who batter, treatment for, 11: 123-138
Minnesota Multiphasic Personality Inventory (MMPI),
    in addictions treatment, 11: 66
    in assessing malingering, 12: 10
    in multicultural assessment, 11: 460-463
    in screening for TMJ, 11: 205-206, 208-209
Mirror, one-way, in parent training, 13: 87-95
M'Naghten rule, 13: 385-388
Multicultural competence in assessment, 11: 455-465
    cultural competence defined, 11: 455-456
    culturally valid assessment techniques, 11: 459-463
        feedback of assessment findings, 11: 463
        moderator variables, 11: 459-460
        selection/interpretation of tests, 11: 460-463
    professional ethics, 11: 463-464
    service delivery styles, 11: 457-459
        African-American, 11: 457
        Asian-American, 11: 458
        Hispanic-American, 11: 458
        Native-American, 11: 458-459
Multiple Personality Disorder,
    malingering in, 12: 9
    treatment innovations for, 13: 21-36
        diagnosis and treatment planning, 13: 23-25
        treatment approaches, 13: 25-33
Muscle relaxation, in chronic pain management, 13: 62

N

Narcissistic personality, 12: 49-64
Native Americans, 12: 437-454
    acculturation, 12: 441-443
    assessment style, 11: 458-459, 12: 447
    clinical suggestions, 12: 449-450
    demographics, 12: 438-439
    diagnosis, 12: 447-448
    ethics, 12: 448
    Indianness, 12: 440-441
    recommendations, 12: 450-451
    research, 12: 439-440
    spirituality, 12: 443-444
    substance abuse, 12: 445-446
    terms, 12: 438
    tests, standardized, 12: 444-445
    treatment, 12: 448
Neuropsychological,
    evaluations, consumer's guide, 12: 592
    tests, malingering on, 12: 11
Neuropsychologists, cross-examination of, 13: 323-338
Neuropsychology of learning, 12: 227-238

Nicotine addiction, treating with 12-Step approach,
    12: 455-474
        emotional recovery, 12: 459-460
        physical recovery, 12: 455-459
        spirituality, 12: 460
        Twelve-Step program strategies, 12: 462-464
        Twelve-Step strategies in other therapeutic settings,
            12: 465-467
Nonsexual dual relationships, 11: 443-454
No-suicide contracts, 12: 279-288

O

Object relations therapy,
    theory of, 11: 64-65
    use of in addiction, 11: 63-74
        treatment process, 11: 66-74
Obsessive compulsive disorder, 12: 69
Oppositionality, Attention-Deficit/Hyperactivity Disorder (ADHD) and, in children, 13: 134
Organic amnesic syndrome, 12: 480
Outplacement firms, consultation to, 11: 425-430
    outplacement considerations, 11: 425-426
    psychologist's role, 11: 426-429
        with employers, 11: 428-429
        with outplacement firms, 11: 429
        with terminated employees and families, 11: 426-428
Over-the-counter drugs, addiction to, 11: 53-61, 12: 488

P

Pain, acute, in children, 12: 193-208
    assessment, 12: 197-201
    clinical issues, 12: 194-197
    definition, 12: 194
    parental involvement, 12: 196
    pharmacological considerations, 12: 195-196
    treatment strategies, 12: 201-204
        behavioral rehearsal, 12: 203-204
        distraction and coaching, 12: 204
        emotive imagery, 12: 203
        hypnosis, 12: 204
        modeling, 12: 203
        positive reinforcement, 12: 203
        relaxation training, 12: 202
Pain, cancer, adjunctive treatment for, 12: 431-436
Pain, chronic, 11: 521-539
    in children, behavioral treatment for, 13: 55-72
    cognitive-behavioral management for, 12: 169-191
    Daily Rating System, 11: 535-536
    McGill Pain Questionnaire, 11: 285-291
    Medication Record, 11: 534
    overview of treatment, 11: 521-523
        acute and chronic pain, 11: 521-522
        chronic pain syndrome, 11: 522
        interdisciplinary treatment, 11: 522-523
        treatment versus management, 11: 523
    Pain Diary, 11: 533, 12: 188
    pain management group, 11: 526-531
        evaluation, 11: 531
        goals, 11: 526-528
        structure, 11: 528-531
    Patient Contract, 11: 532
    patient groups, 11: 288
    psychosocial assessment, 11: 524-526
Panic attack disorder, 12: 65-67, 597-600
    assessment, 12: 116-119

Panic attack disorder *(Continued)*
    behavioral treatment for, 12: 115-133
        outcome data, 12: 119-120
        treatment management, 12: 129-130
        treatment strategies, 12: 120-128
    interoceptive exposure for, 12: 329-336
    self-monitoring, 12: 117-118
    syndrome description, 12: 115-116
Paraprofessional counselors, 11: 431-440
    development, 11: 432-436
        selection, 11: 434
        three models, 11: 432-434
        training, 11: 435-436
    effectiveness, 11: 431-432
    supervision, 11: 437-438
Parent training programs,
    for Attention-Deficit/Hyperactivity
        Disorder (ADHD) children, 13: 132
    consumer satisfaction measures for, 12: 377-382
    one-way mirror in, 13: 87-95
        first session, 13: 89
        guidelines for interventions, 13: 89-92
        setup, 13: 88-89
        termination, 13: 92
        training issues, 13: 93-94
Pharmacological treatment,
    of anxiety and alcoholism, 11: 80-82
    of anxiety disorders, 12: 75-76
Play therapy,
    for children with chronic illness, 11: 87-97
    parent training for, 11: 92-93
Possibility therapy, 12: 99-113
Postpartum depression, 11: 39-51
    etiology, 11: 41
    support organizations, 11: 51
    syndromes, 11: 39-40
    therapy issues and techniques, 11: 46-49
        attachment issues, 11: 49
        body image, 11: 48
        control/perfectionism, 11: 46-47
        dysfunctional family of origin, 11: 47
        financial stress, 11: 48
        guilt, 11: 48
        insomnia, 11: 48-49
        loss, 11: 47-48
        marital discord, 11: 47
        physical stresses, 11: 47
        social support, 11: 46
        uninvolved husband, 11: 46
    therapy options, 11: 41-46
        couples therapy, 11: 41-44
        group therapy, 11: 44-46
        individual therapy, 11: 44-46
Post-Traumatic Stress Disorder, 12: 69-70
    in adolescents, 13: 375
    cognitive-behavioral treatment for crime victims,
        11: 23-38
    in incest victims, 13: 37-54
    individualized treatment for, 12: 529-543
        person-event model, 12: 529
        three-tier model, 12: 529-537
        treatment, 12: 537-539
    malingered, 12: 8
    in rape victims, 11: 325-333
Prescription drugs, addiction to, 11: 53-61, 12: 484-488
Preteen girls, group treatment for abused, 11: 109-122
Projective tests, malingering on, 12: 11
Prolonged exposure treatment, 11: 24-25
PTSD (*see* Post-Traumatic Stress Disorder)

R

Rape victims, 11: 325-333
Rational-emotive therapy for, satanism, 11: 193-199
Rehabilitation counseling, 11: 363-386
    assessment forms, 11: 351-362
Relationship, therapist-client, 12: 49-64
Role conflicts for psychotherapists, 11: 443-454
Rorschach, malingering on, 12: 11

S

Satanism, treatment of, 11: 187-201
    case examples, 11: 197-200
    definition, 11: 187-188
    incidence, 11: 191-192
    misperceptions, 11: 192-193
    treatment, 11: 193-197
        adult survivors, 11: 195-197
        dabblers, 11: 194
        deeply involved satanists, 11: 193-194
        ritualistic abusers of children, 11: 194
    types of activities, 11: 188-191
        adult survivors, 11: 191
        ritualistic abuse, 11: 189-190
        satanist groups, 11: 190-191
        solitary satanists, 11: 190
        teenage satanism, 11: 188-189
Scale of Feelings and Behavior of Love, 11: 303-314
Scale of Marriage Problems, 11: 293-302
Secrecy in marriage, 12: 133-137
Serious mental illness,
    case management for, 11: 505-519
    family issues, 11: 389-402
Sexual abuse,
    hypnosis and, 12: 519-527
    imagery rescripting for, 13: 73-85
    possibility therapy for, 12: 99-113
        dissociation, disowning, and devaluing, 12: 100-102
        intrusion and inhibition, 12: 102-103
        treatment guidelines, 12: 105-113
    of preteen girls, 11: 109-122
    prevention in correctional facilities, 11: 413-423
        proposed program, 11: 416-420
        sexual offending, 11: 413-414
        traditional approaches, 11: 415-416
Sexual harassment and discrimination, 12: 263-276, 13: 237-253
    definitions, 13: 238-240
    effects of, 12: 265-266
    history, 12: 264
    presentation, 12: 268-269
    prevalence, 12: 264-265
    psychological issues, 13: 242-243
    recommendations, 12: 269-272
    responsibilities of employers, 13: 249-251
    roles for the practitioner, 13: 244-249
    severity, 12: 264
    types of sex discrimination, 12: 263-264
    typical responses, 12: 267-268
    workplace abuse, other types of, 12: 266-267
Sexuality, adolescents, and AIDS, myths about, 13: 431-441
Short-term psychotherapy, models of, 12: 250-253
Sifneos' Short-Term Anxiety-Provoking Psychotherapy, 12: 73
Simple phobia, 12: 68-69
Social phobia, 12: 67-68

Solution-focused therapy for chronic problems, 12: 85-97
    backing off, 12: 93-94
    EARS sequence, 12: 92-93
    exception questions, 12: 89-91
    maintaining progress, 12: 91-92
    miracle question, 12: 88-89
    new problems, 12: 94-95
    pre-session change, 12: 87-88
    relapses, 12: 94
    treating the system, 12: 95
State-Trait Anger Expression Scale (STAXI) used in screening for TMJ, 11: 205-206, 208-209
Stockholm Syndrome theory, Graham's, 13: 401-417
Storytelling in families, 12: 147-154
    benefits, 12: 148
    techniques, 12: 149-153
    types, 12: 149
Stress and intimidation, influence of on children's memory, 12: 42-43
Stress inoculation training, 11: 25-26
Structured Interview of Reported Symptoms (SIRS), 12: 12
Strupp's Time-Limited Dynamic Psychotherapy, 12: 75
Subpoenas, responding to, 11: 221-226
    professional liability, 11: 224-225
    purpose, 11: 222-223
        involving clients, 11: 222-223
        involving practitioner, 11: 223
    recordkeeping issues, 11: 224
    responses, 11: 223-224
    types of, 11: 221-222
Substance abuse,
    adolescent, 13: 97-121, 378-379
        assessment, 13: 97-101
        maintenance of behavior change, 13: 114-115
        treatment, 13: 101-114
    AIDS and, 11: 541-552
        assessment issues, 11: 542-547
        referral, 11: 549-550
        treatment issues, 11: 547-549
    dependent patients and, 13: 142
    elderly and, 12: 477-496
        caregiver attitudes, 12: 478
        common drugs of abuse, 12: 484-488
        drug response, 12: 481-482
        dual diagnosis, 12: 492-494
        identifying at-risk patients, 12: 482-484
        intervention, 12: 488
        organically induced mental conditions, 12: 478-480
        scope of the problem, 12: 477-478
        terms, 12: 480-481
        treatment, 12: 488-492
    Native Americans and, 12: 445-446
    over-the-counter drugs, 11: 53-61, 12: 488
    prescription drugs, 12: 484-488
    and suicide risk, 12: 282
Suicide in elderly, 13: 154
Suicide prevention in correctional facilities, 11: 467-480
    intervention, 11: 472-475
        crisis intervention, 11: 473
        detoxification, 11: 474
        first aid/medical services, 11: 474
        manipulation, 11: 475
        monitoring and supervision, 11: 473
        no-suicide contract, 11: 474
        psychiatric intervention, 11: 474
        psychological autopsies, 11: 474-475
        psychological support services, 11: 474
        social contact, 11: 473

Suicide prevention in correctional facilities *(Continued)*
    risk identification, 11: 468-472
        general risk factors, 11: 469
        jails, 11: 468
        mental, affective, psychological context, 11: 469-471
        prisons, 11: 468-469
        stress, 11: 468
    training, 11: 475-477
        attitude, 11: 476
        intervention, 11: 477
        risk identification, 11: 476
        training resources, 11: 477
Suicide risk, 12: 277-293
    assessment, 12: 278-279
    clinical dilemma, 12: 278
    no-suicide contracts, 12: 279-288
        alternatives, 12: 287-288
        contraindications, 12: 281-287
        definition, 12: 279-280
        functions, 12: 280-281
Sutter-Eyberg Student Behavior Inventory, 11: 261-266, 268

T

Teenage mothers, groups for, 13: 377-378
"Tell Me a Story" (TEMAS) in multicultural assessment, 11: 461-463
Temporomandibular joint disorder (TMJ), 11: 203-217
    case examples, 11: 211-213
    diagnostic interview, 11: 206-208
    practical aspects, 11: 213
    psychological diagnoses, 11: 206
    psychological testing, 11: 209
    research, 11: 203-204
    team approach, 11: 205
    TMJ Interview Points, 11: 215
    treatment, traditional, 11: 204-205
    Wharton Scale, 11: 208, 214
Testimony, neurologists, cross-examining, 13: 323-338
Testing, liability in computerized, 11: 251-257
Therapist-client relationship, 12: 49-64
Therapy, marital, 13: 309-322, 359-368
    for postpartum depression, 11: 41-44
    predivorce stage, group treatment for, 13: 309-322
    Scale of Feelings and Behavior of Love, 11: 303-314
    Scale of Marriage Problems, 11: 293-302
Thought stopping, in chronic pain management, 13: 65
Time-limited group treatment with separated couples, 13: 309-322

TMJ Interview Points, 11: 215
Tourette's syndrome, Attention-Deficit/Hyperactivity Disorder (ADHD) and, 13: 135
Transference, 12: 49-64, 13: 49-51
Traumatic brain injury (TBI), 11: 173-174
Traumatic brain injury (TBI) in children, 12: 581-594
    age, effects of, 12: 584-585
    definition, 12: 582
    evaluation of, 12: 587-589
    how TBI occurs, 12: 583-584
    needs of, 12: 585-587
    neuropsychological evaluations, consumer's guide, 12: 592
    past history of TBI, 12: 589-590
    prevalence, 12: 582-583
    psychosocial and behavioral problems, 12: 590-591
Twelve-Step program for nicotine addiction, 12: 455-474

V

Victims,
    crime, 11: 23-38
    rape, 11: 325-333
    of sexual abuse, 11: 109-122
Violence Attitudes Scale (VAS), 13: 279-291
    applications, 13: 283-284
    development of, 13: 280
    standardization and cross-validation of, 13: 281
    theoretical underpinnings of, 13: 281
Violence, marital, 13: 5-19 *(see also* Abuse)
    assessment of, 13: 6-8
    clinical issues for therapists, 13: 14-15
    Domestic Violence Blame Scale (DVBS), 13: 265-278
    prevalence of, 13: 5-6
    research on interventions for, 13: 15-16
    treatment of, 13: 8-13

W

Wharton Scale (for TMJ patients), 11: 208, 214
Witness, expert, 11: 222-223
    in assessing malingering, 12: 12
    in custody disputes regarding sexual abuse allegations, 12: 16-17
Women, battered, 13: 401-417 *(see also* Abuse)
    group treatment for, 13: 10
Workplace abuse and discrimination, 12: 263-276, 13: 237-253

INFORMATION FOR CONTRIBUTORS

The editors of *Innovations in Clinical Practice* welcome the opportunity to review manuscripts that are consistent with the goals of the series. Manuscripts will be reviewed only if they are not simultaneously under consideration elsewhere. While we will attempt to handle all manuscripts with care, it is important to note that we assume no responsibility for unsolicited manuscripts. Any obligations we make to contributors are specified by written agreement after manuscript acceptance, and we may reserve the right to accept or reject manuscripts at our discretion. All submissions should be accompanied by the author's current vita or a brief letter outlining the author's professional experience and training relevant to the topic. Accepted manuscripts are subject to editing.

MANUSCRIPT SUBMISSION

Interested contributors should submit an original and two copies of double-spaced manuscripts with a vita or letter describing their relevant experience to: Senior Editor, *Innovations in Clinical Practice*, Professional Resource Exchange, Inc., P.O. Box 15560, Sarasota, FL 34277-1560. Receipt of all manuscripts will be acknowledged and authors will be contacted again and notified of our editorial decision following review. Contributions not accepted for publication can be returned only if authors include a large, self-addressed envelope with sufficient postage.

MANUSCRIPT PREPARATION

Brief contributions are preferred, and unsolicited manuscripts should generally not exceed 25 double-spaced typed pages. Each manuscript should begin with a title page that includes the name(s), address(es), and telephone number(s) of the author(s). The second page should have the title of the paper centered at the top, but should not contain the names of the author(s). No abstract is required. Manuscripts should generally follow the style specified by the current *Publication Manual of the American Psychological Association* (1994). There is, however, an exception in that each manuscript should include a "Resource" instead of a "Reference" section and "Reference Notes." The use of footnotes is discouraged. Contributors may refer to the contents of the present volume for a general sense of the style that should be followed. Three levels of headings should be used to facilitate the organization of contributions: (a) a centered main heading, (b) a flush side heading, and (c) an indented side heading. Manuscripts should be written in a concise, professional, but readable manner. Writing in the first person, for example, is quite acceptable. Sexist language should be avoided.

ASSESSMENT INSTRUMENTS AND FORMS

The *Innovations* volumes contain informal clinical assessment instruments and checklists. We do not usually publish formal psychological tests. Assessment instruments are designed to help the clinician be more thorough in collecting information. Contributors of assessment instruments should write for the special instructions that pertain to this type of material.

CONTINUING EDUCATION AVAILABLE FOR HOME STUDY

Innovations in Clinical Practice: A Source Book is available as a formal home study continuing education program. This best-selling, comprehensive source of practical clinical information is complemented by examination modules which may be used to earn continuing education credits.

Credits may be obtained by successfully completing examinations based on those contributions in each volume which have been selected by the editorial advisory board. Each of these contributions explores a timely topic designed to enhance your clinical skills and provide the knowledge necessary for effective practice. After studying these selections, a multiple-choice examination is completed and returned to the Professional Resource Exchange for scoring. Upon passing the examination (80% of test items answered correctly), your credits will be recorded and you will receive a copy of your official transcript.

At the time of publication of this volume, continuing education modules are available for Volumes 9 through 12 of *Innovations in Clinical Practice*. Each module contains examination materials for 20 credits (equivalent to 20 hours of continuing education activity). The Volume 13 module will be available in December 1994 and will also earn 20 credits. The cost of each module is under $50 (see the order form on the next page).

The *Innovations in Clinical Practice* Continuing Education Program is one of the most efficient ways to stay current on new clinical techniques and obtain formal credit for your study. If your professional associations and state boards do not currently require formal CE activities, you may still wish to consider this program as an excellent means of receiving feedback on your professional development. This self-study program is . . .

- *Relevant* - selections are packed with information pertinent to your practice.
- *Inexpensive* - typically less than half the cost of obtaining credits through workshops and these expenses are still tax deductible as a professional expense.
- *Convenient* - study at your own pace in the comfort of your home or office.
- *Useful* - the volume will always be available as a practical reference and resource for day-to-day use in your professional practice.
- *Effective* - as a means of staying up to date and obtaining feedback on your knowledge acquisition and professional development. In most states with continuing education requirements, credits earned from American Psychological Association (APA) approved sponsors are automatically approved for licensure renewal. Consult your profession's state board for their policies regarding the status of programs offered by APA approved sponsors.

Specific learning objectives and faculty credentials are available upon request.

The Professional Resource Exchange, Inc. is approved by the American Psychological Association to offer continuing education for psychologists. The Professional Resource Exchange maintains responsibility for the program. The Professional Resource Exchange, Inc. is also recognized by the National Board for Certified Counselors to offer continuing education for National Certified Counselors. We adhere to NBCC Continuing Education Guidelines (Provider #5474). Florida provider #CM-069-95.

Innovations in Clinical Practice: A Source Book (Vol. 13)

ORDER FORM

I want to order *Innovations in Clinical Practice: A Source Book.* Please send me:

Deluxe Binder Editions
  Volume(s) (circle volume numbers wanted) $54.95 each   1 2 3 4 5 6 7 8 9 10 11 12 13 $_____

Hardbound Editions
  Volume(s) (circle volume numbers wanted) $49.95 each   4 5 6 7 8 9 10 11 12 13 $_____

Continuing Education Modules (circle volumes wanted) $45.00 each   9 10 11 12 13 $_____

                            Subtotal .... $_____

                Florida Residents: Please add 7% sales tax .... $_____

Shipping/Handling - For 1 book or CE module in US add $4.25; orders over $60 in US, add 7% of subtotal;
               foreign orders add 10% of subtotal .... $_____

Total Order (Orders from Individuals & Private Institutions Must Be Prepaid) .... $_____

Check or money order enclosed (US funds only)_____
Please charge my: American Express ☐   MasterCard ☐   Visa ☐   Discover ☐

Credit Card Number:_____   Expiration Date:_____

Telephone: (____)____-_____ Profession:_____   Highest Degree:_____

Signature:_____

SHIP TO: _____

(please print)   _____

                 _____

                 _____

Please make check payable to Professional Resource Press and mail your order to:

Professional Resource Press / PO Box 15560 / Sarasota, FL 34277-1560

Phone Orders (American Express/MasterCard/Visa/Discover) call **1-800-443-3364** weekdays,
9:00-5:00 Eastern Time or use our **FAX**: 1-813-366-7971

We usually ship in-stock items within 2 working days. Items ordered prior to publication will be shipped within 15 days after publication. If shipment will be delayed 30 days over normal shipping time, you will be notified and a refund will be made if desired. Thirty day return privilege if not satisfied. Availability and prices on all products are subject to change without notice.

Note: Volume 9-12 Modules each earn 20 CE Credits. The Volume 13 Module will be available in December, 1994. The Modules for Volumes 1-8 have been discontinued and the Volume 9 Module is available only while supplies last. In order to participate in these CE programs, you must purchase a Module and either purchase or have access to the corresponding *Innovations* volume.

Revised: October, 1994